Instructor Resources

Classroom Preparation Resources (Learning Object Gallery)

► Find assets such as **videos, animations, Images** and more!

► **Add selected resources** to presentations that can be shown online or exported to PowerPoint™ or HTML pages

► Organized by topic and **fully searchable** by type and keyword

► **Upload your own resources** to keep everything in one place

► **Rate resources** and view other instructor ratings!

► Pearson Nursing Question Bank

► Even **more** accessible with both pencil and paper and online delivery options

  ► NCLEX® style questions included

  ► **Complete rationales** for both correct and incorrect answers mapped to learning outcomes

Book-specific resources also available to instructors including:

► Instructor's Manual and Resource Guide

  ► Image Library

  ► Test Review PowerPoints

  ► Online Analysis of Exercise Results

  ► Learning Outcomes

  ► Lesson Plans

  ► Concepts for Lecture

  ► Suggestions for Classroom and Clinical Activities

  ► Answer Key to Test Your Knowledge Questions

► Lecture Note PowerPoints

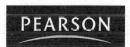

MORE information and purchasing options on these and other Pearson products: Visit nursing.pearsonhighered.com

Brief Contents

Electronic Health Records and Nursing

Richard Gartee • Sharyl Beal, RN, MSN

Pearson

Boston   Columbus   Indianapolis   New York   San Francisco
Upper Saddle River   Amsterdam   Cape Town   Dubai   London   Madrid   Milan
Munich   Paris   Montreal   Toronto   Delhi   Mexico City   Sao Paulo
Sydney   Hong Kong   Seoul   Singapore   Taipei   Tokyo

Publisher: Julie Alexander
Publisher's Assistant: Regina Bruno
Senior Acquisitions Editor: Kelly Trakalo
Assistant Editor: Lauren Sweeney
Development Editor: Michael Giacobbe
Director of Marketing: David Gesell
Senior Marketing Manager: Phoenix Harvey
Marketing Specialist: Michael Sirinides
Marketing Assistant: Crystal Gonzalez
Senior Managing Editor: Patrick Walsh
Production Project Manager: Yagnesh Jani
Senior Operations Supervisor: Ilene Sanford
Senior Art Director: Maria Guglielmo
Cover Designer: Wanda Espana
Lead Media Project Manager: Rachel Collett
Full-Service Project Management: Peggy Kellar, Aptara®, Inc.
Composition: Aptara®, Inc.
Printer/Binder: Courier/Kendallville
Cover Printer: Lehigh-Phoenix Color/Hagerstown

EXCEL®, Windows 2000®, Windows XP®, Windows Vista®, and Windows 7® are a registered trademarks of Microsoft Corporation
Google™ is a trademark of Google, Inc.
ICNP® is a registered trademark of the International Council of Nurses
IQmark™ is a trademark of Midmark Diagnostics Group
LOINC® is a registered trademark of the Regenstrief Institute
Lotus 1-2-3® is a registered trademark of International Business Machines, Corp.
MEDCIN® is a registered trademark of Medicomp Systems, Inc.
NextGen® is a registered trademark of NextGen Healthcare Information Systems, Inc.
SNOMED® and SNOMED CT® are registered trademarks of the College of American Pathologists
UMLS® and Unified Medical Language System® are registered trademarks of the National Library of Medicine
WebMD and WebMD Health are trademarks of WebMD, Inc.
All trademarks used in this book are the property of their respective owners.

Credits and acknowledgments borrowed from other sources and reproduced, with permission, in this textbook appear on the appropriate page within text.

Library of Congress Cataloging-in-Publication Data available upon request.

10 9 8 7 6 5 4 3 2

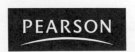

www.pearsonhighered.com

ISBN 10:   0-13-138372-8
ISBN 13: 978-0-13-138372-2

Richard Gartee is the author of seven college textbooks on health information technology, computerized medical systems, managed care, and electronic health records. Before becoming a full-time author and consultant, Richard spent 20 years in the design, development, and implementation of two of the preeminent practice management and electronic health records systems.

Richard also served as a liaison to other companies in the medical computer industry as well as Blue Cross/Blue Shield, a U.S. Department of Commerce International Trade Mission, and various universities.

Richard is a current or past member of many of the professional organizations and national standards groups mentioned in this book:

▶ American Health Information Management Association (AHIMA)

▶ Healthcare Information Management Systems Society (HIMSS)

▶ American National Standards Institute (ANSI) X12n Committee for Development of Electronic Claims Standards

▶ Health Level Seven (HL7) Committee for Development of Claims Attachment Standards

▶ Workgroup for Electronic Data Interchange (WEDI) Task Force for Development of Electronic Remittance Guidelines

▶ A faculty member/speaker at the Medical Records Institute international Electronic Health Records Conference (TEPR) for 12 years

Sharyl Beal is a Registered Nurse with a Master's of Science of Nursing from the University of Michigan and a subspecialty in Nursing Informatics. Sharyl has over 35 years of nursing experience. She served as a Certified Oncology Nurse and a department head for 16 years before moving into her current position as Clinical Information Systems Project Manager at a 500-bed hospital in the Midwest. She has been involved in creating and implementing electronic medical records for the nursing and ancillary departments for the last 18 years as well as training the nurses and physicians to use the clinical systems.

For Mom

Acknowledgments

This book was made possible by the contribution of many individuals and several of the most prominent commercial EHR vendors, whom we would like to thank and acknowledge here.

We first would like to thank Peter S. Goltra, David Lareau, and Roy Soltoff of Medicomp Systems, Inc.

Peter S. Goltra is the father of the Medcin nomenclature. He is the founder and CEO of Medicomp Systems, which he established in 1978 to develop advanced documentation and diagnostic tools for use at the point of care. His honors include an award from the American Medical Informatics Association for contributions to the field of medical informatics.

David Lareau is chief operating officer of Medicomp Systems, Inc. In addition to his COO duties, David is the leading proponent of the Medcin nomenclature, having personally presented it to thousands of key EHR developers and decision makers during his tenure.

Roy Soltoff is the director of software development for Medicomp Systems. Mr. Soltoff has been involved in software development since 1964. He joined the Medicomp development staff in 1992 and has been responsible for significant advances in clinical user interface design and the nursing plan of care module.

We would also like to thank Luann Whittenburg, RN, MSN, Nancy Kaufmann, Director of Nursing, and Kimberly Freese Beal, M.D., for their advice on several of the exercises, and Jim O'Connor, M.D., for his advice on asthma codes. The textbook was greatly enhanced by our acquaintance with Dr. Virginia K. Saba, the developer of the Clinical Classification System nursing terminology, and with EHR experts Dr. Allen R. Wenner and Dr. John Bachman.

Special thanks go to the many individuals who shared their firsthand experiences in real-life stories and allowed them to be used in this book. Their unique perspectives help the student understand the relationship of the conceptual to the practical. We would like to thank Richard A. Gartee, Luann Whittenburg, RN, MSN, Sandra Hillard, RN, Jayne Deal, RN, David Robbins, RN, BSN, Marney Thompson, RN, Sharron Carr, ARNP-BC, Kourtnie Sitarz, RN, Xiaoqiu Hu, RN, MSN, Karen L. Smith, MD, and Primetime Medical who contributed the real-life story of Mr. John Gould.

We are also indebted to the following commercial EHR vendors for allowing their copyrighted work to be reprinted herein. In alphabetical order:

Allscripts, LLC; Carestream Health, Inc.; Medfusion, Inc.; Medicomp Systems, Inc.; Midmark Diagnostics Group; NextGen Healthcare; Primetime Medical Software & Instant Medical History; and Welch Allyn.

Also thanks to Dr. Michael Lukowski for allowing us to reproduce his GYN form; and Susan Majors at Success EHS for contributing the pediatric forms for the well-child exercises in Chapter 12.

Finally, we would like to acknowledge the help of all our editors who assisted us with this work.

Thank You

We would like to thank the academic nursing educators who took time to review and comment on this book. We would also like to recognize the work of the numerous experts who consulted on the development of the Medcin nomenclature. These clinicians did not review the exercises in this book, but they did review the medical accuracy of the Medcin nomenclature that underlies this entire work.

Academic Reviewers

Eva Beliveau, RN, MSN
Northern Essex Community College
Lawrence, MA

Charlene M. Chapman, RN, BSN
Pennsylvania Institute of Technology
Media, PA

Debbie Freyman, RN, MSN, MA
National Park Community College
Springs, AR

Nancy Kaufmann, BSN, MEd, MSN
St. Louis College of Health Careers
Fenton, MO

Carol A. Kilmon, PhD, RN
The University of Texas at Tyler
Tyler, TX

Mary K. Pabst, PhD, RN
Elmhurst College
Elmhurst, IL

Marisue Rayno, RN, MSN, Ed Dc
Luzerne County Community College
St. Nanticoke, PA

Sally J. Schultz RN, MSN
Fox Valley Technical College
Appleton, WI

Doris Stone, MAHSM, MAHRD, MSN, EdD
Jefferson Community & Technical College
Louisville, KY

Patricia Durham-Taylor, RN, PhD
Truckee Meadows Community College
Reno, NV

Leanne M. Waterman, MS, RN, FNP, CNS
Onondaga Community College
Syracuse, NY

Medcin Consulting Editors

Robert G. Barone, MD
Clinical Assistant Professor of Ophthalmology
Cornell University Medical College

J. Gregory Cairncross, MD
Professor, Departments of Clinical Neurological
   Sciences and Oncology
University of Western Ontario and London
   Regional Cancer Centre

Richard P. Cohen, MD
Clinical Associate Professor of Medicine
Cornell University Medical College

Bradley A. Connor, MD
Clinical Assistant Professor of Medicine
Cornell University Medical College

David R. Gastfriend, MD
Assistant Professor in Psychiatry
Harvard Medical School

Stephanie M. Heidelberg, MD
Medical Director, Adult, Older Adult Programs
American Day Treatment Centers

Edmund M. Herrold, MD, PhD
Associate Professor of Medicine
Cornell University Medical College

Allan N. Houghton, MD
Professor of Medicine and Immunology
Cornell University Medical College

Ralph H. Hruban, MD
Associate Professor of Pathology
The Johns Hopkins School of Medicine

Mark Lachs, MD, MPH
Assistant Professor of Medicine
Cornell University Medical College

Fredrick A. McCurdy, MD, PhD
Associate Professor of Pediatrics
University of Nebraska College of Medicine

Paul F. Miskovitz, MD
Clinical Associate Professor of Medicine
Cornell University Medical College

Preeti Pancholi, PhD
Staff Scientist, Department of Virology and Parasitology
Kimball Research Institute

Louis N. Pangaro, MD
Associate Professor, Clinical Medicine
F. Edward Herbert School of Medicine

Edward J. Parrish, MD, MS
Assistant Professor of Medicine
Cornell University Medical College

William B. Patterson, MD, MPH
Assistant Professor of Environmental Health
Boston University School of Public Health

David Posnett, MD
Associate Professor of Medicine
Cornell University Medical College

Calvin W. Roberts, MD
Professor of Ophthalmology
Cornell University Medical College

Ronald C. Silvestri, MD
Assistant Professor of Medicine
Harvard Medical School

Michael Thorpe, MD
Musculoskeletal Radiology Fellow
The Hospital for Special Surgery

Anshu Vashishtha, MD, PhD
Adjunct Faculty Member
Laboratory of Bacterial Pathogenesis and Immunology
The Rockefeller University

H. Hallett Whitman, III, MD
Clinical Assistant Professor of Medicine
Cornell University Medical College

E. David Wright, MD
Clinical Assistant Professor of Medicine
Department of Dermatology
University of Virginia Health Sciences Center

Joseph Zibrak, MD
Assistant Professor of Medicine
Harvard Medical School

Preface

Almost daily the media make us aware that healthcare is transitioning from paper charts to electronic health records (EHR). Government incentive programs have increased the rate at which this is occurring and have set a target date of 2015 to complete the transition. The EHR revolution will impact all of nursing practice; every nurse is going to need to understand and be able to efficiently use electronic health records.

The National League for Nursing (NLN) recognized that if nurses are to become effective users of the electronic health records, nurses need to be educated. The NLN called for reform to nursing education to promote quality education that prepares technology-savvy nurses who can use electronic health records. The NLN Board of Governors (2008) issued a position statement calling for both prelicensure and graduate nursing education programs to provide EHR education and hands on experiences for students.

Adhering to this NLN mandate, this book takes an innovative "learn by doing" approach, providing the learner with a thorough understanding of the EHR that is continuously reinforced by actual EHR experiences. Using the combination of textbook and software, we are creating educated nursing students that understand and are comfortable with computerized health records before they ever enter the workplace.

An article in the American Nurses Association (ANA) *Online Journal of Issues in Nursing* stated, "We, nurses, need to make two decisions: First, we need to decide what data should be included in the electronic record, and secondly, we need to decide what terminology should be used to record this data so that the meaning of the data is clear and consistent" (Thede, 2008).

As authors, we couldn't agree more. In this book you will learn about electronic health records, how to use them, and what benefits are derived from an EHR that uses standardized nomenclature and nursing terminology systems. The hands-on exercises in the text use real EHR software to transform theoretical EHR concepts into practical understanding.

Over the course students will explore the application of EHR in different nursing practices: inpatient, outpatient, home care, nursing home, pediatric, hypertension clinics, and others. However, the purpose of this book is to not to teach nursing practice, but rather to illustrate the successful use of EHR to support nursing practice. This course will build, through practical experience in the classroom, an understanding and a level of comfort with computerized medical records that can be applied in a variety of nursing circumstances.

For too long the idea of teaching EHR has been assumed to be a nursing informatics program at the postgraduate level. The NLN position is clear: teach EHR to all nursing students. Our intended audience is students in undergraduate nursing programs, although nursing informatics students who have not used an actual EHR will benefit from our practical approach as well.

For working nurses, the thought of the impending transition to an EHR is scary. There is a strong interest on the part of working nurses who foresee the impending arrival of EHR in their workplace for a continuing education course to prepare them, and this book is easily adapted to that type of course as well.

Throughout the text we have endeavored to be consistent with other Pearson nursing textbooks by referring to those who are the recipients of nursing care as clients. However, there are several exceptions: quoted material where a regulation or author used the term *patient*, screens or field names in software, government programs such as the Patient-Centered Medical Home, and nursing home residents.

It is our hope that our practical approach to teaching Electronic Health Records and Nursing will prepare you, the learner, for a bright future in nursing.

References

Board of Governors, National League for Nursing. (2008, May 9). Position statement: Preparing the next generation of nurses to practice in a technology-rich environment. Retrieved May 19, 2011, from http://www.nln.org/aboutnln/positionstatements/informatics_052808.pdf

Thede, L. (2008, Aug 18). The electronic health record: Will nursing be on board when the ship leaves? *OJIN: The Online Journal of Issues in Nursing*, *13*(3). Retrieved May 19, 2011, from http://www.nursingworld.org/MainMenuCategories/ANAMarketplace/ANAPeriodicals/OJIN/Columns/Informatics/ElectronicHealthRecord.aspx

The Development and Organization of the Text

This book is organized to provide learners with a comprehensive understanding of the history, theory, and functional benefits of Electronic Health Records. Each chapter builds on the knowledge acquired in previous chapters.

Chapter 1: Electronic Health Records—An Overview provides a foundation for student learning, introducing concepts and topics that are explained in depth in subsequent chapters. The chapter begins with a definition of Electronic Health Records, discusses why they are important, what forces in our society and what federal laws are driving their adoption. Illustrated scenarios compare the workflow of a medical office using paper charts versus one using electronic charts, and the differences between inpatient and outpatient settings. Additional topics include how a medical practice is changed by adoption of an EHR and what constitutes meaningful use of an EHR. The chapter is illustrated with numerous photos of nurses using different types of computers to document at the point of care.

Chapter 2: Functional EHR Systems explains that the format EHR data is stored in determines the potential uses of EHR data to improve care and safety. Chapter 2 describes the various forms of EHR data and the value of using standardized codes for that data. Guided exercises provide the students with an opportunity to explore a component found in most EHR systems—Document Imaging. Major EHR and nursing terminologies are discussed. The student not only achieves knowledge of standardized nomenclatures and their history, but also their importance in enabling different healthcare systems to exchange data. Functional benefits of an EHR such as trending changes in clients' health, generating medical alerts and decision support such as the drug interaction checking feature of electronic prescription writing software, are also covered.

Chapter 3: Learning Medical Record Software introduces the Medcin Student Edition software, which will be used for the remainder of the book. In a series of brief hands-on exercises, the student becomes familiar with EHR concepts, learns to navigate the software, and creates an actual encounter note.

Chapter 4: Increased Familiarity with the Software reinforces the student's computer skills with additional hands-on exercises. Students also learn how to save their work as printed encounters or output encounter notes to PDF or XPS files.

Chapter 5: Data Entry at the Point of Care stresses the importance of entering data at the time of the encounter, not after the fact. Students learn how to increase data entry speed by using EHR features of Lists and Forms.

Chapter 6: Electronic Nursing Care Plans introduces students to standard, individual, and interactive nursing plans of care. Students learn to create and document nursing care plans in the EHR using the Clinical Care Classification System for nursing, which follows the ANA nursing process steps.

Chapter 7: Understanding Electronic Orders introduces students to computerized order entry and electronic prescriptions that are now required in all certified EHR systems. The workflows of paper versus electronic order systems are compared and "closed loop safe medication administration" is emphasized. Hands-on exercises are used for each feature. ICD-9-CM codes are introduced and compared with ICD-10, the future standard. Students continue to build EHR computer skills learning how to search the EHR nomenclature and prompt for diagnosis-based order protocols.

Chapter 8: Problem Lists, Results Management, and Trending expands on concepts introduced in Chapters 1–7. Hands-on exercises allow students to experiment with other methods of documenting the encounter and introducing the concepts of problem lists, pending orders, and electronic results. Students gain firsthand experience trending changes in clients' health by learning to graph lab test results and vital signs.

Chapter 9: Data Entry Using Flow Sheets and Anatomical Drawings teaches the concept of flow sheets and provides students hands-on experiences using several types of flow sheets. Additionally, students learn to annotate medical illustrations electronically to document observations in the EHR and for client education.

Chapter 10: Subacute Care, Nursing Homes, and Home Care introduces students to seven types of long-term care that often follow discharge from an acute care facility. The chapter focuses on the nurse's role in home care and nursing home resident assessments. Hands-on exercises provide students experience with the Resident Assessment Instrument MDS 3.0 and the home health OASIS-C.

Chapter 11: Using the Internet to Expedite Care includes a thorough discussion of the Internet's impact on healthcare, the practice of medicine online, telemedicine, and teleradiology. Hands-on exercises include online nursing research, data entry of symptoms and history using the Internet, and the newest innovation, E-visits, and what is necessary for secure online communications.

Chapter 12: Using the EHR for Prevention and Health Maintenance focuses on preventative care with hands-on exercises on pediatric wellness visits, immunizations, and preventative care screening. Students extend their understanding of trending by learning to create growth charts and to graph additional types of data. The chapter also covers the Patient-Centered Medical Home concept, and personal health records.

Learning Made Easy

A Unique Approach to Learning Electronic Health Records

This textbook–software package introduces learners to the electronic health record (EHR) through practical applications and guided exercises. The textbook, Online Student Resources website, and Medcin Student Edition software combination provides a complete learning system. Chapters integrate the history, theory, and benefits of EHR with the opportunity to experience the EHR environment firsthand by completing guided exercises and critical thinking exercises using the Student Edition software. Each chapter builds on the knowledge acquired in previous chapters.

Applying Theory to Practice

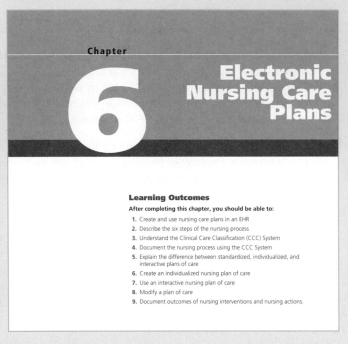

Chapter

6

Electronic Nursing Care Plans

Learning Outcomes

After completing this chapter, you should be able to:

1. Create and use nursing care plans in an EHR
2. Describe the six steps of the nursing process
3. Understand the Clinical Care Classification (CCC) System
4. Document the nursing process using the CCC System
5. Explain the difference between standardized, individualized, and interactive plans of care
6. Create an individualized nursing plan of care
7. Use an interactive nursing plan of care
8. Modify a plan of care
9. Document outcomes of nursing interventions and nursing actions.

▲ **LEARNING OUTCOMES** Each chapter begins with a list of learning outcomes that highlight the key concepts contained in that chapter.

◄ **NOTES** Note boxes found within the chapters explain key terms that are used within the text and provide additional information about the software.

► **ALERTS** Alert boxes found within the chapters caution or remind learners about information related to using the software.

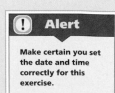

① Alert

Make certain you set the date and time correctly for this exercise.

Note

EHR

The acronym EHR is commonly used as shorthand for Electronic Health Records, and will be used in the remainder of this book.

▼ **ACRONYMS** Acronyms and their definitions are provided in a quick reference on the inside back cover.

Acronyms Used in This Book			
ABG	Arterial Blood Gas	DME	Durable Medical Equipment
ABN	Advance Beneficiary Notice	DOD	Department of Defense
ABN	Abnormal	DTaP	Diphtheria, Tetanus, Pertussis (vaccine)
ADL	Activities of Daily Living	DUR	Drug Utilization Review
ADT	Admission, Discharge and Transfer	DTV	Deep Vein Thrombosis
AHIMA	American Health Information Management Association	Dx	Diagnosis
		ECG or EKG	Electrocardiogram
AHRQ	Agency for Healthcare Research and Quality	EDI	Electronic Data Interchange
ALOS	Average Length of Stay	EHR	Electronic Health Record
AMA	Against Medical Advice	EMS	Emergency Medical Services
AMI	Acute Myocardial Infraction	ENT	Ears, Nose, Throat
ANA	American Nurses Association	EPHI	Protected Health Information in Electronic form
ANSI	American National Standards Institute	EPs	Eligible Professionals
ARRA	American Recovery and Reinvestment Act	ER	Emergency Department or Emergency Room
ADHD	Attention Deficit Hyperactivity Disorder	FDA	Food and Drug Administration
BID	Twice Daily	FS Form	Flow Sheet (based on a) Form
BIPAP	Bilevel Positive Airway Pressure	FS Hx	Family and Social History
BMI	Body Mass Index	GI	Gastrointestinal
BMP	Basic Metabolic Panel	GNA	Geriatric Nursing Assistants
BP	Blood Pressure	H&P	History and Physical
CAA	Care Area Assessment	HAC	Hospital Acquired Condition
CAT	Computerized Axial Tomography	HCAHPS	Hospital Consumer Assessment Healthcare Providers and Systems
CBC	Complete Blood Count		
CC	Chief Complaint	HDL-C	High-Density Lipoprotein (cholesterol test)
CCC	Clinical Care Classification system	HF	Hearth Failure
CCHIT	Certification Commission for Healthcare Information Technology	HEENT	Head, Eyes, Ears, Nose, (Mouth), and Throat
		HepB	Hepatitis B (vaccine)
CCU	Critical Care Unit	HHA	Home Health Agency
CDC	Centers for Disease Control and Prevention	HHS	U.S. Department of Health and Human Services
CDISC	Clinical Data Interchange Standards Consortium	Hib	Haemophilus influenzae type B (vaccine)
		HIE	Health Information Exchange
CDR	Clinical Data Repository	HIM	Health Information Management
CHF	Congestive Heart Failure	HIMSS	Health Information Management Systems Society
CIS	Clinical Information Services		
CMS	Centers for Medicare and Medicaid Services	HIPAA	Health Insurance Portability and Accountability Act
CNA	Certified Nursing Assistant		
CPOE	Computerized Provider Order Entry	HITECH	Health Information Technology for Economic and Clinical Health
CPR	Cardio-Pulmonary Resuscitation		
CPRI	Computer Based Patient Record Institute	HL7	Health Level 7
CPRS	Computerized Patient Record System	HPI	History of Present Illness
CQM	Clinical Quality Measures	Hx	History
CRNA	Certified Registered Nurse Anesthesiologist	ICD-9-CM	International Classification of Diseases, ninth revision, with clinical modifications
CT	Computed Tomography	ICD-10	International Classification of Diseases, tenth revision
CVA	Cerebrovascular Accident		
CVP	Cerebral Vascular Pressure	ICNP	International Classification for Nursing Practice
DAW	Dispense As Written	IMH	Instant Medical History

◀ **REAL-LIFE STORY** Each chapter features a Real-Life Story told by a nurse or client about their experiences with EHR. These vignettes help learners connect chapter content to real life in the hospital or clinic.

Real-Life Story

Nurse Who Uses Flow Sheets and Trending

By Kourtnie Sitarz, RN

Kourtnie Sitarz is a registered nurse working in a community health system in the Midwest. Kourtnie worked as a staff nurse on a pulmonary medical unit before joining the informatics department.

I began my career in healthcare when I was only 18 as a pharmacy technician in a small retail pharmacy. I had just started taking general education classes at the nearby community college, but was still undecided on my major. Because I was working in a pharmacy, it was natural for me to start taking classes with a major in mind. A pharmacy technician position opened up at a local hospital, so I decided to take it, figuring it would help open my eyes to the other world of pharmacy—the clinical pharmacist.

It wasn't long before I realized I was more interested in what the nurses were doing on the units, and began dreading having to go back to my little area so far away from the nurses and clients. Luckily, the classes I had taken in preparation for a career as a pharmacist were above and beyond what I needed for the nursing program. On those rare occasions of downtime, I would hold out as long as I could to document hoping the electronic system could become available so I wouldn't have to document on paper. It was also difficult for me to find the multiple tests and labs on paper, let alone trend them. Electronic medical records put all the information I needed to see the full picture of my client, not only from this visit but from past visits, at my fingertips in a centralized location.

My background as a pharmacy technician, coupled with my nursing degree, as well as my love of electronic medical records, opened a door for me I never realized existed. I was asked to join the Clinical Information Systems Department of my hospital as a clinical systems analyst. When I was asked to consider bidding on the job, I honestly had no idea what the position involved. As a nurse, I never thought about how the screens I documented on or the orders I entered into the system were developed. They were just there, and that was all I needed to know.

As a clinical systems analyst, my responsibility is to be the "voice of nursing in IT". It doesn't make sense for a person who has never taken care of a client to decide how a nurse should document client care. That is where I come in. As one of my fellow nurses during a monthly orders and documentation workgroup, attend a monthly meeting to minimize medication error, teach classes to help familiarize staff with our IT solutions, and act as the voice of the registered nurse while evaluating new IT solutions. Knowing I am able to be the voice of my fellow registered nurses, as well as shape how nurses care for clients using IT solutions, is the most rewarding part of my job.

▶ **CHAPTER SUMMARY** Summaries at the end of each chapter synthesize key points for students and include a reference table of exercises that cover specific EHR skills.

Chapter One Summary

Electronic Health Records are the portions of a client's medical records that are stored in a computer system as well as the functional benefits derived from having an electronic health record.

The IOM set forth eight core functions that an EHR should be capable of performing:

▶ **Health information and data** Provide improved access to information needed by care providers, using a defined data set that includes medical and nursing diagnoses, a medication list, allergies, demographics, clinical narratives, laboratory test results, and more.

▶ **Result management** Electronic results for better interpretation, quicker recognition and treatment of medical problems; reduces redundant testing and improves care coordination among multiple providers.

▶ **Order management** CPOE systems improve workflow, eliminate lost orders and ambiguities caused by illegible handwriting, monitor for duplicate orders, and reduce the time required to fill orders.

▶ **Decision support** Includes prevention, prescribing of drugs, diagnosis and management, and detection of adverse events and disease outbreaks.

Computer reminders and prompts improve preventive practices in areas such as vaccinations, breast cancer screening, colorectal screening, and cardiovascular risk reduction. Computer reminders and real-time audit tracking alert nurses and other care givers to avoid errors or omissions in standards of care.

▶ **Electronic communication and connectivity** Among care partners, enhances patient safety and quality of care, especially for patients who have multiple providers.

▶ **Patient support** For example, patient education and home monitoring by patients using electronic devices.

▶ **Administrative processes and reporting** Increases the efficiency of healthcare organizations and provide better, timelier service to patients.

Practice Opportunities

Guided Exercise 47: Writing Prescriptions in an EHR

In this exercise you will learn to use the Student Edition prescription writer to enter orders that a nurse has received by phone from the doctor. It is necessary for the nurse to enter the prescription, because the hospital's closed loop medication safety policy prevents the automated medication system from dispensing drugs without an order and the doctor does not have remote access to his EHR to write the prescription himself.

Case Study

You will recall from the previous chapter that Eleanore Nash is a 42-year-old female admitted for bacterial pneumonia. She is unable to sleep and informs the nurse that she is in pain from too much coughing. The nurse administers the pain scale and determines the client is at level 7. The nurse contacts Eleanore's physician, who orders Tylenol No. 3 and Ambien. The nurse will write the prescription and the doctor will cosign the order later, usually within 24 hours or in accordance with the facility policies.

▶ Figure 7-18 Select patient Eleanore Nash on ADT tab.

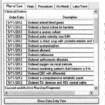

▶ Figure 7-19 Clinical orders for Eleanore Nash.

Step 1

If you have not already done so, start the Student Edition software.

Click on the ADT tab at the bottom of your screen, and then locate and click on **Eleanore Nash**, as shown in Figure 7-18.

Locate and click on the button labeled "Review Plan of Care."

Step 2

The nurse reviews the clinical orders in the plan of care as shown in Figure 7-19 to determine if pain medication has been ordered. Notice that a stronger pain medication is not listed in the clinical orders.

Locate the button labeled "Show Data Entry View" below the left pane, and click on it.

◀ **GUIDED EXERCISES** Guided hands-on exercises using a step-by-step approach allow the students to learn by doing. The companion Medcin® Student Edition software provides a computer experience similar to that of an actual medical facility.

▼ **CRITICAL THINKING EXERCISES** Hands-on critical thinking exercises challenge learners to extend what they have learned through their completion of the guided exercises by applying their knowledge in a new way.

Critical Thinking Exercise 36: Using a Form and a List

In this exercise, you will use both the form and the list from the previous exercises. Using what you have learned so far, document Mr. Green's hospital admission.

Case Study

Charles Green is a 33-year-old male with a complaint of a new-onset, frequent cough that is progressively worse, especially at night. His chest hurts when he coughs and sometimes he vomits because of the coughing. Mr. Green was previously seen at his doctor's office and diagnosed with acute sinusitis. His condition has deteriorated. He is being admitted to the hospital for acute bronchitis.

179

▶ **TEST YOUR KNOWLEDGE** Open-ended study questions at the end of each chapter allow learners to test their knowledge and think critically. Answers are available to instructors.

Chapter 9 | Data Entry Using Flow Sheets and Anatomical Drawings 385

Test Your Knowledge

1. What were the two chronic diseases for which Mr. Daniels was being monitored?
2. Why did the hypertension and diabetes forms create different flow sheets?
3. Why were some items already filled in when you loaded the second form?
4. What form did you use to record dietary orders?
5. What is a flow sheet?
6. What does it mean to cite a finding?
7. What does it mean to create a flow sheet from a form.
8. Describe how to create a problem-oriented flow sheet.
9. Describe how to create a flow sheet for a nursing plan of care.
10. Describe how to cite a finding from a flow sheet.
11. Name two medical specialties that typically incorporate annotated drawings in an encounter note.
12. If you click the date of a flow sheet column when the Cite button is off, what data is displayed?
13. If you click the date of a flow sheet column when the Cite button is on, what data is displayed?
14. How do you print an annotated drawing?
15. You should have produced narrative documents for four clients and two annotated drawings. If you have not already done so, hand these in to your instructor with this test. These will count as a portion of your grade.

Ask your instructor for answers to Test Your Knowledge

nursing.pearsonhighered.com

Prepare for success with animated examples, practice questions, challenge tests, and interactive assignments.

Comprehensive Evaluation of Chapters 1–6

This comprehensive evaluation will enable you and your instructor to determine your understanding of the material covered so far. Complete both the written test and the two exercises provided below. Depending on the time provided, it may be necessary to do this in two separate sessions. Your instructor will advise you. Do not begin the hands-on exercise if there will not be enough class time to complete it.

Part I—Written Exam

You may run the Student Edition software and use your mouse on the screen to answer the following questions. You will also need access to the Internet to answer some of the questions.

Give a brief description of the purpose of each of the following coding systems:

1. Medcin _____
2. CCC _____
3. Explain the difference between an EHR nomenclature and a billing code set.
4. Which screen do you use to set the reason for the visit?
5. How do you load a form?
6. How do you load a list?

Write the meaning of each of the following acronyms:

7. ROS _____
8. Hx _____
9. HPI _____

◀ **COMPREHENSIVE EVALUATION** Learners will test their mastery of the material through two comprehensive evaluations found at the midpoint and end of the text. Each evaluation includes a written exam and hands-on critical thinking exercises using the software and the Internet.

Visualizing the Electronic Health Record

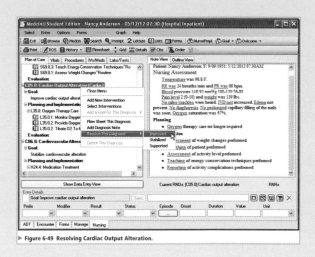

▶ Figure 6-49 Resolving Cardiac Output Alteration.

◀ **SCREEN CAPTURES** Easy-to-follow, step-by-step screen captures of the computer screens from the Medcin software illustrate the steps of the exercise. They serve as a ready reference to help learners orient themselves and assess their progress as they master content.

▼ ▶ **FIGURES AND TABLES** Numerous figures throughout the text help learners visualize workflow scenarios and technical concepts. Photographs of nurses using various types of EHR systems and medical devices make it easy to see the practical applicability in the real world.

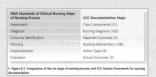

▶ Figure 6-2 Comparison of the six steps of nursing process and CCC System framework for nursing documentation.

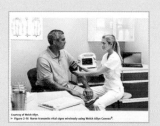

Courtesy of Welch Allyn.
▶ Figure 2-16 Nurse transmits vital signs wirelessly using Welch Allyn Connex®.

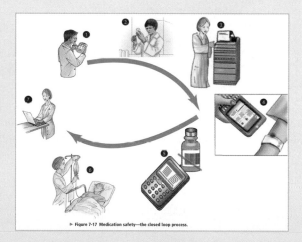

▶ Figure 7-17 Medication safety—the closed loop process.

The Medcin Student Edition Software

▶ The Medcin Student Edition contains the entire Medcin nomenclature used in professional EHR systems and the entire CCC terminology for nursing. Medcin is the licensed core technology in many prominent EHR systems. Because the leading EHR systems for medical offices use the Medcin nomenclature as the technology underlying commercial EHR systems, students in most cases may apply skills they acquire in this course directly to an EHR application in a clinic. Those systems may not be identical to the student software, but they will seem very familiar to someone who has completed this course.

▶ Hands-on exercises are short and have been designed to be completed in a normal class time.

▶ Multiuser software allows multiple students to work simultaneously and keeps each student's work separate.

▶ All work is printed and no exercise requires saving. This allows students from multiple classes to share the same computer and avoids complications caused by saving and backing up databases. Printouts or file output from the exercises automatically include the student's login name or student ID.

▶ The printers will use the standard Windows system, and any compatible printer should work.

▶ For distance learning, the software allows the student to "print" to a file that will output the exercise document into a file in either PDF or XPS format. The output file can then be e-mailed or given to the instructor, who may open and view the student's work with Adobe Reader or an ordinary web browser such as Microsoft Internet Explorer.

▶ All schools will receive Medcin Student Edition software they can install on the school network and computer lab workstations. Software may be installed in two ways: schools with networked computer labs can install a networked client/server system, or schools can install it locally on each student workstation.

▶ Students may download the individual workstation version and install it on their own (Windows-based) computer as well. This is ideal for distance learning students or those who wish to work outside the classroom.

Software Requirements

To complete the exercises in this book, you will need access to the Medcin Student Edition software. If you are taking this course in a classroom, the software will already be installed. If you are in a distance learning program or working independently, you will need to download and install the software on a computer running the Windows operating system. Directions to download and install the software are found on the Online Student Resources website, which is described on the inside cover of this book.

To complete the exercises in Chapters 2, 10, 11, and both comprehensive evaluations, you will also need access to the Internet and a web browser.

Minimum Workstation Requirements

Processor: 200 mHz Pentium
Operating system: Windows XP, Windows Vista, Windows 7 (or later)
RAM: 64 megabytes (free, not counting OS)
Number of colors: 256 (8-bit color)
Display size (pixels per inch): 800 × 600 (1024 × 768 recommended)
Internet Explorer version 6 or later
Microsoft.Net Framework version 2.0 or later

You must have a mouse with at least two buttons that respectively perform the left-click and right-click functions.

Notice

The Medcin Student Edition software is licensed only for educational purposes, to allow the student to perform exercises in the textbook.

By using this program, a healthcare provider agrees that this product is not intended to suggest or replace any medical decisions or actions with respect to the patient's medical care and that the sole and exclusive responsibility for determining the accuracy, completeness, or appropriateness of any diagnostic, clinical, billing, or other medical information provided by the program and any underlying clinical database resides solely with the healthcare provider. Licensor assumes no responsibility for how such materials are used and disclaims all warranties, whether expressed or implied, including any warranty as to the quality, accuracy, or suitability of this information and product for any particular purpose.

Contents

Chapter 3   Learning Medical Record Software   70

Chapter 7   Understanding Electronic Orders   248

Chapter 8   Problem Lists, Results Management, and Trending   301

Chapter 12

Using the EHR for Prevention and Health Maintenance   464

Comprehensive Evaluation of Chapters 7–12   495

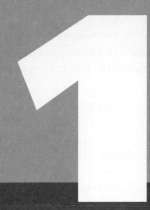

Chapter

1

Electronic Health Records—An Overview

Learning Outcomes

After completing this chapter, you should be able to:

1. Define electronic health records

2. Understand the core functions of an electronic health record as defined by the Institute of Medicine

3. Discuss social forces that are driving the adoption of electronic health records

4. Describe federal government strategies to promote electronic health record adoption

5. Explain why electronic health records are important

6. Describe the flow of medical information into the chart

7. Compare the workflow of an office using paper charts with an office using an electronic health record

8. Contrast inpatient and outpatient charts

9. Explain why client encounters should be documented at the point of care

10. Compare various types of electronic health record computers such as workstation, laptop, and Tablet PC

Evolution of Electronic Health Records

The idea of computerizing clients' medical records has been around for more than 30 years, but only in the past decade has it become widely adopted. Prior to the electronic health record (EHR), a client's medical records consisted of handwritten notes, typed reports, and test results stored in a paper file system. Although paper medical records are still used in many healthcare facilities, the transition to EHR is underway.

Beginning in 1991, the IOM (which stands for the Institute of Medicine of the National Academies) sponsored studies and created reports that led the way toward the concepts we have in place today for electronic health records. Originally, the IOM called them *computer-based patient records* (Dick & Steen, 2000). During their evolution, the EHR have had many other names, including *electronic medical records*, *computerized medical records*, *longitudinal patient records*, and *electronic charts*. All of these names referred to essentially the same thing, which in 2003, the IOM renamed as the *electronic health records*, or EHR.

> **Note**
>
> **EHR**
>
> The acronym EHR is commonly used as shorthand for Electronic Health Records, and will be used in the remainder of this book.

Institute of Medicine (IOM)

The IOM report (Dick & Steen, 2000) put forth a set of eight core functions that an EHR should be capable of performing:

Health information and data This function provides a defined data set that includes such items as medical and nursing diagnoses, a medication list, allergies, demographics, clinical narratives, and laboratory test results. Further, it provides improved access to information needed by care providers when they need it.

Result management Computerized results can be accessed more easily (than paper reports) by the provider at the time and place they are needed.

▶ Reduced lag time allows for quicker recognition and treatment of medical problems.

▶ The automated display of previous test results makes it possible to reduce redundant and additional testing.

▶ Having electronic results can allow for better interpretation and for easier detection of abnormalities, thereby ensuring appropriate follow-up.

▶ Access to electronic consults and patient consents can establish critical links and improve care coordination among multiple providers, as well as between provider and patient.

Order management Computerized provider order entry (CPOE) systems can improve workflow processes by eliminating lost orders and ambiguities caused by illegible handwriting, generating related orders automatically, monitoring for duplicate orders, and reducing the time required to fill orders.

▶ CPOE systems for medications reduce the number of errors in medication dose and frequency, drug allergies, and drug–drug interactions.

▶ The use of CPOE, in conjunction with an EHR, also improves clinician productivity.

Decision support Computerized decision support systems include prevention, prescribing of drugs, diagnosis and management, and detection of adverse events and disease outbreaks.

▶ Computer reminders and prompts improve preventive practices in areas such as vaccinations, breast cancer screening, colorectal screening, and cardiovascular risk reduction.

Electronic communication and connectivity Electronic communication among care partners can enhance patient safety and quality of care, especially for patients who have multiple providers in multiple settings that must coordinate care plans.

▶ Electronic connectivity is essential in creating and populating EHR systems with data from laboratory, pharmacy, radiology, and other providers.

▶ Secure e-mail and web messaging have been shown to be effective in facilitating communication both among providers and with patients, thus allowing for greater continuity of care and more timely interventions.

▶ Automatic alerts to providers regarding abnormal laboratory results reduce the time until an appropriate treatment is ordered.

▶ Electronic communication is fundamental to the creation of an integrated health record, both within a setting and across settings and institutions.

Patient support Computer-based patient education has been found to be successful in improving control of chronic illnesses, such as diabetes, in primary care.

▶ Examples of home monitoring by patients using electronic devices include self-testing by patients with asthma (spirometry), glucose monitors for patients with diabetes, and Holter monitors for patients with heart conditions. Data from monitoring devices can be merged into the EHR, as shown in Figure 1-1.

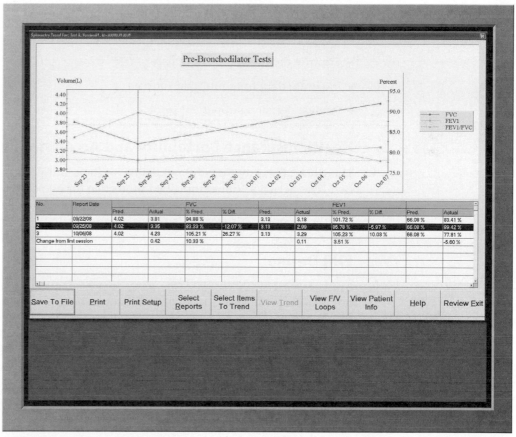

Courtesy of Midmark Diagnostics Group.
▶ **Figure 1-1 Data from digital spirometer transfers to EHR.**

Administrative processes and reporting Electronic scheduling systems increase the efficiency of healthcare organizations and provide better, timelier service to patients.

▶ Communication and content standards are important in the billing and claims management area.

▶ Electronic authorization and prior approvals can eliminate delays and confusion; immediate validation of insurance eligibility results in more timely payments and less paperwork.

▶ EHR data can be analyzed to identify patients who are potentially eligible for clinical trials, as well as candidates for chronic disease management programs.

▶ Reporting tools support drug recalls.

Reporting and population health Public and private sector reporting requirements at the federal, state, and local levels for patient safety and quality, as well as for public health, are more easily met with computerized data.

▶ Eliminates the labor-intensive and time-consuming abstraction of data from paper records and the errors that often occur in a manual process.

▶ Facilitates the reporting of key quality indicators used for the internal quality improvement efforts of many healthcare organizations.

▶ Improves public health surveillance and timely reporting of adverse reactions and disease outbreaks.

Later in this chapter, we will discuss initiatives by the U.S. government to encourage the development of healthcare information technology. It will become apparent how the IOM definitions of core functions influenced and were adapted into the framework proposed by the government.

Computer-based Patient Record Institute (CPRI)

Another early contributor to the thinking on EHR systems was the Computer-based Patient Record Institute (CPRI), which identified three key criteria for an EHR:

▶ Capture data at the point of care

▶ Integrate data from multiple sources

▶ Provide decision support

Health Insurance Portability and Accountability Act (HIPAA)

The HIPAA Security Rule did not define an EHR, but perhaps it broadened the definition. The Security Rule established protection for *all* personally identifiable health information stored in electronic format. Thus, everything about a client stored in a healthcare provider's system is protected and treated as part of the client's EHR.

EHR Defined

In *Electronic Health Records: Changing the Vision*, authors Murphy, Waters, Hanken, and Pfeiffer define the EHR to include "any information relating to the past, present or future physical/mental health, or condition of an individual which resides in electronic system(s) used to capture, transmit, receive, store, retrieve, link and manipulate multimedia data for the primary purpose of providing healthcare and health-related services" (Murphy et al., 1999, p. 4). The EHR can include dental health records as well.

The core functions defined by the IOM and CPRI suggest that the EHR is not just what data is stored, but what can be done with it. In the broadest sense, *Electronic Health Records are the portions of a client's medical records that are stored in a computer system as well as the functional benefits derived from having an electronic health record.*

Social Forces Driving EHR Adoption

Visionary leaders in medical informatics have been making the case for the EHR for a long time. However, the combination of several important reports caught the public's attention and set in motion economic and political forces that are driving the transformation of our medical records systems.

Health Safety

The IOM published a report that stated the following: "Healthcare in the United States is not as safe as it should be—and can be. At least 44,000 people, and perhaps as many as 98,000 people, die in hospitals each year as a result of medical errors that could have been prevented, according to estimates from two major studies.

"Beyond their cost in human lives, preventable medical errors exact other significant tolls. They have been estimated to result in total costs (including the expense of additional care necessitated by the errors, lost income and household productivity, and disability) of between $17 billion and $29 billion per year in hospitals nationwide. Errors also are costly in terms of loss of trust in the healthcare system by patients and diminished satisfaction by both patients and health professionals.

"A variety of factors have contributed to the nation's epidemic of medical errors. One oft-cited problem arises from the decentralized and fragmented nature of the healthcare delivery system—or 'non-system,' to some observers. When patients see multiple providers in different settings, none of whom has access to complete information, it becomes easier for things to go wrong" (Kohn, Corrigan, & Donaldson, 1999, p. 5).

These statements got the attention of the press and public. They also got the attention of 150 of the nation's largest employers.

Health Costs

Employers who sponsored employee health insurance programs had become frustrated by the increasing costs of health insurance benefits for which they had little or no say about the quality of care. Following the release of the IOM report, these employers formed the Leapfrog group.

A study by the Center for Information Technology Leadership found more than 130,000 life-threatening situations caused by adverse drug reactions alone. The study suggested that $44 billion could be saved annually by installing computerized physician order entry systems in ambulatory settings.

Leapfrog created a strategy that tied purchase of group health insurance benefits to quality care standards. It also promoted CPOE as a means of reducing errors.

Changing Society

Changes in the way we live have also made paper medical records outdated. In an increasingly mobile society, clients relocate and change doctors more frequently, thus needing to transfer their medical records from previous doctors to new ones. Additionally, many clients no longer have a single general practitioner who provides their total care. Increased specialization and the development of new methods of diagnostic and preventive medicine require the ability to share exam records among different specialists and testing facilities.

The Internet, one of the strongest forces for social change in the past decade, also affects healthcare. Consumers are becoming accustomed to being able to access very sensitive information securely over the web. They are beginning to ask, "If I can write checks and use Internet banking securely; if I can trade stocks and see my brokerage account; if I can check in for my airline flight and print my boarding passes; why can't I see my lab test result online?"

One solution is personal health records (PHR), secure web sites that allow clients to keep their own medical records online and enable them to control who has access. One advantage of an online PHR is that is available everywhere. Wherever clients travel and need medical care, they can retrieve their own records using the Internet. PHR will be explored further in Chapter 12.

Another important aspect of the World Wide Web is client accessibility to medical information and research. There are literally millions of health-related pieces of information on the web. Clients are arriving at their doctor's office armed with questions and sometimes answers. Medical information previously unavailable to the average consumer is now as easy to access as searching Google™ or WebMD®.

A small but growing number of medical offices are creating interactive web sites that actually allow the client to request an appointment time or a prescription renewal. In a number of states it is even possible for clients and doctors to conduct the medical visit via the Internet. These are called "E-visits" and will be discussed further in Chapter 11.

Critical Thinking Exercise 1: EHR News

1. The topic of EHR is frequently in the news. Describe something you have read or seen on television about EHR and how it may impact you.

Government Response

The response to the IOM report was swift and positive, within both the government and private sectors. Almost immediately, President Bill Clinton's administration issued an executive order instructing government agencies that conduct or oversee healthcare programs to implement proven techniques for reducing medical errors and creating a task force to find new strategies for reducing errors. Congress appropriated $50 million to the Agency for Healthcare Research and Quality (AHRQ) to support a variety of efforts targeted at reducing medical errors.

President George W. Bush followed through by establishing the Office of the National Coordinator for Health Information Technology (ONC), under the U.S. Department of Health and Human Services (HHS) to "develop, maintain, and direct the implementation of a strategic plan to guide the nationwide implementation of interoperable health information technology in both the public and private healthcare sectors that will reduce medical errors, improve quality, and produce greater value for healthcare expenditures" (Exec. Order No. 13,335, 2004).

President Barack Obama identified the EHR as a priority for his administration and signed into law the Health Information Technology for Economic and Clinical Health (HITECH) Act. The act promotes the widespread adoption of EHR and authorizes Medicare incentive payments to doctors and hospitals using a certified EHR and eventually financial penalties for physicians and hospitals that do not (American Recovery and Reinvestment Act, 2009). Note that the HITECH Act is contained within the American Recovery and Reinvestment Act (ARRA), therefore you may see reference to it by the ARRA designation as well.

Office of National Coordinator for Health Information Technology

David J. Brailer, MD, PhD, the first National Coordinator, acted quickly. Ten weeks after his appointment, the ONC delivered a framework for strategic action outlining 4 goals and 12 strategies for national adoption of health information technology (Brailer, 2004). The document outlined a vision for consumer-centric and information-rich healthcare derived from the widespread adoption of health information technology and set a 10-year time frame for that to happen.

Strategic Framework

The framework as first published listed four major goals and a corresponding set of strategies. These were:

Goal 1: Inform Clinical Practice This goal centered largely on efforts to bring EHR directly into clinical practice. The goal was to reduce medical errors and duplicative work, and enable clinicians to focus their efforts more directly on improved patient care. Three strategies for realizing this goal are:

▶ Strategy 1. Incentivize EHR adoption.

▶ Strategy 2. Reduce risk of EHR investment for clinicians who purchase EHR to reduce risk, failure, and partial use of EHR.

▶ Strategy 3. Promote EHR diffusion in rural and underserved areas.

Goal 2: Interconnect Clinicians   Interconnecting clinicians allows information to be portable and to move with consumers from one point of care to another. This will require an interoperable infrastructure to help clinicians get access to critical healthcare information when their clinical or treatment decisions are being made. The three strategies for realizing this goal are:

► Strategy 1. Foster regional collaborations.

► Strategy 2. Develop a national health information network.

► Strategy 3. Coordinate federal health information systems.

Goal 3: Personalize Care   Consumer-centric information helps individuals manage their own wellness and assists with their personal healthcare decisions. The three strategies for realizing this goal are:

► Strategy 1. Encourage use of PHR.

► Strategy 2. Enhance informed consumer choice to select clinicians and institutions based on what they value, including but not limited to the quality of care that providers deliver.

► Strategy 3. Promote use of telehealth systems.

Goal 4: Improve Population Health   Population health improvement by the collection of timely, accurate, and detailed clinical information to allow for the evaluation of healthcare delivery and the reporting of critical findings to public health officials, clinical trials and other research, and feedback to clinicians. Three strategies for realizing this goal are:

► Strategy 1. Unify public health surveillance architectures.

► Strategy 2. Streamline quality and health status monitoring.

► Strategy 3. Accelerate research and dissemination of evidence.

Federal Health IT Strategic Plan 2008–2012

In June of 2008, the ONC published an update to the strategic framework called the Federal Health IT Strategic Plan (Brailer, 2008). The plan had two goals, patient-focused healthcare and population health, with four objectives under each goal. The themes of privacy and security, interoperability, IT adoption, and collaborative governance recur across the goals, but they apply in very different ways to healthcare and population health.

Goal 1: Patient-focused Healthcare   Enable the transformation to higher quality, more cost-efficient, patient-focused healthcare through electronic health information access and use by care providers, and by patients and their designees.

► Objective 1.1—Privacy and Security: Facilitate electronic exchange, access, and use of electronic health information while protecting the privacy and security of patients' health information.

► Objective 1.2—Interoperability: Enable the movement of electronic health information to where and when it is needed to support individual health and care needs.

► Objective 1.3—Adoption: Promote nationwide deployment of EHR and PHR that put information to use in support of health and care.

► Objective 1.4—Collaborative Governance: Establish mechanisms for multi-stakeholder priority setting and decision making to guide development of the nation's health IT infrastructure

Goal 2: Population Health   Enable the appropriate, authorized, and timely access and use of electronic health information to benefit public health, biomedical research, quality improvement, and emergency preparedness.

▶ Objective 2.1—Privacy and Security: Advance privacy and security policies, principles, procedures, and protections for information access and use in population health.

▶ Objective 2.2—Interoperability: Enable the mobility of health information to support population-oriented uses.

▶ Objective 2.3—Adoption: Promote nationwide adoption of technologies and technical functions that will improve population and individual health.

▶ Objective 2.4—Collaborative Governance: Establish coordinated organizational processes supporting information use for population health.

Achievement of the eight objectives was tied to measurable outcomes, describing 43 strategies that needed to be done to achieve the objectives. Each strategy was associated with a milestone against which progress could be assessed. The plan included a set of illustrative actions to implement each strategy.

The HITECH Act

In passing the HITECH Act (American Recovery and Reinvestment Act, 2009), the federal government showed that it firmly believes in the benefits of using EHR. The act encouraged the widespread adoption of EHR by authorizing Medicare to make incentive payments to doctors and hospitals that use a certified EHR. These incentives are intended to drive adoption of EHR in order to reach the goal of every American having a secure EHR. To achieve this vision of a transformed healthcare system that health information technology can facilitate, there are three critical short-term prerequisites:

▶ Clinicians and hospitals must acquire and implement certified EHR in a way that fully integrates these tools into the care delivery process.

▶ Technical, legal, and financial supports are needed to enable information to flow securely to wherever it is needed to support healthcare and population health.

▶ A skilled workforce is needed that can facilitate the implementation and support of EHR, exchange of health information among healthcare providers and public health authorities, and the redesign of workflows within the healthcare settings.

Providers that implement and have a meaningful use of a certified EHR prior to 2015 are eligible for incentives. This means that a practice adopting an EHR actually gets paid more than a practice continuing to use paper charts.

After 2015, Medicare will begin to administer financial penalties for medical practices and hospitals that do not use an EHR. These will involve reducing the provider's payments by 1 percent per year for up to five years. By 2020, a provider still using paper charts will have payments reduced by 5 percent.

Critical Thinking Exercise 2: Compare ONC and HITECH

1. Compare the HITECH requirements with the goals and strategies of the original Strategic Framework discussed earlier.

Strategic Plan Update 2011–2015

The HITECH Act requires the ONC, in consultation with other appropriate federal agencies, to update the 2008–2012 Strategic Plan (discussed above). The 2008–2012 plan is intended "to guide the nationwide implementation of interoperable health information technology in both the public and private healthcare sectors that will reduce medical errors, improve quality, and produce greater value for healthcare expenditures (Brailer, 2008, pp. iii–iv).

The HITECH Act requires that the update include specific objectives, milestones, and metrics with respect to the following:

1. The electronic exchange and use of health information and the enterprise integration of such information.

2. The use of an EHR for each person in the United States by 2014.

3. The incorporation of privacy and security protections for electronic exchange of an individual's individually identifiable health information.

4. Establishing security methods to ensure appropriate authorization and electronic authentication of health information and specifying technologies or methodologies for rendering health information unusable, unreadable, or indecipherable.

5. Specifying a framework for coordination and flow of recommendations and policies under this subtitle among the Secretary, the National Coordinator, the HIT Policy Committee, the HIT Standards Committee, and other health information exchanges and other relevant entities.

6. Methods to foster the public understanding of health information technology.

7. Strategies to enhance the use of health information technology in improving the quality of healthcare, reducing medical errors, reducing health disparities, improving public health, increasing prevention and coordination with community resources, and improving the continuity of care among healthcare settings.

8. Specific plans for ensuring that populations with unique needs, such as children, are appropriately addressed in the technology design, as appropriate, which may include technology that automates enrollment and retention for eligible individuals.

Meaningful Use of a Certified EHR

The HITECH Act specifies the following three components of Meaningful Use:

1. Use of certified EHR in a meaningful manner

2. Use of certified EHR technology for electronic exchange of health information to improve quality of healthcare

3. Use of certified EHR technology to submit clinical quality measures (CQM) and other such measures selected by the Secretary of Health and Human Services

The key terms here are *meaningful use* and *certified EHR*. What is meaningful use and what is a certified EHR?

Meaningful Use

CMS officially published the Electronic Health Record Incentive Program Final Rule July 28, 2010, which finalized the incentive program and defined the criteria for determining "meaningful use" (U.S. Department of Health and Human Services, 2010a).

Requirements for meaningful use incentive payments were implemented over a multi-year period, in three stages. Stage 1, spanning the years 2011 and 2012, set the baseline for electronic data capture and information sharing. Stage 2 (scheduled to begin in 2013) and Stage 3 (scheduled for 2015) will continue to expand on this baseline and be developed through future rule making.

The 2011–2012 meaningful use requirements include a "core" group of requirements that must be met, plus an additional 5 that providers choose from a list of ten. The requirements for hospital and eligible professionals differ.

Eligible Professionals   For Eligible Professionals (EPs), there are a total of 25 meaningful use objectives. Twenty of the objectives must be completed to qualify for an incentive payment. Fifteen are core objectives that are required, and the remaining 5 objectives may be chosen from the list on the right.

EPs Core Requirements (all 15 must be met)	**Additional EPs Objectives (choose 5, at least one with asterisk*)**
CPOE	Drug-formulary checks
E-Prescribing	Incorporate clinical lab test results as structured data
Report ambulatory clinical quality measures	Generate lists of patients by specific conditions
Implement one clinical decision support rule	Send reminders to patients per patient preference for preventive/follow-up care
Provide patients with an electronic copy of their health information, upon request	Provide patients with timely electronic access to their health information
Provide clinical summaries for patients for each office visit	Use certified EHR technology to identify patient-specific education resources and provide to patient, if appropriate
Drug–drug and drug–allergy interaction checks	Medication reconciliation
Record demographics	Summary of care record for each transition of care/referrals
Maintain an up-to-date problem list of current and active diagnoses	Capability to submit electronic data to immunization registries/systems*
Maintain active medication list	Capability to provide electronic syndromic surveillance data to public health agencies*
Maintain active medication allergy list	
Record and chart changes in vital signs	
Record smoking status for patients 13 years or older	
Capability to exchange key clinical information among providers of care and patient-authorized entities electronically	
Protect electronic health information	

Eligible Hospitals   For Hospitals, there are a total of 24 meaningful use objectives. Fourteen are core objectives that are required, and the remaining 5 objectives may be chosen from the list on the right.

Hospitals Core Requirements (all 14 must be met)	**Additional Hospital Objectives (choose 5, at least one with asterisk*)**
CPOE	Drug-formulary checks
Drug-drug and drug-allergy interaction checks	Record advanced directives for patients 65 years or older
Record demographics	Incorporate clinical lab test results as structured data
Implement one clinical decision support rule	Generate lists of patients by specific conditions
Maintain up-to-date problem list of current and active diagnoses	Use certified EHR technology to identify patient-specific education resources and provide to patient, if appropriate
Maintain active medication list	Medication reconciliation
Maintain active medication allergy list	

Record and chart changes in vital signs

Record smoking status for patients 13 years or older

Report hospital clinical quality measures to CMS or States

Provide patients with an electronic copy of their health information, upon request

Provide patients with an electronic copy of their discharge instructions at time of discharge, upon request

Capability to exchange key clinical information among providers of care and patient-authorized entities electronically

Protect electronic health information

Summary of care record for each transition of care/referrals

Capability to submit electronic data to immunization registries/systems*

Capability to provide electronic submission of reportable lab results to public health agencies*

Capability to provide electronic syndromic surveillance data to public health agencies*

Certified EHR

Under the CMS EHR incentive programs, eligible healthcare providers must adopt and meaningfully use a "certified EHR" that has been certified by an ONC Authorized Testing and Certification Body (ONC-ATCB). To synchronize the two regulations, the ONC published the Health Information Technology: Initial Set of Standards, Implementation Specifications, and Certification Criteria for Electronic Health Record Technology Final Rule (U.S. Health and Human Services, 2010b) on the same date as the CMS Final Rule.

The ONC certification criteria represent the minimum capabilities an EHR needs to include and have properly implemented in order to achieve certification. They do not preclude developers from including additional capabilities that are not required for the purposes of certification.

Even prior to the HITECH Act, various leaders in health information technology recognized the need to create a credible authority for certification of EHR systems. Goal 1: Strategy 2 of the original Strategic Framework called for a mechanism to reduce the risk to providers adopting an EHR. The Certification Commission for Healthcare Information Technology (CCHIT®) was formed to do just that.

The history of CCHIT:

▶ 2004: organized by leading health information associations, the American Health Information Management Association (AHIMA), the Healthcare Information and Management Systems Society (HIMSS), and the National Alliance for Healthcare Information Technology, to examine and certify Health IT products.

▶ 2005: awarded a three-year contract by the HHS to develop certification criteria and an inspection process for EHR systems.

▶ 2006: began certifying ambulatory EHR systems.

▶ 2007: began certifying inpatient EHR systems.

▶ 2009: became an independent nonprofit organization.

▶ 2010: applied to become an ONC Authorized Testing and Certification Body

▶ 2011: began usability testing for ambulatory EHR systems.

The CCHIT Certified® program is an independently developed certification that includes a rigorous inspection of an EHR's integrated functionality, interoperability, and security using criteria developed by CCHIT's broadly representative, expert work groups.

The CCHIT inspection process is based on real-life medical scenarios designed to test products rigorously against the complex needs of healthcare providers. As part of the process, successful use is verified at live sites (Certification Commission for Health Information Technology, 2010).

The 2011 CCHIT certification criteria specifically align with those required to meet the ARRA/HITECH meaningful use criteria, with the intention that a provider using a CCHIT Certified EHR will be in compliance with eligibility requirements.

The ONC will recognize Authorized Testing and Certification Bodies in addition to CCHIT.

Clinical Quality Measures (CQM)

CMS has specified a number of clinical quality measures for meaningful use. Eligible Professionals must report on 3 required core or alternate core CQM and 3 additional CQM selected from a list of 38. Hospitals must report on 15 CQM.

To ensure EHR systems can support these CQM reporting requirements, ONC certification requires an EHR designed for an inpatient setting to be tested and certified to all of the clinical quality measures specified by CMS. An EHR designed for an ambulatory setting must be tested and certified as including at least 9 clinical quality measures specified by CMS—all 6 of the core (3 core and 3 alternate core) clinical quality measures specified, and at least 3 of the 38 additional measures. Of course, EHR developers may include as many clinical quality measures above that requirement as they see fit.

Why Electronic Health Records Are Important

Historically, a client's medical records consisted of handwritten notes, typed reports, and test results stored in a paper file system. A separate file folder was created and stored at each location where the client was examined or treated. X-ray films and other radiology records typically were stored separately from the chart, even when they were created at the same medical facility.

These are some of the drawbacks to paper records: Handwritten records often are abbreviated, cryptic, or illegible. When information is to be used by another medical facility, the charts must be copied and faxed or mailed to the other facility. Even single healthcare organizations with multiple facilities must transport the chart from one location to another when a client is seen at a different clinic than usual. Paper records are not easily searchable. For example, if a provider is notified that all clients on a particular drug need to be contacted, the only way of finding those clients is literally to open every chart and look at the medications list.

Certainly, improved legibility, the ability to find, share, and search client records, are strong points for an EHR. There are additional benefits from an EHR that take the delivery of care to levels that cannot be achieved with paper records. Four examples of this are: health maintenance, trend analysis, alerts, and decision support. These will be covered in more detail in Chapter 2.

However, there are the additional criteria. The IOM report calls for *electronic communication and connectivity among care partners* and the second goal of the ONC strategic framework is to *interconnect clinicians*. The need for EHR and better connectivity between EHR systems is examined in the Real-Life Story: Where's My Chart?

Critical Thinking Exercise 3: When the Chart Is Lacking

Read the Real-Life Story: "Where's My Chart?" and answer the following questions:

1. What are the dangers to the client of a provider who has no access to paper charts?

2. What is the likelihood of the second incident of the pulmonary embolism being overlooked?

3. How would client care be improved if the various EHR systems had been able to exchange records electronically?

Real-Life Story

Where's My Chart?

A 63-year-old man went to his doctor's office in Kentucky complaining of chest pains and tightness in his chest. He was immediately transferred to the local hospital, where a stress test and cardiac catheterization confirmed he had had a heart attack. He was hospitalized overnight.

Early retirement from his stressful job as well as a regimen of exercise, diet, beta blockers, aspirin therapy, and other medications proved successful. He moved from Kentucky to Florida and tried unsuccessfully to have his medical records concerning the previous heart attack transferred to his new doctor in Florida. The ECG and stress tests were repeated in Florida. Finally, after two years, the records from Kentucky arrived.

In subsequent years, he moved twice more but, wiser now, he took copies of his medical records with him. He continued a normal and active life until age 77, when he slipped in his workshop and broke his right knee. With his leg in a cast he was less active; a blood clot formed and broke free.

Three weeks after he broke his knee, he went to the doctor's office with what he described as very severe flu symptoms, extreme fatigue, a bad cough, and sharp pains in his back when he moved or coughed. The doctor sent him to the emergency room, where he was diagnosed with a pulmonary embolism in the lower lobe of the right lung. He was hospitalized and put on a therapy of blood thinners.

At age 79, he was continuing to lead an active lifestyle, but he was experiencing occasional sharp, brief, chest pain and brief dizziness. His doctor scheduled a stress test and cardiac catheterization at a cardiac center connected to the hospital. A blockage was discovered and a double bypass surgery was performed at the same hospital. The client tolerated the surgery well and recovered quickly.

However, one of the veins used in the bypass operation had been harvested from the leg that had the previous broken knee. Three weeks after he was discharged, he passed out and fell. He was taken by ambulance to the ER at the same hospital where he had had his surgery and where he had been hospitalized for the previous pulmonary embolism. Here is what happened:

▶ When the ambulance crew arrived at the house, they took a medical history from the client and his wife. They gave him oxygen and transported him to the hospital.

▶ When the ambulance arrived at the hospital, the nurses and ER staff again took a medical history from the client and client's family.

▶ The client's primary care physician had a complete medical history of the client, including copies of his records dating back to his heart attack in Kentucky, but the hospital system was not connected with the physician's office system.

▶ The client reported that he had just had surgery at the same hospital only three weeks before. The hospital system surely had his medical history, but the ER was on a different system and the ER doctors did not have access to the records.

▶ Although the ER was in the same hospital as the cardiac lab, the ER doctors did not have access to those records, either.

▶ The client told the ER staff he thought the symptoms felt similar to his previous experience with a pulmonary embolism, but even though the ER was in the same hospital where the client was hospitalized for a pulmonary embolism two years before, the ER doctors did not have access to the records from his past condition.

▶ A CAT scan was ordered based on client history of the embolism provided by a family member, not his medical record.

▶ After waiting in the ER for 14 hours, he was hospitalized with two pulmonary embolisms, one in each lung.

Seven days later, the client was discharged from the hospital. He has fully recovered and is doing fine.

This is not the story of poor medical care or a bad hospital. The hospital is affiliated with a major teaching hospital and is as good as or better than most. This is a story of the unfortunate state of medical records. Paper records are not accessible and can take months to transfer. The lack of timely copies of existing records often causes tests to be reordered or the obvious conditions to be overlooked. Electronic records are better, more accessible, but even the most sophisticated systems do not necessarily have the infrastructure in place to communicate with other EHR systems even in the same community or, as in this case, not even in the same facility!

Flow of Clinical Information into the Chart

Whether medical records are paper or electronic, the clinician's exam notes are usually documented in a defined structure organized into four components:

▶ Subjective

▶ Objective

▶ Assessment

▶ Plan

Charts in this format are referred to as SOAP notes; the acronym represents the first letter of the words *subjective*, *objective*, *assessment*, and *plan*. Guided Exercises throughout this book will frequently follow the SOAP format.

However, the EHR requires not only computers and software, but also change in the way providers work. To understand this, let us compare the workflow in a medical office using paper charts with a medical office using an EHR system.

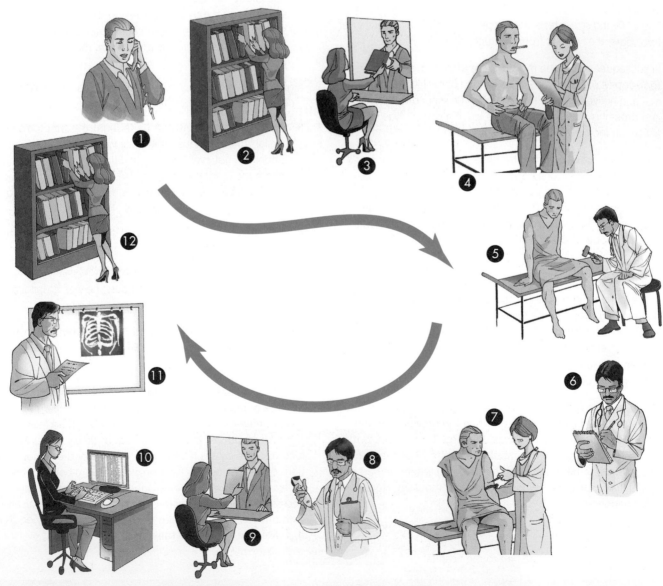

▶ Figure 1-2 Workflow in a medical office using paper charts.

Workflow of an Office Using Paper Charts

Follow the arrows in Figure 1-2 as you read the following description of a workflow in a primary care medical practice using paper charts.

❶ An established client phones the doctor's office and schedules an appointment.

❷ The night before the appointment, the client charts are pulled from the medical record filing system and organized for the next day's clients.

❸ On the day of the appointment, the client arrives at the office and is asked to confirm that insurance and demographic information on file is correct.

The client is given a clipboard with a blank medical history form and asked to complete it. The form asks the reason for today's visit and asks the client to report any previous history, any changes to medications, new allergies, and so on.

❹ Client is moved to an exam room and is ask to wait.

Subjective—The client is asked to describe in his or her own words what the problem is, what the symptoms are, and what he or she is experiencing.

A nurse reviews the form that the client completed, and may ask for more detail about the reason for the visit, which usually is called "the chief complaint." The nurse writes the chief complaint on a form that is placed at the front of the chart along with the updated client form. The nurse takes the vital signs and records them on the form. Vital signs are "objective" data.

❺ The clinician (doctor or nurse practitioner) enters the exam room and discusses the reason for the visit and reviews the symptoms, and may add to the "subjective" portion of the note.

Objective—The clinician performs a physical exam and makes observations about what he or she finds.

Assessment—Applying his or her training to the subjective and objective findings, the clinician arrives at a decision of what might be the cause of the client's condition, or what further tests might be necessary.

Plan of Treatment—The clinician prescribes a treatment, medication, or orders further tests. Perhaps a follow-up visit at a later date is recommended. A note will be made in the chart of each element of the plan.

❻ If medications have been ordered, a handwritten prescription will be given to the client or phoned to the pharmacy. A note of the prescription will be written in the client's chart.

The clinician marks one or more billing codes and one or more diagnosis codes on the chart and leaves the exam room.

❼ If lab work has been ordered, a nurse, medical assistant, or phlebotomist will obtain the necessary specimen and send the order to the lab.

❽ At many practices, the clinician creates the exam note from memory, either handwriting in the chart or dictating the subjective, objective, assessment, plan, and treatment information.

❾ When the client is dressed, the client will be escorted to the check-out area. The nurse or staff may give the client education material or medication instructions.

If x-rays or other diagnostic tests have been ordered at another facility, the office staff may call on behalf of the client and schedule the tests.

If a follow-up visit has been indicated, the client will be scheduled for the next appointment.

❿ The dictated notes are later transcribed and returned to the clinician to review before being permanently stored in the chart.

⓫ If lab, x-ray, or other diagnostic tests have been ordered, the results and reports are subsequently sent to the practice either by fax or on paper a number of days later. When received, they are filed in the client's chart and the chart is sent to the clinician for review.

⓬ The paper chart is filed again. Note that the chart may have to be pulled and re-filed each time a new document, such as the transcription or lab report, was added, which required the provider's review.

One obvious downside to a paper chart is accessibility. If the client chart is needed for a follow-up visit or by another provider, it is possible that it has not been returned to the file room while it is pending dictation or while the provider is reviewing test results.

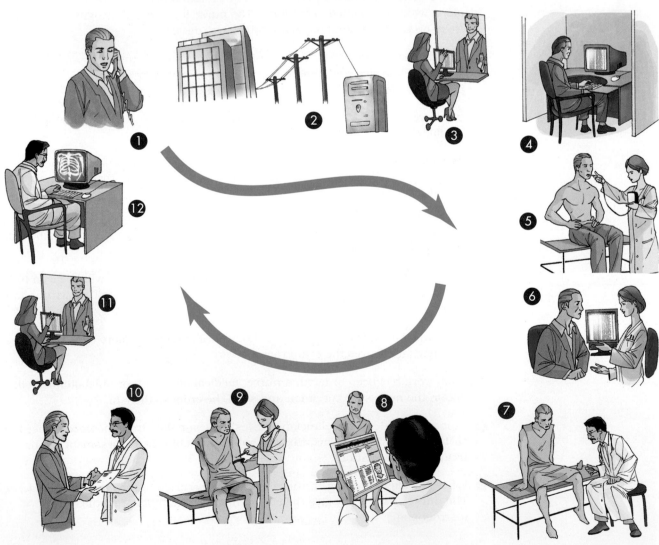

▶ Figure 1-3 Workflow in a medical office fully using an EHR.

Workflow of an Office Fully Using an EHR

Follow the arrows in Figure 1-3 as you read the following description of a workflow of a client visit to an office that fully uses the electronic capabilities that are available in EHR systems today, including client participation in the process and the capabilities of the Internet.

❶ An established client phones the doctor's office and schedules an appointment.

> **Internet alternative:** Clients are increasingly able to request an appointment and receive a confirmation via the Internet.

❷ The night before the appointment, the medical office computer electronically verifies insurance eligibility for clients scheduled the next day.

❸ On the day of the appointment, the client arrives at the office and is asked to confirm that the demographic information on file is still correct.

❹ A receptionist, nurse, or medical assistant asks the client to complete a medical history and reason for today's visit using a computer in a private area of the waiting room. The client completes a computer-guided questionnaire concerning his symptoms and medical history.

> **Internet alternative:** Some medical practices allow clients to use the Internet to complete the history and symptom questionnaire before coming to the office.

❺ When the client has completed the questionnaire, the system alerts the nurse that the client is ready to move to an exam room.

The nurse measures the client's height and weight and records it in the EHR. Using a modern device, vital signs for blood pressure, temperature, and pulse are recorded and wirelessly transferred into the EHR.

❻ *Subjective:* The nurse and client review the client-entered symptoms and history. Where necessary, the nurse edits the record to add clarification or refinement.

The clinician enters the exam room and discusses the reason for the visit and reviews with the client the information already in the chart.

❼ *Objective:* The clinician performs the physical exam. The clinician typically makes a mental provisional diagnosis. This is used to select a list or template of findings to quickly record the physical exam in the EHR.

The EHR present a list of problems the client reported in past visits that have not been resolved. The clinician reviews each, examining additional body systems as necessary, and marks the improvement, worsening, or resolution of each problem.

> **Assessment:** Applying his or her training to t he subjective and objective findings, the clinician arrives at a decision of one or more diagnoses, and decides if further tests might be warranted.

❽ *Plan of treatment:* The clinician prescribes a treatment and/or medication; in addition, the clinician may order further tests using the EHR.

If medication is to be ordered, the provider writes the prescription electronically. The prescription is compared with the client's allergy records and current drugs. The clinician is advised if there are any contraindications or potential problems. The prescription is compared with the formulary of drugs covered by the client's insurance plan and the physician is advised if an alternate drug is recommended (thereby avoiding a subsequent phone call from the pharmacist to revise the prescription). The prescription is then transmitted directly to the patient's pharmacy.

A built-in function of the EHR accurately calculates the correct evaluation and management code used for billing. The billing code is confirmed by the clinician and automatically transferred to the billing system.

When the visit is complete, so is the encounter note. The clinician signs the note electronically at the conclusion of the visit.

9 If lab work has been ordered, a nurse, medical assistant, or phlebotomist will obtain the necessary specimen and the order is sent electronically to the lab.

10 *Client education:* Because of the efficiency of the EHR system, the provider has more personal time with the client for counseling or client education. In many systems the provider can display and annotate pictures of body areas for client education, and print them so that the client can take them home.

When the client is dressed, he or she is given client education material, medication instructions, and a copy of the notes from the current visit. Allowing the client to take away a written record of the visit enables better compliance with the plan of care and recommended treatments.

11 The client is escorted to the check-out area.

If x-rays or other diagnostic tests have been ordered at another facility, the office staff may call on behalf of the client and schedule the tests.

If a follow-up visit has been indicated, the client will be scheduled for the next appointment.

12 If lab tests were ordered, the results are sent to the ordering provider electronically, are reviewed on screen, and automatically merged into the EHR.

If radiology or other diagnostic reports are sent to the practice electronically as textreports, they are imported into the EHR and can be reviewed by the clinician.

Accessibility is not a problem in the EHR system because there is no chart to "re-file." Multiple providers can access the client's chart, even simultaneously; for example, a nurse could be entering vital signs in the chart while another provider is reviewing the previous lab results.

Critical Thinking Exercise 4: Think About Workflow

Having compared the two workflow scenarios, we see the immediate advantages of the EHR for the client and clinician. Think about the workflow of the office that used paper charts (refer to Figure 1-2 if necessary.) Answer the following questions about the first workflow:

1. What was the nurse doing at the time of the client interaction?

2. Could the nurse have recorded this data in a computer?

3. Could the nurse have saved time later?

4. Could the data be entered by someone other than the caregiver?

    The client completed a form concerning any previous history, any changes to medications, new allergies, and so on.

5. Could the client have used a computer, or could the form have been designed to be read by a computer?

6. Could the client have completed the information before the visit?

    The nurse recorded various health measurements (vital signs) in the exam room.

7. Could the nurse have recorded the "chief complaint" or the vital signs in a computer instead of on a paper chart?

8. Were any of the instruments used capable of transferring their measurements to a computer system?

   During the physical exam, the clinician made observations and an assessment. This was later dictated from memory, subsequently transcribed by a typist, and finally reviewed and signed by the provider.

9. Is the time it would take to record the observations and assessment in the exam comparable to the time it takes to dictate and review the transcribed notes later?

   The provider prescribed medications and ordered tests.

10. Would the time spent entering the prescriptions on a computer justify the benefits of electronic prescribing?

11. Are results available electronically from laboratories that the medical practice uses?

12. Would ordering a test electronically improve the matching of results to orders when the tests were completed?

Inpatient Charts versus Outpatient Charts

The previous figures illustrated the differences between two medical clinics, one using a paper chart and another using an EHR. The differences between a hospital using a paper chart and a hospital fully using electronic records are even more significant. However, there are also differences in the type of chart an inpatient facility uses and the overall workflow process. In this section we are going to compare inpatient and outpatient charts.

Although some clients are admitted to the hospital through the emergency department or by transfer from another facility, most client admissions begin in the registration department. As depicted in Figure 1-4, the steps involved in an inpatient admission and discharge include the following:

❶ When the client arrives, client demographic and insurance information is collected or updated, and an account is set up for the client stay. Even if the client has been an inpatient previously, a new account is created (although previous clients will use their existing medical record number).

❷ An admitting and/or attending doctor is assigned to the client. A physician is required to perform a complete history and physical on an inpatient within 24 hours of the admission. In an outpatient facility, no such time limit is imposed on when or what type of physical is performed.

❸ The doctor orders tests, medications, and procedures.

❹ The doctor reviews the results of tests and diagnostic procedures when they are ready.

❺ Nurses provide most of the client care, administer medications, take samples for tests, measure vital signs, perform nursing assessments and nursing interventions, coordinate the care of interdisciplinary providers, manage the client care orders, provide essential client education, enable coordination of care for the discharge plan, and enter nursing notes into the chart.

❻ When a client leaves an inpatient facility, there is also a formal discharge process. Normally, the physician performs a final examination of the client and writes a

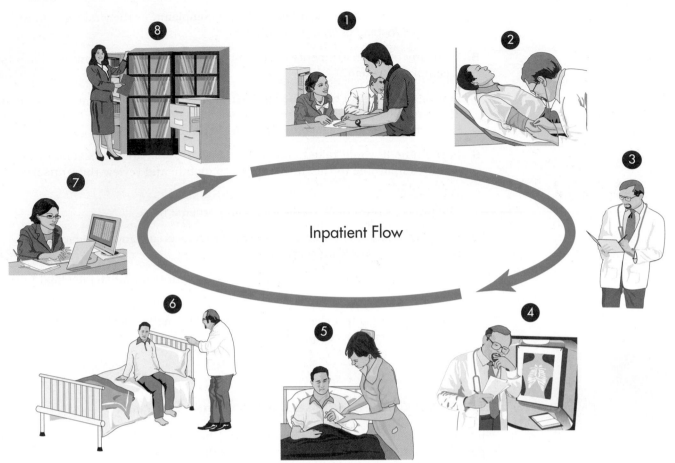

► **Figure 1-4 Flow of an inpatient from admission through discharge.**

discharge order. Discharge does not necessarily mean the client goes home. Clients may be discharged to a skilled nursing facility or a rehabilitation facility for further care. Clients who leave without a doctor's order are discharged AMA (against medical advice).

❼ Following discharge, the Health Information Management (HIM) department examines the client's chart to determine if it has any missing or unsigned documents (called chart deficiencies). When the chart is complete, it is sent to the billing department where the proper billing codes are assigned.

❽ In a facility using paper charts, the last step is to file the chart.

There are also several significant differences in the content and purpose of a client chart used in an acute care facility and that used by a medical office: the amount of information gathered about each client and the number of individuals who will need access to it. Figure 1-5 highlights some of the differences between inpatient and outpatient charts.

In an ambulatory setting such as a medical office, the client visits the office a number of times over a period of months or years. Although items produced outside of each visit, such as lab results and consult reports, are also integrated into the client's chart, the most important element of the outpatient chart is the provider's notes about each visit. The clinician reviews previous notes on each subsequent visit, using them to follow-up on past ailments and to measure the client's progress in managing chronic problems.

The medical chart is primarily used by the doctor and nurse, but is also used briefly by the administrative staff to prepare billings following each visit. The focus of the chart is the longitudinal care of the client. As such, it usually contains all records of the client's visits and any reports or results received from other providers.

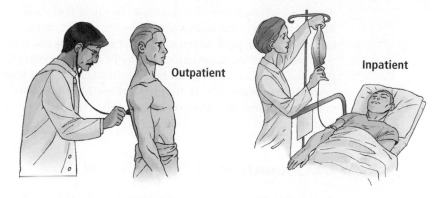

Most physician offices have a single chart for the patient. Notes for each visit, test results, and any other reports are added to the chart.	Most hospitals start a new chart each time a patient is admitted. Information from previous stays in the hospital is linked to the patient ID, but the current chart contains only information related to the current stay.
The quantity of data in an outpatient chart is relatively low by comparison.	The quantity of data in an inpatient chart is likely to be much larger. Vital signs are taken and nurses' notes are added numerous times per day; dietitians, respiratory therapists, and other providers add to the chart; there are typically many more orders for labs, medications, and so on.
The central element in the chart is the physician's exam note.	Physician exams tend to be brief; the main focus of the chart is the physician orders and nurse's notes indicating the patient's response.

▶ **Figure 1-5 Contents typical of acute care versus ambulatory charts.**

The inpatient chart, however, focuses on the treatment of a specific ailment or condition for which the client was hospitalized. Data are gathered more frequently during the inpatient's stay, resulting in a substantially large amount of information gathered during a short period of time. In most hospitals, a new chart or medical record is started for each hospital stay. Although records from previous hospitalizations are available for reference, they are not incorporated into the current chart, except as described in the admitting physician's history and physical notes.

Because a large number of caregivers are involved with the client's stay in an acute care facility, there are a larger number of individuals with a legitimate need to access a client's record than in an ambulatory care setting. These caregivers include not only nurses and physicians, but other specialists that may consult on the case; radiologists, respiratory therapists, dietitians, and in many hospitals, even the hospital pharmacists have access to records when consulting with the ordering physicians about the medications being prescribed.

These differences between an acute care chart and a medical office chart are consistent whether the facility uses paper or electronic charts. However, another difference between the inpatient and outpatient EHR is the system itself. In most systems designed for physicians' offices, the data typically is received and stored by the EHR software in a single electronic medical record system. Most hospitals have a large number of departments using computer systems from many different vendors. The hospital EHR may not necessarily merge the data from these systems into a single EHR. Often the hospital EHR allows the clinician to view data in these other systems through an interface but does not necessarily store the data in a single EHR. When disparate hospital systems are not able to share data, the clinicians may need to access more than one computer system to view the client data.

These same challenges are compounded in other types of care settings, such as nursing homes, extended care facilities, assisted living facilities, and home care. Many of these settings continue to be reliant on paper charts with little or no access to the latest care information of recent hospital or office visits. Although many home health agencies do have electronic records systems, few function with real-time connectivity. Often the nurses or other home care providers document using a portable computer that must be downloaded for permanent storage at the end of the day. Just as the home care or alternate care settings experience a delay in receiving updated patient information from the physician's office or hospital care settings, there is a similar obstacle to the physician or hospital receiving information from these alternate care settings. This lack of timely and effective information sharing impacts the continuity of client care in all care settings and results in a barrier to client care.

Documenting at the Point of Care

A goal of using an EHR system is to improve the accuracy and completeness of the client record. One way to achieve this is to record the information in the EHR at the time it is happening. This is called *point-of-care documentation.* In a physician's office, this means completing the SOAP note before the client ever leaves the office. In an inpatient setting, this means that nurses enter vital signs and nursing notes at bedside, not at the end of their shift. Figure 1-6 shows a nurse entering notes while seeing the client.

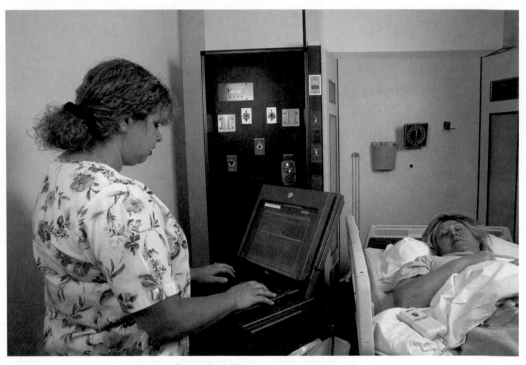

▶ **Figure 1-6 Nurse enters data at client's bedside.**

Real-time data entry into the EHR creates greater accessibility to the client's information, which supports improved decision making and collaboration between physicians, nurses, and other members of the healthcare team. No longer are key pieces of information isolated to the nurse's clipboard until the paper record is available. Without an EHR, the person with the paper record may or may not have the most up-to-date client data upon which decisions are being made.

Documenting at the point of care in an outpatient setting means when the visit is complete, the note is complete. The clinician can then provide not only education materials for clients to take home, but also can actually print a copy of the finished note. Giving clients a copy of the notes from that day's visit ensures that they will remember the key elements of their plan of treatment. They also will have a clearer understanding of their condition as well as information on any tests that may have been ordered or performed.

Leading EHR experts, Allen R. Wenner, an MD in Columbia, South Carolina, and John W. Bachman, an MD, professor of Family Medicine at the Mayo Medical School in Rochester, Minnesota, wrote: "Documenting an encounter at the point of care is the most efficient method of practicing medicine because the physician completes the medical record at the time of a patient's visit. Dictation time is saved and the need for personal dictation aides is eliminated. Thus, point-of-care documentation is less expensive than traditional dictation with its associated high cost of transcription. In addition, the physician can sign the note immediately.

"Patient care is improved because the patient can leave with a complete copy of the medical record, a step that stimulates compliance. The delivery process is improved with point-of-care documentation because referrals can be accomplished with full information available at the time that the referral is needed. For these benefits to occur, the clinical workflow changes to improve efficiency, increase data accuracy, and lower the overall cost of healthcare delivery" (Wenner & Bachman, 2004, pp. 297–319. © 2004 Springer Science + Business Media, Inc., New York).

Dr. John Bachman, MD, has formulated what he refers to as Bachman's Rule and Bachman's Law:

Bachman's Rule: "A patient who has a copy of a note is impressed by the fact that all the information they provided and were given is included for them to review. It also is useful in that it has immunizations prevention information and instructions. Outcome studies have shown it to be helpful in compliance and improvement of health; crossing the Quality Chasm."

Bachman's Law: "A clinician who gives a patient a copy of their note has all their work complete. Consequently there is no dictation, rework, signing, or any activity of maintaining the administrative workflow. This saves a great deal of money and means the workflow systems are extremely efficient."

Underscoring doctors Bachman and Wenner are the CMS regulations for meaningful use, which require eligible professionals to provide clinical summaries to clients' each office visit.

The availability of information from the EHR during the client encounter is an invaluable tool in counseling and client education. The clinician has access to graphs, medical images, test results, and anatomical drawings, all of which are useful in explaining something related to the client's condition or to illustrate an upcoming procedure. Using a Tablet PC, the nurse in Figure 1-7 is able to access the results of the client's most recent electrocardiogram wirelessly and explain them to the client.

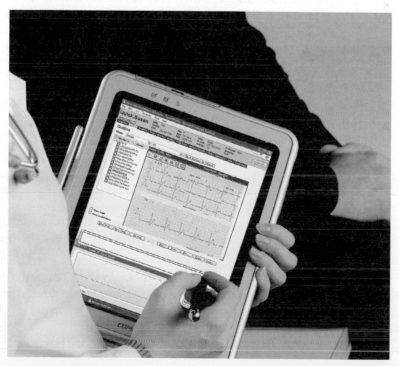

Courtesy of Allscripts, LLC.

▶ **Figure 1-7 Using a Tablet PC, nurse discusses ECG results with client.**

As stated earlier, adopting an EHR may change the way doctors and nurses work. Experience has shown that clients react favorably to the use of a computer during the exam, especially when they are part of the process, able to see the screen, and able to participate in the review of their information (Wenner & Bachman, 2004, pp. 297–319. © 2004 Springer Science + Business Media, Inc., New York).

Figure 1-8, provided by Dr. Wenner, lists the stages of change resulting from adoption of an EHR. Wenner and Bachman believe clients will help the clinician when they are given some degree of control, as reflected in points 2 and 3.

▶ **Figure 1-8 Stages of change in EHR adoption.**

Stages of Change in EHR Technology Adoption			
Stage	Technology Adoption	Medical Records	Medical Practice
Stage I	Do it the old way	The paper chart used and viewed as an historical document by physicians	Health care providers are the center of health care
Stage II	Adopt technology but continue to do it the old way	Transcribing dictation onto paper, using the EHR for data storage only managed by staff	Providers continue to dominate medical decisions and maintain all health care data
Stage III	Change the workflow to leverage the technology Paperless medical office	Use EHR at the point-of-care with providers and patients participating to allow real-time continuity of care	Patients and providers will share decision making as health care information is available to both

Nurses experience a similar challenge adapting their workflow to effectively include the computer technology into their client care, while maintaining their focus on the client and not the computer. As the nurse develops competency in informatics, the nurse finds that the EHR becomes a tool to facilitate and communicate client care across the healthcare team and across the continuum of care. Early electronic programs development facilitated documentation of the client assessment or offered care planning documentation, but only marginally support documentation of the full nursing process into the EHR. Advances in the development of EHR in the past decade have begun to reflect the work of nursing theorists, nursing research, and nursing involvement in health policy and the computer program development that enables nursing electronic documentation in the variety of client settings where nursing care is provided.

The EHR system strives to improve healthcare by giving the provider and client access to complete, up-to-date records of past and present conditions; it also enables the records to be used in ways that paper medical records could not. The sooner the data is entered, the sooner it is available for other providers and the client. Chapters 2–12 will explore how data is entered in the EHR and focus on ways EHR systems speed up data entry, enabling nurses to achieve point-of-care documentation in real time.

This need for real-time documentation poses special challenges in the inpatient setting where the nurse may be juggling the needs of five or more clients simultaneously. Similarly, the nurses must include in their documentation of the full nursing process to affirm care delivery that complies with a varied of safety standards such as the national patient safety goals and documentation standard from the state and federal oversight agencies and private insurers.

The nursing documentation in the EHR also needs to reflect the standards of practice for their area of nursing specialty. Although the EHR puts the client's complete information at a single computer point, it is imperative for the nurse to develop a core competency to use the EHR effectively.

The Physical Clinic and Clinician Mobility

J. Peter Geerloffs, MD, chief medical officer at Allscripts, coined the acronym IDDUINEM, which stands for "If doctors don't use it, nothing else matters." This means, of course, that the EHR has to be designed and deployed in a way that enables clinicians to make it a part of their workflow. The same rule applies for nurses.

One factor that influences the ability of a nurse or other provider to document at the point of care is the availability of a computer when and where it is needed. Let us examine how the medical facility's choice of computers, devices, and technology can affect the successful adoption of an EHR. The following section will provide you with an idea of the types of computers you will find in a hospital, clinic, or medical office.

EHR on Computer Workstations

The most common type of computer in a healthcare facility is a workstation wired to the LAN. In hospitals you will find computer workstations everywhere. In medical offices and clinics, they are used in the billing, nursing, and lab areas. In some offices, you will find them in the exam room, and in a comparatively few offices you will find them in the waiting room or a subwaiting area for clients to use.

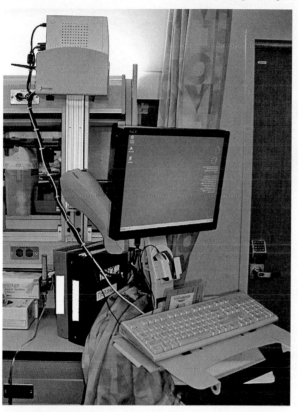

Computer workstations are cheap, reliable, dependable, and usually situated in one location. You are probably working on one right now. They are easier for the IT department to manage and usually easier to upgrade when necessary.

Workstations take up more space, requiring extra room for the keyboard and mouse. Most medical facilities were built long before anyone thought about nurses and other providers using computers. Many nursing stations are already filled and have only a small counter or writing area. Sometimes, workstations are mounted on flexible telescoping mounts to make access easier. Figure 1-9 shows and example of an adjustable workstation mounted in a hospital pediatrics unit.

Certainly workstations at fixed locations will be the right choice for some of the personnel who input data in the EHR. Whether they make sense at the point of care depends on the setting. In a hospital it typically wouldn't make sense to put a computer in every inpatient's room. Hospitals tend toward some of the more portable devices discussed below. However, in a medical office with a smaller number of exam rooms, workstations will frequently be used if the room has enough free space to install one.

Photo by Richard Gartee.

▶ **Figure 1-9 Nursing Workstation in a pediatric unit.**

Although workstations can pose a security risk when left unattended, that is easily handled through any number of biometric, or smart card, and auto sign-off solutions. With these solutions, the screen blanks or the EHR is logged off whenever an authorized user is not present. An ID badge or other device has a computer chip imbedded in it that can be detected by the workstation. Biometric solutions usually involve a pad on the keyboard or mouse that reads and authenticates a user's fingerprint.

One final advantage of the workstation is that it can support a substantially higher screen resolution (finer picture) than any other device. This makes it the only viable choice for radiologists and others who "read" diagnostic quality images of x-rays, CAT scans, as shown in Chapter 2, Figure 2-15.

Of course, the EHR is actually on a network server somewhere else. Workstations and other devices are connected to the network. This can be done with cables that have been wired in the building walls or through "wireless" access points that connect to the network through high-frequency radio signals. One advantage of a workstation is that it is ideally suited to a wired network connection. These are usually much faster and less subject to failure.

EHR on Laptop Computers

A laptop computer, as shown in Figure 1-10, packages the screen, keyboard, mouse, and computer in one unit, about the size of an 8″ × 11″ notebook. These provide mobility for nurses to stay connected and take their work from room to room.

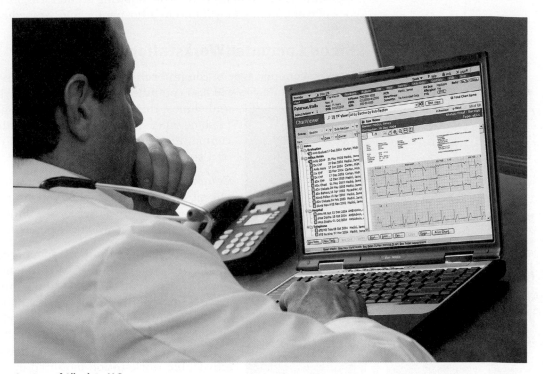

Courtesy of Allscripts, LLC.

▶ **Figure 1-10 Laptop computers with Wi-Fi connectivity provide portability.**

Although laptops can be connected to a wired network fairly easily, it is usually bothersome to have to plug the computer in and log on to the network each time you enter a room. For this reason, most laptops use a wireless standard called "Wi-Fi," which stands for "wireless fidelity," to connect to the network. Wi-Fi capability is standard on many laptop computers.

Wireless networking, however, works only for very short distances; therefore, it requires infrastructure in the medical facility. Transmitters and receivers called "access points" must be installed throughout the building in close enough proximity that the laptop (or other wireless device) can always find the radio signal.

There are some concerns that wireless access points can be used by unauthorized computers to enter the network, or that wireless transmissions containing EPHI (protected health information in electronic form) can be intercepted. However, medical systems installed by qualified installers use secure authentication and encryption techniques that effectively protect the EHR and client data.

Laptops also are more troublesome for the IT department to manage and update, and laptops eventually become obsolete because they have only limited capability for hardware upgrades. Laptops have other issues as well. Typically they run on batteries. This means after 2 to 4 hours of use, the batteries need to be recharged. Although laptop computers have A/C adapters, most users do not like having to plug them in every time they come into a room. The small appearance of a laptop is deceptive. They typically weigh from 3.5 to 9 pounds; after carrying it all day, that weight feels quite heavy.

Being mobile, laptops also are more susceptible to being dropped, lost, or damaged. The keyboards are smaller and the built-in pointing devices that replace the mouse take some getting use to. However, laptops typically have high-resolution screens and will usually run any program that will run on a workstation.

One choice for facilities with space limitations is to combine the laptop with a portable cart, as shown in Figure 1-11. The cart can be easily rolled from room to room and provides a stable and comfortable work area for the nurse. If the laptop has Wi-Fi connectivity, there is nothing to plug in. Also, if the batteries begin to run low, the A/C adapter-battery charger is usually right on the back of the cart. You also may have seen computer carts used on hospital floors, where they are affectionately known as "computers on wheels."

EHR on a Tablet PC

The Tablet PC (shown earlier in Figure 1-7) offers the size and portability (and drawbacks) of a laptop computer. However, it offers one feature that many providers really like. Users can move and click the mouse by just touching the screen with a special stylus supplied with the Tablet PC. EHR systems that involve primarily opening lists and clicking findings with a mouse work well on a Tablet PC.

If 95 percent of the charting is done with a mouse, then a Tablet PC is ideal. However, a Tablet PC typically does not have a keyboard for touch typing. Most have a small area of the screen that can be used as a keyboard. Typing is done by clicking the mouse over each letter of the alphabet. This technique is serviceable for a word or two but painful for a nurse who uses a lot of free text.

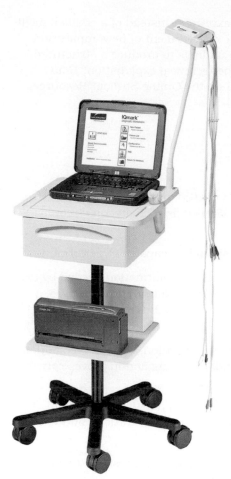

Courtesy of Midmark Diagnostics Group.
▶ **Figure 1-11 Laptop on computer cart.**

To compensate for the lack of a keyboard, the Tablet PC has two other features. One is handwriting recognition, which allows you to hand print characters on the screen, and then a few seconds later it will convert them into typed characters. The other is speech recognition, which is built into the Tablet PC operating system. Spoken words are recorded and then processed with special software to produce a text note. Both of these features require you to train the computer to recognize your handwriting or speech patterns. For some nurses, these features work relatively well; others find that the error rate is too high.

Speech Recognition

Speech recognition is a useful computer tool that is frequently used in specialties such as radiology and pathology, as it allows providers to document their observations, while they use the mouse for a different application such as the manipulation of x-rays or diagnostic images. Modern voice recognition software can also recognize verbal commands to operate the software. This allows the radiologist or pathologist to open orders, save reports, zoom images, or change contrast without using his or her hands. In nursing, speech recognition can be used to add free-text comments to findings in the codified medical record.

Speech recognition software recognizes the patterns in your speech as words and turns them into text. But does speech recognition work? Most people speak at least 160 words per minute but type fewer than 40 words a minute, so speech recognition should be a lot faster. Speech recognitions systems can achieve up to 99 percent accurate recognition, but most people seem to average about 95 percent. This means that dictated notes will have one or more errors that must be corrected. The time spent backing up and making corrections slows down the overall rate of efficiency. The good news is that speech recognition systems improve as they are used. Each time the speaker makes a correction, the system learns a little more about the speaker's voice patterns. Recognition is also improved by use of a special medical language model, which recognizes medical terms that might not be in a generic speech recognition product.

Historically, these systems were used to produce a text report instead of a codified medical record. That problem has been overcome with the development of new applications that match the spoken text to Medcin nomenclature findings to produce a structured note. To learn how speech recognition works, read the technical explanation, *How Speech Recognition Software Works*, which is located on the Online Student Resources web site (access details provided on the inside cover).

Chapter One Summary

Electronic Health Records are the portions of a client's medical records that are stored in a computer system as well as the functional benefits derived from having an electronic health record.

The IOM set forth eight core functions that an EHR should be capable of performing:

▶ **Health information and data** Provide improved access to information needed by care providers, using a defined data set that includes medical and nursing diagnoses, a medication list, allergies, demographics, clinical narratives, laboratory test results, and more.

▶ **Result management** Electronic results for better interpretation, quicker recognition and treatment of medical problems; reduces redundant testing and improves care coordination among multiple providers.

▶ **Order management** CPOE systems improve workflow, eliminate lost orders and ambiguities caused by illegible handwriting, monitor for duplicate orders, and reduce the time required to fill orders.

▶ **Decision support** Includes prevention, prescribing of drugs, diagnosis and management, and detection of adverse events and disease outbreaks.

Computer reminders and prompts improve preventive practices in areas such as vaccinations, breast cancer screening, colorectal screening, and cardiovascular risk reduction. Computer reminders and real-time audit tracking alert nurses and other care givers to avoid errors or omissions in standards of care.

▶ **Electronic communication and connectivity** Among care partners, enhances patient safety and quality of care, especially for patients who have multiple providers.

▶ **Patient support** For example, patient education and home monitoring by patients using electronic devices.

▶ **Administrative processes and reporting** Increases the efficiency of healthcare organizations and provide better, timelier service to patients.

▶ **Reporting and population health** Facilitates the reporting of key quality indicators and timely reporting of adverse reactions and disease outbreaks.

The CPRI identified three key criteria for an EHR:

▶ Capture data at the point of care

▶ Integrate data from multiple sources

▶ Provide decision support

The ONC created a strategic framework for achieving widespread adoption of EHR within 10 years. The framework was revised for 2008–2012, and again for 2011–2015.

The HITECH Act provides CMS incentives for providers to use a certified EHR.

ONC seeks to reduce the risk of EHR investment by establishing Authorized Testing and Certification Bodies to certify EHR systems.

An encounter document is organized into four components:

► Subjective

► Objective

► Assessment

► Plan

EHR systems strive to improve healthcare by giving the provider and client access to complete, up-to-date records of past and present conditions.

Documenting at the point of care means the providers (clinicians, nurses, and medical assistants) record findings at the time of the encounter, not after they have left the client.

Implementing an EHR requires changes in the way that providers work. The choice of computers, devices, and technology can affect the successful adoption of an EHR. One aspect, how much space is available, may determine the type of device to use. The second aspect is the mobility of the clinicians. The third aspect is what type of clinician–client interaction the clinicians hope to achieve. These factors determine how and where to use computers to achieve point-of-care EHR.

Each of the devices we discussed had advantages and disadvantages:

► Computer workstations are cheap, reliable, dependable, and easier for the IT department to manage, and can be upgraded when necessary. But they take up more space and may not fit in the exam rooms.

► A laptop computer packages everything in a unit about the size of a notebook. They provide mobility for clinicians who want to take their work from room to room. But they require a wireless network to gain that mobility and they have limited battery life.

► The Tablet PC offers the size and portability of a laptop computer and users can move and click the mouse by just touching the screen with a special stylus. However, in tablet mode, it does not have a keyboard, so it is less desirable when there is a lot of keyboard input. It works well for EHR systems that primarily involve opening lists and clicking findings with a mouse. Similar to laptops, it requires a wireless network and has a limited battery life.

► Speech recognition software can interpret the sound waves of speech and match them to vocabulary words, converting speech to text.

References

American Recovery and Reinvestment Act of 2009, Title XIII Health Information Technology for Economic and Clinical Health, Pub. L. 111-5 (February 17, 2009).

Brailer, D. J. (2004, July 21). *The decade of health information technology: Delivering consumer-centric and information-rich healthcare.* Washington, DC: U.S. Department of Health and Human Services.

Brailer, D. J. (2008). *The ONC-coordinated federal health IT strategic plan: 2008–2012.* Washington, DC: Office of National Coordinator for Health Information Technology.

Certification Commission for Health Information Technology. (2010). *CCHIT Certified® 2011 certification handbook.* Chicago, IL: Author.

Dick, R. S., & Steen, E. B. (2000). *The computer-based patient record: An essential technology for health care.* Washington, DC: Institute of Medicine, National Academy Press. (Originally published 1991, revised 1997)

Exec. Order No. 13,335, 69 Fed. Reg. 24,059 (April 27, 2004).

Kohn, L. T., Corrigan, J. M., & Donaldson, M. S. (Eds.). (1999). *To err is human: Building a safer health system.* Washington, DC: Committee on Quality of Healthcare in America, Institute of Medicine.

Murphy, G., Waters, K., Hanken, M. A., & Pfeiffer, M. (Eds.). (1999). *Electronic health records: Changing the vision.* Philadelphia: W. B. Saunders Company.

U.S. Department of Health and Human Services, 42 CFR 412, 413, 422, and 495. Medicare and Medicaid Programs; Electronic Health Record Incentive; Final Rule 75(144) Fed. Reg. 44,314 (July 28, 2010a).

U.S. Department of Health and Human Services, 45 CFR 170; Medicare and Medicaid Programs; Electronic Health Record Incentive; Final Rule 75(144) Fed. Reg. 44,314 (July 28, 2010b).

Wenner, A. R., & Bachman, J. W. (2004). Transforming the physician practice: Interviewing patients with a computer. In M. J. Ball, C. A. Weaver, & Joan M. Kiel (Eds.), *Healthcare information management systems: Cases, strategies, and solutions* (3rd ed., pp. 297–319). New York: Springer Science + Business Media, Inc.

Test Your Knowledge

1. What does the acronym EHR stand for?

2. What is the definition of an EHR?

3. Explain the benefits of EHR over paper charts.

4. Describe what points of the workflow are different between offices using a paper and an electronic chart.

5. Name at least three forces driving the change to EHR.

6. What are the four goals of the Strategic Framework created by the Office of the National Coordinator for Health Information Technology?

7. Describe at least three differences between inpatient and outpatient EHR systems.

8. Explain why documenting at the point of care improves healthcare.

9. What is the HITECH Act?

10. What is the name of an organization that certifies EHR systems?

11. What three benefits of electronic results identified by the IOM report?

12. List the eight core functions that an EHR should be capable of performing.

13. List the three criteria of an EHR defined by CPRI.

14. How can the universal implementation of EHR in all settings help drive improvements in healthcare in general?

15. How can the EHR impact the nurse–physician working relationship?

Ask your instructor for answers to Test Your Knowledge

nursing.pearsonhighered.com

Prepare for success with animated examples, practice questions, challenge tests, and interactive assignments.

Chapter

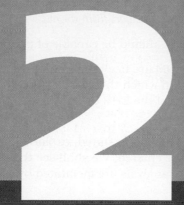

Functional EHR Systems

Learning Outcomes

After completing this chapter, you should be able to:

1. Compare different formats of EHR data

2. Describe the importance of codified EHR

3. Have an understanding of prominent EHR code sets such as SNOMED-CT, MEDCIN, LOINC, and CCC

4. Explain different methods of capturing and recording EHR data

5. Catalog and retrieve documents and images from a digital image system

6. Discuss the exchange of data between EHR and other systems

7. Discuss the benefits of client-entered data

8. Describe the functional benefits from a codified EHR

9. Compare different formats of lab result data

10. Discuss alert systems and drug utilization review

11. Describe two important components of health maintenance

12. Provide examples of EHR decision support

Format of Data Determines Potential Benefits

Chapter 1 identified the EHR as the portions of the client's medical record stored in the computer system, *as well as the functional benefits derived from them.*

The IOM defined eight core functions that an EHR should be capable of performing.

Four of the *functional benefits* identified by the IOM are health maintenance, trend analysis, alerts, and decision support. The form in which the data is stored determines to what extent the computer can use the content of the EHR to provide additional functions that improve the quality of care.

This chapter will examine the forms in which EHR data is stored, explore how functional benefits are derived from it, and how data may be entered. We shall see that health information exchange, trending, alerts, and data analysis are facilitated by adherence to coding standards.

EHR Data Formats

The various ways in which medical records data are stored in the database may be broadly categorized into three forms:

Digital images This form of EHR data can be retrieved and displayed by the computer, but a human is required to interpret the meaning of the content. This category may be subcategorized into:

> **Diagnostic images** such as digital x-rays, CAT scans, digital pathology, and even annotated drawings

> **Scanned documents** such as paper forms, old medical records, letters, or even sound files of dictated notes

Text files The second type of data includes word processing files of transcribed exam notes and text reports. It is principally obtained in the EHR by importing text files from outside sources.

Discrete data This third form of stored information in an EHR is the easiest for the computer to use. It can be instantly searched, retrieved, and combined or reported in different ways. Discrete data in an EHR may be subcategorized into:

> **Fielded data** in which each piece of information is assigned its own position in a computer record called a "field." The meaning of the information is inferred from its position in the record. For example, a record of the client's medical problem might look like this:

> "knee injury", "20120331", "improved", "20120428"

> The fields in this example are surrounded by quotation marks. The computer would be programmed to look for the name of the problem in the first field, the date of onset in the second field, the status of the problem in the third field, and the date of the last exam in the fourth field.

> **Coded data** is fielded data that also contains codes in addition to or in place of descriptive text. Codes eliminate ambiguities about the clinician's meaning.

> A codified EHR record of the same knee problem might look like this:

> "8442", "knee injury", "20120331", "improved", "20120428"

Limitations of Certain Types of Data

An EHR certainly offers improved accessibility to client records as a functional benefit regardless of the format of its data. However, to achieve its full functional benefits, the computer must be able to quickly and accurately identify the information contained within the records.

Digital image data can be retrieved and displayed by the computer, but a human is required to interpret the meaning of the content. Although this is beneficial for sharing diagnostic images, if the bulk of the EHR is simply scanned paper documents, only one or two of the IOM criteria defined in Chapter 1 are satisfied.

Text data are useful for nurses to read and can be searched by the computer for research purposes. However, text data is seldom used for generating alerts, trend analysis, decision support, or other real-time EHR functions, because the search capability is slow and the results often ambiguous.

Fielded data is the most common way to store information in computers and EHR systems. It is fast and efficient and uses very little storage space. However, unless the fielded data is also codified, the meaning of the data can be ambiguous.

Within nursing, many different terms are used to describe the same symptom, condition, or observation. Additionally, clinicians often use short abbreviations to document their observations in a client chart. This makes it difficult for a computer to compare notes from one provider to another. For example, nurses on two different shifts might record a knee injury problem differently:

> Nurse 1: "twisted his knee"

> Nurse 2: "knee sprain"

A search of medical records by the description "knee injury" might not find the records created by either nurse.

Coded data is when a code is stored in the medical record in addition to the text description—the record is then considered codified. The EHR system can instantly find and match the desired information by code regardless of the clinician's choice of words. A codified EHR is more useful than a text-based record because it precisely identifies the clinician's finding or treatment.

EHR data stored in a fielded, codified form adds significant value, but if the codes are not standard it will be difficult to exchange medical record data between different EHR systems or facilities. Remember, the exchange of data is one of the eight core functions defined by the IOM. Using a national standard code set instead of proprietary codes to codify the data will better enable the exchange of medical records among systems, improve the accuracy of the content, and open the door to the other functional benefits derived from having an electronic health record.

Standard EHR Coding Systems

EHR coding systems are called *nomenclatures*. EHR nomenclatures differ from other code sets and classification systems in that they are designed to codify the details and nuance of the client–clinician encounter. EHR nomenclatures are different from billing code sets in this respect. For example, a procedure code used for billing an office visit does not describe what the clinician observed during the visit, just the type of visit and complexity of the examination. EHR nomenclatures need to have a lot more codes to describe the details of the encounter; for this reason, they are said to be more *granular*. Two prominent nomenclatures for EHR records are SNOMED-CT® and MEDCIN®. Another prominent coding system, LOINC®, is used for lab results.

Unfortunately, many hospital systems use none of these standard systems, having instead developed internal coding schemes applicable only to their facilities. These work within the organization but create problems when trying to integrate other software or exchange data with other facilities. As discussed in the previous chapter, the HITECH Act contains a federal mandate for the exchange of data with other facilities.

Furthermore, there is an international recognition of global challenges and opportunities for testing improvements in evidenced-based practice, contributing to improved public health worldwide and describing clients' health status, nursing interventions, and care outcomes. To create an EHR that is able to receive, create, and compare medical information from numerous sources, it is necessary to adopt a coding system that is used by many providers—in other words, a national standard. The challenge to nursing is not only the adoption of a codified language of nursing documentation, but also a national or international standard.

Prominent EHR Code Sets

EHR nomenclatures have hundreds of thousands of codes to represent not only procedures and diseases but also symptoms, observations, history, medications, interventions, and a myriad of other details. The level of granularity determines how fine a level of detail is represented by a code in the nomenclature.

However, too much granularity can make a code set difficult to use at the point of care. The point of care is when both the clinician and client are present. Extremely granular code sets, called *reference terminologies*, are impractical for a provider to use at the point of care. Designed for data analysis, these code sets often are applied to the medical records after the fact for a specific research project.

To balance the need for granularity with the practical requirements of point-of-care documentation, EHR nomenclatures use the concept of *findings*, or codified observations, which are medically meaningful to the clinician. Although some systems of clinical vocabulary are just "data dictionaries" that are used to standardize medical terms, EHR nomenclatures precorrelate those terms into clinically relevant findings.

For example, a clinical vocabulary will have the terms *eye*, *arm*, *leg*, *chest*, *nostril*, *left*, *right*, *red*, *yellow*, *radiating*, *discharge*, and *pain*. These terms could be combined in many ways, some of them meaningless. Findings are less granular than individual terms but combine those terms in ways that are clinically relevant. For example, "chest pain radiating to the left arm" uses one coded finding to record five clinical terms as a meaningful symptom.

Findings are often linked to other findings, whereas codes in classification code sets are usually only related to the root code of the group that the code is in.

For example, the finding of abdominal pain is related to more than 550 diagnosis codes, whereas a specific diagnosis code for peptic ulcer is not related to any other diagnosis code.

Conversely, in an EHR nomenclature the diagnostic finding of peptic ulcer is related to 168 other findings (one of which is abdominal pain).

Linked or indexed findings in an EHR nomenclature enable clinicians to quickly locate related symptoms, elements of the physical exam, assessments, and treatments when documenting the client's condition.

EHR users tend to locate findings by the description, not by the code. EHR nomenclature code numbers are typically invisible to the user.

A feature unique to EHR nomenclatures is that they often include internal cross-references to other standard code sets. These tables help the EHR to communicate with other systems. Code sets not designed for an EHR do not typically contain a map to other code sets with their structure.

The following sections will provide a brief history and purpose of several of the most prominent coding standards you are likely to encounter or use in an EHR.

SNOMED-CT   SNOMED stands for Systematized Nomenclature of Medicine; CT stands for Clinical Terms. SNOMED-CT is a merger of SNOMED, a medical nomenclature developed by the College of American Pathologists, and the "Read Codes," developed by Dr. James Read for the National Health Service in the United Kingdom.

SNOMED-CT includes cross-references to map SNOMED-CT to other standard code sets, including those discussed below.

SNOMED-CT Structure   The SNOMED-CT Core terminology contains over 364,400 healthcare *concepts*, organized into 18 hierarchical categories. The data structure of SNOMED-CT is complex. Concept names, descriptions, and synonyms number more than 984,000.

SNOMED Concepts have descriptions and Concept IDs (numeric codes). The concepts are arranged in the following hierarchies:

- Finding
- Disease
- Procedure and intervention
- Observable entity
- Body structure
- Organism
- Substance
- Pharmaceutical/biological product
- Specimen
- Physical object
- Physical force
- Events
- Environments and geographical locations
- Social context
- Context-dependent categories
- Staging and scales
- Attribute
- Qualifier value

SNOMED-CT has approximately 1,450,000 semantic relationships in the nomenclature. There are two types of relationships between SNOMED-CT concepts: *Is-A* relationships and *Attribute* relationships.

Is-A relationships connect concepts within a single hierarchy. For example, the disease concept Bronchial Pneumonia *Is-A* Pneumonia (also a disease concept).

Attribute relationships, however, connect concepts from two different hierarchies. For example, the disease concept Bronchial Pneumonia has the associated *Attribute* Inflammation (which is from a different hierarchy, morphology.)

MEDCIN   MEDCIN is a medical nomenclature and knowledge base developed by Medicomp Systems, Inc., in collaboration with physicians on staff at Cornell, Harvard, Johns Hopkins, and other major medical centers. The nursing codes in MEDCIN are the result of collaboration with Virginia Saba, developer of the CCC system described later in this chapter.

The purpose of the MEDCIN nomenclature and the intent of the design differentiate it from other coding standards. SNOMED-CT and other coding systems were designed to classify or index medical information for research or other purposes. MEDCIN was designed for point-of-care use by the provider. MEDCIN is not just a list of medical terms, but rather a list of *findings* (clinical observations) that are medically meaningful to the clinician.

MEDCIN includes cross-references to map MEDCIN to SNOMED-CT as well as other standard code sets that will be discussed later in this book. These include: ICD-9-CM, ICD-10, CPT-4, LOINC, CCC, and RxNorm drug codes.

MEDCIN Structure   The MEDCIN nomenclature consists of 277,000 clinical concepts or "findings" divided into six broad categories:

► Symptoms

► History

► Physical Examination

► Tests

► Diagnoses

► Therapy

MEDCIN differs from other EHR coding systems in that the nomenclature is not just a codified list of findings. The MEDCIN nomenclature is available in a "knowledge base" with a diagnostic index of more than 68 million links between clinically related findings. This "knowledge" enables an EHR system based on MEDCIN to quickly find other clinical "findings" that are likely to be needed; this in turn reduces the time it takes to create encounter or nursing notes.

This difference means a clinician selects less individual codes to document the complete client encounter. For example, SNOMED-CT has a code for "arm" and a code for "pain"; MEDCIN has a "finding" for "arm pain." MEDCIN often has additional findings that infer important nuances; for example, the "finding" for "arm tenderness" might more accurately describe the client's symptom than arm pain.

SNOMED-CT is often referred to as a "reference terminology." It provides very granular coding that normalizes data for research and reporting. Its structure provides millions of semantic links based on a term, word, or concept. Figure 2-1 shows the SNOMED-CT finding Asthma with its various Is-A relationships.

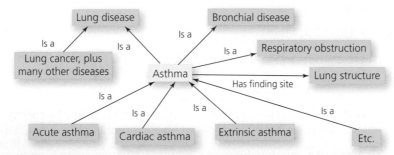

► **Figure 2-1 SNOMED-CT links for the term "Asthma."**

Figure 2-1 and Figure 2-2 compare the structure of SNOMED-CT and MEDCIN using the finding for asthma. As you can see from the comparison, the MEDCIN knowledge base relates asthma to 279 total direct links (only 70 are shown in Figure 2-2). Each of these has relevancy to point-of-care use for a client with asthma. SNOMED-CT links include obvious links to asthma but not directly to the symptoms, tests, or therapy. Links in Figure 2-1 also connect to lungs and other lung diseases not related to asthma. Such associations are sometimes useful when coding records for research but can make it difficult for the clinician to use such a system while seeing the client.

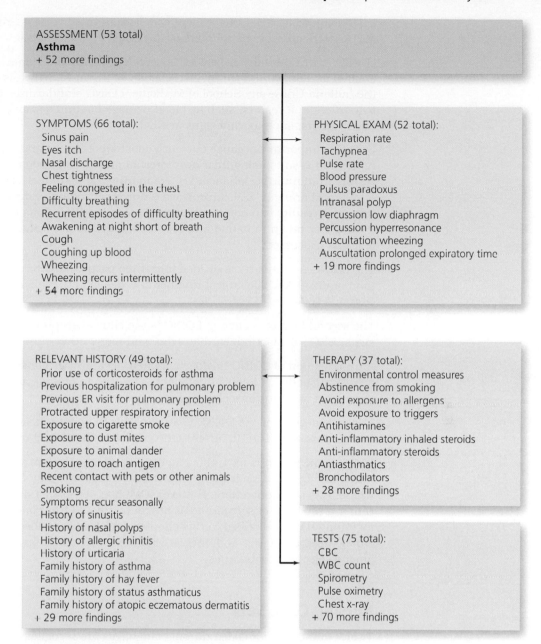

ASSESSMENT (53 total)
Asthma
+ 52 more findings

SYMPTOMS (66 total):
 Sinus pain
 Eyes itch
 Nasal discharge
 Chest tightness
 Feeling congested in the chest
 Difficulty breathing
 Recurrent episodes of difficulty breathing
 Awakening at night short of breath
 Cough
 Coughing up blood
 Wheezing
 Wheezing recurs intermittently
 + 54 more findings

PHYSICAL EXAM (52 total):
 Respiration rate
 Tachypnea
 Pulse rate
 Blood pressure
 Pulsus paradoxus
 Intranasal polyp
 Percussion low diaphragm
 Percussion hyperresonance
 Auscultation wheezing
 Auscultation prolonged expiratory time
 + 19 more findings

RELEVANT HISTORY (49 total):
 Prior use of corticosteroids for asthma
 Previous hospitalization for pulmonary problem
 Previous ER visit for pulmonary problem
 Protracted upper respiratory infection
 Exposure to cigarette smoke
 Exposure to dust mites
 Exposure to animal dander
 Exposure to roach antigen
 Recent contact with pets or other animals
 Smoking
 Symptoms recur seasonally
 History of sinusitis
 History of nasal polyps
 History of allergic rhinitis
 History of urticaria
 Family history of asthma
 Family history of hay fever
 Family history of status asthmaticus
 Family history of atopic eczematous dermatitis
 + 29 more findings

THERAPY (37 total):
 Environmental control measures
 Abstinence from smoking
 Avoid exposure to allergens
 Avoid exposure to triggers
 Antihistamines
 Anti-inflammatory inhaled steroids
 Anti-inflammatory steroids
 Antiasthmatics
 Bronchodilators
 + 28 more findings

TESTS (75 total):
 CBC
 WBC count
 Spirometry
 Pulse oximetry
 Chest x-ray
 + 70 more findings

▶ **Figure 2-2 MEDCIN links for the term "Asthma."**

The MEDCIN knowledge base also includes 600,000 synonyms for findings allowing a finding to be looked up by several different terms. The MEDCIN knowledge base includes each finding selected by the clinician in a readable narrative text. EHR applications using the MEDCIN nomenclature can store medical information as coded data elements and still generate readable exam notes from the same data.

An EHR system based on MEDCIN enables the provider to select fewer individual codes and to quickly locate other clinical "findings" that are likely to be needed. This difference reduces the time it takes to create accurate notes and this makes it possible to complete the client note at the time of the encounter.

Many experts feel that for point-of-care documentation, medical nomenclatures such as MEDCIN are the key to successful adoption of an EHR by clinicians. MEDCIN is used in many commercial EHR systems as well as by the Department of Defense at all military medical facilities worldwide. Because of this, MEDCIN has been selected as the

EHR nomenclature for the student exercises in this textbook. You will learn more about MEDCIN in subsequent chapters of this book.

LOINC   LOINC stands for Logical Observation Identifiers Names and Codes. LOINC was created and is maintained by the Regenstrief Institute, which is closely affiliated with the Indiana University School of Medicine. LOINC standardizes codes for laboratory test orders and results, such as blood hemoglobin and serum potassium, and clinical observations, such as vital signs or EKG.

LOINC is important because currently most laboratories and other diagnostic services report test results using their own internal proprietary codes. When an EHR receives results from multiple lab facilities, comparing the results electronically is like comparing apples and oranges. LOINC provides a universal coding system for mapping laboratory tests and results to a common terminology in the EHR. This then makes it possible for a computer program to find and report comparable test values regardless of where the test was processed.

The LOINC terminology is divided into three portions: laboratory, clinical (nonlaboratory), and HIPAA. The largest number of codes is in the laboratory section, which contains codes in 14 categories.

The second largest section of LOINC is the clinical section, which includes codes for vital signs, EKG, ultrasound, cardiac echo, and many other clinical observations.

A third section of LOINC has been created to categorize codes for a HIPAA claims attachment transaction. Claims attachments are used to provide additional information to support an insurance claim.

The wide acceptance of LOINC is attributable in part to its adoption by HL7 (discussed later in this chapter). HL7 uses LOINC codes in its clinical messages.

UMLS   UMLS stands for Unified Medical Language System®. It is maintained by the National Library of Medicine (NLM). Because students may find mention of UMLS elsewhere, it is mentioned here. However, UMLS is not itself a medical terminology, but rather a resource of software tools and data created from many medical nomenclatures, including those described in this chapter. UMLS is described as a "meta-thesaurus." It can be used to retrieve and integrate biomedical information and provide cross-references among selected vocabularies.

Nursing Code Sets

Twelve standards for coded nursing languages are recognized by the American Nurses Association today for use in the assessment, diagnosis, intervention, and outcome of nursing care. Using a commonly understood codified structure enables nurses to create and communicate a client plan of care that is evidence based, facilitates documentation of the practice of nursing in the EHR, and permits data sharing to improve client care outcomes. This is not a comprehensive explanation of all 12 coding structures, but does represent some of those that may be found in EHR systems today.

Clinical Care Classification System (CCC)   The Clinical Care Classification system (CCC) was developed by Virginia Saba at Georgetown University. It can be used to document client care in hospitals, home health agencies, ambulatory care clinics, and other healthcare settings. Developed from government-funded research, it was originally known as the Home Health Care Classification system, but CCC is applicable to clinical care as well as other healthcare services.

The CCC system provides standardized coding concepts for nursing diagnoses, outcomes, nursing interventions, and actions in two interrelated taxonomies. CCC defines 21 Care Components that provide a framework to interrelate the 182 CCC Nursing Diagnoses and 198 CCC Nursing Interventions.

The CCC system offers a unique approach to documenting the nursing process in an EHR by correlating the six steps of the CCC system with the six steps of the nursing process. The CCC codes have been integrated into the Medcin nomenclature and will be used for this course. CCC codes are also integrated into UMLS, SNOMED-CT, and LOINC.

NANDA-I   NANDA-I stands for the North American Nursing Diagnosis Association International. The NANDA-I Taxonomy is a system of classification of 206 Nursing Diagnoses that have been grouped into 13 domains of nursing practice. They offer a clearly understood language to enable the professional nurse to identify and prioritize nursing diagnosis to plan interventions that are based on best practice but individualized to the client's responses to health problems or life processes. It is available in 11 international languages, is HL7 (Health Level 7) and ISO (International Organization for Standardization) compatible, included in UMLS, and available in SNOMED-CT. This association's body of work facilitates all forms of nursing communications and guides the process of professional nursing practice for assessing and treating the nursing diagnosis. The NANDA-I Taxonomy supports the development of EHR and enables the collection, retrieval, and analysis of nursing data to promote education, research, and evidence based standards of care.

NIC and NOC   NIC stands for Nursing Interventions Classification. It is a code set designed for documenting nursing interventions in any clinical setting. NIC was first published in 1992 and is updated every four years. The system consists of numeric codes for 514 interventions, which are grouped into 30 classes and seven domains that span all nursing specialties. The seven domains are: Basic Physiological, Complex Physiological, Behavioral, Safety, Family, Health System, and Community. Their design is for use at the point of care to document care planning and nursing practices.

NOC stands for Nursing Outcomes Classification and includes a comprehensive list of nursing outcomes. It is used to document the effect of nursing interventions on client progress. It can be used to measure the quality of care, cost efficiency, and progress of treatment. It is a structure of 330 numerically coded outcomes (311 individual, 10 family, and 9 community level outcomes). The NOC codes are grouped into 31 classes and seven domains corresponding to those identified in NIC.

NIC and NOC codes were developed in the University of Iowa, College of Nursing, and are owned by Elsevier Science.

ICNP®   ICNP stands for International Classification for Nursing Practice. It is the result of a project by the International Council of Nurses, to create an organizing structure into which other nursing terminologies can be mapped. It was intended to facilitate the comparison of nursing data gathered from multiple systems. However, ICNP has evolved into a separate coding system attempting to unify other systems. It uses numeric codes to represent concepts in three areas—Nursing Phenomenon, Nursing Actions, and Outcomes, which are similar to the concepts of nursing diagnosis, interventions, and outcomes.

One factor that differentiates ICNP from other systems is that it has merged the two different taxonomies used for nursing diagnosis and nursing interventions into one classification, which can be used to represent diagnoses, interventions, and outcomes.

Omaha System   The Omaha System is a standardized terminology recognized by the American Nurses Association as a standard language system to support nursing practice. It has been in development since the 1970s and is one of the oldest systems for nursing documentation. It often is used in community-based nursing such as visiting nursing associations. It is no longer under copyrights, but when used the terms and structure must be used as published. It is included in the U.S. Department of Health and Human Services interoperability standards for electronic health records, and is integrated into LOINC and SNOMED-CT. It is recognized by HL7, congruent with ISO, and being mapped to the ICNP.

NMDS   NMDS stands for Nursing Minimum Data Set. It was originally developed as the result of conferences held at the University of Illinois College of Nursing in Chicago in 1977 and at the University of Wisconsin—Milwaukee School of Nursing in 1985 in an attempt to define the minimum set of basic data elements for nursing use in the EHR. It has label and conceptual definitions of the essential, specific elements that are used on a regular basis by the majority of nurses in a variety of settings. The elements are arranged into three categories: nursing care, patient or client demographics, and service elements. NMDS is intended to standardize the collection of essential nursing data and can be used to capture nursing data for comparison of client outcomes.

PNDS   PNDS stands for Perioperative Nursing Data Set and was developed by the Association of Perioperative Registered Nurses in the early 1990s. Like other nursing systems, it codifies nursing diagnoses, interventions, and outcomes, but this system is focused on the special needs and level of detail required to document perioperative nursing.

PNDS is used by nurses in hospital perioperative settings to document the client experience from preadmission to discharge. PNDS consists of 74 nursing diagnoses, 133 nursing interventions, and 28 nurse-sensitive client outcomes. PNDS is incorporated into SNOMED-CT.

PCDS   PCDS stands for Patient Care Data Set. PCDS was developed by Judy Ozbolt at the University of Virginia as a comprehensive catalog of terms used in client care records at nine hospitals. PCDS was officially adopted as one of the standards by the American Nurses Association in 1998.

PCDS is different from the other classifications that have been previously described. Where CCC was based on home care nursing, the Omaha System on community-based nursing, and PNDS on perioperative needs, PCDS has a much stronger acute care origin. PCDS also includes terms for 363 problems, 311 goals, and 1357 client care orders. PCDS is organized into 22 care components (the CCC components plus one as Immunology and Metabolism were divided into separate components). However, "the Patient Care Data Set has been developed primarily not as a classification system for clinical terms but as a data dictionary defining elements to be included in and abstracted from clinical information systems" (Ozbolt, 1997, p. 884).

Real-Life Story

A Nurse's Experiences with Development of Health Data Standards

By Luann Whittenburg, RN, MSN

I started my career in informatics by being exposed to healthcare data standards when I represented the Military Health System (MHS) at an American National Standards Institute (ANSI) Health Informatics Standards Board meeting in Washington, DC. My role was to recommend the health data standards and code sets used to integrate and exchange the health data for the 9.4 million MHS beneficiaries across federal agencies using metadata standards maintained by ANSI Standard Development Organizations.

I learned from this initial meeting that there were few implemented data exchange standards across the county; through a series of health data interoperability meetings, I began to understand the importance of health data exchange standards to nursing. The American Nurses Association (2009) position statement on EHR states the public has a right to expect health information and data centered on patient safety and improved health outcomes. The promotion of standards-based EHR for efficient and effective nursing communication and decision making contributes to being able to tell the story of the contribution of nursing to healthcare outcomes. I decided at that moment informatics should be my nursing career focus with a specialization in healthcare data standards and terminologies designed for electronic processing.

This was my opportunity to explore and analyze health information management within one of the largest health data system in the world, so I studied technology asset management, continuity of operations, health information standards, data models, and the validation of clinical requirements in the electronic health record for patient care documentation. I became certified in health informatics, and after the MHS received Federal Health Architecture awards, I was asked to speak about Military Health System Enterprise Architecture at national health technology conferences. I also continued my education by becoming a board-certified family nurse practitioner and began to represent the Department of Defense (DOD)/Health Affairs as a U.S. delegate to the ISO.

My activities with ANSI and ISO focused on metadata within the U.S. Health Information Knowledgebase, a metadata repository of health data elements used in health applications and standards development through a public/private partnership among the DOD/Health Affairs, the Veterans Health Administration, and the Centers for Disease Control and Prevention, and other healthcare organizations. Through participation in ISO, I learned how to apply national standards development to global health information interoperability specifically in pharmacy and medication business exchanges. I supported the development of the ISO Technical Report (TR25257) for the International Coding of Medicinal Products and focused the MHS functional requirements for population health applications in patient safety and quality. My responsibilities in health information and data management increased; I became more involved in international and national health information exchanges and was elected, in 2005, ISO TC215: Health Informatics Pharmacy and Medications Workgroup Vice-Convenor.

With the goal of informatics to improve healthcare practice through the use of technology, the integration of the first national nursing terminology, the CCC, as recognized by the Department of Health and Human Services, engages the nursing process framework in the implementation of EHR systems. The benefits of using a coded, standardized nursing terminology are:

- Increases productivity through standardized documentation

- Results in standardized, consistent, health data for interventions and research

- Reduced healthcare cost from improved, documented outcomes by intervention

- Health data for cross-organization comparisons

- Accelerated healthcare software development

- Reduced level of effort in unnecessary computer system data element development

- Earlier return on investment on information technology design and development costs

I am optimistic that the use of electronic documentation for nursing supported by the CCC System will ensure standardized quality nursing data in EHR.

Capturing and Recording EHR Data

The value of having an EHR is evident, but how does the data get into the EHR? Thus far we have discussed three forms of EHR data. In subsequent chapters of this book we will explore how nurses and nurse practitioners create codified EHR. But before we move on, let us briefly examine how digital image data and text file data are added to the EHR and used. We will also discuss additional sources of EHR data that can be imported directly into the system.

Digital Image Systems

As discussed previously, digital image data may be subcategorized into diagnostic images and scanned document images. Even with the implementation of a codified EHR, there will always be some paper documents. Obviously there are all the old paper charts of established clients, but there is also a continuing influx of referral letters and other medical documents from outside sources.

Many healthcare organizations choose to bring paper documents into the EHR as scanned images. Although document images do not offer all the benefits of a codified medical record, they do provide widespread accessibility and a means to include source documents for a complete electronic chart.

Most document image systems have a computer program to associate various ID fields and key words with scanned images. This is called *cataloging the image*. Catalog data adds the capability to search for the electronic document images in multiple ways.

Guided Exercise 5: Exploring a Document Imaging System

In this exercise you will experience how an imaging system works. You will need access to the Internet for this exercise. If you have not already done so, complete the student registration for the Online Student Resources website provided on the inside cover of this textbook.

Step 1

Start your web browser program and follow the steps listed inside the cover of this textbook to log in.

When the welcome page is displayed, click on the link "**Exercises and Activities**" or select it from the drop-down list and click on the button labeled "Go."

Step 2

A menu on the left of the screen will list various activities and exercises. Locate and click on the link **Exercise 5**.

Information about the exercise will be displayed.

Locate and click the link "Click here to start the Document/Image System program."

A screen similar to Figure 2-3 will be displayed.

The Document/Image System Window
As you proceed through the following steps, you will be introduced to names, functions, and components of the Document/Image System window. This program

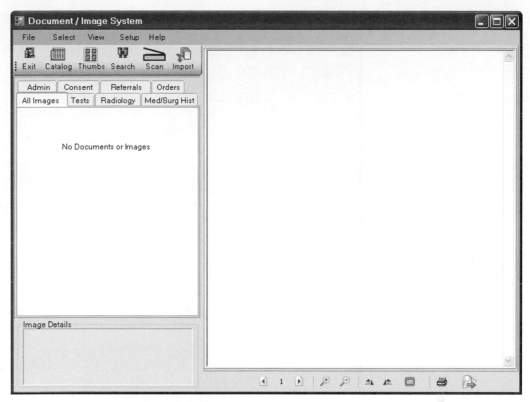

▶ **Figure 2-3 Document/Image System window.**

simulates many of the features typically found in an EHR document/image management system.

The Menu Bar   At the top of the screen, the words "File," "Select," "View," "Setup," and "Help" are the menus of functions typically found in document image software. We call this the *Menu bar.* When you position the mouse over one of these words and click the mouse once, a list of functions will drop down below the word.

Once a menu list appears, clicking one of the items will invoke that function. Clicking the mouse anywhere except on the list will close the list. Certain items on the menu are displayed in gray text. These items are not available until a client or document has been selected. The Setup and Help options are not available in this simulation.

Step 3

Position the mouse pointer over the word "Select" in the Menu bar at the top of the screen and click the mouse button once. A list of the Select menu functions will appear as shown in Figure 2-4.

Step 4

Move the mouse pointer vertically down the list over the word "Patient" and click the mouse to invoke the Patient Selection window shown in Figure 2-5.

Step 5

Find the client named Raj Patel in the Patient Selection window. Position the mouse pointer over the client's name and double-click the mouse. (*Double-click* means to click the mouse button twice, very rapidly.)

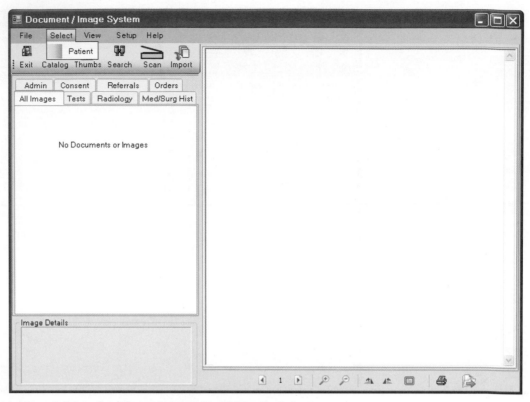

▶ **Figure 2-4 Document/Image System after clicking the Select menu.**

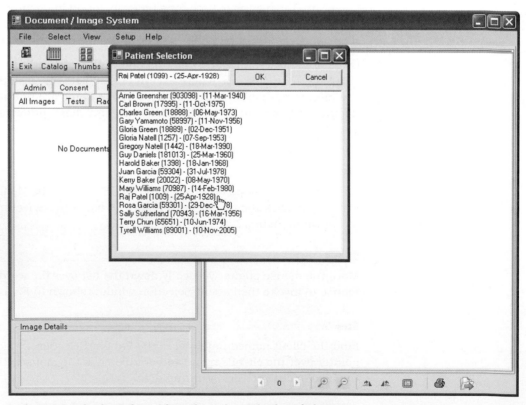

▶ **Figure 2-5 Selecting Raj Patel from the Patient Selection window.**

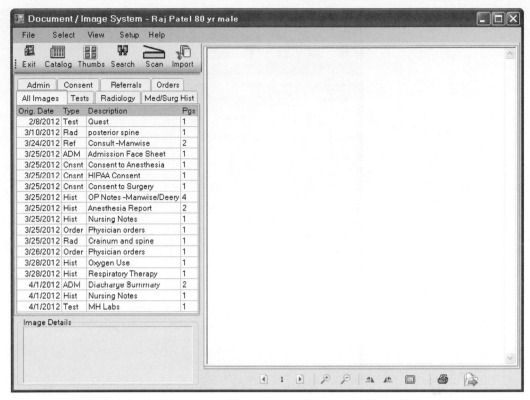

▶ Figure 2-6 Left pane displays catalog list of documents and images for Raj Patel.

Once a client is selected, the client's name, age, and sex are displayed in the title at the top of the window.

Compare your screen to Figure 2-6 as your read the following information:

The Toolbar

Also located at the top of your screen are a row of icon buttons called a *Toolbar*. The purpose of the Toolbar is to allow quick access to commonly used functions. Most Windows programs feature a Toolbar, so you may already be familiar with the concept.

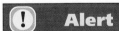 **Alert** All instructions in these exercises refer to the simulation window. Because you are running this simulation inside a browser, be careful to use the Menu bar and Toolbar inside the simulation window, not the Menu bar or Toolbar of your Internet browser program.

The Catalog Pane

The middle portion of the screen is divided into two window panes. The left pane (just below the Toolbar) is where a list of cataloged documents display once a client is selected. At the top of the Catalog pane there are eight tabs. These look like tabs on file folders. The tabs are used to limit the list to images by category, making it easier to find a specific type of image quickly. The initial tab is "All Images," listed in date order.

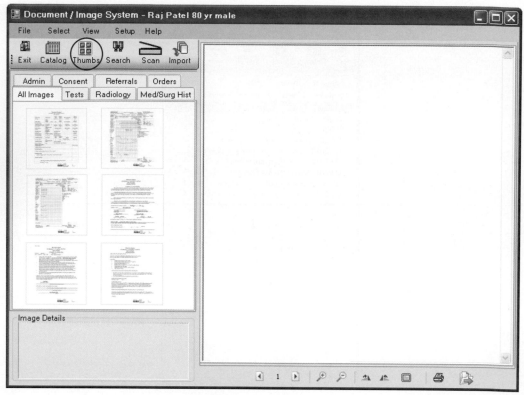

▶ **Figure 2-7 Catalog pane displaying thumbnails of images.**

Step 6

Locate the Toolbar in the Document/Image System window. The first icon is labeled "Exit" and it will close the simulation program and return you to the Online Student Resources web page. Do not click it yet.

The next two buttons are used to change display of items in the Catalog pane from a list to thumbnails. Thumbnails are small versions of the document or image.

Position your mouse pointer over the "Thumbs" icon on the Toolbar (circled in Figure 2-7) and click your mouse.

Compare your screen to Figure 2-7.

Now position your mouse pointer over the "Catalog" icon on the Toolbar and click your mouse. Your screen should again resemble Figure 2-6.

Step 7

Locate the tab labeled "Med/Surg Hist" above the Catalog pane. Position your mouse pointer over it and click your mouse. The list should now be shorter as it is limited to items cataloged in the category of Medical/Surgical History.

Step 8

Locate the catalog item "Anesthesia Report" and click on it. Compare your screen to Figure 2-8 as you read the following information.

The Image Viewer Pane
The right pane of the window will dynamically display the corresponding image for a catalog entry that is clicked.

▶ **Figure 2-8 Catalog on Med/ Surg tab, Anesthesia Report, displayed in Image Viewer pane.**

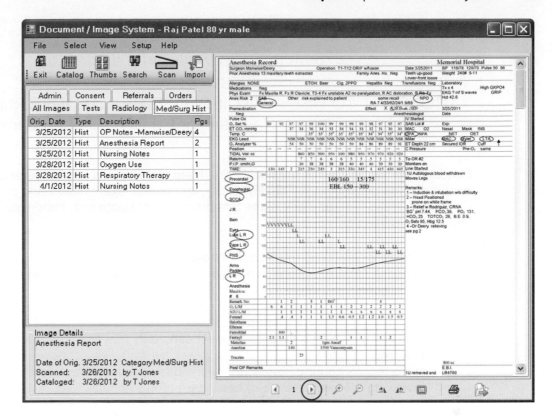

Image Details

Just below the Catalog pane is a gray panel that displays information about a selected catalog item such as the user who scanned the document, relevant dates, and a longer description of the item.

Image Tools

Just below the Image Viewer pane is a row of icon buttons used to change the displayed image. These include the ability to page through multipage documents, enlarge or reduce the displayed image.

Step 9

Locate the image tools buttons just below the viewer pane. The first three icons become active whenever a multipage document is selected. The Anesthesia Report has two pages. Locate and click on the Next page button (circled in red in Figure 2-8). The button displays the next page of a multipage document. The numeral between the two buttons is the page number currently displayed. Your screen should now display the second page of the report and the Image Tool should display the numeral two.

The Previous page button is the first icon in the image tools. Locate it and click on it.

The Image Tool area should now display numeral one, and the Image Viewer should again display the first page of the report.

The next two icons resemble magnifying glasses. One includes a plus sign—this is the Zoom In tool; it enlarges the text in the viewer. The other magnifying glass has a minus sign—this is the Zoom Out tool; it reduces the enlarged view to show more of the page in the viewer.

Locate and click on the Zoom In icon to see how this works.

Cataloging Images

The process of scanning documents or importing scanned images into an image system includes not only capturing the image but tying it to the correct client and entering data

Memorial Hospital
876 Memory Ln, Anywhere, ID 83776
(208) 378-5555
CONSENT TO USE AND DISCLOSE HEALTH INFORMATION
for Treatment, Payment, or Healthcare operations

I understand that as part of my healthcare, Memorial Hospital originates and maintains health records describing my health history, symptoms, examination and test results, diagnoses, treatment, and any plans for future care or treatment. I understand that this information serves as:

- a basis for planning my care and treatment
- a means of communication among the many health professionals who contribute to my care
- a source of information for applying my diagnosis and surgical information to my bill
- a means by which a third-party payer can verify that services billed were actually provided
- and a tool for routine healthcare operations such as assessing quality and reviewing the competence of healthcare professionals

I understand and have been provided with a *Notice of Privacy Practices* that provides a more complete description of information uses and disclosures. I understand that I have the right to review the notice prior to signing this consent. I understand that Memorial Hospital reserves the right to change their notice and practices and prior to implementation will mail a copy of any revised notice to the address I've provided. I understand that I have the right to object to the use of my health information for directory purposes. I understand that I have the right to request restrictions as to how my health information may be used or disclosed to carry out treatment, payment, or healthcare operations and that Memorial Hospital is not required to agree to the restrictions requested. I understand that I may revoke this consent in writing, except to the extent that the hospital and its employees have already take action in reliance thereon.

 I request the following restrictions to the use or disclosure of my health information:

Signature of Patient or Legal Representative Witness

Date Notice Effective Date or Version

___X_ Accepted _____ Denied

Signature: _____Raj Patel_____   Date: ____3-24-2011_____

Patient: Patel, Raj
Med Rec #:   837155

▶ **Figure 2-9 HIPAA Consent Form with barcode.**

in the computer about the document such as the date, provider, type of image, and so on. This is called *cataloging the image*. Figure 2-10, shown later, is an example of an image catalog system.

Document images are scanned and cataloged into the EHR by many different people, including nurses, medical assistants, and personnel in the client registration and Health Information Management departments. During scanning and cataloging, quality control is most important. Once a document has been scanned and cataloged, the original may be shipped to a remote storage facility or shredded. In either case, the original document may no longer be available for comparison. Although the scanned document image is stored safely on the computer, if it has been incorrectly cataloged it may not be easy to locate.

For the most part, the catalog data is entered by hand, but in some instances the image cataloging can be automated. Here are some examples of automated image cataloging:

Paper forms can include a barcode to identify catalog data; the scanning software interprets the barcode and automatically creates the catalog record. For example, Figure 2-9 shows a HIPAA authorization form that was printed for the client's signature. The form includes a barcode identifying the client, date, and document type, allowing automatic cataloging of the signed copy when it is scanned by the Document/Image System.

Another type of technology uses Optical Character Recognition (OCR) software to recognize text characters in images. Some document imaging systems can be programmed to find and use the text contained in the scanned document to populate the fields in the catalog records. Typically, only a few types of documents are processed this way, as each document type requires custom programming. However, when an organization images thousands of the same type of document, it can be worth it. For example, your bank keeps an image of the front and back of each check it processes. Because the account number and check number are in a consistent place at the bottom of the check, the bank computers can automatically catalog each image to the correct account as it is scanned.

Guided Exercise 6: Importing and Cataloging Images

In this exercise you will catalog a scanned document and two diagnostic images for a client. You will need access to the Internet for this exercise.

Step 1

If you are still logged in from the previous exercise, proceed to Step 2; otherwise, start your web browser program and follow the steps listed inside the cover of this textbook to log in.

When the welcome page is displayed, click on the link "**Exercises and Activities** or select it from the drop-down list and click on the button labeled "Go."

Step 2

Locate and click on the link **Exercise 6**. Information about the exercise will be displayed.

Locate and click the link "Click here to start the Document/Image System program."

The document image system screen will be displayed. (Refer to Figure 2-3 for an example.)

Position your mouse pointer over the word "Select" in the Menu bar at the top of the screen and click the mouse button once.

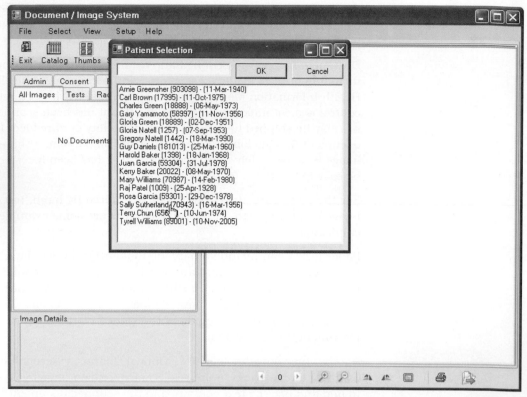

▶ **Figure 2-10 Selecting Sally Sutherland from the Patient Selection window.**

Move the mouse pointer vertically down the list over the word "Patient" and click the mouse to invoke the Patient Selection window shown in Figure 2-10.

Step 3

Find the client named **Sally Sutherland** in the Patient Selection window. Position the mouse pointer over the patient name and double-click the mouse.

Once a patient is selected, the client's name, age, and sex are displayed in the title at the top of the window. The Catalog pane displays the message "No Documents or Images" because Sally has no documents or images in the catalog.

Step 4

Because you may not have a scanner connected to your computer, you are going to import a file that has already been scanned but not yet cataloged.

Locate and click on the Toolbar button labeled "Import."

The "Open Media File" window, displaying available files, will open. Compare your screen to Figure 2-11.

Step 5

Locate and click on the thumbnail image of the **radiologist report document** (suth70943rpt.tif)

Locate and click on the button labeled "Open."

Compare your screen to Figure 2-12.

Step 6

The imported file displays in the Image Viewer pane and data entry fields replace the catalog list. The fields shown in Figure 2-12 are the minimum for most Document/Image systems. The actual fields in a catalog record will differ by software vendor or medical facility.

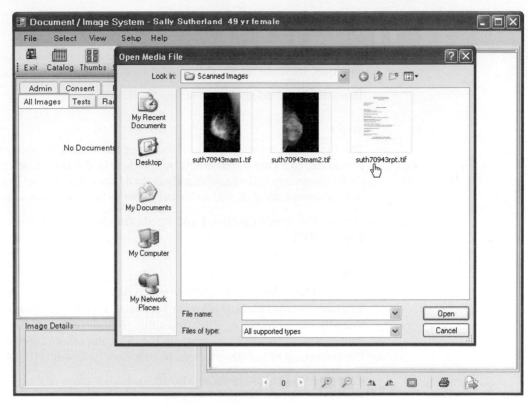

► Figure 2-11 Open Media window displays after the clicking Import icon.

The image you have imported should be the radiologist's report. The Catalog pane reminds you that it has not been saved into the client's EHR.

The first two fields in the catalog pane are determined automatically because the Document/Image System recognizes that you have imported the file and that you

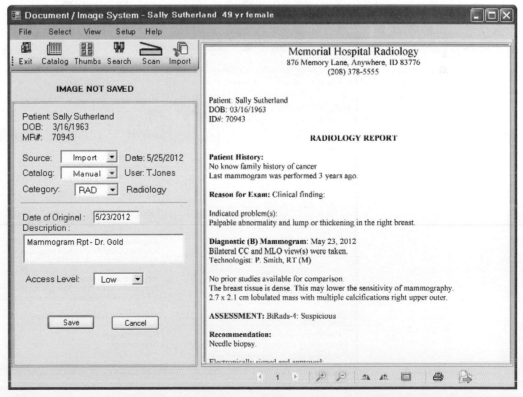

► Figure 2-12 Data Entry fields in Catalog pane; Image Viewer displays imported Radiology report.

are performing a manual entry of the catalog data. Other options for these fields are "Scanned" image and "Automatic" cataloging (e.g., from a barcode).

The Category field uses short mnemonic codes to represent longer category names, for example, HIST for "Medical/Surgical History," or RAD for "Radiology."

The Category field is already set to "RAD."

Step 7

The first field you will enter is the date of the original document; this is for reference purposes, to locate a document by the date of the report, letter, surgery, and so on. Note that the system will automatically record other dates, such as the date of the scan, the date it was cataloged, and so forth. These other dates are used for audit purposes.

Look at the image displayed and locate the date of the report, May 23, 2012. Enter **5/23/2012**.

Step 8

The final field you must complete is the description. Although the field can hold a lengthy description, only the first portion of it is displayed in the catalog list, which is used by others at the healthcare facility to find the document/image. Therefore, when cataloging documents and images, the most important information should be placed at the beginning of the description. In this case, you will type: **Mammogram Rpt - Dr. Gold**

Compare your fields to those shown in the left pane of Figure 2-12. If everything is correct, click on the button labeled "Save."

Step 9

The Catalog pane will now display your cataloged listing (as shown in Figure 2-13).

Now catalog the corresponding diagnostic images.

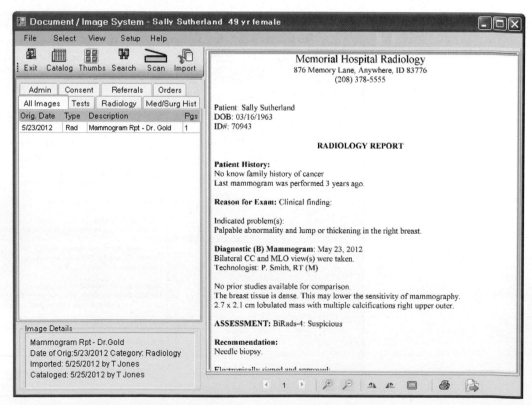

▶ **Figure 2-13 Cataloged mammogram report.**

Locate and click on the Toolbar button labeled "Import." The Open Media window (shown in Figure 2-11) will be displayed.

Click on the **center** Thumbnail (the mammogram image "suth70943mam2.tif").

Locate and click on the button labeled "Open."

Step 10

Enter the catalog data in the Catalog entry fields as follows:

Date: **5/23/2012**

Description: **Mammogram right breast w/abnormality**

Click the button labeled "Save."

Compare your screen to Figure 2-14.

The Catalog pane will now display two listings.

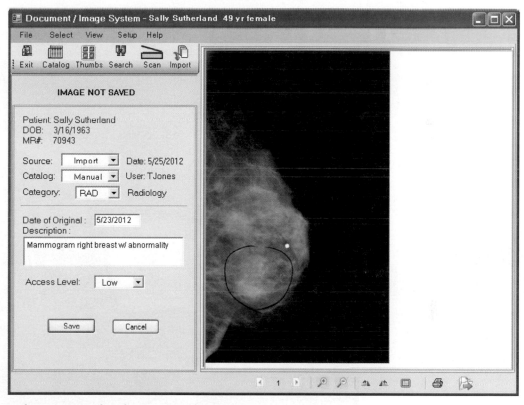

▶ **Figure 2-14 Cataloged mammogram image.**

Step 11

Catalog the other mammogram image by clicking the Toolbar button labeled "Import." When the Open Media window appears, click on the **left** Thumbnail (the mammogram image "suth70943mam1.tif).

Locate and click on the button labeled "Open."

Enter the catalog data in the Catalog entry fields as follows:

Date: **5/23/2012**

Description: **Mammogram left breast**

Click the button labeled "Save." The Catalog pane will now display three listings.

The exercise is concluded. You may exit and close your browser.

Picture Archival and Communication System (PAC)

In the previous exercise you imported diagnostic images (mammograms) into the EHR. At many facilities, digital images such as x-rays and CAT scans reside on a separate Picture Archival and Communication System (PAC). These images can be associated with the radiology report in the EHR and appear to be part of the EHR record, even though they are on a separate system. In those facilities, the diagnostic image is not actually imported into the EHR, but rather linked to the client EHR record.

Importing Text to the EHR

The second form of data we discussed is text data—that is, data that consists of words, sentences, and paragraphs, but is not fielded data. Frequently this type of data comes from word processing files that result from transcribed dictation. A good example of this is the radiologist's report. A radiologist is a specialist who interprets diagnostic images. Radiologists often dictate their impressions of a study (as shown in Figure 2-15). Their dictation is later typed by a medical transcriptionist. The word processing file containing the radiology report can be imported directly into the EHR, eliminating the steps of printing and scanning.

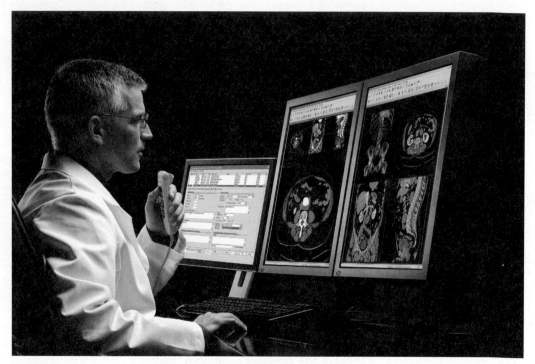

Photo provided courtesy of Carestream Health, Inc.
▶ **Figure 2-15 Radiologist dictates report while interpreting radiology study on a PAC system.**

Many radiology departments have implemented voice recognition software that immediately converts the dictated words into a digital word processing file for inclusion in the EHR. This technology decreases the delay of making diagnostic reports available to support clinical decisions regarding diagnosis and treatment.

Eventually, a healthcare facility implementing an EHR will need to bring old paper charts into the Document/Image System. If the facility has retained word processing files of transcribed dictation, importing them as EHR text records instead of scanning the printed pages from the paper chart increases the amount of the EHR that is text data and reduces the number of pages to be scanned.

Although imported text data are not codified like those created when clinicians enter actual data, they may be preferable to a scanned image for two reasons. First, the text records are searchable by computer. Second, text data can be dynamically reformatted for display on smaller devices such as mobile phones, images of scanned documents cannot.

For example, a text document viewed on a small device such as a mobile phone might display in a font suitable for that device. If the same document were a scanned image, it might be too small to read, thus requiring the clinician to zoom the image and making it cumbersome to read.

Importing Coded EHR Data

As we have already learned, the very best form of EHR data is fielded, codified data. In addition to the coded data that will be created by the clinician using an EHR, many other sources of codified data can be imported. Importing coded data produces a better EHR and eliminates the need to re-key data or scan reports into the chart.

For example, electronic lab order and results systems can be interfaced to send the orders and merge test results directly into the EHR. The numerical data that makes up many lab results lends itself to trend analysis, graphs, and comparison with other tests. The ability to review and present results in this manner allows providers to see the immediate, tangible benefits of using an EHR and improves client care.

Other sources of EHR data available for import into the EHR include vital signs when they are measured with modern electronic devices (as shown in Figure 2-16). Similarly, glucose monitors and Holter monitors are devices that gather and store data about the client. Most of these medical devices have the ability to transfer the data they have collected to a computer.

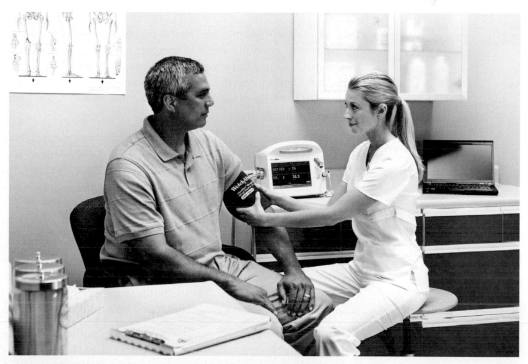

Courtesy of Welch Allyn.
▶ Figure 2-16 Nurse transmits vital signs wirelessly using Welch Allyn Connex®.

When clinicians use the EHR to write prescriptions, the orders are also automatically recorded in the EHR as part of the workflow. This keeps a record of the client's past prescriptions and makes renewing prescriptions much faster for the provider.

HL7 Health Level 7 (HL7) is a nonprofit organization and the leading messaging standard used by healthcare computer systems to exchange information. The organization is comprised of healthcare providers, institutions, government representatives, and software developers. HL7 uses a consensus process to arrive at specifications acceptable to every-one involved. The HL7 specifications are updated regularly and released as new versions.

Hospitals and other large healthcare organizations often have many different computer systems created by unrelated vendors. These systems generate various portions of the client's medical data. HL7 is used to translate and interface that data into the main EHR system.

The simplest act of transferring client information from the admissions office to the radiology department or hospital pharmacy would not be easy without HL7. If you work in a hospital, your hospital probably uses HL7. As a part of this course, it is not necessary to delve into the specific structure or flow of HL7 messages, but it is helpful to understand its advantages and limitations.

HL7 specifications are independent of any application or vendor; therefore, applications that can send and receive HL7 messages can potentially exchange information. That is its advantage and importance to an EHR system.

HL7 has been successful because it is very flexible both in its structure as well as its support for multiple coding standards. However, when a message is received, the codes and terms used by the other system may not match those used by the EHR. That is its disadvantage.

To overcome this problem, segments of the HL7 message that contain coded data also contain an identifier indicating which coding standard is being used. A special computer program called an HL7 translator is used to match the codes in the message with the codes in the EHR. The translator also can reconcile differences between HL7 versions from multiple systems.

DICOM   DICOM stands for Digital Imaging and Communications in Medicine. It is the standard used for medical images, such as digital x-rays, CT scans, MRIs, and ultrasound. Other uses include the images from angiography, endoscopy, laparoscopy, medical photography, and microscopy. It was created by the National Electrical Manufacturers Association and is the most widely used format for storing and sending diagnostic images.

DICOM is the standard for communication between diagnostic imaging equipment and the image processing software. The standard also defines the specification for a file that contains the actual digital image. A DICOM file includes a "header" that contains information about the image, dimensions, type of scan, image compression, and so on, as well as client information such as ID number or name. DICOM compatible software is required to view the image.

CDISC   A subgroup of HL7 is CDISC, which stands for Clinical Data Interchange Standards Consortium. CDISC originated as a special interest group of the Drug Information Association, but became its own entity and formed an alliance with HL7. Although the focus of HL7 is to facilitate message standards for a broad range of healthcare, CDISC has a specific focus on clinical drug trials.

CDISC standards enable sponsors, vendors, and clinicians to acquire and exchange data used in clinical trials. Because the FDA is the agency to whom the final results are submitted, the standard is very focused on following the FDA requirements. However, the commitment of CDISC to HL7 will eventually make it easier to use EHR data in clinical trial studies. It is mentioned here because you may encounter CDISC if you work at a healthcare facility that participates in clinical trials.

Biomedical Devices   Biomedical devices can output important and useful medical information that can be received and stored as data in the EHR. However, the type of data and method of communicating between the device and EHR often are proprietary to the particular device. Therefore, HL7 is often used to exchange demographic information between the device and the EHR system.

Still, the advantage of having the data in the EHR is so strong as to warrant the additional interfaces. Many of the monitoring, point-of-care testing, and biomedical devices in hospitals have the capability of exporting data to the EHR. Examples include instruments for measuring vital signs and cardiac and arterial blood gas monitors. Today, many of these devices have wired or wireless telemetry to transmit their information to nurse stations and into the EHR.

A similar capability is available in systems used in medical offices and for home monitoring such as the spirometer data shown in Chapter 1, Figure 1-1. Other examples include electrocardiograms, ultrasound, and the vital signs device shown earlier.

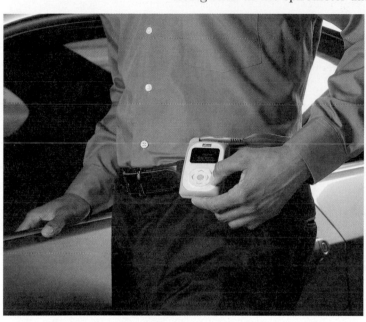

Courtesy of Midmark Diagnostics Group.

▶ **Figure 2-17 An IQholter™ worn by the client gathers cardio data.**

Telemonitors Many clients with chronic conditions are monitored at home using devices such as blood pressure monitors, glucose meters, and Holter monitors. Some of these devices store the readings and transfer the data to the provider's system either by using a modem and phone line or by downloading from the device during a client encounter. For blood pressure monitoring, if the device does not store the readings, the client may keep a log, which is then entered into the client's medical record during the clinic visit.

One example of a telemonitor is the Holter monitor, a device that the client wears for 24 to 72 hours to measure and record information about the client's heart. The data is then transferred either remotely or in person to the healthcare provider's computer, where it is reviewed. Figure 2-17 shows a client wearing a Holter monitor.

When a client is seen in a clinic, measurements of vital signs, a glucose test, or even an ECG reflect only the client's condition at that particular time. The advantage of telemonitoring is that it allows the provider to study these values measured many times over the course of the client's normal daily activity.

RHIO One of the issues discussed in Chapter 1 was that many clients no longer see a single doctor, so their records reside at many separate facilities. Regional Health Information Organizations (RHIO) and the Office of National Coordinator for Health Information Technology's development of a national health information network (NHIN) are both examples of projects to enable to electronic transfer of health records between providers.

Although it may take considerable time to create a true NHIN, many areas of the nation are attempting to create state or local versions. RHIO stands for regional health information organization. The Health Information Management Systems Society (HIMSS) defines a RHIO as a "neutral organization that adheres to a defined governance structure which is composed of and facilitates collaboration among the stakeholders in a given medical trading area, community or region through secure electronic health information exchange to advance the effective and efficient delivery of healthcare for individuals and communities" (Health Information Management Systems Society, 2005).

RHIOs encourage the exchange of a client's health information across medical practices and facilities that are owned by different entities for the better well-being of the client. The formation and operation of a RHIO must overcome numerous obstacles. These include technical, economic, and political issues:

Technical: Interfacing systems from different vendors in a hospital is not an easy task, but at least it is managed by one Information Technology (IT) department and shares a common network. The level of difficulty becomes multiplied when unrelated hospitals and physician practices—each with numerous systems—attempt to translate data and share a common network.

Economic: The translation of data from one system to another requires an interface engine and possibly a regional MPI (master person index). Who bears the cost of the networking, interface programming, and maintenance of the translation and MPI systems? Also, many RHIOs operate on a volunteer basis, but require a paid IT director, employed by the RHIO, not one of its members.

Political: Some participants in the RHIO are business competitors who may be leery about what data is shared and whether it can be analyzed to reveal their client or case mix, volume of business, and so on. Additionally, state laws may affect who can participate in the RHIO and whether members can be in bordering states.

Client-Entered Data

Numerous studies (cited in Chapter 11) have shown that client-entered data also can become a significant contributor to the EHR, for some of the following reasons:

▸ Only the client has the information about what symptoms were present at the outset of the illness.

▸ Only the client knows the outcome of medical treatment of those symptoms.

▸ The client is also the source of past medical, family, and social history.

▸ Client-entered data is a more accurate reflection of a client's complaints.

▸ Clients who can review their histories are better prepared for the visit.

A computer program such as Instant Medical History™ allows clients to enter their history and symptom information on a computer in the waiting room or via the Internet, before seeing the nurse. Clients do not access the actual EHR, but use a separate program that is linked to the EHR. The client-entered data is reviewed by the nurse during the encounter before being merged into the EHR. You will have an opportunity to explore this concept yourself in Chapter 11.

Provider-Entered Data

Finally, the surest source of reliable, coded EHR data is that entered by the providers (doctor, nurse, and medical assistant) during the client encounter using a standardized nomenclature. That process will be the subject of Chapters 3–12 of this book.

Functional Benefits from Codified Records

Because coded EHR data is nonambiguous, the computer can use it for trend analysis, alerts, health maintenance, decision support, orders and results, administrative processes, and population health reporting. We will now explore four of the functional benefits that can be derived from using a codified EHR.

Trend Analysis

In healthcare, laboratory tests are used to measure the level of certain components present in specimens taken from the client. When the same test is performed over a period of time, changes in the results can indicate a *trend* in the client's health.

With a paper chart, the clinician must page through the reports and mentally remember the values to compare them. When a health record is electronic, it is easier to compare data from different dates, tests, or events. When the data is fielded and coded, it is possible to generate graphs and reports that support trend analysis.

To experience the differences in forms of data, we will compare a client's lab results that have been stored in each of the three data formats that we discussed earlier in this chapter.

Critical Thinking Exercise 7: Retrieving a Scanned Lab Report

In this exercise you will use what you have learned in Guided Exercise 5 to locate information from a recent lab report for a client.

Step 1

Start your web browser program and follow the steps listed inside the cover of this textbook to log in as you did in Guided Exercise 5. Locate and select Exercise 7.

Locate and click the link to start the Document/Image System program.

Step 2

Select **Raj Patel**

Step 3

On **February 8, 2012**, the facility received the results of a lab test performed by **Quest** laboratories. The lab report was scanned and cataloged in Raj Patel's chart.

Locate the catalog entry for this lab report and click on it to display the report.

Step 4

When the report is displayed in the Image Viewer, locate the results for the test component "Triglycerides" and write down the value on a sheet of paper with your name and today's date.

You may need to use the Zoom In button to read the value accurately.

Step 5

Close your browser window and give your paper to your instructor.

This is an example of data in the format of a digital image. As you can see, the lab data are present in the EHR, but requires a human to locate and read the data values.

Lab Report as Text Data   If a lab results report was received as a text file, it might resemble Figure 2-18. The file could be imported into the EHR, but because the data is

```
Raj Patel: M: 3/5/1932:

Doctor's Laboratory
3/10/2012 11:30AM

Tests
Blood Chemistry:                    Value          Normal Range
Total plasma cholesterol level      215 mg/dl       140 - 200
Plasma HDL cholesterol level        40 mg/dl         30 - 70
Plasma LDL cholesterol level        98 mg/dl         80 - 130
Total cholesterol/HDL ratio         5.4              4 - 6

Hematology:                         Value          Normal Range
INR                                 2.1             25 - 40
```

▶ **Figure 2-18 Text-based lab results.**

not fielded or codified, a computer might have difficulty accurately parsing the data in the report; however, it could easily search text records and locate those that contained the word *cholesterol*. This could be useful to quickly locate records of previous tests containing the same word.

Coded Lab Data   If the test result data is fielded and coded, the computer can find matching results in the data and generate a cumulative summary report or a graph, making it easier to compare test results from different times and dates.

The cumulative summary report shown in Figure 2-19 has three sections of results: blood gases, whole blood chemistries, and general chemistry. Within each section are the results from tests performed five different times; the date and time is printed above each column of data.

```
************************************* Blood Gases *************************************

DATE:              [-------------------- 03/26/2012 --------------------]  03/25/2012
TIME:          2132        1920        1720        1506        1615       NORMAL       UNITS

pH-Arterial    7.30 L      7.36        7.38        7.47 H      7.48 H     7.35-7.45
PCO2-Arterial  47.4 H      41.1        38.3        34.8 L      33.0 L     35-45        mm Hg
PO2-Arterial   90.2        189.0 H     187.0 H     188.0 H     227.0 H    90-105       mm Hg
HCO3-Arterial  22.8        22.8        22.0        24.9        24.4       21-27        mEq/L
Base Excess-A                                      1.7         1.6        0-3          mEq/L
Base Deficit-A 3.2 H       1.9         2.3                                0-3          mEq/L
O2 Sat Dir-A   96.0        99.3 H      99.5 H      99.6 H      99.9 H     95-99        % Saturation
O2 Content-A   15.9        15.3        14.6 L      10.3 L      14.4 L     15-17        vol %
Hemoglobin-BG  12.0        10.8        10.3        7.2         10.1                    g/dL
CarboxyHb-A    1.1 H       1.0 H       1.2 H       0.9         1.6 H      0.0-0.9      % Saturation
MetHb-A        0.9         0.4         0.7         0.4         0.8        0.0-0.9      % Saturation
FIO2                       .55         .56         0.54        .65                     %


*********************************** Whole Blood Chemistries ***********************************

DATE:               [---------------------03/26/2012----------------------]  03/25/2012
TIME:         2209      2132      1920      1720      1506      1615      NORMAL      UNITS

Sodium-WB                         142       142       142       139       135-145     mEq/L
Potassium-WB  3.5                 3.3       3.0 L     2.9 L     2.7 L     3.3-4.6     mEq/L
Calcium Ionized         1.21      1.05      0.99 L    1.07      1.08      1.05-1.30   mmol/L
Lactic Acid-WB          1.3       0.8       1.1       0.8       0.5       0.3-1.5     mmol/L
Glucose-WB              197 H     156 H     165 H     118 H     90        65-99       mg/dL
Hematocrit-WB           37        34 L      32 L      22 L      31 L      36-46       %


************************************* General Chemistry *************************************

DATE:       04/01/2012 [---- 03/30/2012 ----] [----------- 03/29/12 -----------] 03/28/2012
TIME:         *0620     0653      0327      1835      0915      0532      2048      NORMAL      UNITS

Sodium        140                                               143                 136-145     mmol/L
PotaSSium     2.7 L     3.0 L               2.9 L     3.0 L     2.7 L               3.3-5.1     mmol/L
Chloride      101                                               100                 98-107      mmol/L
Carbon Dioxide 32 H                                             36 H                22-30       mmol/L
Urea Nitrogen 10                                                7                   6-20        mg/dL
Creatinine    0.54                                              0.60                0.40-0.90   mg/dL
Glucose       115 H                                             96                  65-99       mg/dL
Calcium       8.4                                               8.0                 8.0-10.6    mg/dL
Magnesium     1.9                                               2.3       1.8       1.5-2.8     mg/dL
Phosphorus Inorg 2.3 L                                          2.8       1.8 L     2.7-4.5     mg/dL
CK Total                          165                                     273 H     30-170      U/L


----------------------------------------------------------------------------------
    H=Abnormal High         L=Abnormal Low         H*=Critical High         L*=Critical Low
  Date Printed: 04/01/2012            Admit Date: 03/25/2012         Discharge Date: 04/01/2012
                              INPATIENT MEDICAL RECORDS COPY                   Page: 1
```

▶ **Figure 2-19 Cumulative summary lab report.**

The report is read from left to right; each row contains the name of the test component followed by result values for each of the five times. The right two columns are informational; they contain the range of values considered normal for each particular test and the unit of measure.

A simple graphing tool can turn numeric data in the EHR into a powerful visual aid that would be impractical to create from a paper chart. Figure 2-20 provides an example of how data from multiple lab tests can be quickly extracted and graphed for the clinician. The value of the total cholesterol results over a three-month period of time is trended with the green line. The reference ranges of normal high (200) and low (140) values are shown in the graph as red and blue lines, respectively.

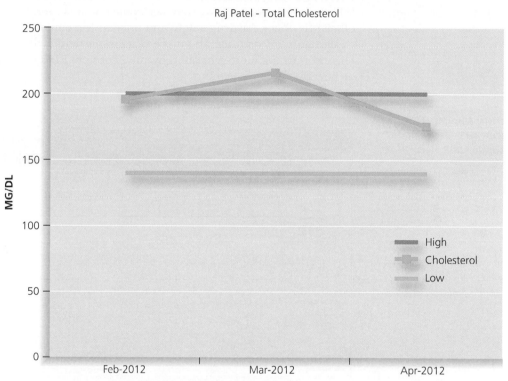

▶ **Figure 2-20 Graph of total cholesterol from codified lab results.**

The computer is able to generate this graph because the data is fielded and the different tests and components have unique codes. From all the possible tests that a client might have had, the computer can quickly find those coded as "total cholesterol." Using a graph, the clinician can easily see the trend of this client's total cholesterol levels.

Trend analysis is not limited to lab test results. Graphs of client weight loss or gain are used as client education tools. Effects of medication can be measured by comparing changes in dosage to changes in blood pressure measurements. Flow sheets (shown later in Chapter 9) are another type of trend analysis tool.

Alerts

One of the important reasons for the widespread adoption of EHR is the potential to reduce medical errors. Paper charts and even electronic charts that are principally scanned images depend on the clinician noticing a risk factor about the client. However, when an EHR consists primarily of fielded and codified data using standard nomenclature, rules can be set up that allow the computer to do the monitoring.

Alert is the term used in an EHR for a message or reminder that is automatically generated by the system. Alerts are based on programmed rules that cause the EHR to alert the provider when two or more conditions are met. For example, an electronic prescription system generates an alert when two drugs known to have adverse interactions are prescribed for the same client.

Alerts can be programmed for just about anything in the EHR. However, the most prevalent alert systems are those implemented with electronic prescription systems. Interactions between multiple prescription drugs, allergic reactions to certain classes of drugs, and health conditions that contraindicate certain drugs can all contribute to suffering, additional illness, and in extreme cases even death.

To prevent this, doctors and nurse practitioners that create prescriptions manually consult the client medication list, allergy list, and the *Physicians' Desk Reference* (for interactions) before writing a prescription. As a further precaution, the pharmacy checks for drug conflicts and provides the client with warning materials about the drug. When prescriptions are written electronically, however, the computer can quickly and efficiently check for drug safety and present the clinician with warnings, alerts, and explanatory information about the risks of particular drugs. Figure 2-21 shows a clinical warning alert generated by the Allscripts EHR system. Let's take a closer look at how this process works.

Courtesy of Allscripts, LLC.

▶ **Figure 2-21 Electronic prescription DUR alert.**

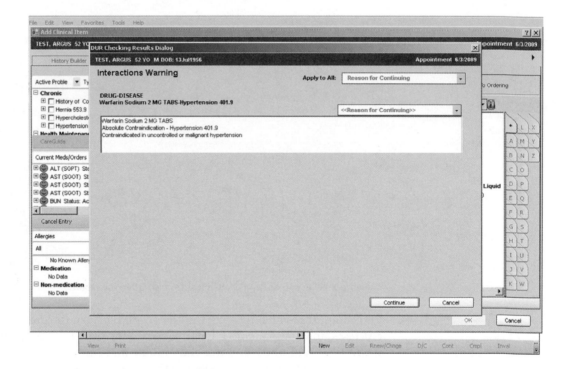

Drug Utilization Review   When the clinician writing an electronic prescription selects a drug and enters the Sig information, the EHR system sends the client's allergy information, past and current diagnoses, and a list of current medications to a drug utilization review (DUR) program that compares the prescription to a database of most known drugs. The database includes prescription drugs as well as over-the-counter drugs, and even nutritional herb and vitamin supplements. The DUR program performs the following functions:

▶ The drug about to be prescribed is checked against the client medication list to determine if there is a conflict with any drug the client is already taking. Certain drugs remain in the body for a period of time after the client has stopped taking it. This latency period is factored in as well.

▶ Ingredients that make up the drug are checked against the ingredients of current medications to see if they conflict or would hinder the effectiveness of the drug.

▶ Drugs are checked for duplicate therapy, which occurs when a client is taking a different drug of the same class that would have the effect of an overdose.

▶ Allergy records are checked for food and drug allergies that would be aggravated by the new drug.

▶ Some drugs cannot be given to clients with certain medical conditions; the client's diagnosis history is checked to see if such a situation would occur.

▶ A client education alert is created when the drug might be affected by certain foods or alcohol interactions.

▶ If the Sig has been entered at the time of the DUR, then it is also checked to see if it matches recommended guidelines for the drug. Too much, too little, too many days, or too many refills could cause overdosing, underdosing (causing it to be ineffective), or abuse.

If the DUR software finds any of these conditions, the clinician is given an alert message explaining the conflict. The clinician can then alter the prescription or select a new drug, having never issued the incorrect one.

Nursing Medication Alerts   EHR systems can also alert the nurse during the administration of medication to ensure the ten rights of medication administration. These systems can also display reminder alerts to the nurse about prescribed limitations for administration. For example, a client may be ordered to receive an antihypertensive drug if the client's blood pressure is above the prescribed threshold. The ten rights and closed loop medication safety will be discussed further in Chapter 7.

Formulary Alerts   Another type of alert found in many EHR prescription systems warns the clinician if the drug about to be prescribed is not covered by a client's pharmacy benefit insurance. This is important because if a client's insurance will not pay for it, the client may choose not to fill the prescription or to take less than the amount prescribed.

Insurance plans provide formularies indicating preferred, nonpreferred, and noncovered drugs. If the clinician prescribes a drug that is not on the list, then when the client tries to have the prescription filled, the pharmacy will call and ask the provider to change it. This causes an inconvenience to the client and wastes the ordering provider's time. Instead, a clinician using an EHR can select from a list of therapeutically equivalent drugs that are on the formulary of the client's insurance plan and avoid writing an incorrect prescription. Figure 2-22 shows an Allscripts Therapeutic Alternatives alert.

Courtesy of Allscripts, LLC.
▶ **Figure 2-22 Electronic prescription formulary alert.**

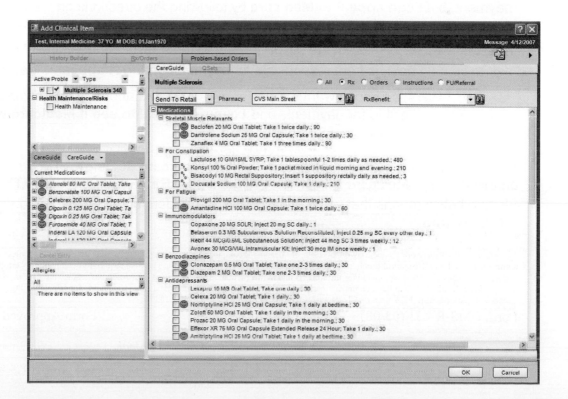

(A) **Notifier(s):**

(B) **Patient Name:**   *(C)* **Identification Number:**

ADVANCE BENEFICIARY NOTICE OF NONCOVERAGE (ABN)

<u>NOTE:</u> If Medicare doesn't pay for *(D)*_____ below, you may have to pay.

Medicare does not pay for everything, even some care that you or your health care provider have good reason to think you need. We expect Medicare may not pay for the *(D)*_____ below.

*(D)*_____	*(E)* Reason Medicare May Not Pay:	*(F)* Estimated Cost:

WHAT YOU NEED TO DO NOW:

- Read this notice, so you can make an informed decision about your care.
- Ask us any questions that you may have after you finish reading.
- Choose an option below about whether to receive the *(D)*_____ listed above.
  Note: If you choose Option 1 or 2, we may help you to use any other insurance that you might have, but Medicare cannot require us to do this.

(G) OPTIONS: Check only one box. We cannot choose a box for you.

❏ **OPTION 1.** I want the *(D)*_____ listed above. You may ask to be paid now, but I also want Medicare billed for an official decision on payment, which is sent to me on a Medicare Summary Notice (MSN). I understand that if Medicare doesn't pay, I am responsible for payment, but **I can appeal to Medicare** by following the directions on the MSN. If Medicare does pay, you will refund any payments I made to you, less co-pays or deductibles.

❏ **OPTION 2.** I want the *(D)*_____ listed above, but do not bill Medicare. You may ask to be paid now as I am responsible for payment. **I cannot appeal if Medicare is not billed**.

❏ **OPTION 3.** I don't want the *(D)*_____ listed above. I understand with this choice I am **not** responsible for payment, and **I cannot appeal to see if Medicare would pay.**

(H) Additional Information:

This notice gives our opinion, not an official Medicare decision. If you have other questions on this notice or Medicare billing, call **1-800-MEDICARE** (1-800-633-4227/**TTY**: 1-877-486-2048).

Signing below means that you have received and understand this notice. You also receive a copy.

(I) **Signature:**	*(J)* **Date:**

According to the Paperwork Reduction Act of 1995, no persons are required to respond to a collection of information unless it displays a valid OMB control number. The valid OMB control number for this information collection is 0938-0566. The time required to complete this information collection is estimated to average 7 minutes per response, including the time to review instructions, search existing data resources, gather the data needed, and complete and review the information collection. If you have comments concerning the accuracy of the time estimate or suggestions for improving this form, please write to: CMS, 7500 Security Boulevard, Attn: PRA Reports Clearance Officer, Baltimore, Maryland 21244-1850.

Form CMS-R-131 (03/08)   Form Approved OMB No. 0938-0566

▶ **Figure 2-23 Sample advance beneficiary notice form.**

Other Types of Alerts   Electronic lab order systems can provide alerts as well. For example, certain tests are not covered by Medicare. CMS requires that clients sign a waiver indicating that they were notified that a test would not be covered. The waiver called an Advance Beneficiary Notice (ABN) is shown in Figure 2-23. When certain tests are ordered, the clinician is alerted if an ABN is required.

Another example is an alert that monitors changes in values of certain blood tests and pages a nurse whenever the value is outside of a certain range. Alerts can also be created to assist busy clinicians and nurses ensure accurate and complete documentation that meets standards of clinical practice. For example, a nurse could receive a reminder alert if a post pain medication record has not been documented in the expected time frame to ensure that the client has received the adequate pain relief. Or physicians can be alerted when a time-limited treatment is due to be ended.

Alerts can be generated by nonactions as well. Task list systems can notify an administrator when medical items are not handled in a timely fashion. CPOE systems can generate alerts when results for a pending test order have not been received within the time frame normally required for that type of test.

Once an EHR system contains codified data, an alert system is just a matter of programming a rule to watch for a certain event or detect a finding with a value above or below the desired limit.

Health Maintenance

One of the best ways to maintain good health is to prevent disease, or if it occurs, to detect it early enough to be easily treated. Two important components of health maintenance are preventive care screening and immunizations.

Preventive Care   The simplest example of health maintenance is a card or letter reminding the client that it is time for a checkup. In a paper-based office, creating this reminder is a manual process. However, when a medical practice has electronic records, preventive screening can become more dynamic and sophisticated.

Health maintenance systems, also known as preventive care systems, can go beyond simple reminders for an annual checkup. When an EHR has codified data, it can be electronically compared with the recommendations of the U.S. Preventive Services Task Force (described further in Chapter 12).

Using a sophisticated set of rules, the EHR software compares the list of tests recommended for clients of a certain age and sex to previous test results stored in the EHR. It also calculates the time since the test was last performed and compares that to the recommended interval for repeat testing. A guideline unique to the client is generated and displayed on the clinician's computer. Using this information, the clinician can order tests, discuss important healthcare options, and recommend lifestyle changes to the client at the point of care. Figure 2-24 shows the Health Maintenance screen from EHR vendor NextGen.

It would be difficult to create standardized rules for the preventive care system if the tests were not coded using a standardized coding system. Preventive care screening guidelines are not limited to lab tests; other examples include mammograms, hearing and vision screening, and certain elements of the physical examination.

Immunizations   The other important component of preventive care is immunizations. Immunization slows down or stops disease outbreaks. Vaccines prevent disease in the people who receive them and protect those who come into contact with unvaccinated individuals.

Immunizations must be acquired over time. Vaccines cannot be given all at once. Several require repeated applications over a period of time, and some, such as the measles vaccine, cannot be given to children under the age of one year. Therefore, the CDC and state health departments have designed a schedule to immunize children and

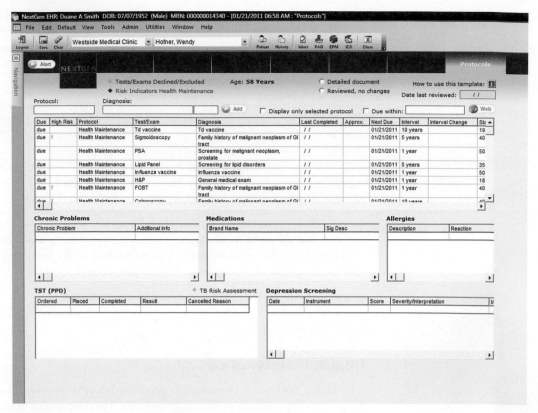

Courtesy of NextGen Healthcare, www.nextgen.com.
▶ **Figure 2-24 Health Maintenance screen.**

adolescents from birth through 18 years of age. The CDC also publishes a recommended immunization schedule for adults. Adult immunizations are different from those given to a child.

Using the codified data in an EHR, computers can compare a client's immunization history with the CDC-recommended vaccines and intervals and identify which immunizations the client needs. EHR systems can also scan the data and generate letters to send to clients who have not been in recently but may need to renew their immunizations.

Decision Support

Physicians and nurses are trained to analyze information from a client's history, physical exams, and test results for a medical decision. They are also accustomed to researching professional literature when faced with an unusual case. However, the quantity of information available to clinicians regarding conditions, disease management, protocols, case studies, and treatments far exceeds their available time to read it.

Decision support refers to the ability of EHR systems to store or quickly locate materials relevant to the findings of the current case. These might include defined protocols, results of case studies, or standard care guidelines prepared by specialists, medical societies, nursing professional organizations, or government organizations.

Decision support is not about "artificial intelligence" replacing a nurse or physician with a computer; it is instead about providing help just when the clinician needs it. There are many examples of decision support systems, but let us look at five:

▶ **Prescriptions:** Decision support can include the drug formularies mentioned earlier. Formularies can be used to look up drugs by name or therapeutic class. Electronic prescription systems provide decision support to the clinician by comparing alternative brands that are therapeutically equivalent. They can also provide information on costs, indications for use, treatment recommendations, dosage, guidelines, and prescribing information. These also offer key points of information to support client education including client-friendly documents.

▶ **Medical references:** Decision support systems can provide quick access to medical references directly from the EHR. This can make access to evidence-based guidelines or medical literature as easy as clicking on a link in the chart.

▶ **Protocols:** Protocols are one form of decision support that can ultimately speed up documentation of the care plan and improve client care. Protocols are standard plans of therapy established for different conditions. With a decision support system, when a client has been diagnosed with a particular condition, the appropriate protocol appears on the EHR screen and all therapies are ordered with a click of the mouse.

▶ **Medication dosing:** Many medications have serious side effects, some of which must be monitored by regular blood tests. When both the medications and lab results are stored in the EHR as codified data, it is possible for decision support software to compare changes in medication dosing with changes in the client's test results. This assists the clinician in adjusting the client's medication levels to obtain the maximum benefit to the client.

▶ **Nursing care planning:** As described earlier, the Medcin knowledge base includes the CCC framework, making it possible to quickly identify intervention and outcome standards based on the nursing diagnosis. The CCC system permits customization to the client's individual needs and generating appropriate nursing order sets to guide the client's care. The nursing plan of care is then stored in the EHR. Nursing Plans of Care will be covered in Chapter 6.

Meeting the IOM Definition of an EHR

The IOM identified eight criteria that define an EHR. The IOM definition of an EHR went beyond a computer that just stores the client's medical record to include *the functional benefits* derived from having an electronic health record.

In Chapter 1 we learned how the ONC strategies, CMS requirements, and EHR certification criteria support the IOM vision of an EHR. In this chapter we explored how the format that the data are stored in determines to what extent the data can be used to achieve that extended functionality. Each of the functional benefits we have discussed—trend analysis, alerts, health maintenance, and decision support—are products of EHR systems that store medical records as codified, fielded data. It is only when these functional benefits are added to the clinical practice that the EHR approaches the vision of the IOM and meets the full CMS "meaningful use" criteria.

Chapter Two Summary

The forms of EHR data are broadly categorized into three types:

1. Digital image data (provides increased accessibility)

2. Text-based data (provides accessibility and text search capability; can be displayed on different devices)

3. Discrete data, fielded and ideally codified (provides all of the above plus the capability to be used for trending, alerts, health maintenance, and data exchange)

Increased benefits of an EHR can be realized when the information is stored as codified data. In addition, codified EHR data that adheres to a national standard enables the exchange and comparison of medical information from other facilities.

A code set designed specifically to record medical observations is referred to as a clinical "nomenclature." Using an EHR nomenclature provides consistency in client records and improves communication between different medical specialties.

EHR nomenclatures differ from other coding standards in several ways:

▶ EHR nomenclatures precorrelate individual terms into clinically relevant "findings" or codified observations that are medically meaningful to the clinician.

▶ Findings are often linked to other findings, which helps the clinician quickly locate associated information and shortens the time required to document the exam.

▶ EHR nomenclatures differ from billing codes in that EHR nomenclatures have many more codes used to describe the detail of the exam such as the symptoms, history, observations, and plan. Billing codes tend to represent simply that the service was rendered.

▶ Reference terminologies designed for research may codify each medical term, but these terms can combine in ways that are not clinically relevant; therefore, these nomenclatures are not easy to use at the point of care.

▶ EHR nomenclatures often include cross-references to other standard code sets. Coding systems not intended for EHR do not typically contain a map to other coding systems.

Several of the most prominent coding standards you are likely to encounter or use in an EHR were discussed in this chapter.

▶ SNOMED-CT is a medical nomenclature developed by the College of American Pathologists and United Kingdom's National Health Service.

▶ MEDCIN is a medical nomenclature and knowledge base used in many commercial EHR systems as well as by the Department of Defense. MEDCIN differs from other EHR coding systems in that MEDCIN was designed for point-of-care use by the clinician, so that each "finding" represents a meaningful clinical observation or term. The MEDCIN findings are linked in a "knowledge base." This enables a clinician to quickly find other clinical "findings" that are likely to be needed. This difference means a provider selects fewer individual codes to complete the client exam note.

▶ LOINC stands for Logical Observation Identifier Names and Codes. LOINC is an important clinical terminology for laboratory test orders and results.

▶ CCC stands for Clinical Classification Codes, a system of codes for nursing that is incorporated into MEDCIN and other EHR nomenclatures.

EHR data may be captured in many ways:

▶ Scanning paper records

▶ Importing diagnostic images in digital format

▶ Importing text or word processing files

▶ Receiving data electronically from other systems using

  ▶ HL7

  ▶ DICOM

  ▶ CDISK

  ▶ RHIO

▶ Biomedical devices

▶ Telemonitoring devices

▶ Clients may enter their own history and symptoms

▶ Providers record the EHR at the point of care

When EHR data is coded, it can be used for:

▶ Trend analysis, the comparison of multiple values or findings over a period of time

▶ Alerts, computer-prompted warnings such as a potential drug interaction or a lab result seriously above or below the expected range

▶ Health maintenance, which creates reminders of health screening, immunizations, and other preventive measures

▶ Decision support, systems to quickly locate materials relevant to the findings of the current case such as defined protocols, standard care guidelines, or medical research

▶ Ease of aggregating data to support medical and nursing research for improvements in client care

References

American Nurses Association. (2009, December 11). *Position statement on electronic health records*. Silver Spring, MD: Author.

Health Information Management Systems Society. (2005, October 21). Definitions and acronyms. Retrieved April 27, 2011, from http://www.himss.org/content/files/RHIO_Definitions_Acronyms.pdf

Ozbolt, J. G. (1997). Multiple attributes for patient care data: Toward a multiaxial, combinatorial vocabulary. In D. L. Masys (Ed.), *Proceedings of the AMIA Annual Fall Symposium* (p. 884). Philadelphia: Hanley & Belfus.

Test Your Knowledge

1. Name three forms of EHR data.
2. Name at least two medical code sets considered national standards.
3. What is a nomenclature?
4. In an EHR, what is meant by the term *finding*?
5. Describe the difference between an EHR nomenclature and a billing code set.
6. What is one advantage of codified data over document imaged data?

Give examples for the following terms:

7. Trend analysis
8. Decision support
9. Alerts
10. Health maintenance
11. List at least two ways codified data in the EHR can be used to manage and prevent disease.
12. Name at least two benefits of having clients entering their own symptoms and history into the computer.
13. Describe two ways decision support can augment nursing practice.
14. Identify two possible nursing alerts that could help improve care to a hospitalized client.
15. What is HL7?

Ask your instructor for answers to Test Your Knowledge

nursing.pearsonhighered.com

Prepare for success with animated examples, practice questions, challenge tests, and interactive assignments.

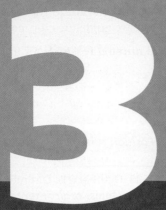

Chapter

3

Learning Medical Record Software

Learning Outcomes

After completing this chapter, you should be able to:

1. Start and stop the Student Edition software

2. Navigate the screen

3. Select a client

4. Create a new encounter

5. Access the Symptoms, History, Physical Exam, Assessment, and Therapy tabs to add appropriate findings in each portion of the exam

6. Select findings for edit and remove findings

7. Add entry details, free text, prefix, and status to findings

8. Enter a chief complaint

9. Enter vital signs

Introducing the Medcin Student Edition Software

In this chapter you will learn to document a client chart using Medcin, one of the standard EHR nomenclatures discussed in Chapter 2. Special Medcin Student Edition software has been created for you to use with this course. It is similar to many commercial software packages that use the Medcin knowledge base for their EHR nomenclature.

The Student Edition software allows you select findings for symptoms, history, physical examination, tests, diagnoses, therapy, nursing diagnosis, nurse interventions, nursing orders, and outcomes to produce medical documents typical of the clinical notes created in a medical facility using EHR software. At the conclusion of certain exercises, you will print or output your work to a file and give it to your instructor.

Because the Student Edition is designed for the classroom, it will be different in some aspects from EHR systems you will encounter when working in a hospital or medical office. Hospital software in particular is often customized by the facility and frequently does not use one of the national standard nomenclatures. However, the concepts, skills, and familiarity with EHR systems you will acquire by practicing with the Student Edition software will transfer directly into the workplace.

About the Exercises in This Book

Exercises in this and subsequent chapters of the book using the software provided will give you practical experience in creating electronic health records. The purpose of the exercises is to teach EHR concepts by providing hands-on experience.

Each set of exercises is designed to illustrate an EHR concept. In some exercises you will be asked to record entries that would normally be reserved for the physician or nurse practitioner. These advance nurse practices are included to demonstrate concepts such as CPOE and to add data necessary to complete an encounter document.

Although the clinical notes produced by the exercises are medically accurate, routine elements of a complete client assessment that should normally be documented are frequently omitted from the exercises. This is done solely to facilitate completion of the exercises in the allotted class time.

EHR Login

In Exercise 9 you will learn to log in to the Student Edition software. Before we do that, let us discuss the most fundamental component of secure EHR systems, your login.

In the Student Edition software your student login is your name or student ID. In a healthcare facility your login will be unique and will provide a permanent record of your use of the system, recording which entries into the client's record were made by you. To protect the integrity of the client's records and your liability for entries made under your "electronic signature," it is imperative that you use the correct log-in and log-off procedures required by the hospital or clinic. Similarly in the classroom, you should always use your own login.

There are several ways healthcare facilities identify authorized users:

▶ Require something known only to that individual, such as a password or PIN.

▶ Require something that individuals possess, such as a smart card, a token, or a key.

▶ Require something unique to the individual such as a biometric. Examples of biometrics include fingerprints, voice patterns, facial patterns, or iris patterns.

Most facilities use one of the first two methods to authenticate the user. Figure 3-1 shows the log-in procedure for a leading commercial EHR system.

As a general practice, users should log off the system when their workstation is unattended. However, there will be times when a nurse may not have the time or will

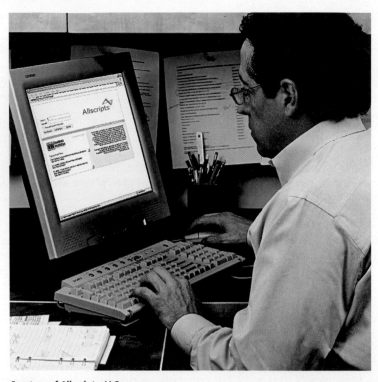

Courtesy of Allscripts, LLC.

▶ **Figure 3-1 A clinician logs in using a unique user ID and secure password.**

not remember to log off a workstation. Automatic logoff is an effective way to prevent unauthorized users from accessing a workstation when it is left unattended for a period of time. Most healthcare systems automatically log the user off after a predetermined period of inactivity. Even though your facility may have automatic logoff, you should not rely on this, but should follow proper log-off procedures whenever you are leaving your workstation unattended.

Critical Thinking Exercise 8: Electronic Signature

Research and answer the following:

1. What is the legal status of the Electronic Signature in the EHR in your state?

2. How can you protect your own electronic signature?

3. Identify potential impacts of a failure to log off or exit from the client record.

Understanding the Software

The following series of exercises is designed to allow you to become familiar with the Student Edition software, the Medcin nomenclature, and the screen navigation controls. Do not worry if you cannot complete all of them in one class period.

Guided Exercise 9: Starting Up the Software

The Student Edition software should have been installed on your school's network computers or on your local workstation. If you are working on your own computer and have not already installed the Student Edition software, you must do so before you can proceed. See the inside cover of this book for information on downloading the Student Edition software.

Step 1

Turn on the computer and wait for the Windows operating system desktop to appear on the screen. If you are using a school computer, you may be required to log in to the school network first; if so, ask your instructor for the correct log-in procedure.

Step 2

Locate the Medcin icon shown in Figure 3-2. If you do not see it on the computer desktop screen, click on the Start Button, and look in Programs or All Programs for the program named "Medcin Student Edition."

▶ **Figure 3-2 The Medcin Student Edition icon.**

Position the mouse pointer over the Medcin icon shown in Figure 3-2 and double-click the mouse button. This will display the Student Edition log-in screen shown in Figure 3-3.

▶ **Figure 3-3 Student Edition log-in screen.**

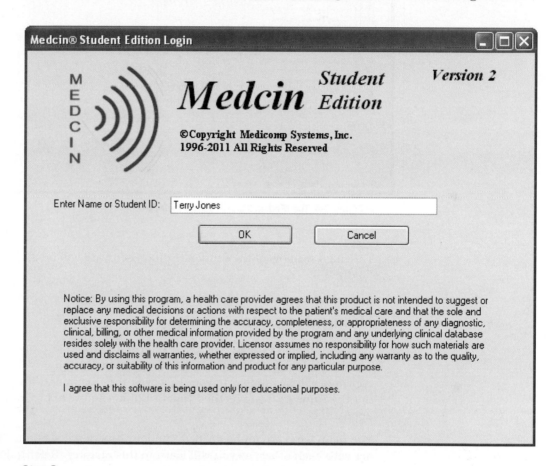

Step 3

Figure 3-3 shows the Medcin Student Edition log-in screen. The screen contains one data entry field and two buttons. The field is used for either the student's name or the student ID, depending on the policy of the school. Confirm with your instructor whether you should use your name or student ID. In the example, the student's name is Terry Jones. Do not type Terry Jones in the field.

Type either your name or student ID into the field.

When your name or ID is exactly as you want it to be, position the mouse pointer over the button labeled "OK" and click the mouse button.

The button labeled "Cancel" is used to cancel the login and close the window.

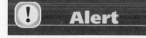

Version 2 of the software is required for this text. If "Version 2" is not displayed in the upper right corner of the log-in screen, stop and inform your instructor at once.

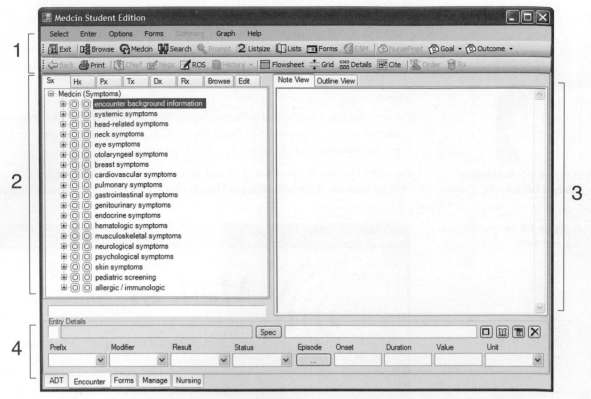

▶ **Figure 3-4 The Medcin Student Edition window.**

The main window of the Student Edition software will be displayed, as shown in Figure 3-4.

Navigating the Screen

This section will explain how the screen is organized and discuss some of the features you will use later. Having completed Exercises 5 through 7 in Chapter 2, some of these concepts will be familiar to you. However, the Document/Image System simulation is not the same software as the Student Edition software program. It is only similar in appearance.

The main window can be divided into four functional sections. These four sections interact with each other, as you will learn in this chapter. Refer to Figure 3-4 and locate each of the sections indicated by the red numerals 1–4.

Section 1: The Menu Bar and Toolbar At the top of the screen, the words "Select," "Enter," "Options, " "Forms," "Summary," "Graph," and "Help" are the menus of functions in the Student Edition software. As you learned in the previous chapter, when you position the mouse pointer over one of these words and click the mouse once, a list of functions will drop down below the word. Once a list appears, moving the mouse pointer vertically over the list will highlight each item. In the Student Edition, highlight refers to a colored rectangle that appears over an item. Clicking on the highlighted item will invoke that function. Clicking the mouse anywhere on the screen other than the list will close the list.

Also located at the top of your screen are two rows of icon buttons called a "Toolbar." The purpose of the Toolbar is to allow quick access to commonly used functions. Toolbar buttons will be identified later in the chapter, as you learn to use them.

Section 2: The Medcin Nomenclature Pane The middle portion of the screen is divided into two window panes. The left pane (shown in Figure 3-4 with the numeral 2) displays the Medcin nomenclature findings you will select from. In the next exercise, you will select a client and learn to navigate the Medcin Nomenclature pane.

At the top of the Nomenclature pane there are eight tabs. These look like tabs on file folders. The first six of these are labeled: Sx (symptoms), Hx (history), Px (physical examination), Tx (tests), Dx (diagnosis, syndromes, and conditions), and Rx (therapy). The tabs are used to logically group the findings into six broad categories. Two additional tabs, labeled "Browse" and "Edit," will be explained later as you use it the software.

Section 3: The Encounter View Pane The right pane of the window (shown in Figure 3-4 with the numeral 3) will dynamically display the encounter note as it is being created. When a healthcare professional selects a finding from the Nomenclature pane, the finding and relevant accompanying text are recorded in the encounter note and displayed in the pane on the right.

Free text also may be entered through the software; it will appear in the Note View pane as well. This will become clearer during subsequent exercises. Because you have not yet selected a client or an encounter, the pane is empty at this time.

There are two tabs on the top of the right pane. The Note View tab displays the encounter note as you create it. The Outline View displays findings that have been selected as well as appropriate ICD-9-CM or CPT-4 codes.

Section 4: Entry Details for a Current Finding The bottom portion of the screen (shown in Figure 3-4 with the numeral 4) consists of two rows of fields that allow the user to add detail to any finding recorded in the right pane. Entry of data in these fields adds informational text to the finding in the encounter note, and in some cases modifies its meaning.

For example, a client-reported symptom of "headaches" could be modified using the Entry Details field labeled "Status" to indicate the condition was "improving." The meaning of the finding could be altered completely by use of the Entry Details field labeled "Prefix" to indicate "family history of." This would indicate that the client did not have this condition, but that it had been a problem for close relatives. Each of the fields in the details section of the screen will be covered in subsequent exercises in this book.

To actually see the interactions of the four sections of the screen, you need to select a patient and create a new encounter. Subsequent exercises will show you how, but first let us discuss exiting the software.

Guided Exercise 10: Exiting and Restarting the Software

There are three ways to exit the Student Edition software. In this exercise, you will practice exiting the software. You will then restart the program to continue with subsequent exercises.

At the top of your screen is a row of words called the Menu bar. Below it are two rows of buttons with icons, called the Toolbar. The first button in the Toolbar is labeled "Exit"; its icon looks like an open door. If you click on the Exit button, the Student Edition program will end and the window will close.

In the upper right corner of the window are three buttons that are standard to all Windows programs. From left to right, these buttons minimize, maximize, and close the window. The close button is red, with a large X. If you click on the close button, the Student Edition program will end and the window will close.

A third way to close the program is explained next.

Step 1

The first word in the Menu bar is "Select." Position the mouse pointer over the word "Select" in the Menu bar at the top of the screen and click the mouse button once. A list of the functions on the Select menu will drop down.

You will notice some of the items in the menu are listed in black text and some of them are in gray. Menu items in gray text indicate a particular function is not applicable to the current state of the encounter note and are therefore not selectable. You may have noticed some of the buttons on the Toolbar also are gray; this is for the same reason.

Step 2

Move the mouse pointer vertically down the list until the Exit function is highlighted. Click the mouse on the word "Exit" to end the program.

Step 3

Start the Student Edition software again by repeating Exercise 9, and logging in.

Note

In subsequent exercises, when you attempt to exit after entering some data, you will receive a warning that you have not printed the encounter. It is permissible to exit without printing *for this chapter only.* In all other chapters you must not exit without printing or you will lose your work.

Guided Exercise 11: Using the Menu to Select a Patient

Once you are logged in, the first step in every encounter is to select the patient.

Step 1

Position the mouse pointer over the word "Select" in the Menu bar at the top of the screen and click the mouse button once. A list of the Select menu functions will appear (see Figure 3-5).

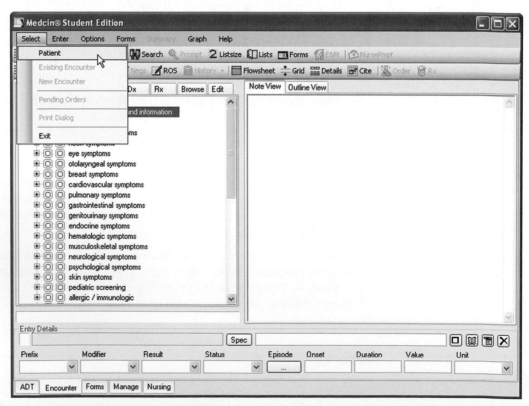

▶ **Figure 3-5 Functions on the Select menu.**

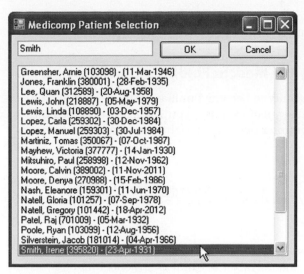

▶ **Figure 3-6 Selecting Irene Smith from the Patient Selection window.**

Step 2

Move the mouse pointer vertically down the list until Patient is highlighted. Click the mouse on the word "Patient" to invoke the Patient Selection window shown in Figure 3-6.

Step 3

The Student Edition Patient Selection window displays a list of all clients in the system, their last name, first name, patient ID number, and date of birth. A field at the top of the window allows you to type the client's last name to quickly find someone in a large list.

Find the client named Irene Smith in the Patient Selection window by typing "Smith" in the field. When you start typing the name, the first surname beginning with an "S" will be highlighted; as you continue to type, the next alphabetical name will be highlighted.

When "Smith, Irene" is highlighted, click the OK button.

Clicking the Cancel button will close the window.

An alternate method of selecting the client is to visually locate the client's name, position the mouse pointer over it, and double-click the mouse button. (*Double-click* means to click the mouse button twice, very rapidly.)

Step 4

Once a patient is selected, the client's name is displayed in the title at the top of the window (see Figure 3-7).

The Medcin Nomenclature (in the left pane) becomes active and the first group of findings (symptoms) is displayed.

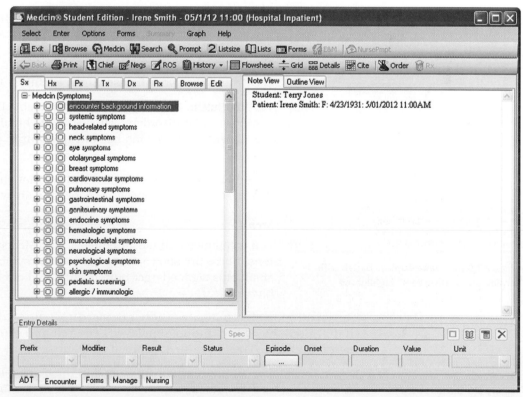

▶ **Figure 3-7 Left pane displays Medcin nomenclature.**

The right pane containing the encounter note is populated with the student's name or ID and the patient's name, sex, and date of birth.

Guided Exercise 12: Navigating the Medcin Findings

In this exercise you will have an opportunity to become familiar with one way to navigate the Medcin nomenclature. In a subsequent exercise, you will learn to record the findings from the left pane into the encounter note in the right pane. In this exercise, you will not yet record any findings.

Step 1

Your screen should resemble Figure 3-7. If it does not, repeat Exercise 11.

Step 2

Look at the list of findings in the left pane. As mentioned earlier, the pane on the left of the screen is used to select findings to document the current client encounter.

The Medcin Nomenclature consists of more than 277,000 findings with 68 million relationships. To make it easy to find what you are looking for, the tabs on the left of the pane categorize findings into six broad groups that follow the order of a typical exam.

Chapter 1 described the standard order of medical exams in a SOAP format. The six tabs on the left pane make it easy to document in that format as follows:

Subjective	Sx	Symptoms
	Hx	History
Objective	Px	Physical Exam
	Tx	Tests (performed)
Assessment	Dx	Diagnosis
Plan	Rx	Therapy, plan, and tests (ordered)

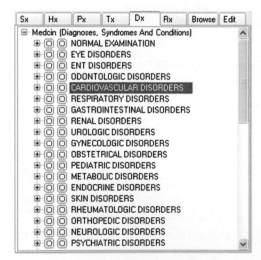

▶ **Figure 3-8 Left pane displays Dx tab with "Cardiovascular Disorders" highlighted.**

If, for example, we wanted to begin by recording the admitting diagnosis, you would click on the tab labeled "Dx" at the top of the left pane.

Step 3

Locate and click your mouse on the Dx tab at this time.

The findings in the left pane should resemble Figure 3-8, except that "cardiovascular disorders" will not be the highlighted finding. Notice that the currently selected tab has the appearance of being slightly raised from the others.

In addition to the tabs, another feature that shortens the list of findings displayed in the nomenclature pane is to show only the main topics.

Step 4

You will notice that most findings in the Medcin list are preceded by buttons. These are shown in Figure 3-9. The symbols on the buttons are a small plus sign, a larger button with a red circle, and a larger button with blue circle.

The small plus sign indicates there are more specific findings hidden from view that are related to the finding displayed. The red and blue buttons are used to record findings. These will be explained in a subsequent exercise.

▶ **Figure 3-9 Buttons used in the Nomenclature pane.**

Locate the finding "Cardiovascular Disorders" in the nomenclature symptoms list (highlighted in Figure 3-8) . Position the mouse pointer over the small plus symbol and click the mouse button once.

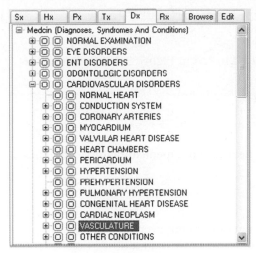

▶ **Figure 3-10 Left pane displays expanded list of findings for Cardiovascular Disorders.**

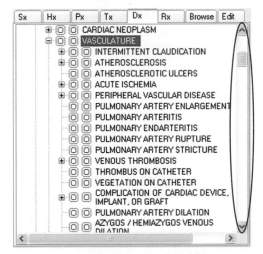

▶ **Figure 3-11 Left pane displays expanded list of findings for Vasculature (scroll bar circled).**

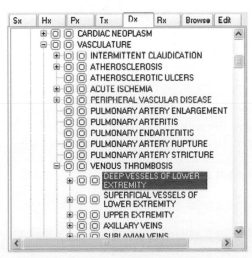

▶ **Figure 3-12 Left pane displays expanded list of findings for Venous Thrombosis.**

Compare the left pane of your screen with Figure 3-10. The list should have expanded to reveal many additional cardiovascular-related findings. Notice that the findings under "Cardiovascular Disorders" are indented.

Notice also that some of the additional findings have small plus symbols as well, for example, "conduction system" and "coronary arteries." This indicates even more specific findings are available for those items. Conversely, findings such as "normal heart" and "prehypertension" do not have the small plus. This means that there are not more specific findings for those items.

Step 5

Position the mouse pointer over the small plus symbol for the finding "vasculature" in the indented list, and click the mouse. The list expands further.

Notice that this time there were too many findings to fit in the space allotted. A light blue scroll bar has appeared on the right side of the pane. You are probably familiar with the concept of scrolling a window.

Step 6

Position the mouse pointer on the light blue scroll bar and hold the mouse button down while you drag the mouse in a downward motion. This action will scroll the list. Continue scrolling the list until you can see all the findings under "vasculature," as shown in Figure 3-11.

Locate the finding "venous thrombosis."

Position the mouse pointer over the small plus symbol for the finding "venous thrombosis" and click the mouse.

Notice that even that finding has a small plus symbol indicating that further detailed findings are available. Compare your list to Figure 3-12.

This type of list is called a *tree* because each indention of the list represents smaller branches of the finding above it. Look again at Figure 3-12; notice how each new level is indented further than the one above it. You may already be familiar with this concept because it is used in many other computer programs, including the Windows operating system.

Each time you clicked on the small plus symbol next to a finding in steps 4 to 6, the list grew. The term we use for this is to say that "the tree has expanded." Also notice that a small minus sign replaced the small plus sign in the button next to the finding that has been expanded.

Step 7

Position the mouse pointer over the small minus symbol next to the finding "vasculature" and click the mouse button again. The expanded list of various types of vasculature-related findings will again be hidden from view. Your screen should once again look like Figure 3-11.

When you clicked on the small minus symbol for the main finding, the number of findings for "vasculature" was reduced back to one. The term we use for this is to say that "the view of the tree has been collapsed." These are the terms that will be used when working with Medcin lists for the remainder of this book.

Guided Exercise 13: Tabs on the Medcin Nomenclature Pane

Step 1

Position the mouse pointer over the Hx tab (circled in red in Figure 3-13) and click the mouse once.

The list will change to that shown in Figure 3-13.

Step 2

Position the mouse pointer over the small plus next to "past medical history" and click the mouse button to expand the list.

Step 3

Position the mouse pointer over the small plus next to "recent events" and click the mouse button to expand the list. Locate the finding "recently high altitude flight" as shown in Figure 3-14).

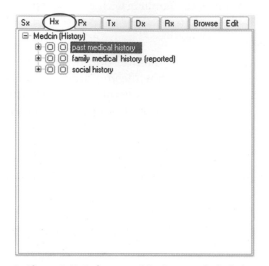

▶ **Figure 3-13 Left pane with History tab circled in red.**

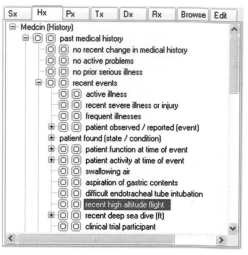

▶ **Figure 3-14 Left pane displays expanded past medical history and recent events.**

Step 4

Position the mouse pointer over the Dx tab and click the mouse once. The display will return to the previous list shown in Figure 3-11.

Step 5

Position the mouse pointer again over the Hx tab and click the mouse once. Notice the list is expanded as when you left it. In most cases, the software will remember how much of the expanded tree was displayed in each tab as well as what finding was highlighted. This feature allows the clinician to easily go back to a previous tab to add another finding, and then return to where she or he left off.

Step 6

Explore each of the remaining sections of the Medcin Nomenclature pane, by clicking on each of the remaining tabs. Take a moment on each tab to look at the type of findings in each tab. Feel free to expand or collapse the list in any of the tabs.

Data Entry of Clinical Notes

The main purpose of EHR software based on the Medcin nomenclature is to document clinical notes in a codified electronic medical record. This is done by selecting the finding from the Medcin nomenclature list in the left pane of the window. The finding and accompanying text are automatically recorded in the encounter note displayed in the right pane of the window. (The note view portion of the screen is indicated by the numeral 3 in Figure 3-4.)

Information is also added to the clinical note by adding or modifying a finding using the Entry Details fields in the bottom portion of the window. (The Entry Details section is indicated in Figure 3-4 by the numeral 4.)

The following exercises are designed to let you explore the interactions of the four sections of the Student Edition window. During the course of these exercises, you will create your first clinical encounter note with the Medcin nomenclature. To keep the exercises short, you will only record a few findings in each tab.

Case Study

The remaining exercises in this chapter concern Irene Smith, an 81-year-old female client who complains of pains in her right leg following an extended airplane flight. She has been admitted to the hospital with a working diagnosis of deep venous thrombosis.

Guided Exercise 14: Creating an Encounter

When a doctor, nurse, or other healthcare provider examines a client in a facility or at home, it is commonly referred to as an *encounter*. Similarly, an outpatient visit to a provider in a medical office or clinic is also called an encounter. Clinical notes documenting the encounter are variously referred to as *exam notes*, *provider notes*, *nurse notes*, or *encounter notes*. Whatever term is used, the encounter note is a record of the findings of an examination or care provided that occurred on a specific date and time. Although a portion of the data may be recorded by the medical assistant, another portion by the nurse, and yet another by a doctor, one completed encounter record should encompass the entire visit. However, when the client returns for another visit, a new encounter is created.

In any type of medical facility it is important to accurately record the date and time of the encounter. In this exercise, you will create a new encounter and learn how to set the date and time of the encounter.

Step 1

The name Irene Smith should be displayed at the top of the Medcin window. If it is not, repeat Guided Exercise 11.

The Select menu (which you have used previously) also has functions to select an existing encounter or create a new encounter. In this exercise, you will create a new encounter.

Position the mouse pointer over the word "Select" in the Menu bar, and click the mouse button. Move the mouse pointer vertically down the list until the item "New Encounter" is highlighted. Click the mouse button.

Step 2

When you create a new encounter, a window is invoked that allows you to set the date, time, and reason for the encounter. The month, day, year, and time will default to current date and time settings in your own computer. Today's month and year are displayed in the calendar on the window. Today's date is outlined in red. Days that occur in the previous and subsequent months are in gray text.

Because it is unlikely that you are doing this exercise on May 1, 2012, you will need to manually set the date and time as instructed in this exercise. The purpose of this exercise is to teach you how to set the date and time using the new encounter window.

Setting the Date to May 1, 2012

Small gray buttons with left and right arrows are located at the top of the calendar window. Clicking the button with the right arrow advances the calendar one month for each click of the mouse. Clicking the button with the left arrow takes the calendar backward one month for each click. If you click on the year, the field will open and small up and down arrows will appear (as shown in Figure 3-15). Clicking on these arrow buttons will allow you to quickly change years without cycling through all the months.

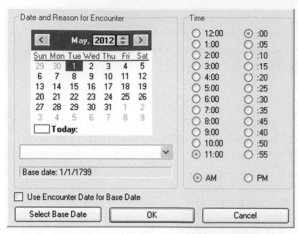

▶ **Figure 3-15 Select New Encounter, set date/time May 1, 2012, 11:00 AM.**

Click the buttons on the top of the calendar until the month **May** is displayed.

If the year 2012 is not currently displayed, click on the year to quickly modify it. Click the up or down arrow button to increase or decrease the year until 2012 is displayed.

Position the mouse pointer over day **1** and click the mouse button. The first day will be highlighted with a blue rectangle.

The time is indicated on the right side of the window by white circles that are filled in the center. For example, in Figure 3-15, the circles next to 11:00 and :00 and :AM are each filled, indicating the time of the encounter will be 11:00 AM.

Select the time by clicking your mouse in the circles next to **11:00** and **:00** and **:AM**. Each of the circles should become filled in.

Step 3

The reason for the encounter is also set in this window. The encounter reason field is located just below the calendar. To view a list of reasons, position the mouse pointer over the button with the down arrow in the right side of the field, and click the mouse. A drop-down list of reasons will appear as shown in Figure 3-16.

In a previous exercise, you learned to scroll a list by holding the mouse button while dragging it down the scroll bar. Using the same technique, you can scroll the list of reasons. Locate the reason "Hospital Inpatient" by scrolling the list until it is displayed. Position the mouse pointer over it and then click the mouse button to select the reason.

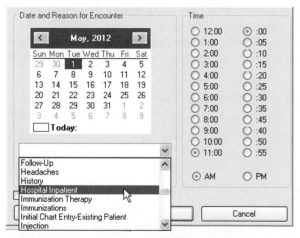

▶ **Figure 3-16 Select Hospital Inpatient from list of reasons for encounter.**

Step 4

Compare your screen to Figure 3-17. Make certain you set the date, time, and reason correctly. If the date, time, or reason needs to be corrected, repeat the previous steps.

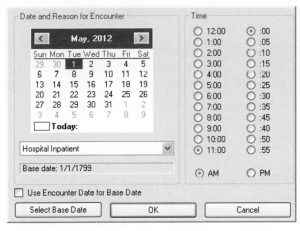

▶ **Figure 3-17 New encounter for a Hospital Inpatient, May 1, 2012,11:00 AM.**

Locate the button labeled "OK" in the bottom of the new encounter window, position the mouse pointer over the OK button, and click the mouse. The "Date and Reason for Encounter" window will close.

Step 5

The encounter date, time, and reason "Hospital Inpatient" should be displayed in the title of the window. The encounter date and time should be recorded in the encounter note in the right pane of the window.

Compare your screen with Figure 3-7; if your screen matches Figure 3-7, you are ready to proceed. If it does not, repeat steps 1 to 4.

Note

Tips for Completing the Exercises

The purpose of this chapter is to help you become familiar with the software and EHR concepts through guided exercises. You will not be able to complete all the exercises in this chapter in one class period.

However, in subsequent class periods, each time you resume work on this chapter you must repeat at least three steps:

1. **Start the Medcin Student Edition software**
2. **Select the patient Irene Smith**
3. **Create a new encounter for hospital inpatient, May 1, 2012 11:00 AM**

In most cases, you will be able to continue with the next guided exercise without repeating preceding ones. When you continue without repeating prior exercises, the encounter note in the right pane of the window will not contain as much information as the figures printed in the textbook.

In Chapter 4 you will create and print an entire encounter note in one session.

Guided Exercise 15: Recording the Admitting Diagnosis

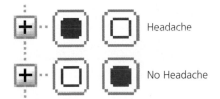

▶ **Figure 3-18 Buttons adjacent to findings fill with color when selected.**

Information is recorded in the encounter note by clicking the mouse on the red or blue buttons adjacent to each finding (shown enlarged in Figure 3-18). Clicking on a button with the red circle will record the finding as it appears in the list and fill in the red circle. Clicking on a button with the blue circle will record the finding in its opposite state and fill in the blue circle. For example, clicking on the button with the red circle next to "Headache" will record that the client has a headache; clicking on the button with the blue circle will record that the client has reported no headache.

When a finding is recorded in the encounter note on the right pane, the description of the finding in the left pane also changes to match the selected state. For example, the finding of Headache becomes "No Headache" when the blue button is selected, as shown in Figure 3-18. Should the finding descriptions in the nomenclature pane become too long, they are displayed truncated with an ellipsis (three dots), which indicates there is more to the description than will fit in the left pane.

Because the description of the findings change when their buttons are clicked, instructions to click a red or blue button identify a finding by its description *before* it is selected, so that you can locate it in the nomenclature pane. Screen figures used for comparison show the description of a finding as it appears *after* being selected.

For the remainder of this book, the buttons used to select findings will simply be referred to as the red button or the blue button.

A finding can be highlighted (surrounded with a blue background) without selecting either the red or blue button by clicking on the description of the finding instead of the buttons. You will learn to highlight a finding later, in Exercise 24.

Using what you have learned in the previous exercises, you are going to record your first finding, the admitting diagnosis.

Step 1

Locate and click on the Dx tab as you did in Exercise 12.

Locate "Cardiovascular Disorders" and click on the small plus sign next to it to expand the tree.

Locate "Vasculature" and click on the small plus sign next to it to expand the tree. Scroll the window until you can see the full list of vasculature findings.

Locate "Venous Thrombosis" and click on the small plus sign next it to expand the tree. Refer back to Figure 3-12 if necessary.

Step 2

Locate and click on the red button next to the finding "Deep vessels of lower extremity."

Compare your screen to Figure 3-19.

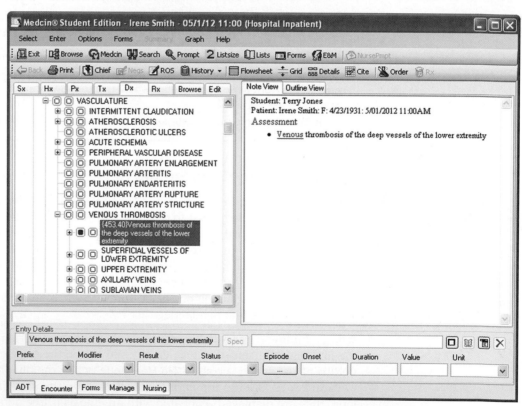

▶ **Figure 3-19 Selected Finding: Venous Thrombosis, deep vessels of lower extremity.**

Step 3

Notice that the finding has been added to the encounter note in the right pane and that the description in the left pane has also changed. Compare its current description to the description of the finding in Figure 3-12.

Remember, instructions to click a red or blue button identify a finding by its description *before* it is selected, so that you can locate it in the nomenclature pane. Screen figures used for comparison show the description of a finding *after* it has been selected.

Guided Exercise 16: Recording Subjective Findings

Step 1

Client-reported symptoms are entered on the Sx tab.

If you are continuing from the previous exercise, position the mouse pointer over the Sx tab and click the mouse once.

If you are beginning a new session, repeat the necessary steps to select a client, select a new encounter, and make sure you are on the Sx tab.

Step 2

The client reports leg pain.

Locate musculoskeletal symptoms and click on the small plus sign to expand the tree.

Scroll the expanded list to locate "legs" and click on the small plus sign to expand the tree.

Position the mouse over the red button for the finding "Pain." Click the mouse button. Compare your screen to Figure 3-20.

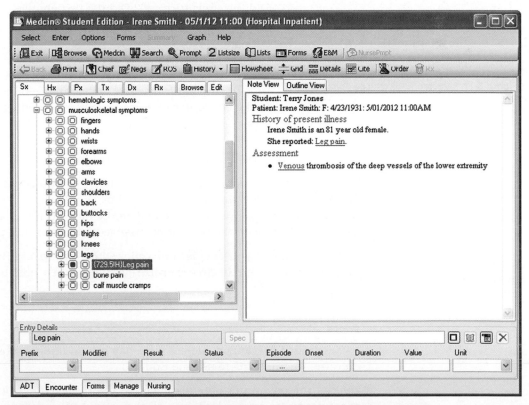

▶ Figure 3-20 Expanded tree for musculoskeletal, leg symptoms—Pain finding selected.

The center of the button should turn red. This indicates that the finding has been selected. The finding description "Pain" has changed to "Leg pain" and the finding should have appeared on the right pane in the encounter note.

When you record the first symptom finding, a section titled "History of present illness" was added to the encounter note as well. The history of present illness section also includes the client's age on the date of the encounter.

Section titles are dynamically added or removed by the software based on the findings selected. Dynamically adding section titles only when they are needed creates a cleaner-looking encounter note without empty sections. For example, if tests are not performed, the right pane does not show an empty section called "Tests."

Step 3

To further explore the operation of the red and blue buttons, position the mouse over and then click on the blue button for "Leg pain" instead. The center of the blue button should fill in and the red button should return to its previous (cleared) state. Also, the text in the encounter note and the finding description will both change to "No leg pain."

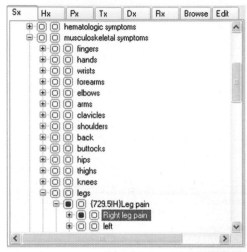

▶ **Figure 3-21 Selected findings: Leg pain and Right.**

Click on the red button to restore the finding back to "Leg pain." Make sure the button is red and the text in the encounter note again reads "Leg pain" before proceeding to step 4.

Step 4

EHR information should be as specific as possible. For example, is the pain in the left, right, or both legs?

Click on the small plus next to "Leg pain" to expand the tree. Locate the finding "Right" and click on the red button.

Did the circle turn red? Did the text change in the encounter note?

Compare your screen to Figure 3-21.

Notice that not only does the software change the description of findings when you select them, but surrounding text is added to the encounter note to automatically construct sentences. In this example, the finding in the encounter note reads: "She reported leg pain in the right leg."

Guided Exercise 17: Removing Findings

In step 3 of the previous exercise, you learned that you could change the state or meaning of a finding that was already recorded by simply clicking your mouse on the opposite color button. In that example, clicking on the blue button changed "Leg pain" to "No leg pain" and clicking on the red button changed it back to "Leg pain."

However, what if you accidentally clicked on the wrong finding? How would you undo it completely? In this exercise, you will learn how to remove findings from the encounter note.

Step 1

As mentioned previously, the left pane has two additional tabs, Browse and Edit. In this exercise, we are going to use the Edit tab.

Look at the encounter note displayed in the right pane. Notice that findings in the encounter note are underlined and the surrounding text is black. The section titles are blue and not underlined. You can click on underlined findings to edit them. You cannot click on section titles or the black text (i.e., you cannot click on text that is not underlined).

In the right pane (encounter note) locate the underlined portion of the symptom finding "in the" and position your mouse pointer over it. The mouse pointer changes into the shape of a hand (as shown in Figure 3-22). While the hand is over the underlined words, click the mouse once. This will select the finding for Edit.

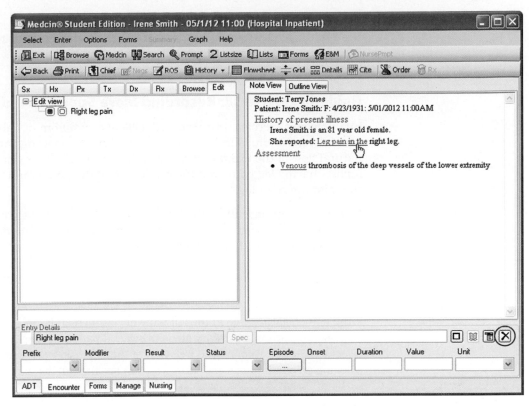

► Figure 3-22 Edit mode with Delete finding button circled in red.

The Edit tab above the Nomenclature pane has been automatically selected and the list in the Nomenclature pane has been limited to the one finding being edited.

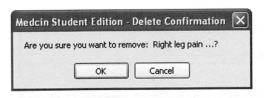

► Figure 3-23 Click OK to confirm removing the finding.

Step 2

Locate the button with an X in the lower right corner of the screen. (It is circled in red in Figure 3-22.) This is the Delete button, which is similar in appearance to the Delete button used in word processors, e-mail, and many other Windows programs. Position your mouse pointer over the Delete button and click once.

A small window called a "dialog" will appear (as shown in Figure 3-23). The dialog is asking you to confirm your intention to remove the finding from the encounter note.

Note this procedure only removes the finding from the current encounter note. Findings will not be deleted from the Medcin nomenclature or previous encounter notes by this procedure.

Click on the OK button.

The finding "Right leg pain" will be removed from the encounter note, but the finding "Leg pain" will remain in the note. The left pane will remain on the Edit tab. This is normal.

Step 3

Practice removing findings by repeating steps 1 and 2 for the "Leg pain" finding.

When you remove the last finding in a section, the section title will be removed automatically. In this case, "History of present illness" and "Irene Smith is 81 year old female" were removed.

Step 4

Restore the Medcin nomenclature list to the left pane by positioning the mouse over the Sx tab and clicking once. This will redisplay the Medcin nomenclature.

Guided Exercise 18: Recording More Specific Findings

In a previous exercise, you recorded a client's symptom of pain in the right by selecting two different findings from the list. There is nothing wrong with doing it that way if the natural flow of the exam progresses in that manner. For example, if when the client reports having leg pain, and the nurse asks if the pain is in both legs, the client says "no, just the right leg."

However, if you have all of the information before selecting the finding, you can simply select the most specific finding and Medcin will add the surrounding text. In this exercise, you will record both pieces of information about the client's symptom by clicking only one finding.

Step 1

If the nomenclature tree in the left pane of your screen is not expanded as in the previous exercise, repeat the necessary steps to select a patient, select a new encounter, and then select the Sx tab. Expand the tree view of "musculoskeletal symptoms," "leg," and "pain" (clicking on small plus signs) until you can see the full list expanded as in Figure 3-21.

Step 2

Position the mouse pointer over the red button for the finding "right" (indented under "pain") and click the mouse.

Compare your screen with Figure 3-24. Did the red button fill in?

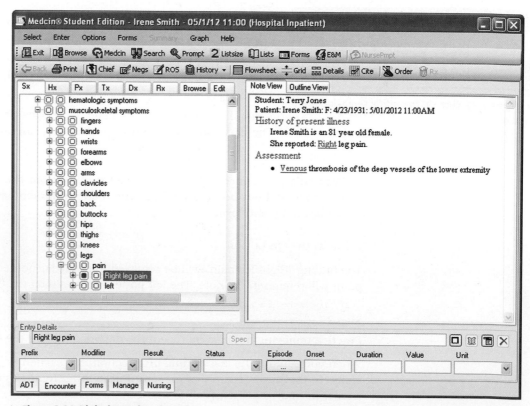

▶ **Figure 3-24 Right leg pain selected.**

Compare the text of the encounter note in Figure 3-22 with the text in the right pane of Figure 3-24. The two notes are different but medically equivalent. Additionally, in the codified EHR, Medcin has taken care of relating the underlying codes.

In the real-world application of electronic medical records, speed of input is important. Use whichever technique accurately documents the exam in the least amount of time. There is no reason to go back and delete the findings as we did in the previous exercise when they are correct. However, when an entire symptom or observation can be documented by selecting a single finding, do so, as you have in this exercise. The purpose of Guided Exercise 17 was to teach you how to remove findings when necessary.

Guided Exercise 19: Recording History Findings

The History tab is used to record the client's past medical, surgical, family, and social history.

Step 1

Position the mouse pointer over the Hx tab and click the mouse once.

Using the skills you have acquired in Exercise 13, navigate the Hx list and expand the tree by clicking on the small plus signs next to "past medical history," and "recent events." The expanded tree in left pane of the window should resemble Figure 3-14.

Step 2

Locate and click on the red button next to the finding "recent high altitude flight."

Compare your screen to Figure 3-25.

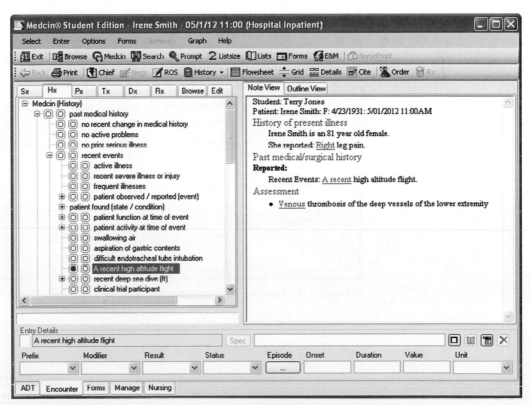

▶ **Figure 3-25 Past medical history, recent events, high altitude flight selected.**

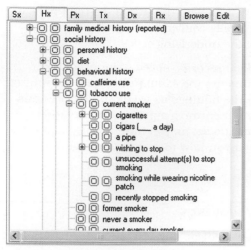

▶ **Figure 3-26 Hx social history, behavioral history, current smoker, expanded.**

Step 3

Scroll to the bottom of the list of history findings.

Locate "social history" and click the mouse on the small plus sign to expand the list.

Locate "behavioral history" and click the mouse on the small plus sign to expand the list.

Locate "tobacco use" and click the mouse on the small plus sign to expand the list.

Locate "current smoker" and click the mouse on the small plus sign to expand the list.

The expanded tree in left pane of the window should resemble Figure 3-26.

Step 4

Position the mouse over the red button next to the finding "cigarettes." Click the mouse button. The circle in the button should turn red and "Behavioral: Cigarette smoking" should appear in the encounter note pane on the right pane.

Compare your screen to Figure 3-27. Note that two new titles were added as well: "Personal history" and "Behavioral."

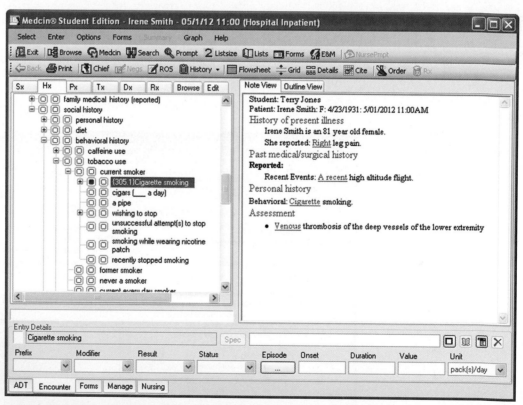

▶ **Figure 3-27 Cigarettes selected; Behavioral: Cigarette smoking added to note.**

Adding Details to the Findings

In addition to the narrative text that the software automatically generates, you also can add further clarification to the encounter note using Entry Details fields.

The section labeled "Entry Details" is located at the bottom of your screen. It was indicated in Figure 3-4 with the numeral 4. The Entry Details section consists of two rows of white boxes. These are the Entry Details fields.

The first row of fields contains the description of the currently highlighted finding, a note field for adding free text about the current finding, and four buttons. You have already used the Delete button (with the X) in a previous exercise. We will discuss and use two other buttons in later exercises.

The second row contains the following fields: "Prefix," "Modifier," "Result," "Status," "Episode," "Onset," "Duration," "Value," and "Unit."

All of the fields in the Entry Details section apply to a single finding, the one currently selected or highlighted.

In the following exercises, you will learn to use the Entry Details fields. Notice the Entry Details fields as you select findings. In some cases, Medcin will automatically set one or more of the fields; other times you will set the field yourself.

Guided Exercise 20: Recording a Value

The Value field can be used to enter a value about any type of finding. For example, the client's weight could be entered for a finding of weight, or the result of a simple blood test performed at the point of care could be entered as a numeric value for the finding "Hematocrit."

The Unit field is related to the Value field in that it describes the unit of measure for the value. In the two previous examples, the unit for weight would be pounds or kilograms, and the unit for the Hematocrit would be percent.

In this exercise, cigarette consumption is measured in packs per day. So the value will be the number of packs client consumed and the unit would be "packs per day."

Step 1

Make sure "Cigarette smoking" is the current finding. If you are beginning a new class, you will need to repeat the previous exercise to add the finding before proceeding.

Step 2

Locate the Value and Unit fields in the Entry Details section at the bottom of the screen. Notice that the Unit field already contains the words "pack(s)/day."

Click your mouse in the Value field and type "**1**" and then press the Enter key on your keyboard.

Compare your screen with Figure 3-28. The text in the encounter note should now read: "Behavioral: Cigarette smoking 1 pack(s)/day."

Guided Exercise 21: Recording Objective Findings

The Px tab is used to record the observations and results of the clinician's physical examination of the client as well as measurements and vital signs recorded during the course of the encounter.

Step 1

Position the mouse pointer over the Px tab and click the mouse once. The Physical Examination list will be displayed. Notice that the list is organized by body systems, essentially in the order that you would perform a head-to-toe exam.

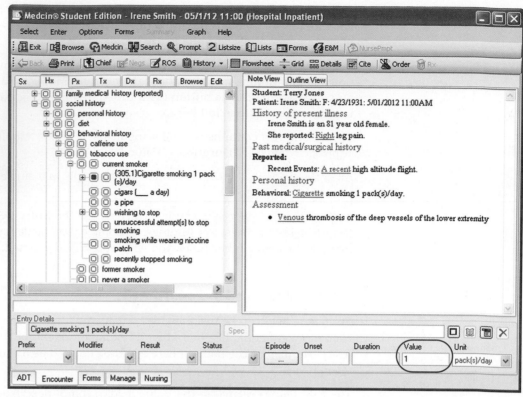

▶ **Figure 3-28 Recording the Value 1 pack per day.**

Step 2

Scroll the list down to Musculoskeletal System and click on the small plus sign next to it, to expand the list. The Nomenclature pane should resemble Figure 3-29.

Step 3

Scroll the expanded list to locate "Leg (Below Knee)" and click on the small plus sign.

Locate and click on the small plus signs next to "Appearance" and "Calf swelling."

Compare your left pane to Figure 3-30.

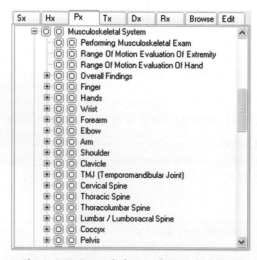

▶ **Figure 3-29 Expanded tree of Musculoskeletal System.**

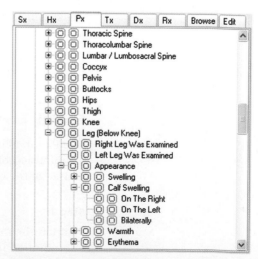

▶ **Figure 3-30 Expanded tree of Leg (Below Knee), Appearance, and Calf Swelling.**

Step 4

Locate and click on the red button next to the following findings:

● (red button) On the Right
● (red button) Warmth
● (red button) Erythema

Compare your screen to Figure 3-31.

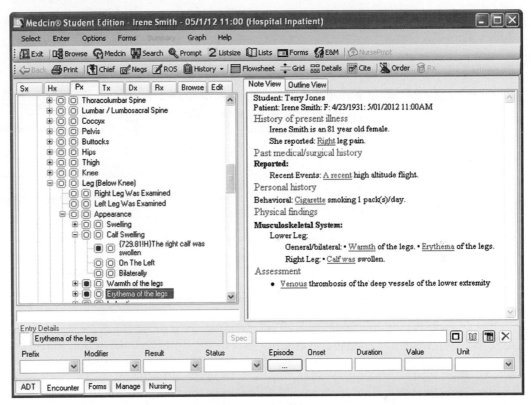

▶ **Figure 3-31 Physical observation of the client's leg (below knee).**

Guided Exercise 22: Adding Detail to Recorded Findings

EHR software must be very flexible because additional observations or information from the client could necessitate going back to any section at any time. In this exercise, you will add status information to the client's reported symptom.

Step 1

Select the finding for Edit by moving your mouse pointer over the underlined word "Right" in "Right leg pain" in the history of present illness section of the right pane. When the mouse pointer changes to a hand, click the mouse button. The left pane should automatically change to the Edit tab. "Right leg pain" is now the current finding.

This step of the procedure is the same one you used in Guided Exercise 17: Removing Findings.

Step 2

The Prefix, Modifier, Result, Status, and Unit fields have buttons next to the field with an arrow pointing down. This type of button indicates there is a drop-down list of items you can choose for that field. You have previously used this type of list to select the reason when creating a new encounter.

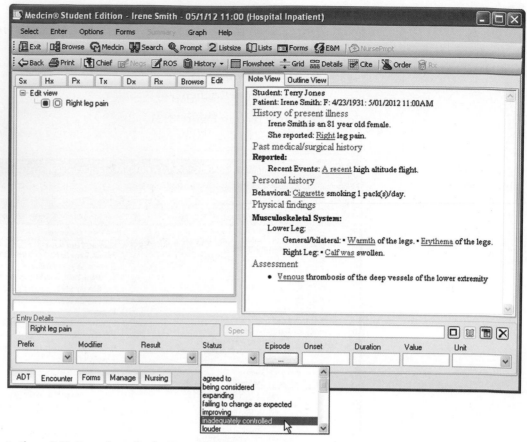

▶ **Figure 3-32 Drop-down list for Status field.**

Locate the Status field in the Entry Details section at the bottom of the screen. Click your mouse on the button with the down arrow in the status field. A drop-down list of phrases (as shown in Figure 3-32) will appear. Do not be concerned if the position of a drop-down list differs from the figures in this book. Drop-down lists may appear either above or below a field, depending on the screen settings of each computer.

Step 3

Position your mouse pointer on the status "inadequately controlled" and click the mouse button. The field will display a portion of the phrase, and the text in the encounter note will change to "Right leg pain which is inadequately controlled."

Using Free Text

In this exercise you will learn how to add your own text into the note. The term for this is "free text," meaning that the text is not codified and might contain anything.

In contrast, the other Entry Details fields (Prefix, Modifier, Result, Status, Episode, Onset, Duration, Value, and Unit) are stored as fielded data. This has the advantage of producing a uniform, searchable EHR throughout the medical practice.

Ideally, the less free text used in the EHR, the better. Still, there are many times when free text is appropriate—for example, adding a nuance to a finding that extends its meaning or entering text that more accurately portrays the client's own words.

Guided Exercise 23: Adding Free Text

In this exercise, the client reports the leg pain is keeping her from sleeping.

Step 1

If you are beginning a new class, you will need to repeat exercises 18 and 22 to add the finding before proceeding.

Step 2

Look at the Entry Details section at the bottom of your screen. There are two long fields in the first row. The gray field on the left contains the description of the finding and cannot be directly edited; the field on the right is used to add free text to the currently selected finding.

Click your mouse in the free-text field. Type "**and keeps her awake**" in the field and then press the Enter key on your keyboard. Compare your screen with Figure 3-33.

► **Figure 3-33 Free text "and keeps her awake" added to note.**

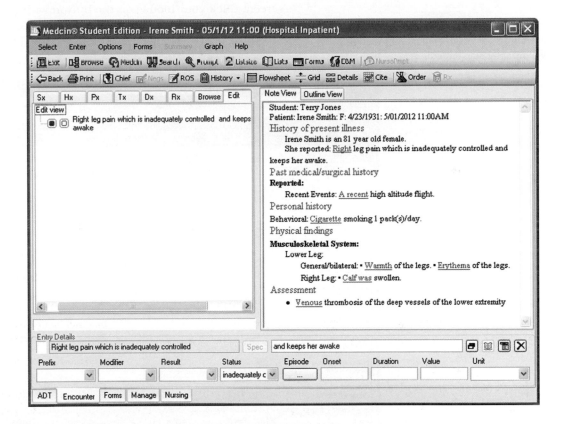

► **Figure 3-34 List of imaging studies.**

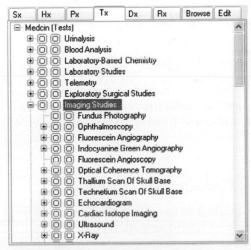

Guided Exercise 24: Using the Tx Tab and Setting the Prefix Field

In this exercise you will learn to use the Tx tab, highlight a finding, and set the Prefix field. The Tx tab lists tests that may be selected as performed, ordered, resulted, or scheduled. If a test has been performed, it will appear in a section of the note labeled "Tests." If a test is ordered but not yet performed, it will appear in the Plan section of the note. The client is scheduled for a venography.

Step 1

Click on the tab labeled "Tx."

Venography is an imaging study.

Locate "Imaging Studies" and click on the small plus sign to expand the tree as shown in Figure 3-34.

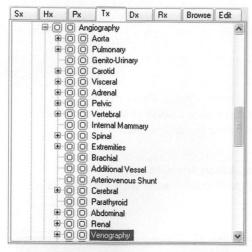

► **Figure 3-35 List of angiography studies with Venography highlighted.**

Step 2

Scroll the list of imaging studies to locate "Angiography." Click on the small plus sign to further expand the tree as shown in Figure 3-35.

Step 3

Scroll the list of angiography studies to locate the finding "Venography."

Highlight the finding by clicking on the description "Venography" (not on the red or blue button) as shown in Figure 3-35.

Locate the Prefix field in the Entry Details section at the bottom of the screen. Click your mouse on the button with the down arrow in the field. A drop-down list of choices (as shown in Figure 3-36) will appear. Scroll the list of prefixes to locate "Scheduled for."

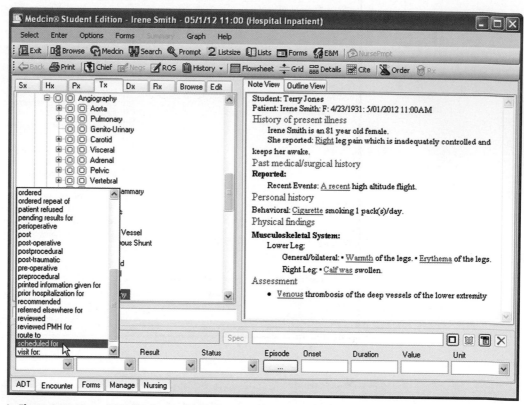

► **Figure 3-36 Drop-down list for Prefix field.**

Position your mouse pointer on the Prefix "scheduled for" and click the mouse button. The field will display the word "scheduled for," and the text "Scheduled for venography" will be recorded in the encounter under the heading "Plan" as shown in Figure 3-37.

Guided Exercise 25: Using the Free-Text Finding Note Window

In Exercise 23, you added free text to a symptom finding. When you have more than a few words of free text to enter, a larger window may be useful as well. In this exercise, you will add free text using the Finding Note window.

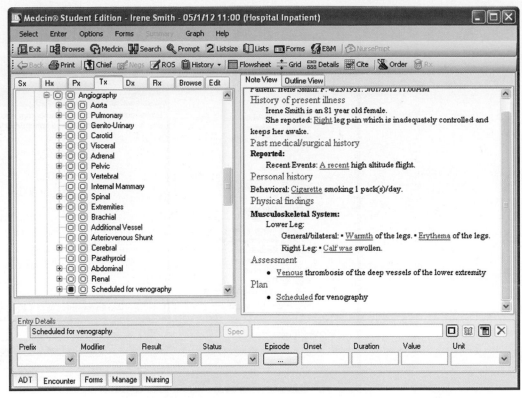

▶ **Figure 3-37 Plan: Scheduled for venography.**

Step 1

Make sure "Scheduled for venography" is the current finding. If you are beginning a new class, you will need to repeat the previous exercise to add the finding and prefix before proceeding.

Step 2

In the lower right corner of your screen are four buttons. You used the Delete button (with the X) in previous exercises. In this exercise you will use the Finding Note button, which is circled in red in Figure 3-38.

Position your mouse pointer on the Finding Note button and click the mouse. A small Finding Note window will be invoked, as shown in Figure 3-38.

Step 3

There are several advantages to entering free text in this window as opposed to in the free-text field in the Entry Details section.

1. The area in the window is larger than the free-text field, making it easier to type longer notes.

2. The window includes a spell checker (the "abc" button in the center of the Finding Note window).

3. The Insert text feature allows frequently used text that has been stored to be inserted as free text whenever appropriate, saving time typing.

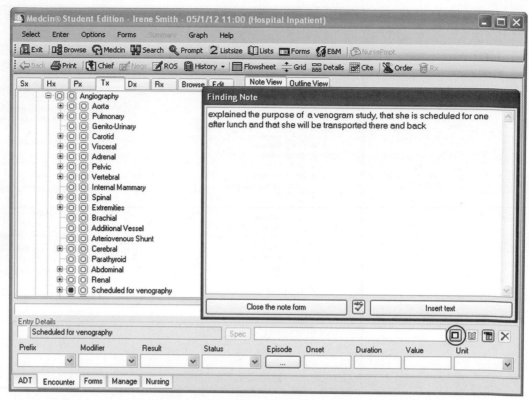

▶ Figure 3-38 Finding Note window used for free text (button circled in red).

Type the following text into the Finding Note window:

"explained the purpose of a venogram study, that she is scheduled for one after lunch and that she will be transported there and back."

When you have finished, click your mouse on the button labeled "Close the note form." This will add your text to the encounter note.

Guided Exercise 26: Recording Nursing Care on the Rx Tab

In this exercise you will record nursing care on the Therapy (Rx) tab. To keep the exercise short, only a few of the actions that a nurse would normally perform have been included.

Generally, findings selected on the Rx tab will appear in the Therapy group if they are performed or administered. The same findings from the Rx tab would appear in the "Plan" group if they are ordered but not yet administered. This will be covered further in Chapter 7 when we discuss orders.

Step 1

Position the mouse pointer on the Rx tab and click the mouse button. The Medcin Therapy list will be displayed.

Step 2

Locate and click on the small plus signs next to "Nursing Care" and "General Care." Scroll the window if necessary to locate and click on the red button next to the following findings:

- (red button) Bed rails check
- (red button) Call light within reach

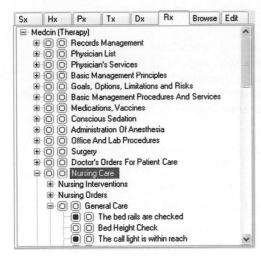

► **Figure 3-39 Selected General Care findings on Rx tab.**

Compare your left pane to Figure 3-39.

Step 3

Scroll to the nomenclature pane downward to locate and click on the following finding:

● (red button) Patient ID bracelet check

Step 4

Scroll to the Nomenclature pane further downward to locate the finding labeled "IV Device." Click on the small plus signs for "IV Device," "Care," and "Administration" to expand the list as it is shown in Figure 3-40).

Locate and click on the blue button next to the following findings:

● (blue button) Phlebitis
● (blue button) Pain

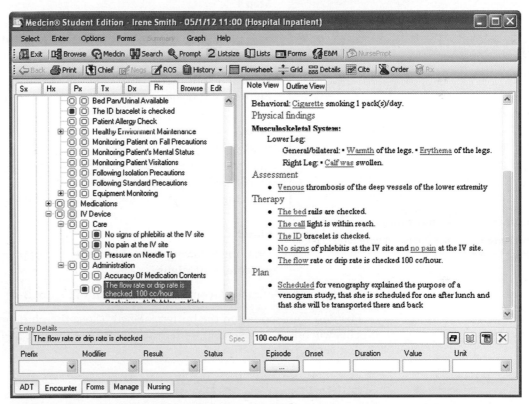

► **Figure 3-40 Selected IV Care findings and Therapy section of note.**

Scroll the window if necessary to locate and click on the red button next to the following finding:

● (red button) Flow Rate or Drip Rate

Step 5

In the free-text field below the right pane, type **100 ml/hour** and press the Enter key. Compare your screen to Figure 3-40. The findings that have been selected from the Nursing Care list on the Rx tab have been documented under the heading "Therapy" in the encounter note.

Introduction to Using Forms

You may have noticed in Exercise 25 that the Finding Note window was called a *form*. Forms make it convenient to enter findings or free text without locating and selecting the finding from the nomenclature. When a form is used, the information is automatically recorded in the proper section of the encounter note. In the following two exercises, you will use forms to add information to the encounter note.

Normally, the items in the next two exercises would have been recorded early in the client encounter; they were placed at the end of the exercises only because of the organization of the chapter.

Guided Exercise 27: Recording the Chief Complaint

Typically, the first thing recorded in the encounter is a description of the client's reason for the encounter. This is called the "Chief complaint." You could locate the finding "Chief complaint" and then enter a free-text note, but because Chief complaint is a standard part of most encounter notes, it is more efficient to provide a form for text entry.

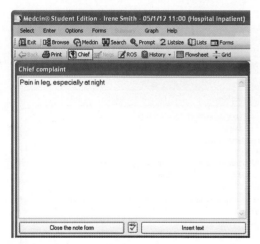

▶ **Figure 3-41 Chief complaint note form invoked from Toolbar.**

Step 1

As we discussed at the beginning of this chapter, there are two rows of icon buttons at the top of your screen called the Toolbar. The purpose of the Toolbar is to allow quick access to commonly used functions.

Locate the button in the Toolbar labeled "Chief" (highlighted orange in Figure 3-41, position your mouse pointer over it, and click your mouse.

Step 2

The Chief complaint window will be invoked. This window looks similar to the Finding Note window in the previous exercise except that when you close the note form, instead of just recording free text, it will automatically associate the text with the finding "Chief complaint."

Step 3

Type the following text into the Chief Complaint window: "**Pain in leg, especially at night**."

When you have finished, compare your screen to Figure 3-41.

Position your mouse on the button labeled "Close the note form" and click the mouse. This will add a new section to the encounter note titled "Chief complaint" followed by the text you typed.

Guided Exercise 28: Recording Vital Signs

Forms are not limited to free text. Many findings can be included on one form, and the form can contain specific Entry Details fields such as Result, Status, Value, and Unit.

A form is frequently used to record vital signs (routine measurements of the body taken at nearly every client encounter). As you will see in this exercise, it is more efficient to enter numerical data using a form than to locate and select findings one at a time and then enter data in the value field for each.

Step 1

At the very bottom of the screen are five tabs labeled "ADT," "Encounter," "Forms," "Manage," and "Nursing." All forms except the Finding Note and Chief complaint windows used in previous exercises are accessed from the Forms tab.

Position your mouse pointer over the tab labeled "Forms" (circled in red at the bottom of Figure 3-42) and click the mouse.

When the tab changes, the familiar Encounter View of the Student Edition will be replaced with an Outline View of the headings that have findings in your encounter note. The Outline View presents the headings as icons of file folders, with small plus signs preceding them. If you click on the small plus signs next to the folders, the tree will expand to show the findings recorded in the encounter under that heading. Because you may not have performed all of the previous exercises in a single class period, your Outline View may not have as much detail as shown in Figure 3-42.

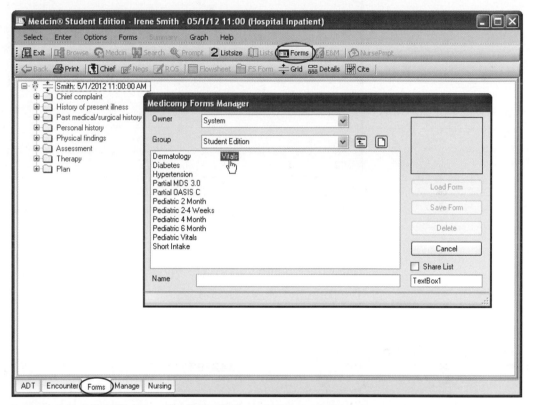

▶ **Figure 3-42 Select Vitals from the list in the Forms Manager window.**

Step 2

Locate and click on the button labeled "Forms" in the top row of the Toolbar at the top of your screen. (The button is circled in red in Figure 3-42.) This will invoke the Forms Manager window shown in Figure 3-42. The Forms Manager lists forms used in the Student Edition.

Locate and click on the form labeled "Vitals" in the Form Manager window as shown in Figure 3-42. This should open the form shown in Figure 3-43.

Note

Systolic and diastolic blood pressure readings are entered in two separate fields. Omit the "/" character when entering blood pressure (BP) in the form.

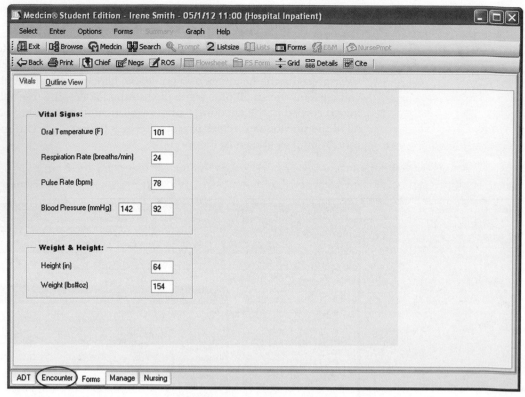

▶ **Figure 3-43 Vital Signs form for Irene Smith; Encounter tab circled in red.**

Enter Irene Smith's vital signs into the corresponding fields. They are as follows:

Temperature:	**101**
Respiration:	**24**
Pulse:	**78**
BP	**142/92**
Height:	**64**
Weight:	**154**

When you have entered all of the vital signs, compare your screen to Figure 3-43 and then click your mouse on the Encounter tab at the bottom of the screen (circled in red in the figure).

The vital signs information will be found in the encounter note on the right pane under the Physical Findings section.

Step 3

Look at the results of the Vital Signs entry as they appear in the encounter note. Also notice that there is a tab on top of the right pane labeled "Outline View." This tab will display the same outline in the right pane as was displayed on the Forms tab.

When you have finished looking at the note, exit the Student Edition software.

By Sandra Hilliard, RN

Sandra Hilliard is a registered nurse in a 500-bed community hospital. Sandra is a member of the nursing user group at her hospital and has been helping to transition the nursing documentation from paper to computers at the hospital where she works. She described her personal experience of changing from paper patient charts to the electronic medical record.

The biggest challenge of computerized charts is overcoming the fear of going into the computer for all the patient information. When I was in college I thought I wanted to be a teacher. So I took a computer class. That made it a lot easier for me to learn the computer system. I see a lot of people who have never used a computer. They are very afraid of making a mistake. Overcoming their fear of the unknown makes it harder for them to learn. They don't want to take the computer into the room to chart, because they aren't comfortable using the computer.

I take the computer in the room, which allows me to chart as I go and I have all the information with me all the time in one spot. Even on bad days, the workflow is better. If I am in the room and need to look something up or chart something that I have observed or done for the patient, I can do the search on the spot. When I leave the room, all my notes are done.

Some of our forms are still in paper. I will be glad when everything is computerized. It is hard to switch back and forth between computer and paper.

It will be really nice when the doctors' notes are in the computer too. It is hard to read different people's handwriting. Most of the orders are put in by CPOE, but there are still a few doctors who don't like to put their own orders in CPOE, even though they are supposed to do it themselves. I challenge them, if they try to give me an order instead of putting it in the computer.

Recently we started charting medications in the computer. I was apprehensive the first day, because I didn't know how it would work into my workflow, but within two days I was comfortable and knew I would never want to go back to paper charting. It is safer. I just log in and review the medication orders. I can take the medications and the computer right to the patient, when I administer them. I just explain to the patient that I'm charting the medications right when I scan them. I would hate to go back to paper.

Visually Different Button Styles

The Medcin Student Edition software has been specially created for this course. Therefore, it will be different in some aspects from EHR systems you will encounter when working in a medical facility, but the concepts, skills, and familiarity with EHR systems you will acquire by practicing with the Student Edition will transfer directly into the workplace.

Many EHR software packages are based on the Medcin Nomenclature. Each vendor has created a unique visual style, and although they share a common nomenclature, the EHR may look quite different.

One difference is the look of the buttons. In many systems, a large plus sign and a large minus sign similar to those shown in Figure 3-44 are used to select findings instead of the red and blue buttons used in the Student Edition. However, as you become familiar with the Student Edition software, you should have no trouble transitioning to a similar Medcin-based EHR in your job.

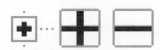

▶ **Figure 3-44 Alternative Select buttons used to select findings in some EHR systems.**

Chapter Three Summary

In this chapter you have learned about the Student Edition software: the menus and Toolbar, the Nomenclature pane, the Note View pane, the Entry Detail fields, as well as the Chief complaint, free-text note, the Outline View, and Vital Signs forms.

As you continue through the course, you can refer to the Guided Exercises in this chapter when you need to remember how to perform a particular task.

Task	Guided Exercise(s)	Page No.
Starting up and exiting the software	9 and 10	72 and 75
Select a patient	11	76
Navigating Medcin findings and tabs	12 and 13	78 and 80
Creating an new encounter. Setting the date, time, and reason for encounter	14	81
Recording findings		
Subjective findings	16	85
History findings	19	89
Objective findings	21	91
Admitting diagnosis	15	83
Nursing care (Therapy tab)	26	98
Removing findings or selecting findings for edit	17	86
Adding details to the findings		
Adding a value	20	91
Adding detail to current findings	22	93
Setting the Prefix field	24	95
Adding free text	23	94
Adding free text using the Finding Note window	25	96
Using the Chief complaint form	27	100
Forms tab, Forms Manager, and the Vital Signs form	28	100

EHR software allows clinicians to document the client encounter by selecting findings for symptoms, history, physical examination, tests, diagnoses, and therapy.

The Medcin Student Edition software has been specially created for this course. Therefore it will be different in some aspects from EHR systems you will encounter when working in a medical facility, but the concepts, skills, and familiarity with EHR systems that you will acquire by practicing with the Student Edition will transfer directly into the workplace.

To more easily understand the Student Edition software, we divided the screen into four sections and discussed each of them.

1. **The Menu bar and Toolbar** are located at the top of the window.

   The menus are Select, Enter, Options, Forms, Summary, Graph, and Help. Within these are lists of functions in the Student Edition software.

   You select a menu item by positioning the mouse pointer over one of these words and click the mouse once; a list of functions will drop-down below the word. Moving the mouse pointer vertically down the list will highlight each item. Clicking on the highlighted item will invoke that function. Clicking the mouse anywhere on the screen other than the list will close the list.

In the Student Edition, *highlight* means a colored rectangle appears over an item or a button on the Toolbar changes color.

The Toolbar is also located at the top of your screen. It consists of two rows of buttons, each containing a small picture called an icon, and a brief label. The purpose of the Toolbar is to allow quick access to commonly used functions. Clicking on a button in the Toolbar invokes a function or feature. The Exit, Chief, and Forms buttons on the Toolbar were used in this chapter.

2. **The Medcin Nomenclature Pane** is located in the left pane of the window.

   The left pane displays the lists of Medcin findings from which you choose when documenting an encounter. On the top of the nomenclature pane there are eight tabs. These look like tabs on file folders. Six of the tabs, labeled "Sx" (symptoms), "Hx" (history), "Px" (physical examination), "Tx" (tests), "Dx" (diagnosis, syndromes, and conditions), and "Rx" (therapy or plan) are used to logically group the findings into six broad categories. An additional tab labeled "Edit" is used when editing a finding that has already been selected. The Browse tab was not covered in this chapter.

3. **The Encounter View Pane** is located in the right pane of the window. It has two tabs labeled Note View and Outline View. When the clinician selects a finding from the Medcin nomenclature list in the left pane, the text for that finding will display in the right pane.

   The Note View tab dynamically displays the findings accompanied by narrative text automatically generated by Medcin. Titles for the sections of the note are also added dynamically as findings are selected.

   The Outline View displays findings that have been selected and appropriate ICD-9-CM codes. The extra narrative text is omitted in the Outline View.

4. **The Entry Details** fields are located at the bottom portion of the screen. The Entry Details section consists of two rows of fields and four buttons that affect only the currently selected finding. Using the Entry Details features, the user can add detail or free text to the finding, or remove a finding from the encounter note.

   The first row has two fields and four buttons. The first field displays the finding description as it appears in the text. The field cannot be directly edited. The second field may be used to add short free text to notes to the finding.

   The four buttons are also located in the first row of fields. The first button invokes the Find Note window, which makes it easier to enter longer free-text notes and includes a spell checker. The second and third buttons were not covered in this chapter. The fourth button deletes the current finding from the encounter note (but not from the nomenclature).

   The fields in the second row are Prefix, Modifier, Result, Status, an Episode button, Onset, Duration, Value, and Unit. The fields add informational text to the finding in the encounter note, and in some cases modifies its meaning. The advantage of these fields over free text is that they allow the EHR to store the status, result, and the like as fielded data that can be used later, which free-text entries do not.

Documenting the Encounter

The first step in every encounter is to select the patient, then open an existing encounter or create a new encounter. In this chapter you learned to select clients and create new encounters.

It is important when creating new encounters to use the exact date, time, and reason given in the exercise.

Selecting patients, encounters, adding chief complaint, notes, and selecting forms open small windows that close when the user is finished.

The left pane displays lists of Medcin findings in a *tree* structure where small plus signs indicate more detailed findings are available. Clicking on the button with the small plus sign expands the list further, like branches on a tree. When the tree is expanded, the button changes from a small plus sign to a small minus sign. If the button with the small minus sign is clicked, the expanded list collapses to its previous size.

Findings are selected by clicking on buttons with red or blue circles in them located next to each finding. When a finding is selected, circles in the button become filled with red or blue and the finding is displayed in the encounter note. The solid colors in the buttons help you quickly identify which findings have already been selected. Generally, the red button records that a client has the condition described in the finding. Clicking the blue button generally records that a client did not have the symptom or the condition described in the finding. The description of the finding in the left pane also changes when a red or blue button is clicked.

Test Your Knowledge

You may run the Medcin Student Edition software and use your mouse on the screen to answer the following questions:

1. Which menu did you use to select the client?

2. Which menu did you use to start a new encounter?

3. Where did you set the label "Hospital Inpatient," which appeared in the title of the window?

The tabs on the left pane of Medcin findings have medical abbreviations. Write the meaning of each of the following:

4. Sx _____

5. Hx _____

6. Px _____

7. Tx _____

8. Dx _____

9. Rx _____

10. What was the client's chief complaint?

11. What was the clinical assessment (her admitting diagnosis)?

12. Describe two ways you enter free-text notes into the encounter record.

13. How did you invoke the Vital Signs window?

14. How do you remove a finding?

15. How did you invoke the Chief complaint window?

Ask your instructor for answers to Test Your Knowledge

nursing.pearsonhighered.com

Prepare for success with animated examples, practice questions, challenge tests, and interactive assignments.

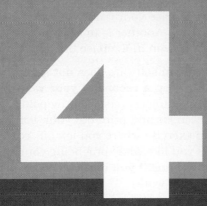

Increased Familiarity with the Software

Learning Outcomes

After completing this chapter, you should be able to:

1. Create a new encounter note
2. Document several different types of hospital admissions
3. Print a copy of the completed encounter note
4. Add results, episodes, onset, duration, and history to findings

Applying Your Knowledge

In this chapter, you will practice documenting encounters using the Student Edition software. One of the goals in this chapter is to increase your familiarity with the software and thereby increase your speed of data entry. Another is to learn how to print your work. You will learn how to use the Print function in Exercise 30.

It is important to remember that the Student Edition software does **not** save your entries to the school's database; therefore, you will **keep a record of your work by printing it**. Whereas in the previous chapter you could stop exercises at any point, in this chapter it is important to complete the entire exercise and print out your work before stopping. You cannot stop and then resume an exercise where you left off. You can print the encounter note at any time and as often as you like while practicing your exercises. However, remember not to quit or exit the program **until you are sure the encounter note has printed**. Once you exit, you will lose your work.

In Chapter 3, you learned the basic layout of the screen and the concepts of creating an encounter note, adding findings, editing findings, and adding details to findings. Detailed instructions for scrolling and navigating the lists, which were provided in the previous chapter, should no longer be necessary. From this point forward, simplified instructions will guide you in areas where you are already familiar with the program. Red or blue circles will be printed in the text as a visual cue to indicate whether to click on a red or blue button to select a finding.

Exercises in this chapter are intended to provide conceptual learning experiences with the software. In order to keep the exercises short many routine nursing orders, interventions and elements of care are omitted. These exercises are intended to increase your familiarity with EHR software, and do not necessarily reflect the entirety of nursing care best practices for any of the exercise cases.

Creating Your First Complete Encounter Note

In Guided Exercise 29, you will apply what you have learned in Chapter 3 to document Irene Smith's admission. In Guided Exercise 30, you will learn to print out your work to hand in to your instructor. You must complete both exercises in a single session. Do not begin Guided Exercise 29 unless you have enough class time remaining to complete both exercises.

Guided Exercise 29: Documenting an Admit for DVT

This exercise is similar but not identical to the cumulative exercises in Chapter 3.

Case Study

Irene Smith is an 81-year-old female client who complains of pains in her right leg following an extended airplane flight. She has been admitted to the hospital with a working diagnosis of deep venous thrombosis (DVT).

Step 1

If you have not already done so, start the Student Edition software.

Locate the Medcin icon shown in Chapter 3, Figure 3-2. If you do not see it on the computer desktop, click on the Start button, and look in Programs or All Programs for the program named "Medcin Student Edition."

Step 2

When the Student Edition login screen is displayed, type into the field either your name or student ID as directed by your instructor.

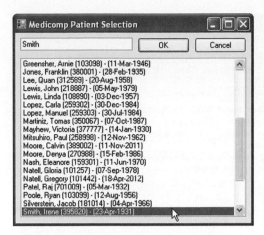

▶ **Figure 4-1 Select Irene Smith from Patient Selection window.**

When your name or ID is exactly as you want it to be, position the mouse pointer over the button labeled "OK," and click the mouse. The Student Edition software window will be displayed.

Step 3

Position the mouse pointer over the word "Select" in the menu at the top of the screen and click the mouse button once. A list of the Select menu options will appear.

Click the mouse on the word "Patient" to invoke the Patient Selection window.

Locate and click on **Irene Smith** as shown in Figure 4-1.

Step 4

Again, position the mouse pointer over the word "Select," and click the mouse button. Move the mouse pointer vertically down the list until the item New Encounter is highlighted. Click the mouse button.

Using what you have learned in the previous chapter, select the reason **Hospital Inpatient** from the drop-down list. If you need assistance setting the encounter reason, refer to Chapter 3, Figure 3-16.

You do not have to set the date or time for this exercise; you may use the current date. However, be certain to set the encounter reason correctly before clicking on the OK button.

The left pane should now display the Medcin Symptoms list and the right pane should display your student ID and Irene Smith's information. Before proceeding, confirm that the client name and the reason for the visit displayed in the title of the window are all correct.

Note

The software calculates the client's age based on the encounter date. In any exercise where you use today's date instead of the date in the book, the date of the encounter and the age of the client will differ from the screen figures in the book. Except for the date and age, you should ensure your work matches the figures.

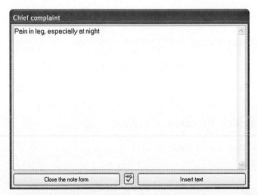

▶ **Figure 4-2 Chief complaint is pain in leg, especially at night.**

Step 5

Enter the Chief complaint by locating the button in the Toolbar labeled "Chief" and clicking on it.

The Chief complaint window will open; type: "**Pain in leg, especially at night**."

Compare your screen to Figure 4-2. If it is correct, click button labeled "Close the note form."

▶ **Figure 4-3 Dx tab: admitting diagnosis DVT.**

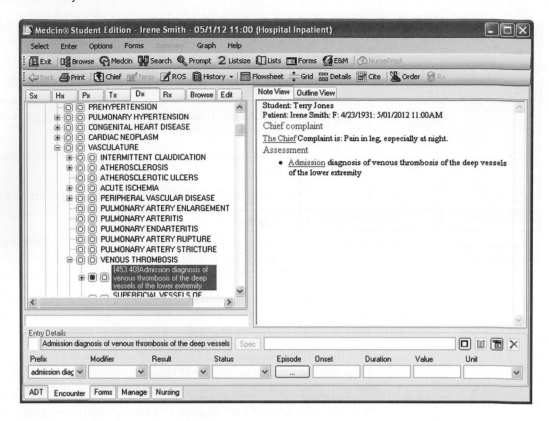

Step 6

Locate and click on the Dx tab at the top of the left pane, as you did in Chapter 3, Exercise 12.

Using the skills you have acquired in the previous chapter, navigate the Dx list.

Locate and click on the small plus signs next to "Cardiovascular Disorders" and "Vasculature" to expand the tree.

Scroll the window until you can see the full list of vasculature findings.

Locate "Venous Thrombosis" and click on the small plus sign next it to expand it as well.

Locate and click on the red button next to the following finding:

● (red button) Deep vessels of lower extremity

Locate the Prefix field and click your mouse on the button with the down arrow in the Prefix field.

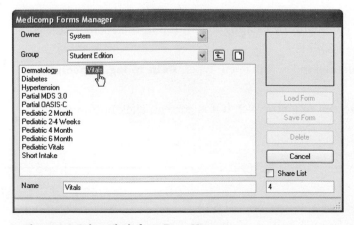

▶ **Figure 4-4 Select Vitals from Form Manager.**

Position your mouse pointer on the Prefix "Admission diagnosis of" and click the mouse button.

Compare your screen to Figure 4-3.

Step 7

Normally, vital signs are recorded early in the initial encounter.

Locate and click on the button labeled "Forms" in the top row of the Toolbar. The tabs at the bottom screen will automatically change to the Form tab. The Forms Manager window will be invoked.

Locate and double-click on the form labeled "Vitals," as shown in Figure 4-4.

▶ **Figure 4-5 Vital Signs form for Irene Smith.**

Medcin® Student Edition - Irene Smith - 05/1/12 11:00 (Hospital Inpatient)

Select   Enter   Options   Forms   Summary   Graph   Help

Exit | Browse | Medcin | Search | Prompt | 2 Listsize | Lists | Forms | E&M | NursePmpt

Back | Print | Chief | Negs | ROS | Flowsheet | FS Form | Grid | Details | Cite

| Vitals | Outline View |

Vital Signs:

Oral Temperature (F)   101

Respiration Rate (breaths/min)   24

Pulse Rate (bpm)   78

Blood Pressure (mmHg)   120   78

Weight & Height:

Height (in)   64

Weight (lbs#oz)   140

ADT   Encounter   Forms   Manage   Nursing

Step 8

Enter Irene Smith's vital signs into the corresponding fields as follows:

Temperature: **101**

Respiration: **24**

Pulse: **78**

BP: **120/78**

Height: **64**

Weight: **140**

When you have entered all of the vital signs, compare your screen to Figure 4-5 and then click your mouse on the Encounter tab at the bottom of the screen.

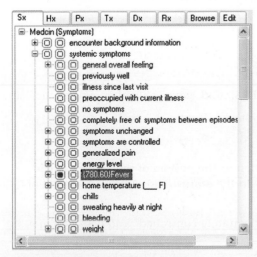

▶ **Figure 4-6 Sx tab: "Fever" selected.**

Notice that the vital signs information has been recorded in the right pane under the Physical Findings section of the encounter note.

Step 9

Locate and click on the Sx tab.

Locate and expand the list of systemic symptoms.

Locate and click on the red button next to the following finding:

● (red button) Fever

Compare your screen to Figure 4-6.

Step 10

Scroll the list down to "Genitourinary symptoms" and click on the small plus sign next to it, to expand the list.

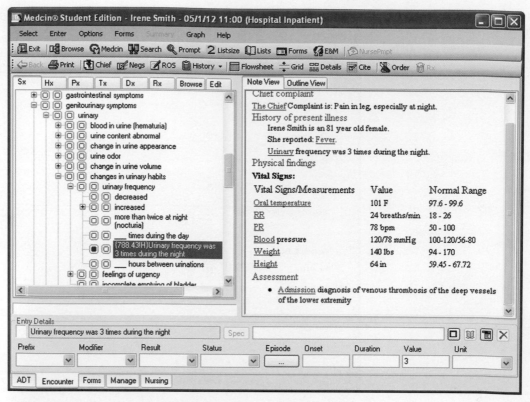

▶ Figure 4-7 Genitourinary symptoms, urinary frequency selected, value is 3.

Locate and click on the small plus signs next to "urinary," "changes in urinary habits" and "urinary frequency," to further expand the list.

Locate and click on the red button next to the following finding:

● (red button) ___ times during the night

Locate the Value field in the Entry Details section at the bottom of the screen.

Click your mouse on the Value field and type the numeral **3**, and then press the enter key on your keyboard.

Compare your screen to Figure 4-7.

Step 11

Scroll the list down to "Musculoskeletal symptoms" and click on the small plus sign next to it, to expand the list.

Locate and click on the small plus signs next to "legs," and "pain," to further expand the list.

Locate and click on the red button next to the following finding:

● (red button) Right

Locate the Status field in the Entry Details section at the bottom of the screen. Click your mouse on the button with the down arrow in the status field. A drop-down list of status phrases will appear.

Position your mouse pointer on the status "inadequately controlled" and click the mouse button.

Compare your screen to Figure 4-8.

► **Figure 4-8 Musculoskeletal symptom is pain in right leg, with Status set.**

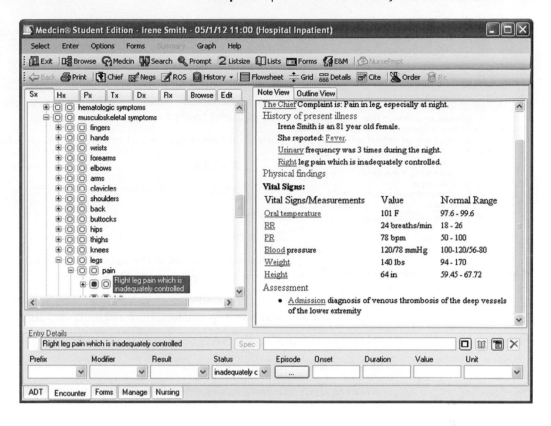

Step 12

Locate the free-text field in the first row of the Entry Details section, under the right pane.

Click your mouse in the free-text field. Type "**and keeps her awake**" in the field and then press the Enter key on your keyboard. Compare your screen with Figure 4-9.

► **Figure 4-9 Free text added to finding.**

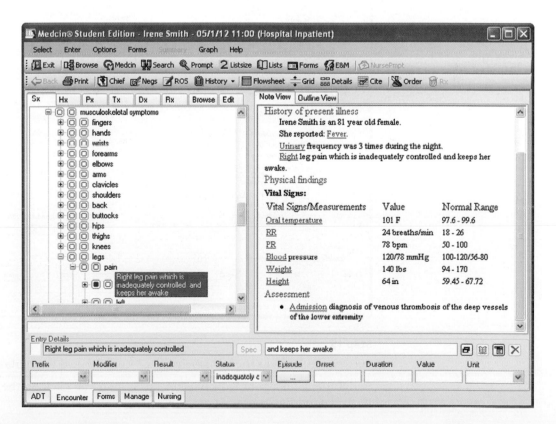

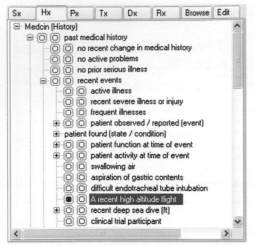

▶ **Figure 4-10 History of recent high altitude flight.**

Step 13

Locate and click on the Hx tab. The three types of history will be displayed.

Using the skills you have acquired in Chapter 3, navigate the Hx list and expand the tree by clicking on the small plus signs next to "past medical history," and "recent events."

Locate and click on the red button next to the finding:

● (red button) Recent high altitude flight

Compare the left pane of your screen to Figure 4-10.

Step 14

The client reports smoking 1 pack of cigarettes a day.

Scroll to the bottom of the list of history findings to locate "social history" and click the mouse on the small plus sign next to it.

Locate and click on the small plus signs next to "behavioral history," "tobacco use," and "current smoker," to further expand the list.

Locate and click on the red button next to the finding:

● (red button) Cigarettes

Locate the Value field in the Entry Details section, type the numeral **1** in the value field, and then press the Enter key on your keyboard.

Compare your screen to Figure 4-11.

▶ **Figure 4-11 Social history, behavioral history, Smoking Cigarettes 1 pack per day.**

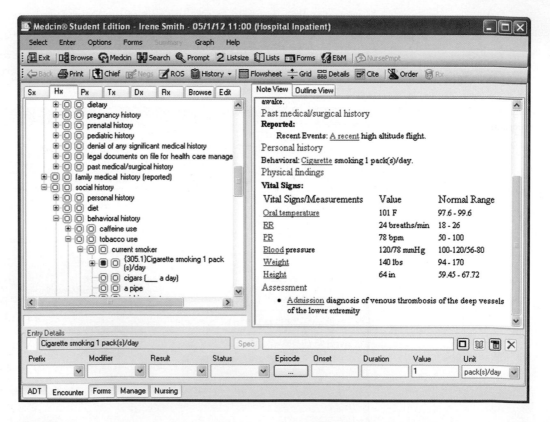

Step 15

Locate and click on the tab labeled "Px." The Physical Examination list will be displayed.

Scroll the list down to Musculoskeletal System and click on the small plus sign next to it, to expand the list.

► **Figure 4-12 Px tab: physical observations of the client's right leg.**

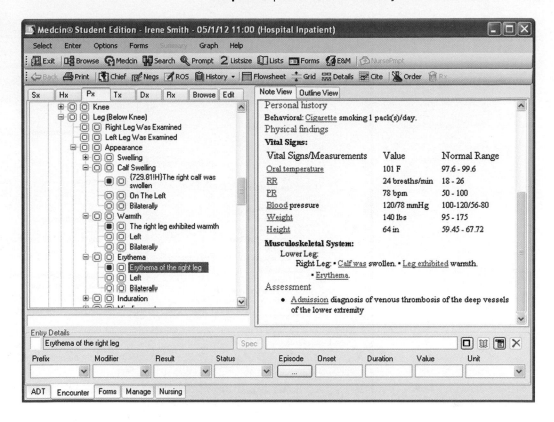

Locate and click on the small plus signs next to "Leg (Below Knee)," "Appearance," and "Calf Swelling."

For each of the following findings, click the small plus sign to expand the tree and then click on the red button next to "Right":

Calf Swelling

● (red button) on the Right

Warmth

● (red button) Right

Erythema

● (red button) Right

Compare your screen to Figure 4-12.

Step 16

The doctor has ordered a venography, which is an imaging study.

Locate and click on the tab labeled "Tx." Categories of tests will be displayed.

Locate Imaging Studies and click on the small plus sign to expand the tree.

Scroll the list of imaging studies to locate Angiography and expand the tree.

Scroll the list of angiography studies to locate and highlight the finding "Venography." Remember that you highlight the finding by clicking on the description (not on the red or blue button).

Locate the Prefix field and click your mouse on the down arrow button in the Prefix field.

Scroll the list of prefixes to locate "Scheduled for" and then click on it.

Compare your screen to Figure 4-13.

▶ **Figure 4-13 Tx tab: client scheduled for venography.**

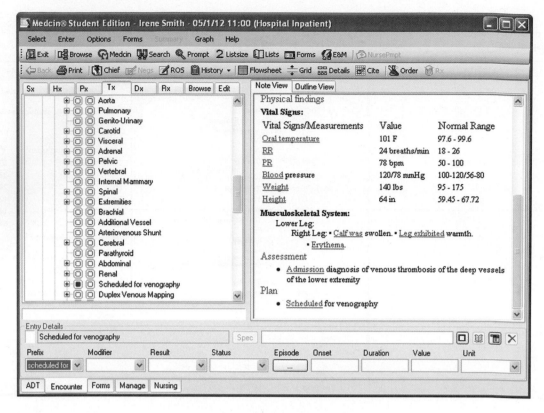

Step 17

Locate and click on the Finding Note button (circled in red in Figure 4-14).

Locate and click on the Finding Note button in the lower right corner of your screen (circled in red in Figure 4-14). A small Finding Note window will be invoked.

Type the following text into the Finding note window:

> "**Explained a venogram to the patient and that transport to the x-ray department is scheduled for after lunch**"

▶ **Figure 4-14 Finding Note window (button circled in red).**

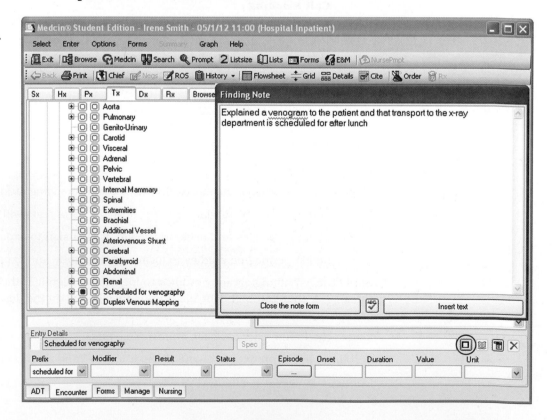

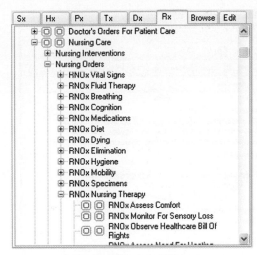

▶ **Figure 4-15 Rx tab: Nursing orders, Nursing therapy lists expanded.**

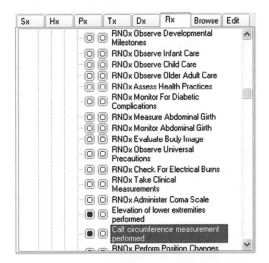

▶ **Figure 4-16 Scrolled list, nursing therapies selected.**

When you have finished, compare your Finding Note window to the one shown in Figure 4-14. If it is correct, click your mouse on the button labeled "Close the note form." This will add your free text to the encounter note.

Step 18

Locate and click on the tab labeled "Rx." The Medcin Therapy list will be displayed.

Locate and click on the small plus signs next to "Nursing Care" and "Nursing Orders."

Locate and click on the small plus sign next to "RNOx Nursing Therapy" as shown in Figure 4-15.

In Medcin, the descriptions of CCC nursing orders have the prefix RNOx. Nursing orders are also referred to as nursing actions. This will be discussed further in Chapter 6.

Scroll a considerable way down the list of nursing therapies to locate and click on the red button next to the following findings:

- (red button) RNOx Elevate lower extremities
- (red button) RNOx Measure calf circumference

Compare your left pane to Figure 4-16.

Step 19

Record the measurements of the client's right and left calf.

Locate and click on the Px tab.

Scroll the left pane upward to locate and expand the tree for "Cardiovascular System."

Locate and click the small plus signs next to "Peripheral Vascular Exam," "Vein Findings," and "Measured Calf Circumference."

To record the calf measurements, click the red button and enter the measurement in the Value field.

Record the right calf measurement. Locate and click on:

- (red button) Right Leg

Type **50** in the Value field; Unit field is set to **cm**.

Record the left calf measurement. Locate and click on:

- (red button) Left Leg

Type **40** in the Value field; Unit field is set to **cm**.

Compare your screen to Figure 4-17.

You have now successfully created your first complete encounter note. However, do not stop or close the program until you complete the following exercise.

Guided Exercise 30: Printing the Encounter Note

The Student Edition software does **not** save your entries to the school's database; therefore, you **will keep a record of your work by printing it**. In this exercise, you will learn to print the encounter note. You will be asked to give your finished printout to your instructor.

You can use either of two methods to print your work, sending the output to a printer or to a file. The method you will use will be based on the policy of your school. Your instructor will tell you which to use. The choice of printer or file is selected from the Print Dialog window.

Step 20

Position your mouse pointer over the menu item Select at the top of the screen and click your mouse button. A list of the Select menu functions will appear (see Figure 4-18).

▶ **Figure 4-17 Px tab: Measurements of right and left calf.**

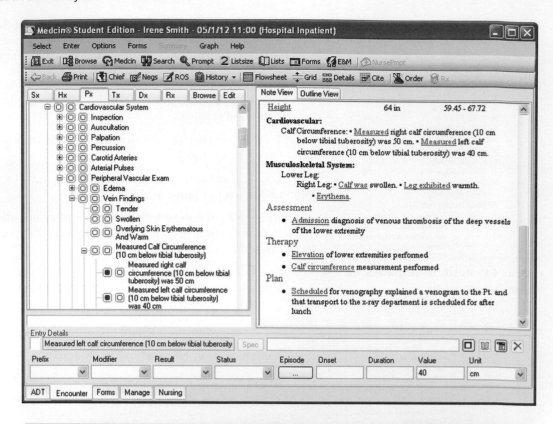

▶ **Figure 4-18 File menu showing print options.**

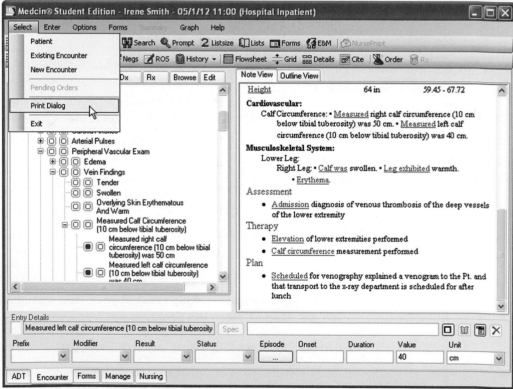

Move the mouse pointer vertically down the list until Print Dialog is highlighted and then click the mouse button. The Print Data window (shown in Figure 4-19) will be invoked.

The two panes on the left of the Print Data window list items that are available for printing. A check box selects the items you wish to print. If the box next to "Current Encounter" does not have a check mark, position your mouse pointer over it and click the mouse button. A check mark should appear in the box.

The right pane displays a preview of what is to be printed.

▶ **Figure 4-19 Print Dialog window.**

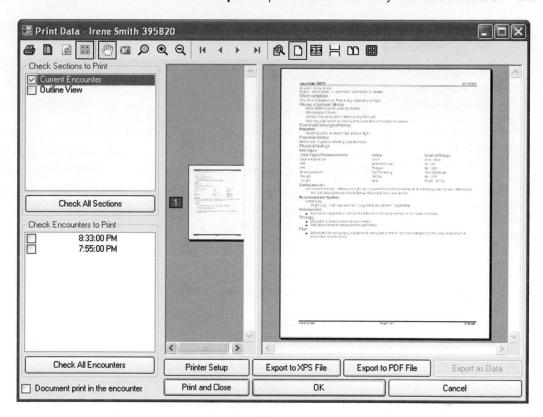

Located below the right pane are two rows of buttons. Those of interest to us are as follows:

Print and Close   Prints the items selected with check marks to a local or networked printer. This produces a paper copy you can hand in to your instructor.

Export to XPS File   Outputs the items selected with check marks to a file on your local computer. The file can be copied to a disk or flash drive, or e-mailed to your instructor.

The XPS file is a Microsoft file that can be viewed with Internet Explorer.

Export to PDF File   Outputs the items selected with check marks to a file on your local computer. The file can be copied to a disk or flash drive, or e-mailed to your instructor.

The PDF file is a file that can be viewed with Adobe Acrobat Reader®.

Your instructor will tell you which method is appropriate for your class.

Step 21: Print a Paper Copy of the Encounter Note

If the instructor wants you to export a file, skip this step and proceed to step 22.

If the instructor wants you to print out a paper copy, locate the button labeled "Print and Close" and click the mouse.

Depending on how your computer is set up, an additional Print window from the operating system may appear. Figure 4-20 shows an example. Yours may be different, but if you see a printer dialog similar to this, verify that the printer name is the printer you want to use and then click your mouse on the button labeled "Print."

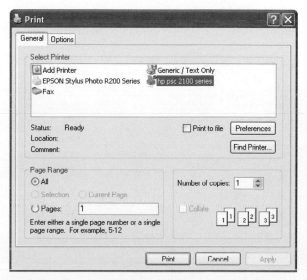

▶ **Figure 4-20 Additional print window from operating system.**

If you need assistance printing, ask your instructor.

Alert

Some printers may close the Print window before the printing has even started. Therefore, do not exit the Student Edition program or go on to another exercise until you have your printout in hand. You could lose your work.

Compare your printout to Figure 4-21. If there are any differences (other than the date and client's age), review the previous steps in the exercise and find your error.

You may print extra copies by repeating steps 20 and 21 before exiting the Student Edition software.

Step 22: Print to a File

Unless the instructor wants you to export to a file, omit this step.

To export to a file instead of printing to paper, click mouse pointer on the appropriate button (either Export to XPS File or Export to PDF File as directed by your instructor).

The action of either button is to create a file on your computer in the directory named My Documents. The file name will include the student name or ID you entered when you logged in plus the date and time. The file name ends in either "XPS" or "PDF."

Irene Smith   Page 1 of 1

Student: *your name or ID here*
Patient: Irene Smith: F: 4/23/1931: 5/01/2012 11:00AM
Chief complaint
The Chief Complaint is: Pain in leg, especially at night.
History of present illness
    Irene Smith is an 81 year old female.
She reported: Fever.
Urinary frequency was 3 times during the night.
Right leg pain which is inadequately controlled and keeps her awake.
Past medical/surgical history
Reported:
Recent Events: A recent high altitude flight.
Personal history
Behavioral: Cigarette smoking 1 pack(s)/day.
Physical findings
Vital Signs:

Vital Signs/Measurements	Value	Normal Range
Oral temperature	101 F	97.6 - 99.6
RR	24 breaths/min	18 - 26
PR	78 bpm	50 - 100
Blood pressure	120/78 mmHg	100 - 120/56 - 80
Weight	140 lbs	95 - 175
Height	64 in	59.45 - 67.72

Cardiovascular:
Calf Circumference: • Measured right calf circumference (10 cm below tibial
tuberosity) was 50 cm. • Measured left calf circumference (10 cm below tibial
tuberosity) was 40 cm.
Musculoskeletal System:
Lower Leg:
Right Leg: • Calf was swollen. • Leg exhibited warmth. • Erythema.
Assessment
    • Admission diagnosis of venous thrombosis of the deep vessels of the lower
      extremity
Therapy
    • Elevation of lower extremities performed
    • Calf circumference measurement performed
Plan
    • Scheduled for venography Explained a venogram to the Patient and that
      transport to the x-ray department is scheduled for after lunch

▶ **Figure 4-21 Printed encounter note for Irene Smith.**

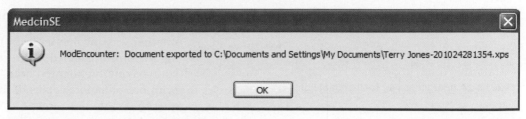

▶ **Figure 4-22 Export to file confirmation.**

When the file has been successfully created, a confirmation similar to Figure 4-22 will be displayed.

Write down the file name shown in the dialog box, then click on the OK button.

Once the file has been created, you can copy it to a disk or e-mail it, as directed by your instructor. Use the computer operating system to locate the file on your computer. It will be located in the directory named "My Documents." Follow your instructor's directions for handing in your file.

The instructor can view or print the student XPS file using Internet Explorer as shown in Figure 4-23. The instructor can view or print the student PDF file using Adobe Acrobat Reader (not shown).

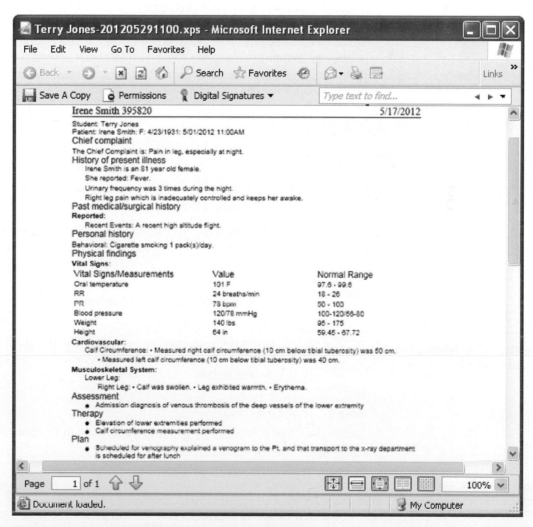

▶ **Figure 4-23 Student XPS file displayed with Internet Explorer.**

Invoking the Print Dialog Window from the Toolbar

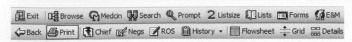

▶ **Figure 4-24 Print button on Toolbar (highlighted).**

Another way invoke the Print Dialog window is by clicking the button labeled "Print" on the Toolbar at the top of your screen (highlighted orange in Figure 4-24). You can print out or export copies of the encounter note as frequently as you like, and at anytime during an exercise.

Creating An Initial Chart Upon Admission

The next exercise will allow you to evaluate your knowledge of the software by using only the features you have learned in Chapters 3 and 4. If you have any difficulty with this exercise, you should review and repeat the exercises in Chapter 3 before continuing with this chapter.

Guided Exercise 31: Documenting an Admit for Transient Ischemic Attack (TIA)

This exercise will allow you to explore several ways of entering medical history related to a hospital admission. You will learn to use a new button on the Toolbar and several additional Entry Detail fields.

Case Study

Franklin Jones is a 77-year-old male, transferred from the emergency department where he was taken by EMS (Emergency Medical Services) following a sudden onset of dizziness and brief loss of consciousness on the golf course. The working diagnosis is transient ischemic attack. He is concerned about having to stay in the hospital because his wife has early stage Alzheimer's disease and he is the primary party responsible for management of their household and finances.

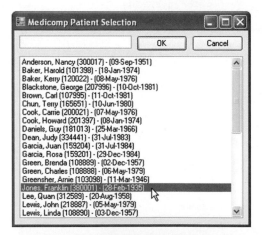

▶ **Figure 4-25 Selecting Franklin Jones from the Patient Selection window.**

Step 1

If you have not already done so, start the Student Edition software.

Click Select on the Menu bar, and then click Patient.

In the Patient Selection window (shown in Figure 4-25), visually locate and double click on **Franklin Jones**.

Alternatively, you can always type the client's *last name, first name* in the field at the top of the window as you did in Chapter 3.

Step 2

Click Select on the Menu bar, and then click New Encounter.

Scroll the drop-down list to locate the reason **Emergency Department**. As in the previous exercise, you may use the current date for this exercise, but be certain that you have selected the correct reason before clicking on the OK button.

Step 3

Enter the Chief complaint by locating the button in the Toolbar labeled "Chief" and clicking on it.

In the dialog window that will open, type:

"Sudden onset of dizziness and weakness with loss of consciousness while golfing. Witness reported the incident lasted less than one minute. Admitted from ER."

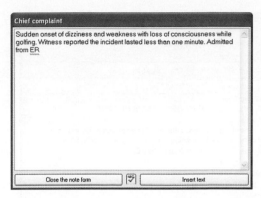

▶ **Figure 4-26 Chief complaint dialog for sudden onset of dizziness.**

Compare your screen to Figure 4-26 before clicking on the button labeled "Close the note form."

Step 4

Locate and click on the Dx tab to record the admitting diagnosis.

Locate and click on the small plus signs next to "Neurologic Disorders" and "CNS Vasculature Disorders" to expand the tree.

Locate and click on the red button next to the following finding:

● (red button) Transient ischemic attack (TIA)

Locate the Prefix field and click your mouse on the button with the down arrow in the Prefix field. Select "Admission diagnosis of" from the drop-down list.

Compare your screen to Figure 4-27.

▶ **Figure 4-27 Admission diagnosis of transient ischemic attack.**

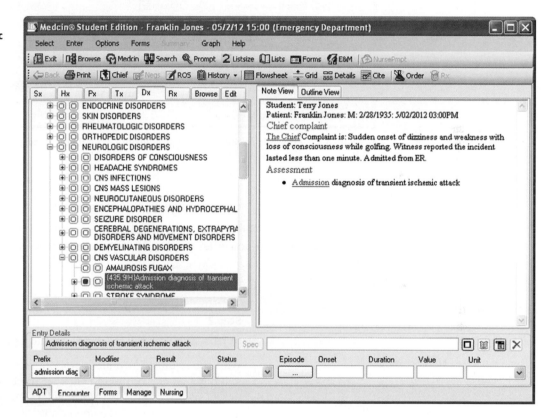

Step 5

The client reports that he is not currently dizzy, but has had previous recurrent episodes.

Locate and click on the Sx tab to record the client's symptoms.

Locate and click on the small plus sign next to neurological symptoms.

Locate and click on the indicated button for the following finding:

● (blue button) Dizziness

The description will change to "No dizziness."

Step 6

In this step you will learn to use a new Toolbar button.

Click on the small plus sign next to "No dizziness."

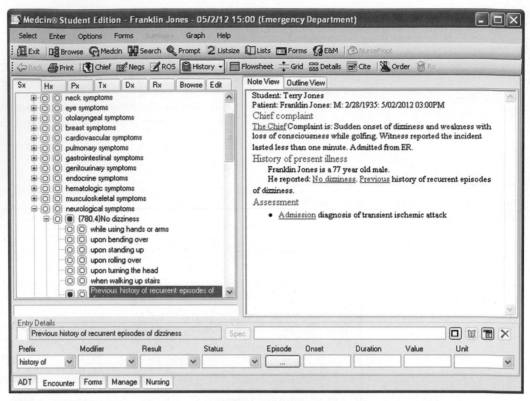

▶ **Figure 4-28 Presently no dizziness, but prior history of dizziness; History button highlighted orange on Toolbar.**

Locate and highlight "recurrent episodes" in the expanded tree.

Locate and click on the button labeled "History" on the Toolbar. (The button is orange in Figure 4-28.) A drop-down list may appear when you click the button. Select "history of" from the list.

Compare your screen to Figure 4-28.

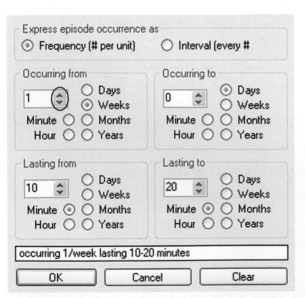

▶ **Figure 4-29 Episode occurring 1/week, lasting from 10 to 20 minutes.**

Step 7

In this step you will learn to use the Episode button.

With the finding "Previous history of recurrent episodes of dizziness" still highlighted, locate and click on the Episode button at the bottom of your screen. The button is located below the label "Episode" and has an ellipsis (three dots) on it.

The Episode window shown in Figure 4-29 will be invoked. It is used to record information about the intervals and repetitions at which findings occur. Take a moment to look at Figure 4-29.

Numbers in the Episode window are increased or decreased by clicking on the up or down arrow buttons (circled in Figure 4-29). These are located next to each numeric field. The units by which time is measured are set by clicking on one of the white circles next to Minutes, Hours, Days, Weeks, Months, or Years.

The window has four sections: "Occurring from," "Occurring to," "Lasting from," and "Lasting to."

Locate the section "Occurring from." Set it to **1** week by clicking on the up arrow button once and then clicking on the circle next to **Weeks**.

Locate the section "Lasting from." Set it to **10** minutes by clicking on the up arrow button ten times and then clicking on the circle next to **Minute**.

Locate the section "Lasting to." Set it to **20** minutes by clicking on the up arrow button twenty times and then clicking on the circle next to **Minute**.

Compare your screen to the Episode window in Figure 4-29. If it is correct, then click on the OK button.

Look at the encounter note in the right pane. Does the text read "Previous history of recurrent episodes of dizziness occurring 1/week lasting 10-20 minutes"?

Step 8

Scroll the left pane as necessary to locate and then click on the indicated button for the following findings:

- (red button) Lightheadedness
- (red button) fainting (syncope)

With the finding "Fainting" still highlighted, click the "History" button on the Toolbar.

Set the duration of his fainting spells using the Episode window, which you have learned in the previous step.

Locate and click on the Episode button at the bottom of your screen.

Locate the section "Lasting from." Set it to **5** minutes by clicking on the up arrow button ten times and then clicking on the circle next to **Minutes**.

Locate the section "Lasting to." Set it to **10** minutes by clicking on the up arrow button twenty times and then clicking on the circle next to **Minutes**.

Compare your screen to Figure 4-30.

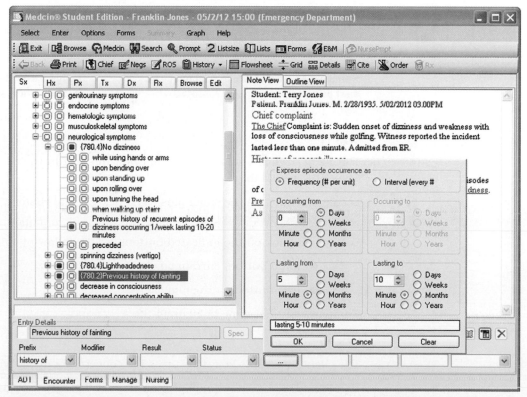

▶ **Figure 4-30 Lightheadedness with previous history of fainting; episodes lasting 5 to 10 minutes.**

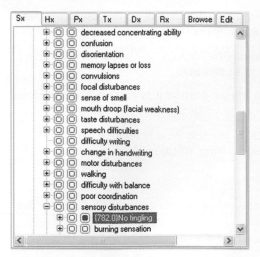

▶ **Figure 4-31 Sensory disturbances—No tingling.**

Click on the OK button to close the Episode window.

Step 9

Scroll the Nomenclature pane downward to locate "sensory disturbances" and click on the small plus sign to expand the tree (as shown in Figure 4-31).

Locate and click on the indicated button for the following finding:

● (blue button) Tingling (paresthesia)

Compare your left pane to Figure 4-31.

Step 10

Scroll the Nomenclature pane to the top of the symptoms list to locate and expand the tree of "Cardiovascular symptoms."

Locate and click on the indicated button for the following finding:

● (blue button) Chest pain

Compare your left pane to Figure 4-32.

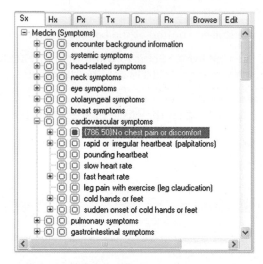

▶ **Figure 4-32 Cardiovascular symptoms—No chest pain.**

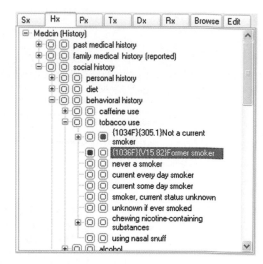

▶ **Figure 4-33 Behavioral history: Not a current smoker; former smoker.**

Step 11

The client does not smoke anymore. Enter this fact in the client's history.
Click on the Hx tab.

Locate and click on the small plus signs next "Social History," "Behavioral History," and "Tobacco use" to expand the tree.

Locate and click on the indicated buttons for the following findings:

● (blue button) current smoker

● (red button) Former smoker

Compare your left pane to Figure 4-33.

Step 12

The client interrupts you, to express his concern about his wife's well-being.

Locate and click on the small plus signs next "family medical history" and "family health status" to expand the tree.

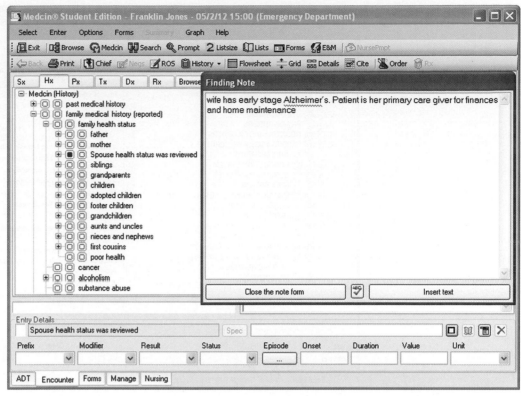

▶ **Figure 4-34 Family history: health status for spouse with Finding Note window.**

Locate and click on the red button for the following finding:

- (red button) Spouse

Locate and click on the Finding Note button (circled in red in Figure 4-14). Type the following text in the Finding Note window:

> **"wife has early stage Alzheimer's. Patient is her primary care giver for finances and home maintenance."**

Compare your screen to Figure 4-34 and then click on the button labeled "Close the note form."

Step 13

The History button on the Toolbar can be used to record any past or current medical conditions of the client that are not part of the current reason for hospitalization. The client reports a 20-year history of hypertension and an acute myocardial infarction in 2009. The ER reported sinus bradycardia upon arrival of the client in the ER.

Locate and click on the Dx tab. If we click on the red or blue buttons for any findings in this tab, they will be recorded as part of the current assessment. However, we will only highlight the following findings and then click the History button on the Toolbar. This will record them in the client's diagnosis history.

Your Dx tab may still be displaying the admitting diagnosis "Transient Ischemic Attack." If your Nomenclature pane is not at the top of the diagnosis list, scroll the pane upward until it is at the top of the diagnosis list.

Locate and click the small plus sign next to "Cardiovascular Disorders."

Locate and highlight the finding "**Hypertension**" and then click on the History button on the Toolbar.

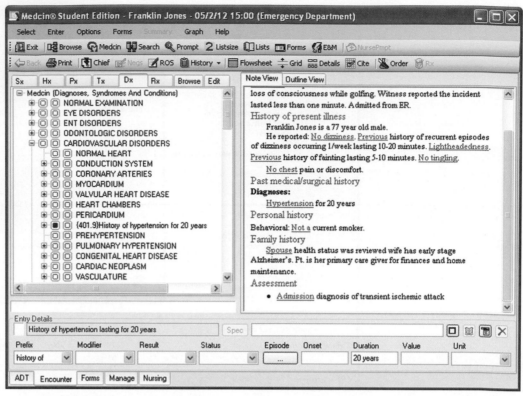

▶ **Figure 4-35 Diagnosis history: Hypertension 20 years.**

Locate the Entry Detail field labeled "Duration," type "**20 years**" in the duration field, and then press the Enter key on your keyboard.

Compare your screen to Figure 4-35.

Step 14

Locate "Conduction System" (which is also in Cardiovascular Disorders, but above Hypertension). Click on the small plus sign next to "Conduction System."

Locate and highlight the finding "**Sinus Bradycardia**" and then click on the History button on the Toolbar.

Locate the free-text field just below the right pane. Click in the field and type:

"**upon arrival in ER with HR 42 BP 90/42**" and then press the Enter key on your keyboard.

Compare your screen to Figure 4-36.

Step 15

Scroll the Dx list downward until you locate "Coronary Arteries." Click the small plus sign to expand the list.

Locate and highlight the finding "**Acute Myocardial Infarction**" and then click on the History button on the Toolbar.

Locate the Entry Detail field labeled "Onset," and type "**2009**" in the onset field, and then press the Enter key on your keyboard.

Compare your screen to Figure 4-37.

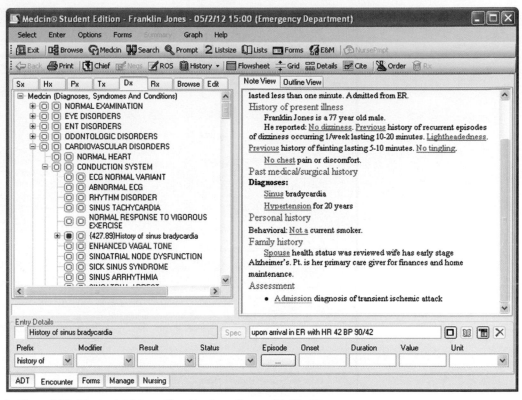

▶ **Figure 4-36 Diagnosis history: Sinus Bradycardia reported by ER.**

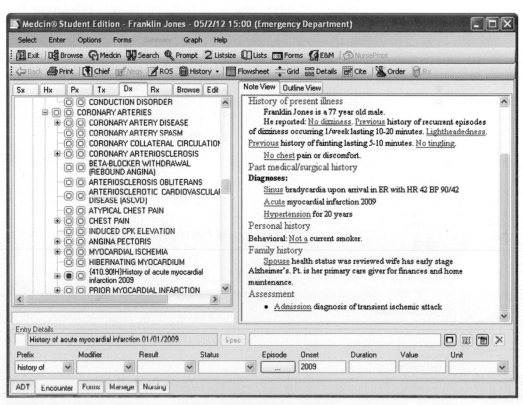

▶ **Figure 4-37 Diagnosis history: Acute Myocardial Infarction 2009.**

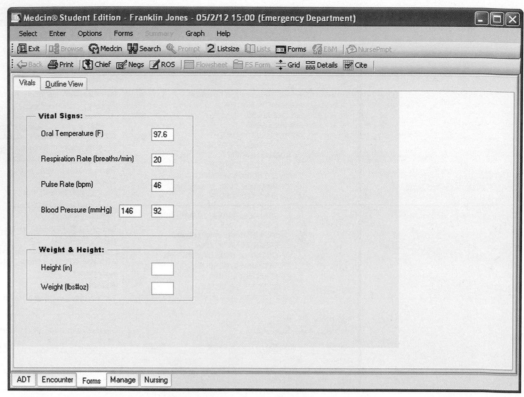

▶ **Figure 4-38 Vital signs for Franklin Jones.**

Step 16

Locate and click on the button labeled "Forms" in the top row of the Toolbar to invoke Forms Manager window. Locate and double-click on the form labeled "Vitals." The form shown in Figure 4-38 will be displayed. Enter Mr. Franklin's vital signs in the corresponding fields as follows:

Temperature: **97.6**

Respiration: **20**

Pulse: **46**

BP: **146/92**

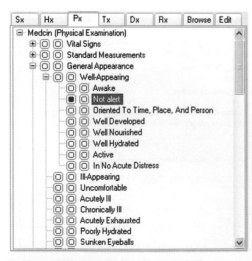

▶ **Figure 4-39 General Appearance, Well-Appearing —Not alert.**

Note that his weight and height were not measured; leave those fields blank. When you have entered the vital signs, compare your screen to Figure 4-38 and then click your mouse on the Encounter tab at the bottom of the screen.

Step 17

Locate and click on the Px tab.

Locate and click on the small plus signs next to "General Appearance," and "Well- Appearing" to expand the tree.

Locate and click on the red button for the following finding:

● (red button) Alert

The description will change to "Not alert." Compare your left pane with Figure 4-39.

Step 18

Scroll the list of Physical findings downward to locate and click on the small plus signs next to "Eyes," and "Pupils."

Locate and click on the blue button for the following finding:

● (blue button) PERRL

Compare your left pane with Figure 4-40.

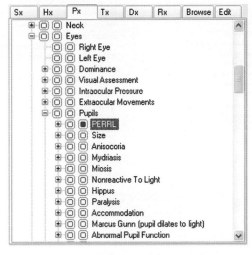

▶ **Figure 4-40 Eyes, Pupils—PERRL (Pupils Equal, Round, and Reactive to Light).**

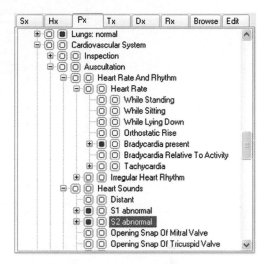

▶ **Figure 4-41 Lungs, Cardiovascular System, Auscultation, Heart Rate Rhythm and Sounds.**

Step 19

Scroll the list of Physical findings downward to locate "Lungs" and "Cardiovascular System." Expand the tree by locating and clicking the small plus signs next to "Cardiovascular System," "Auscultation," "Heart Rate and Rhythm," "Heart Rate," and "Heart Sounds."

When the cardiovascular portion of your list is expanded as shown in Figure 4-41, you will be able to quickly locate and click on the indicated buttons for the following findings:

● (blue button) Lungs

● (red button) Bradycardia

● (red button) S1

● (red button) S2

Compare your left pane with Figure 4-41.

Step 20

In this step you will learn to set the Result field.

Scroll the list of Physical findings downward to locate and click on the small plus sign next "Neurological System" to expand the tree.

Locate and highlight the finding "**Cognitive Functions**."

Locate the Entry Details field labeled "Result" and click on the down arrow button in the Result field. Select **Normal** from the drop-down list as shown in Figure 4-42.

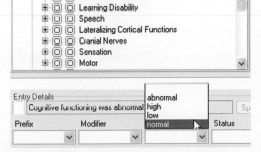

▶ **Figure 4-42 Neurological System, Cognitive Functions; set Result field to normal using drop-down list.**

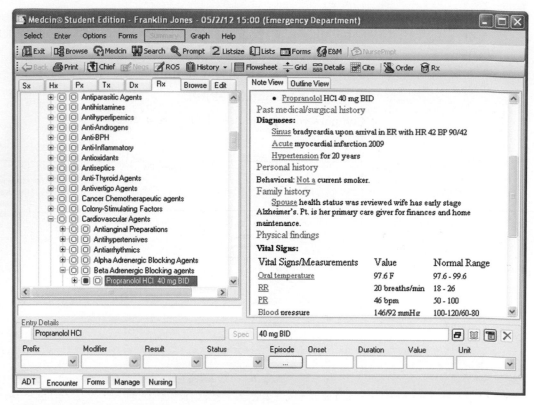

▶ **Figure 4-43 Current medication: Propranolol HCL 40 mg BID.**

Step 21

The client is currently taking the prescription drug Inderal, which is listed in the nomenclature under its generic name "Propranolol HCL."

Locate and click on the Rx tab.

Locate and click on the plus sign next to "Medications and Vaccines."

Scroll the list of medications downward to locate "Cardiovascular Agents," click on the small plus sign, and then on the small plus sign next "Beta Adrenergic Blocking agents."

Locate and click on the red button for the following finding:

- (red button) Propranolol HCL

Click in the free-text field just below the right pane; type "**40 mg BID**" and then press the Enter key on your keyboard.

Compare your screen to Figure 4-43.

Step 22

Remain on the Rx tab to record several nursing care orders.

Scroll the Rx list downward until you can see Nursing Care and then click on the small plus signs next to "Nursing Care," "Nursing Orders," and then "RNOx Cognition."

Locate and click on the red buttons for the following findings:

- (red button) RNOx Assess Perceptions
- (red button) RNOx Assess Cognitive Ability
- (red button) RNOx Monitor Level of Consciousness
- (red button) RNOx Follow-up of counseling service

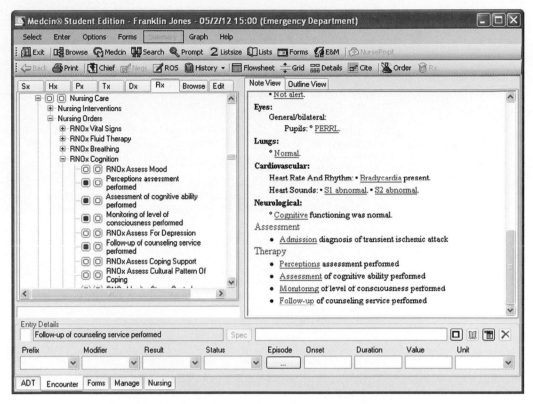

▶ **Figure 4-44 RNOx Cognition Nursing Orders selected on Rx tab.**

Compare your screen to Figure 4-44.

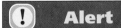 **Alert**

Do not close or exit the encounter until you have a printed copy in your hand. You will lose your work if you exit before printing.

Step 23

Print your completed encounter note.

Click on the Print button on the Toolbar at the top of your screen to invoke the Print Data window.

Look at the upper left pane of the window. If the box next to "Current Encounter" does not have a check mark, position your mouse pointer over it and click the mouse button. A check mark should appear in the box.

Click on one of the buttons labeled "Print and Close," or "Export to XPS File," or "Export to PDF File," as directed by your instructor.

Compare your printout or file output to Figure 4-45. If it is correct, hand it in to your instructor. If there are any differences (other than the date and client's age), review the previous steps in the exercise and find your error.

Once you have successfully completed this exercise, you should be comfortable with the general process of locating findings and expanding the tree to view additional findings.

Franklin Jones   Page 1 of 1

Student: *your name or ID here*
Patient: Franklin Jones: M: 2/28/1935: 5/02/2012 03:00PM
Chief complaint
The Chief Complaint is: Sudden onset of dizziness and weakness with loss of
consciousness while golfing. Witness reported the incident lasted less than one
minute. Admitted from ER.
History of present illness
     Franklin Jones is a 77 year old male.
He reported: No dizziness. Previous history of recurrent episodes of dizziness
occurring 1/week lasting 10-20 minutes. Lightheadedness. Previous history of
fainting lasting 5-10 minutes. No tingling. No chest pain or discomfort.
Current medication
     • Propranolol HCl 40 mg BID
Past medical/surgical history
Diagnoses:
Sinus bradycardia upon arrival in ER with HR 42 BP 90/42
Acute myocardial infarction 2009
Hypertension for 20 years
Personal history
Behavioral: Not a current smoker. Former smoker.
Family history
Spouse health status was reviewed wife has early stage Alzheimer's. Patient is
her primary care giver for finances and home maintenance.
Physical findings
Vital Signs:

Vital Signs/Measurements	Value	Normal Range
Oral temperature	97.6 F	97.6 - 99.6
RR	20 breaths/min	18 - 26
PR	46 bpm	50 - 100
Blood pressure	146/92 mmHg	100 - 120/60 - 80

General Appearance:
     • Not alert.
Eyes:
General/bilateral:
Pupils: ° PERRL.
Lungs:
       ° Normal.
Cardiovascular:
Heart Rate And Rhythm: • Bradycardia present.
Heart Sounds: • S1 abnormal. • S2 abnormal.
Neurological:
              ° Cognitive functioning was normal.
Assessment
     • Admission diagnosis of transient ischemic attack
Therapy
       • Perceptions assessment performed
       • Assessment of cognitive ability performed
       • Monitoring of level of consciousness performed
       • Follow-up of counseling service performed

▶ **Figure 4-45 Printed encounter note for Franklin Jones.**

Real-Life Story

A Nurse's Notes

By Sharyl Beal, RN, MSN

Sharyl Beal is a registered nurse with a master's degree in nursing and a subspecialty in nursing informatics. Sharyl has over 35 years nursing experience. She served as a nurse and a department head for 16 years before becoming a clinical systems analyst at a 500-bed hospital in the Midwest, where she was involved in creating and implementing electronic medical records for the nursing and ancillary departments, as well as training the nurses and doctors to use the clinical systems. She is currently a project manager in the Clinical Information Systems department and is co-author of this book.

Our hospital has successfully transitioned all nursing units to computerized charts. We rolled it out very slowly, one unit at a time, taking three years to implement all the areas. Today, all inpatient units are online, including our behavioral health units. We do not print nursing notes—everyone works online. These are some of my experiences and observations from this project.

We did medical/surgical units first because it is the broadest definition and fits the majority of clients. When that model was in operation, we went to the next unit and asked, "With this as a model, what do we need to do to make it work for you?" We did a fair amount of redesign as we added units, including descriptors for procedures that had not been necessary for another unit. Charting screens were structured to facilitate efficiency and provide evidence to meet regulatory requirements and best practice standards.

The first thing we did for all departments was to spend considerable time flowcharting all their processes: how they get their clients, how they communicate about their clients, with whom, what it looks like. We created a "life in the day of" scenario for every skill level in the unit, then we designed their charting based on their client population and the model of care used in that department.

The last unit to go online was Behavioral Health. Behavioral Health was challenging because this department's charts contain more abstract observations describing mental reactions, emotional reactions, and so on. But the most problematic unit was the Obstetrics (OB) Department.

OB charting is not difficult, but it is very meticulous. Our OB Department had a lot of rules and regulations about what had to be charted and how it was to be worded. The hospital legal department had to review all of our designs before the nurses could begin using them; they then reviewed samples of what was actually being documented once the department went online. We had to do some redesign to let the nurses better describe all of the requirements.

That was our design process; implementation was another matter. Our methodology of bringing one unit online at a time

allowed us to provide plenty of support when the unit went online. I think that was key. Clinical Informatics personnel were scheduled in shifts that overlapped the nursing shifts. We were in the unit, with the nurses, 24 hours a day for the first two weeks. Whenever new users were struggling, someone was right at their elbow to calmly guide them through, to make sure they were successful. Even with that level of support, there were some concerns that remained constant through the last unit of the rollout.

Nurses are very accustomed to being in control, confident in their expertise and their skills. When their documentation becomes computerized, all of a sudden everything they know has to be translated through the structure of a computer screen. The most common reaction when we rolled out charting into a new unit was that the nurses were extremely apprehensive their first day of charting. The universal complaint was that they could not sleep the night before.

My experience was that at the end of the first day they were still not feeling good about it, but when they came back the second day they had figured out how to get through it and they had very few questions. By the third day, they were usually doing very well. They still did not feel confident about finding the information, but they knew they could do it.

The nurses' biggest fear was that they would spend all their time taking care of the computer instead of their clients. They verbalized that idea for months afterwards, but that was not reality. Research has repeatedly shown that nurses spend 50 to 70 percent of their time documenting. In short, nurses already spend an enormous amount of their work life documenting, but it takes them a long time to feel like they are spending less time on the computer than on their clients. Their other fear was that they would miss care or fail to document something. This was especially true when they began electronically charting medication administration.

The real issue was that they felt like they were cut off from the information; they could not just flip open a chart and see what they were looking for. They had to remember how to find it and that was time out of their day. I have had them cry; I have had them yell, venting their frustration. But the good part was that they were all in the same boat together, so their peers readily understood what they were going through and we used peer "superusers" to help each other learn.

The nurses who had the easiest time transitioning were nurses who were accustomed to taking the time to write everything down as they went through their workday. The majority of nurses do not do that. Most nurses have notes stuffed in their pockets and tons of information in their head. They tend to store it up and write it all down when they come back from lunch at the end of their shift. When they try to follow that same model with a computer, but they are not yet comfortable with the computer, it is twice as hard because they have a lot to remember and they have to figure out what to do with it. Nurses who normally charted as their day progressed did not have to remember as much, so they seemed to learn faster.

In nursing school, students have to chart as it happens—instructors insist on it. This meant that nurses who just came out of nursing school had an advantage because they came to the job with good habits. Additionally, most of the new nurses grew up with computers and were more familiar with them.

We found that the ancillary departments—respiratory therapy, physical therapy, dietary, and so on—were also easy to implement. Their documentation is much more concrete, limited in its focus, so it was much easier to adapt from paper to computer. They were almost self-sufficient from the very beginning.

The doctors, however, were another story. We had to spend time up front making sure the doctors can get the information, and most doctors cannot give up enough time in their day to learn a computer. The nurses trained for 8 hours on the computer but the doctors only for about 15 minutes. We balanced this by trying to be attentive to any doctor who came on the floor. We would often say, "Let me help you find the information. The nurses are now charting on the computer. As of today you are not going to find that information on a piece of paper." We don't print anything. The doctors have adapted to the readily available information so well that on the rare occasion when we have downtime, it is usually the physicians who are the most upset.

It is important for the nursing leadership to dedicate time to learning the system so its members fully understand why the switch to computers is happening and what the benefits are. Then when their staff is apprehensive or when the physicians are frustrated because the nurses have not charted, there is reinforcement from the management that computerized charting is an expectation and during the week of initial use they "staff up" their units to support the new learners.

This point was illustrated in two of the units we rolled out. In one unit, the leadership was very computer savvy and expected the staff to do well. Leadership members held reinforcing in-service programs every 10 days and they would have us talk about specific areas where they thought their staff was weak in charting. Because the nurse manager was so proactive, that whole area adapted very easily; as a result, the physicians also adapted very easily.

In another unit where the nurse manager was not very computer savvy, the manager's apprehension reinforced that of the staff. For that reason, our team found the staff learning process took longer. Although this unit has been online for long time, there is still a core group of nurses who have not incorporated point-of-care charting into their nursing practice, because their leaders did not require it of them; they have continued to struggle with almost all aspects of the EHR.

One final benefit of an involved leadership is that it results in better charting. When we did the first units, the implementation team spent a lot of time reading the documentation for quality, to see if the nurses forgot to chart something, and so on. However, as the rollout continued throughout the hospital, the implementation team could not really spend a lot of time reviewing. You really need the people who know the client population of the unit, the leaders, the managers, or supervisors to be spending some time each day randomly selecting charts created by their nurses, reading them, and helping their nurses understand if they are not doing it thoroughly enough. Once the unit is implemented, they can use query reports to help them monitor, but the key is timely feedback. This not only improves the quality of the charts but also helps the staff get better at it quickly.

Critical Thinking Exercise 32: Documenting an Admit for the Cath Lab

This exercise will help you evaluate how well you can use the Student Edition software to document an encounter. The exercise provides step-by-step instructions, but does not provide screen figures for reference. The exercises in Chapters 3 and 4 covered each feature used in this exercise. If you have difficulty at any step during this exercise, refer to the Chapter 3 or Chapter 4 summaries, where a table lists each feature and the corresponding exercise for that feature.

Case Study

Linda Lewis is a 53-year-old female who has no prior cardiac history, but has recently been experiencing chest pain and shortness of breath on exertion especially when walking up stairs or inclines. She is being admitted as a short stay for a cardiac catheterization procedure, as a follow-up to an ECG with some abnormal findings. She has been referred by her primary care physician. She has a strong family history of cardiovascular disease and cancer.

Step 1

If you have not already done so, start the Student Edition software.

Click Select on the Menu bar, and then click Patient.

In the Patient Selection window, locate and click on **Linda Lewis**.

Step 2

Click Select on the Menu bar, and then click New Encounter.

Select the reason **Cath Lab** from the drop-down list.

Make sure you have selected the reason correctly. You may use the current date for this exercise.

Step 3

Enter the Chief complaint by locating the button in the Toolbar labeled "Chief" and clicking on it. In the dialog window that will open, type:

> **"Patient states she is here for a cardiac catheterization because she had chest pain and is short of breath when walking, especially on stairs or even low inclines**."

Click on the button labeled "Close the note form."

Step 4

Enter the client's vital signs using the Vitals form.

Locate and click on the button labeled "Forms" in the Toolbar at the top of your screen to invoke the Forms Manager window and then click on the Form name "Vitals" in the list.

Enter Linda's vital signs in the corresponding fields as follows:

Temperature:	**97.8**
Respiration:	**18**
Pulse:	**78**
BP:	**120/87**
Height:	**65**
Weight:	**152**

When you have entered all of the vital signs, click your mouse on the Encounter tab at the bottom of the screen.

Step 5

Enter the client's symptoms using the list of findings on the Sx tab.

Locate and click on the small plus signs next to "Systemic Symptoms," and "General overall feeling" to expand the tree.

Locate and click on the indicated buttons next to the following findings:

- (red button) Feeling fine
- (blue button) Previously well

Step 6

Scroll the list of Sx findings downward to locate "Cardiovascular Symptoms" and click on the small plus sign to expand the tree.

Locate and click on the small plus signs next to "Chest pain," and "Location" to further expand the tree.

Locate and click on the indicated button for the following findings:

- (red button) reported as pain
- (red button) centrally (substernal)
- (blue button) radiating

The description for radiating will change to "chest pain does not radiate."

Step 7

Scroll the list further downward. Locate and click on the small plus signs next to "Accompanied by," "Made worse by," and "Relieved by."

Locate and click on the indicated button for the following findings:

- (red button) difficulty breathing
- (red button) exertion
- (red button) rest

Step 8

Scroll the list further downward to locate and click on the small plus sign next to "Nitroglycerine."

Locate and click on the blue button for the following finding:

- (blue button) in under 5 minutes

Scroll the list if necessary to locate and click the red button for the following:

- (red button) rapid or irregular heartbeat (palpitations)

Locate and click on the Entry Details Episode button; the Episode window will be displayed.

Locate the section "Lasting from" and set it to **1 minute**.

Locate the section "Lasting to" and set it to **5 minute**.

Step 9

Click on the Hx tab.

Locate and click on the small plus sign next to Past Medical History.

Locate and click on the red button next to the following findings:

- (red button) No recent change in medical history
- (red button) no prior serious illness

Scroll the list further downward to locate and expand "Medical."

Locate and click on the indicated button for the following finding:

- (blue button) infections

Step 10

Locate and click on the small plus signs next to "Allergy," "Drugs," and "Antibiotic Agents" to expand the tree further.

Locate and click on the red button next to the following finding:

- (red button) Cephalosporins

Step 11

Scroll the list to locate and click on the small plus signs next "Reported prior tests," and "Chest x-ray."

Locate and click on the blue button for the following finding:

- (blue button) normal film

Locate the free-text field under the right pane and type **1 week ago**, and then press the Enter key on your keyboard.

Locate and click on the small plus sign next to "Prior ECG."

Locate and click on the red button for the following finding:

- (red button) abnormal

Locate and click in the free-text field, type **1 week ago**, and then press the Enter key on your keyboard.

Step 12

Scroll the list to locate and click on the small plus signs next to "Family Medical History" and "Family health status."

Locate and click the small plus sign next to "Father," and then click on the finding:

- (red button) deceased

Locate the Entry Details Onset field. Type **1999** in the Onset field and then press the Enter key on your keyboard.

Locate and click the small plus sign next to "Mother," and then click on the finding:

- (blue button) Alive

Step 13

Scroll the list downward to locate and click on the following findings:

- (red button) Cancer
- (red button) Heart disease

Step 14

The client has never smoked. Enter this fact in the client's History.

Scroll the list to locate and click on the small plus signs next "Social History," "Behavioral History," and "Tobacco use" to expand the tree.

Locate and click on the red button for the following finding:

- (red button) never a smoker

Step 15

Locate and click on the Px tab.

Locate and click on the small plus signs next to "General Appearance," and "Well-Appearing" to expand the tree.

Locate and click on the blue button for the following findings:

- (blue button) Awake
- (blue button) Alert
- (blue button) In No Acute Distress

Step 16

Scroll the list further downward to locate and expand "Lungs."

Locate and click on the indicated button for the following findings:

- (blue button) Respiration rhythm and depth

Step 17

Scroll the list further downward to locate and expand "Cardiovascular system."

Locate and click on the small plus signs next to "Auscultation," and "Heart Rate and Rhythm," to further expand the tree.

Locate and click on the indicated button for the following findings:

- (red button) Heart Rate and Rhythm
- (red button) Irregular Heart Rhythm

Step 18

Scroll the list further downward to locate and click the indicated buttons for the following finding:

- (blue button) Abdomen

Step 19

Click on the Dx tab.

Locate and click on the small plus signs next to "Cardiovascular Disorders," and "Conduction system" to expand the tree.

Locate and highlight "**Abnormal ECG**."

Click on the down arrow in the Prefix field and select the prefix "Referral diagnosis of" from the drop-down list.

Locate and highlight "**Rhythm disorder**."

Click on the History button on the Toolbar and select "history of" from the drop-down list.

Step 20

Click on the Rx tab.

Locate and click on the small plus signs next to "Nursing Care," and "Nursing Interventions," and "RNRx Tissue perfusions," to expand the tree.

Locate and click on the indicated buttons for the following findings:

- (red button) RNRx Circulatory care
- (red button) RNRx Neurovascular care

Click in the free-text note field below the right pane, type "**post catheterization**," and press the Enter key.

Step 21

Scroll the list further downward to locate and click on the plus signs for "IV Device," and "Care."

Locate and click on the indicated buttons for the following findings:

- (red button) Care
- (blue button) Phlebitis
- (blue button) Pain
- (blue button) Pressure at needle tip

Scroll the list further downward to locate and click on the plus sign for "Administration."

Locate and click on the red button for the following finding:

- (red button) Insertion site intact

Step 22

Scroll to the bottom of the list to locate and click on the plus signs for "Management of patient visit," "Disposition of patient," and "Discharge to."

Locate and click on the indicated button for the following finding:

- (red button) Home

 Alert   **Do not close or exit the encounter until you have a printed copy in your hand. You will lose your work if you exit before printing.**

Step 23

Print your completed encounter note.

Click on the Print button on the Toolbar at the top of your screen to invoke the Print Data window.

Be certain there is a check mark in the box next to "Current Encounter" and then click on the appropriate button to either print or export a file, as directed by your instructor.

Compare your printout or output file to Figure 4-46. If it is correct, hand it in to your instructor. If there are any differences (other than the date and client's age), review the previous steps in the exercise and find your error.

▶ **Figure 4-46 Printed encounter note for Linda Lewis.**

Linda Lewis   Page 1 of 1

Student: *your name or ID here*
Patient: Linda Lewis: F: 12/03/1957: 5/03/2012 06:00AM
Chief complaint
The Chief Complaint is: Patient states she is here for a cardiac catheterization because she had chest pain and is short of breath when walking, especially on stairs or even low inclines.
Referred here
Referral diagnosis of abnormal electrocardiogram.
History of present illness
    Linda Lewis is a 54 year old female.
She reported: Not feeling fine. Previously well.
Chest pain or discomfort reported as pain and substernally. Chest pain does not radiate. Chest pain and dyspnea, worse by exertion, and relieved by rest. Chest pain not relieved by nitroglycerin in under five minutes. Palpitations lasting 1-5 minutes.
Past medical/surgical history
Reported:
No recent change in medical history and no prior serious illness.
Medical: No infections.
Tests: A chest x-ray was normal 1 week ago. An ECG was abnormal 1 week ago.
Diagnoses:
Rhythm disorder
Personal history
Behavioral: Never a smoker.
Family history
Father deceased 1999
Mother is alive
Cancer
Heart disease.
Physical findings
Vital Signs:

Vital Signs/Measurements	Value	Normal Range
Oral temperature	97.8 F	97.6 - 99.6
RR	18 breaths/min	18 - 26
PR	78 bpm	50 - 100
Blood pressure	120/87 mmHg	100 - 120/56 - 80
Weight	152 lbs	98 - 183
Height	65 in	59.84 - 68.11

General Appearance:
    ° Awake. ° Alert. ° In no acute distress.
Lungs:
    ° Respiration rhythm and depth was normal.
Cardiovascular:
Heart Rate And Rhythm: • Abnormal. • Heart rhythm irregular.
Abdomen:
    ° Normal.
Therapy
    • Circulatory care
    • Neurovascular care post catheterization
    • IV therapy care. No signs of phlebitis at the IV site, no pain at the IV site, and no pressure on the needle tip.
    • The IV tube insertion site is intact.
    • Disposition - discharged home.
Allergies
An allergy to cephalosporins.

Chapter Four Summary

In this chapter you have performed exercises intended to increase your familiarity with the Student Edition software and thereby increase your speed of data entry. You have also learned to print out encounter notes or export them as files. You can print the encounter note at any time and as often as you like while practicing your exercises. However, remember not to quit or exit the program **until you are sure the encounter note has printed**. Once you exit, you will lose your work.

As you continue through the course, you can refer to the Guided Exercise 30 in this chapter if you need to remember how to print or export a file. You can also repeat any of the exercises in this chapter to increase your skills using the software. You should not proceed with the remainder of the text until you can perform the exercises in this chapter with ease.

In these and many subsequent exercises, you are permitted to use the current date instead of setting it to a specific date. Remember when you do that, the date of the encounter and the client's age will differ from the samples printed in the book. However, all of the other items in your printout or file should match the figures in the book.

As you continue through the course, you can refer to the Guided Exercises in this chapter when you need to remember how to perform a particular task that you learned in this chapter.

Task	Guided Exercise(s)	Page No.
Printing or exporting an XPS or PDF file of the encounter note	30	117
History (Toolbar button)	31 (step 6)	123
Entry Detail fields:		
Episode (occurring, lasting from/to)	31 (step 7)	124
Duration	31 (step 13)	127
Onset	31 (step 15)	128
Result	31 (step 20)	131

Test Your Knowledge

1. Why is it important to print your work before exiting?

2. What does the Export PDF button do?

3. What does the Episode button do?

4. What year did Franklin Jones have an acute myocardial infarction (AMI)?

5. What Entry Details field was used to record the date of Franklin's AMI?

6. On what tab do you record a client's tobacco habits?

7. How many packs a day does Linda Lewis smoke?

8. What imaging study was scheduled for Irene Smith?

9. When is it more useful to use the Finding Note window instead of the free-text field?

10. What was the assessment (admission diagnosis) for Franklin Jones?

11. What was Franklin Jones's concern about his wife?

12. What Entry Details field was used to record that his cognitive functioning was normal?

13. What is the effect of using the History button on the Toolbar to record a diagnosis?

14. For which client did the nurse order follow-up of counseling service?

15. You should have produced three narrative documents of client encounters, which you printed. If you have not already done so, hand it in to your instructor with this test. The printed encounter notes will count as a portion of your grade.

Ask your instructor for answers to Test Your Knowledge

nursing.pearsonhighered.com

Prepare for success with animated examples, practice questions, challenge tests, and interactive assignments.

Chapter

5

Data Entry at the Point of Care

Learning Outcomes

After completing this chapter, you should be able to:

1. Load and use Lists of findings to speed up data entry
2. Describe Review of Systems
3. Change symptoms from History of Present Illness to Review of Systems
4. Know how to quickly record "pertinent negatives"
5. Understand and use Forms
6. Use Lists and Forms together

Why Speed of Entry Is Important in the EHR

A recent survey of nurses conducted by Jackson Healthcare (2010) found that nurses in a hospital setting spent 25 percent of their time on indirect patient care activities. The report stated that the majority of that time was spent on documentation. In Chapter 2, EHR expert Dr. Allen Wenner estimated that in a medical office, up to 67 percent of the nurse or clinician's time with the client is spent entering the client's symptoms into the visit documentation.

There is no question that symptoms, history, orders, observations, assessments, and all other aspects of client care must be documented. The accuracy of nursing documentation and efficiency of workflow can be improved by documenting at the time of the encounter, rather than after the nurse has left the client. Previous chapters have referred to this as "point-of-care" or "real-time" data entry—that is, to document the visit completely before the nurse leaves the client.

Speed of entry is important because the less time it takes to record the nurse's notes, the more time a nurse has available for client care. Real-time data entry is important because the chart is always up-to-date. Accuracy is improved because nothing is forgotten. Documenting at the point of care allows the nurse to ask the client to elaborate or clarify any point of concern. Best of all, when the nurse leaves the client's room, the nursing notes are done. No longer will the nurse spend the final hours of every shift finishing up "paperwork." The documentation becomes a part of the client care, rather a task to be completed before the nurse's shift ends. More importantly, health information about the client is available for other caregivers, physicians, and ancillary care givers instead of in the nurse's memory or pocket.

To document in real time, a nurse must be able to quickly navigate and enter findings. To help the nurse accomplish this, an EHR must present the finding the nurse requires when it is needed. In this chapter we are going to look at several approaches that EHR systems use to help accomplish this.

Lists and Forms Speed Data Entry

As you have seen from the exercises in the previous chapters, completely documenting the encounter could take quite a bit of time. Those exercises documented relatively simple encounters with findings that were fairly easy to locate and omitted many routine findings to keep the exercises short. However, in the real world client's often have multiple problems, more complex history and symptoms. Is there a faster way to find what you are looking for than just scrolling the navigation list and expanding the trees? Yes!

EHR vendors work constantly with EHR users to devise means to locate and present findings when they are most likely needed. The Student Edition software provides examples of a few of the ways that EHR systems do this. In this chapter, you will learn about two features that help doctors, nurses, and other care team members to enter data more quickly. These are Lists and Forms.

Lists and Forms are two approaches to point-of-care data entry that are used extensively in nearly every EHR system. These are templates to display findings that are most frequently needed for typical cases, allowing the encounter to be documented with minimal navigation or searching.

Shortcuts That Speed Documentation of Typical Cases

Both inpatient and outpatient facilities see a lot of individuals with similar conditions. There are several reasons for this:

▶ The top 10 diseases cause the highest proportion of hospitalizations.

▶ Geographic location or environmental factors may cause a facility to see more cases of a particular nature than similar facilities in another region.

▶ There can be seasonal increases of certain illnesses such as influenza and other upper respiratory infections.

▶ A clinic or hospital may focus on certain diseases or clients of a certain age. For example, an oncology center sees only cancer cases; a children's hospital focuses on children's diseases.

▶ In outpatient clinics the specialty of the physicians may limit the type of cases they treat. For example, a pulmonary specialist sees primarily respiratory cases, nephrologists see clients with kidney problems, and a pediatric clinic sees children.

▶ Nurses routinely need the same findings to document the admission and create care plans for clients with similar conditions.

It is therefore logical to create shorter, quicker methods of entering the data. One frequently used approach is to created templates based on the admitting diagnosis or type of ailment.

The Concept of Lists

You may not have heard the term *Lists* used in the context of an EHR, but the concept should be very familiar to you because you have been scrolling and navigating the list of findings since Chapter 3. Now, imagine that you are a nurse in a pediatric office that sees many children with earaches (otitis media) and that each time the chief complaint was an earache the system could magically present the findings that you needed to document the visit. That is the idea behind lists. Of course, lists do not magically appear. They are created by clinicians, nurses, and the hospital Clinical Information Services (CIS) staff. However, the effort expended to create a list is saved again and again when subsequent clients are seen for the same or similar reasons.

The advantage of using these short lists is that they are used just like browsing the full Medcin Nomenclature except that only the desired subset is shown. The list can (and usually does) contain findings in every tab, which means that time savings are realized all the way through the encounter. If only certain therapies or certain drugs are used for a particular condition, then when the clinician clicks the mouse on the Rx tab, only those items are shown. When using a list, if there is a finding that is needed but is not on the list, the nurse can switch to the full nomenclature hierarchy to select the finding and then switch back to continue using the list.

Although lists are sometimes limited to one particular condition such as otitis media, this is not a rule; it is a convenience factor because shorter lists mean less scrolling. Lists are flexible and can contain as many findings as necessary to document a typical encounter.

With some types of symptoms, the assessment could be one of several possible diagnoses. For example, adult upper respiratory infections could be the result of rhinitis, sinusitis, or bronchitis. Therefore, a list with more findings reduces the possibility that the nurse will need to switch to browsing the full nomenclature.

A good example of a multiple diagnosis type of list is the one for Adult Upper Respiratory Infections (URI) used in the next exercise. Because a client could be admitted for several possible infections such as bronchitis, influenza, or pneumonia, it is helpful that the list includes a larger number of relevant findings.

Guided Exercise 33: Using an Adult URI List

During the cold and flu season, many clients may require treatment for upper respiratory infections. Therefore, a list of findings for adults presenting with symptoms of URI can really speed up the documentation process. In this exercise, you will learn how to use the List feature as well as several additional buttons on the Toolbar.

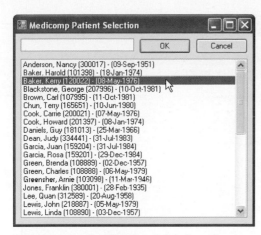

▶ **Figure 5-1 Selecting Kerry Baker from the Patient Selection window.**

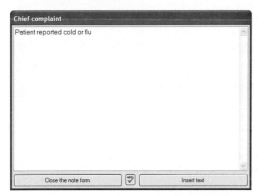

▶ **Figure 5-2 Chief complaint dialog for client-reported cold or flu.**

Case Study

Kerry Baker is a 35-year-old female who presented to the ER with complaints of cold and flu-like symptoms including sinus pain and nasal stuffiness and discharge. She reported having a recent cold, but is not taking medications at this time. She is being admitted for acute bronchitis and influenza.

Step 1

If you have not already done so, start the Student Edition software.

Click Select on the Menu bar, and then click Patient.

In the Patient Selection window, locate and click on **Kerry Baker** as shown in Figure 5-1.

Step 2

Click Select on the Menu bar, and then click New Encounter.

Use the current date and time for this encounter. Select the reason **Emergency Department**. Click on the OK button.

Step 3

Enter the Chief complaint by locating the button in the Toolbar labeled "Chief" and clicking on it.

In the dialog window that will open, type "**Patient reported cold or flu.**"

Compare your screen to Figure 5-2 before clicking on the button labeled "Close the note form."

Step 4

In this exercise, the nurse will begin by recording Kerry's vital signs using the Vitals form (as you have in previous exercises).

Enter Kerry's vital signs in the corresponding fields on the Form as follows:

Temperature:	**100**
Respiration:	**16**
Pulse:	**78**
BP:	**120/80**
Height:	**60**
Weight:	**100**

When you have finished, compare your screen to Figure 5-3 and, when it is correct, click on the Encounter tab at the bottom of the screen.

Step 5

As the client reported cold or flu symptoms, we will use a List created for this type of condition.

Locate and click on the Lists button in the Toolbar at the top of your screen (highlighted orange in Figure 5-4). The icon resembles an open book. The List Manager window will be invoked.

▶ **Figure 5-3 Vital Signs form for Kerry Baker.**

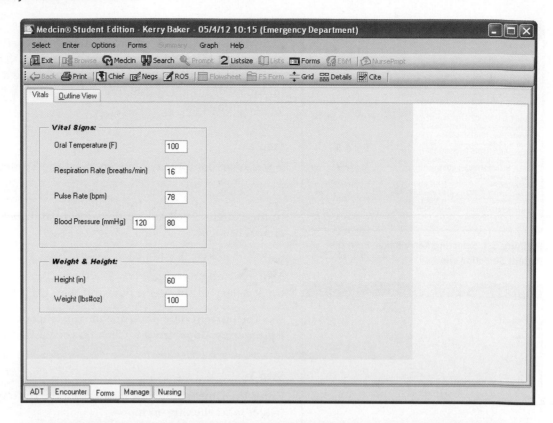

▶ **Figure 5-4 Select Adult URI from Lists Manager window (invoked by Lists button).**

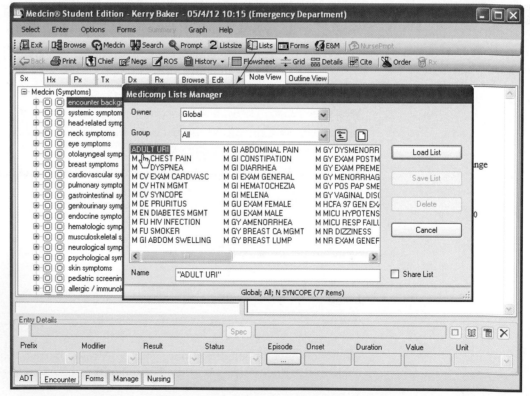

The List Manager displays the various Lists available to healthcare providers in the facility. Two fields at the top of the screen organize the display of List names, filtering them by Owner and Group.

As we discussed earlier in this section, clinicians also can create personal copies of Lists customized to their specialty. The Owner field allows clinicians to quickly find their customized Lists by changing the field from "Global" to "Personal."

Lists also can be assigned to Groups, which helps to organize them by department, body system, disease, type of exam, or any other criteria the facility desires. The Group field allows a user to quickly find a list by limiting the display to a desired group. Note that the Student Edition has two groups, "All" and "Student Edition."

Locate and highlight the list named Adult URI, which is the first list in the window. Click your mouse on the button labeled "Load List."

Step 6

Notice that the normal display of the Medcin Nomenclature in the left pane has been replaced with a list of symptoms that clients with upper respiratory infections are likely to report. Notice that the title of the first line "Templates (Symptoms)" indicates that the findings are limited by a List (referred to in the left pane as a Template). You will also notice a special HPI button next to each finding—this will be explained in a moment.

Locate and click on the following symptom findings:

- (red button) feeling poorly or tired
- (red button) chills
- (red button) sinus pain
- (red button) nasal discharge
- (red button) nasal passage blockage (stuffiness)
- (red button) difficulty breathing (dyspnea)
- (red button) cough
- (red button) coughing up sputum
- (red button) muscle aches

Compare your screen to Figure 5-5. Before proceeding, notice that symptoms reported by the client have been documented in "History of Present Illness," or "HPI" (circled in red in Figure 5-5).

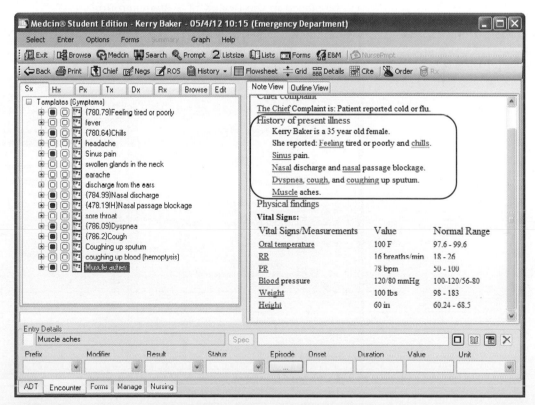

▶ **Figure 5-5 Symptoms on the Adult URI List (Template)—HPI circled in red.**

Step 7

Review of Systems (ROS) is a way of organizing an exam by body systems starting from the head down. You should already be familiar with the body systems from anatomy and physiology classes. The body systems in a standard ROS are:

- ▶ Constitutional symptoms
- ▶ HEENT (head, eyes, ears, nose, mouth, throat)
- ▶ Cardiovascular
- ▶ Respiratory
- ▶ Gastrointestinal
- ▶ Genitourinary
- ▶ Musculoskeletal
- ▶ Integumentary (skin and/or breast)
- ▶ Neurological
- ▶ Psychiatric
- ▶ Endocrine
- ▶ Hematologic/lymphatic
- ▶ Allergic/immunologic

Typically, you will document the symptoms directly related to the Chief complaint in the HPI. The remainder of the symptoms review is usually documented as a "Review of Systems."

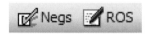

▶ **Figure 5-6 Auto Negative (Neg) and Review of Systems (ROS) buttons.**

The Toolbar at the top of your screen has a button that can be used to change the way symptom findings are grouped from HPI into a ROS. The button on the right in Figure 5-6, labeled "ROS," toggles between on and off. When you click on the ROS button, it changes from blue to orange, which indicates the ROS grouping is on. If you click on the button again, it will change back to its original color, indicating that the ROS grouping is off.

Locate and click on the ROS button. It will turn orange as shown in Figure 5-7. When you click on symptom findings while the ROS button is orange, the selected symptom will be placed in the Review of Systems group.

▶ **Figure 5-7 Symptom: No Headache in Review of systems group (circled in red).**

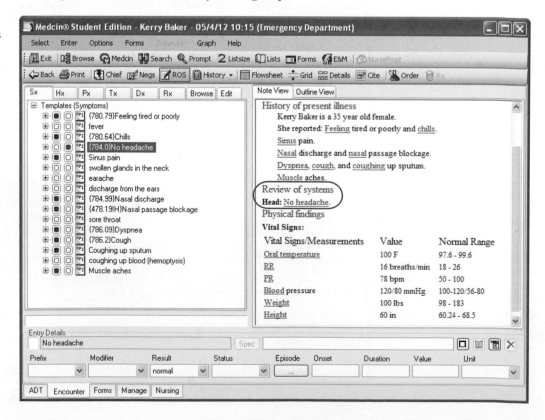

Step 8

Verify the ROS button is orange, then locate and click on the following finding:

● (blue button) headache

Compare your screen to Figure 5-7. Notice that the finding "No headache" was placed in a new group "Review of systems" that was created in the note (shown circled in red).

Step 9

Frequently, most of the symptoms in the ROS will be negative, as they were not reported by the client in the HPI. Using a List such as Adult URI, you could quickly go down the list clicking a blue button on each of the remaining findings. However, that would still be a lot of mouse clicks.

Fortunately, the Toolbar has another button, labeled "Negs" for "Auto Negatives," that is used to speed up the documentation process. When the nurse has clicked a red or blue button for all the relevant positive findings, the remainder of the list can be set to "within normal limits" with one click on the "Negs" button on the Toolbar. (It is the button on the left in Figure 5-6.)

The purpose of Auto Negatives is not to shortcut the exam process but to speed up the documentation of the encounter. Nurses find they can review systems much more quickly than they can document each finding. The Auto Negatives feature allows them to document this portion of the assessment in fewer clicks.

The Auto Negative feature selects the "normal" button (usually the blue button) for all displayed findings that are not already set. The user can modify any finding after the process is finished. Because all the findings displayed in the current tab are automatically selected, the Auto Negative feature works best with Lists or Forms because the List is already limited to findings that the clinician would normally use in a particular type of encounter.

Locate and click on the button labeled "Negs" in the Toolbar at the top of your screen. The icon resembles a box with a teal check mark. The Negs button is highlighted in Figure 5-8.

▶ **Figure 5-8 Auto Negative button quickly completes multiple findings.**

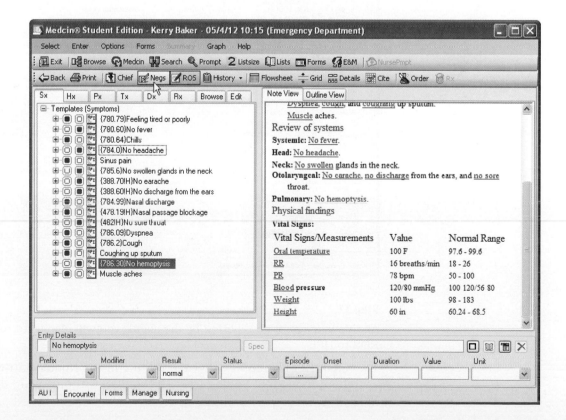

All symptoms that have not previously been selected have automatically had their blue buttons selected. Notice how quickly the documentation process was completed.

Compare the encounter notes on your screen with Figure 5-8. (You may need to scroll the right pane upward to see the full effect.) Notice that the three findings with red buttons were not altered.

The Auto Negative function will record the findings according to the state of the ROS button. Because the ROS button was on, the additional symptoms were recorded in the Review of Symptoms group, not the HPI group.

Step 10

Although all unselected symptoms findings were set by the Auto Negative feature, they can be changed by the user at any time during the encounter. Kerry mentions that she has had a mild fever. You note that Ms. Baker's temperature is 100°F. Therefore, you will change the finding.

Locate and click the red button for the following finding:

- (red button) No fever

This will change the button from blue to red and the description will change to "Fever." With the finding still highlighted, locate the Entry Details field "Modifier" and click your mouse on the down arrow button to display a drop-down list (as shown in Figure 5-9). Scroll the list of modifiers until you locate the word "**Mild**," then click on it.

▶ **Figure 5-9 Modifying the finding "Fever."**

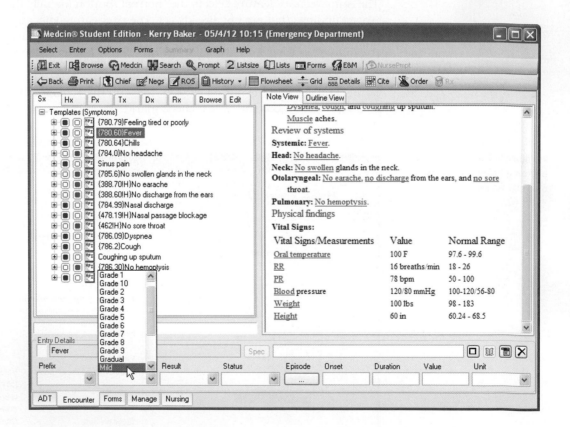

Step 11

As this is a symptom reported by the client, you will also want to change "Fever" from ROS to HPI.

The small HPI button next to each finding in the Nomenclature pane is used to switch an individual finding from HPI to ROS without using the ROS button on the Toolbar.

The differences between the actions of these two buttons are as follows:

▶ The ROS button on the Toolbar applies to all symptoms selected while the button is on (orange).

▶ The HPI/ROS button on an individual finding affects only the selected finding and only affects it when the Toolbar ROS button is off (blue).

▶ The HPI/ROS button on individual findings is only available on the Sx tab, and only when a List is loaded.

▶ The ROS button on the Toolbar is available anytime you are on the Sx tab.

Locate and click on the ROS button on the Toolbar, to turn it off. The button should no longer be orange.

Locate the finding of "Fever" in the Nomenclature pane and click the small HPI button next to it. The button is circled in Figure 5-10.

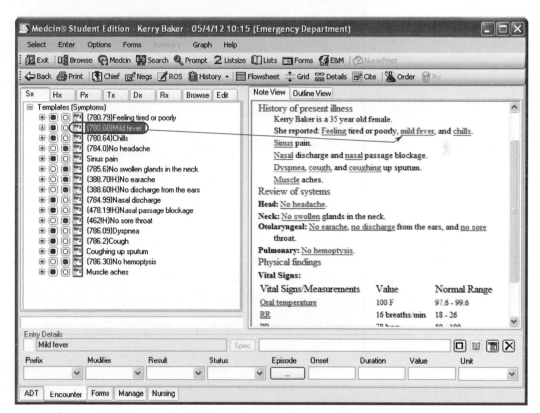

▶ **Figure 5-10 HPI/ROS button (circled in red) changes finding to a different group.**

Look at the button. Did it change? Look at the encounter note. Did "Mild Fever" move from the Review of systems group to the History of present illness group?

If "Mild Fever" did not change groups, repeat step 11, being certain that the ROS button on the Toolbar is off (blue).

Step 12

Next, click on the Hx tab to enter the client's history. Note that the "Negs" button is grayed out. This is because the Auto Negative function is only available on the Sx (Symptoms) and Px (Physical Exam) tabs.

You will recall from previous exercises how many items are typically in the Hx tab, but because you are using a list, only those items related to Adult URI are displayed. This makes navigation of the list quicker because the list is shorter. Locate and click on the buttons indicated for the following History findings.

- (red button) recent upper respiratory infection (URI)
- (blue button) allergies
- (blue button) taking medications
- (blue button) current smoker

Compare your left pane to Figure 5-11. If it is correct, scroll the encounter note (right pane) upward far enough to see both groups of history. Note that even though the findings were listed together in the left pane, they were actually from three different history groups: Past Medical History, Social (Behavioral) History, and Allergies. Note that Allergy findings are in their own group at the very bottom of the note and not shown in the figure. Scroll your right pane downward to locate the Allergies group.

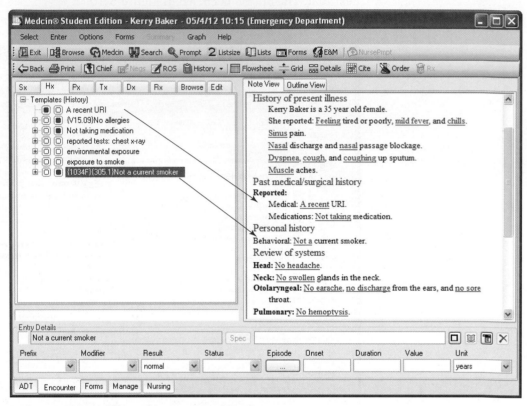

► **Figure 5-11 Two different history groups from List.**

This is an example of how lists can present together findings that are normally located very far apart in the expanded tree.

Step 13

Click on the Px tab to document the physical exam.

Locate and click on the buttons indicated for the following Physical Exam findings.

- (blue button) Both tympanic membranes were examined
- (red button) Nasal discharge purulent
- (red button) Sinus tenderness

Locate the button labeled "Negs" in the Toolbar. Notice the "Negs" button in the Toolbar that was grayed out in the previous tab is again available when you are on this tab. The Negs button is available only on the Sx and Px tabs.

Click on the "Negs" button.

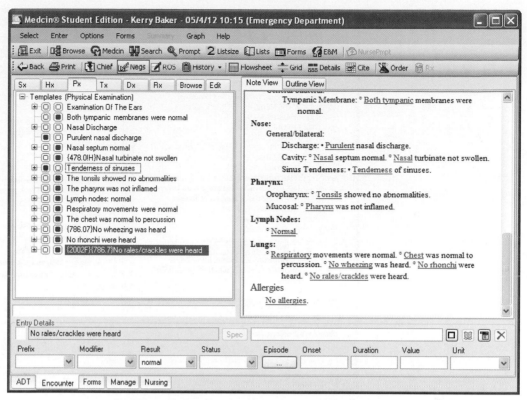

▶ **Figure 5-12 Physical exam completed using Neg button (highlighted).**

Compare your screen to Figure 5-12. Notice that the first and third findings (ears and nasal discharge) were not set. This because the Auto Negative feature correctly determined that the tympanic membrane finding was an examination of the ears, and the purulent discharge finding was a refinement of the nasal discharge finding.

Step 14

The client is being admitted for acute bronchitis and Type A influenza.

Click on the Dx tab and notice that the Adult URI list contains diagnoses that are most likely to be present in cases of upper respiratory infections.

Locate the finding **"Acute Bronchitis"** and highlight it.

Locate the Prefix field at the bottom of the screen, click the down arrow, and select "Admission diagnosis of" from the drop-down list.

Locate the finding **"Influenza"** and highlight it.

Locate the Prefix field at the bottom of the screen, click the down arrow, and select "Admission diagnosis of" from the drop-down list.

Locate and click on the small plus sign next to Respiratory Alteration.

Locate and click on the following Nursing Diagnoses findings:

- (red button) RNDx Respiratory Alteration
- (red button) RNDx Airway clearance impairment
- (red button) RNDx Breathing pattern impairment

Compare your screen to Figure 5-13.

Step 15

Click on the Rx tab and again appreciate the fact that the tab contains types of treatments most likely to be prescribed for adult upper respiratory infections.

▶ **Figure 5-13 Clinical assessments and nursing diagnosis.**

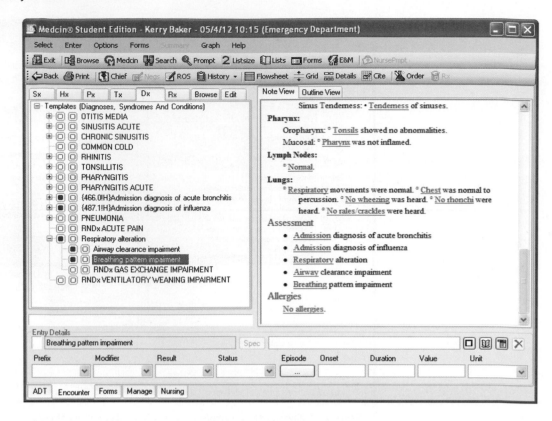

The admitting doctor has ordered fluids and an antibiotic.

Locate and highlight "**ordered Antibacterial Amoxicillin**," and then locate and click the down arrow button in the Prefix field. Select the prefix "**Administered**" from the drop-down list as shown in Figure 5-14.

▶ **Figure 5-14 Amoxicillin administered.**

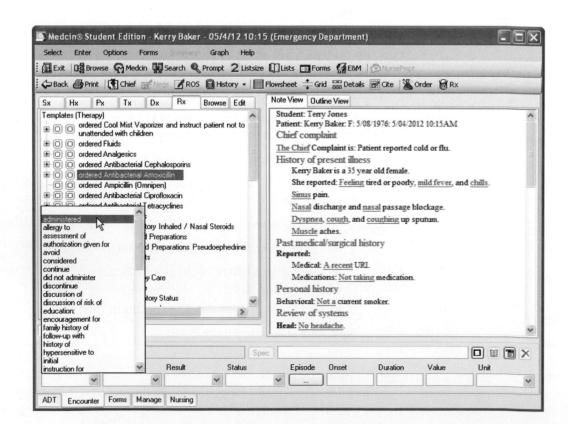

Step 16

Scroll the list downward to locate and click on the indicated buttons for the following nursing actions:

- (red button) RNOx Monitor Lung sounds
- (red button) RNOx Assess sputum appearance
- (red button) RNOx Monitor oxygen saturation
- (red button) RNOx Encourage coughing and deep breathing

Compare your screen to Figure 5-15.

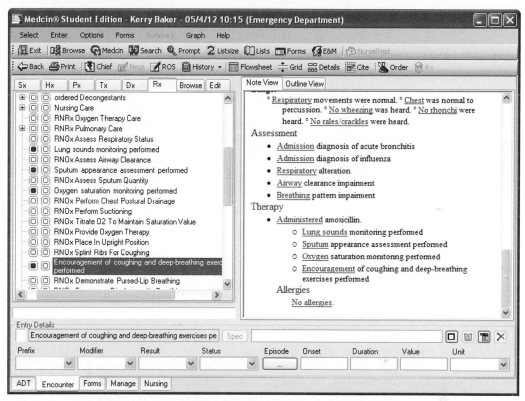

▶ **Figure 5-15   Nursing orders for Kerry Baker.**

In this exercise you learned to use the List feature as well as the ROS and Auto Negative buttons. You also learned to use the Modifier field and the individual ROS/HPI button.

Step 17

Click on the Print button on the Toolbar at the top of your screen to invoke the Print Data window.

Be certain there is a check mark in the box next to Current Encounter and then click on the appropriate button to either print or export a file, as directed by your instructor.

Compare your printout or file output to Figure 5-16. If it is correct, hand it in to your instructor. Note your printer may produce two pages. If there are any differences (other than the date, the pagination, or the client's age), review the previous steps in the exercise and find your error.

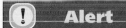 **Alert**

Do not close or exit the encounter until you have a printed copy in your hand. You will lose your work if you exit before printing.

Kerry Baker   Page 1 of 1

Student: *your name or id here*
Patient: Kerry Baker: F: 5/08/1976: 5/04/2012 10:15AM
Chief complaint
The Chief Complaint is: Patient reported cold or flu.
History of present illness
    Kerry Baker is a 35 year old female.
    She reported: Feeling tired or poorly, mild fever, and chills. Sinus pain.
    Nasal discharge and nasal passage blockage. Dyspnea, cough, and coughing up
    sputum. Muscle aches.
Past medical/surgical history
Reported:
    Medical: A recent URI.
    Medications: Not taking medication.
Personal history
    Behavioral: Not a current smoker.
Review of systems
Head: No headache.
Neck: No swollen glands in the neck.
Otolaryngeal: No earache, no discharge from the ears, and no sore throat.
Pulmonary: No hemoptysis.
Physical findings
Vital Signs:

Vital Signs/Measurements	Value	Normal Range
Oral temperature	100 F	97.6 - 99.6
RR	16 breaths/min	18 - 26
PR	78 bpm	50 - 100
Blood pressure	120/80 mmHg	100 - 120/56 - 80
Weight	100 lbs	98 - 183
Height	60 in	60.24 - 68.5

Ears:
    General/bilateral:
    Tympanic Membrane: ° Both tympanic membranes were normal.
Nose:
    General/bilateral:
    Discharge: • Purulent nasal discharge.
    Cavity: ° Nasal septum normal. ° Nasal turbinate not swollen.
    Sinus Tenderness: • Tenderness of sinuses.
Pharynx:
    Oropharynx: ° Tonsils showed no abnormalities.
    Mucosal: ° Pharynx was not inflamed.
Lymph Nodes:
    ° Normal.
Lungs:
    ° Respiratory movements were normal. ° Chest was normal to percussion.
    ° No wheezing was heard. ° No rhonchi were heard. ° No rales/crackles were
    heard.
Assessment
    • Admission diagnosis of acute bronchitis
    • Admission diagnosis of influenza
    • Respiratory alteration
    • Airway clearance impairment
    • Breathing pattern impairment
Therapy
    • Administered amoxicillin.
    • Lung sounds monitoring performed
    • Sputum appearance assessment performed
    • Oxygen saturation monitoring performed
    • Encouragement of coughing and deep-breathing exercises performed
Allergies
    No allergies.

▶ **Figure 5-16 Printed encounter note for Kerry Baker.**

Critical Thinking Exercise 34: Using Syncope List for a TIA Case

Now that you have learned that the Lists and Auto Negative feature can help you enter EHR data more quickly, prove it to yourself with this exercise.

In Chapter 4 you documented the admission of a client with a working diagnosis of transient ischemic attacks (TIA) by navigating the entire nomenclature. In this exercise you will discover how a using a List can expedite documenting the admission for a similar case, but this time using what you have learned about lists, you are going to time yourself.

Case Study

Victoria Mayhew is a 82-year-old female admitted for syncope probably TIA after experiencing a sudden loss of consciousness for under 5 minutes as reported by her daughter who accompanied her to the hospital. For approximately 20 minutes following this episode, she experience mild confusion, difficulty talking, and doesn't recall the incident at all. There doesn't seem to be any residual effects except mild confusion to the situation. She has diagnostic tests ordered, and has been placed on Telemetry. She will need to be on safety precautions for ambulation, though her current neurological and musculoskeletal statuses are intact.

Step 1

Look at the clock and write down the current time.

If you have not already done so, start the Student Edition software.

Click Select on the Menu bar, and then click Patient.

In the Patient Selection window, locate and click on **Victoria Mayhew**.

Step 2

Click Select on the Menu bar, and then click New Encounter.

Use the current date and time. Select the reason **Hospital Inpatient**. Click on the OK button.

Step 3

Enter the Chief complaint by locating the button in the Toolbar labeled "Chief" and clicking on it.

In the dialog window that will open, type "**Daughter reported patient fainted without warning while sitting in a chair, followed by 20 minutes of confusion with difficulty talking**."

Click on the button labeled "Close the note form."

Step 4

The nurse begins the encounter by recording Victoria's vital signs using the Vitals form.

Enter Victoria's vital signs in the corresponding fields on the Form as follows:

Temperature:	**98.2**
Respiration:	**18**
Pulse:	**72**
BP:	**140/96**
Height:	**60**
Weight:	**120**

When you have finished, click on the Encounter tab at the bottom of the screen.

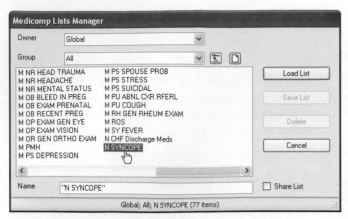

▶ **Figure 5-17 Select N Syncope list from the List Manager.**

Step 5

Because her daughter reported that Victoria fainted, we will use a List created for this type of encounter (syncope).

Locate and click on the Lists button in the Toolbar at the top of your screen (highlighted orange in Figure 5-4).

Scroll the List Manager window to the end of the list to locate and highlight the list named **N Syncope** as shown in Figure 5-17). Click your mouse on the button labeled "Load List."

Step 6

You can verify that the list has been loaded because the first line of the Sx tab in the left pane should read: "Templates (Symptoms)" and there should be an HPI button next to each symptom finding.

Verify the **List Size** is **2**. If it is not, click the ListSize button on the Toolbar repeatedly until the List Size is 2.

Locate and click on the following symptom findings:

- (red button) fainting (syncope)
- (red button) difficulties in speech

Locate the Status field at the bottom of the screen, click the down arrow, and select **improving** from the drop-down list. The description should change to "Speech difficulties which is improving."

Notice that Symptoms recorded in the right pane have been documented in "History of Present Illness" section of the encounter note.

Step 7

Verify that the ROS button on the Toolbar at the top of your screen is blue (off).

Locate and click on the following finding:

- (blue button) difficulty breathing (dyspnea)

Locate and click on small HPI icon button next to the finding "No dyspnea."

The icon should change to "ROS" and the finding in the encounter note (right pane) should move to the "Review of systems" group.

Step 8

Locate and click on the small plus sign next to "Symptoms" at the top of the list.

Locate and click on the following symptom finding:

- (blue button) Head-related symptoms

The description will change to "No head symptoms."

Step 9

Locate and click on the small plus sign next to "Encounter background information" near the top of the list.

Locate and click on the following symptom findings:

- (red button) Family history reviewed

Scroll the list if necessary, to locate and click on the small plus signs next to "Patient accompanied," and "by family member."

Locate and click on the following symptom findings:

- (red button) daughter

Step 10

Click on the Hx tab.

Locate and click on the following history finding:

- (red button) reported previous cardiac problems

Click in the free-text field below the right pane, type **MI 5 years ago**, and then press the Enter key on your keyboard.

Step 11

Locate and click on the following history findings:

- (blue button) taking medication
- (blue button) reported trauma head

Step 12

Click on the Px tab.

Locate and click on the following findings:

- (blue button) Evidence of head injury
- (blue button) Examination of the Lungs
- (blue button) Examination of the Cardiovascular system

Step 13

Locate and click on the small plus signs next to "Examination of the Neurological system," "Level of Consciousness," "Cognitive Functions," and "Orientation" to expand the list.

Beginning beneath Level of Consciousness, work your way down the expanded list locating and clicking the indicated buttons for the following neurological findings:

- (blue button) Drowsy
- (blue button) Confusion
- (blue button) Person
- (blue button) Place
- (blue button) Time
- (blue button) Date
- (red button) Situation

With situation still highlighted, click in the free-text field below the right pane, type: **patient doesn't recall incident** and then press the Enter key on your keyboard.

Step 14

Modify the finding "No Confusion."

Locate the finding "No confusion" in the right pane, note view. Move your mouse over the underlined finding until the mouse pointer changes into the shape of a hand and then click the mouse.

Confirm that the finding "No Confusion" is displayed the left pane on the Edit tab. Modify the finding by clicking the red button.

- (red button) Confusion

Locate the Modifier field at the bottom of the screen, click the down arrow, and select **Mild** from the drop-down list. The description should change to "mild confusion was observed."

Step 15

Click on the Dx tab.

Locate the finding "**Transient Ischemic Attack**" and highlight it.

Locate the Prefix field at the bottom of the screen, click the down arrow and select "Admission diagnosis of" from the drop-down list.

Step 16

Record the Nurse Assessments. The bottom two findings on the Dx tab are Nursing Diagnosis.

Locate and click on the small plus sign next to "RNDx Cerebral Alteration."

Locate and click on the following findings:

- (red button) RNDx Injury Risk
- (red button) RNDx Cerebral alteration
- (red button) RNDx Confusion

Step 17

Click on the Rx tab.

Locate and click on the small plus sign next to "Rn General Care."

Locate and click on the red button for the following findings:

- (red button) Monitor Vital signs
- (red button) Assess perceptions
- (red button) Bed rails check
- (red button) Call light within reach
- (red button) Bed pan/urinal available
- (red button) Patient ID bracelet check
- (red button) Patient allergy check
- (red button) Monitoring patient on fall precautions
- (red button) Monitoring Patient's Mental Status

Step 18

Scroll the list downward to locate and click on the small plus sign next to "Equipment monitoring."

Locate and click on the red button for the following findings:

- (red button) Telemetry Equipment

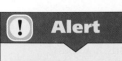

Alert

Do not close or exit the encounter until you have a printed copy in your hand. You will lose your work if you exit before printing.

Step 19

Look at the clock and write down the time you completed the encounter note.

Were you surprised how quickly you completed the complete encounter note?

Click on the Print button on the Toolbar at the top of your screen to invoke the Print Data window.

Be certain there is a check mark in the box next to Current Encounter and then click on the appropriate button to either print or export a file, as directed by your instructor.

Compare your printout or file output to Figure 5-18. If it is correct, hand it in to your instructor. If there are any differences (other than the date or client's age), review the previous steps in the exercise and find your error.

Victoria Mayhew   Page 1 of 1

Student: *your name or id here*
Patient: Victoria Mayhew: F: 1/14/1930: 5/04/2012 04:00PM
Chief complaint
The Chief Complaint is: Daughter reported patient fainted without warning while sitting in a chair, followed by 20 minutes of confusion with difficulty talking.
History of present illness
    Victoria Mayhew is an 82 year old female.
    She reported: Family history reviewed.
    Patient accompanied by daughter.
    Fainting. Speech difficulties which is improving.
    No head symptoms.
Past medical/surgical history
Reported:
    Medical: Cardiac problems MI 5 years ago.
    Medications: Not taking medication.
    Physical Trauma: No trauma to the head.
Review of systems
Pulmonary: No dyspnea.
Physical findings
Vital Signs:

Vital Signs/Measurements	Value	Normal Range
Oral temperature	98.2 F	97.6 - 99.6
RR	18 breaths/min	18 - 26
PR	72 bpm	50 - 100
Blood pressure	140/96 mmHg	100 - 120/56 - 80
Weight	120 lbs	94 - 170
Height	60 in	59.45 - 67.72

Head:
    Injuries: ° No evidence of a head injury.
Lungs:
    ° Normal.
Cardiovascular:
    ° System: normal.
Neurological:
    • Mild confusion was observed. • Disorientation to situation patient doesn't recall incident. ° No drowsiness was observed. ° No disorientation to person. ° No disorientation to place. ° No disorientation to time. ° No disorientation to date.
Assessment
    • Admission diagnosis of transient ischemic attack
    • Injury risk
    • Cerebral alteration
    • Confusion
Therapy
    • Vital signs monitoring performed
    • Perceptions assessment performed
    • The bed rails are checked.
    • The call light is within reach.
    • A bed pan/urinal is available.
    • The ID bracelet is checked.
    • The patient's allergies are checked in the chart.
    • The patient is on fall precautions and is being monitored.
    • The patient's mental status is being monitored.
    • The telemetry equipment is being monitored.

▶ **Figure 5-18 Printed encounter note for Victoria Mayhew.**

The Concept of Forms

In this chapter, you experienced the value in using predesigned lists for specific conditions such as Adult URI and TIA. The other type of template that can speed up data entry is called a Form. You already have worked briefly with Forms, because the Vital Signs screen is actually a form.

Forms are templates that display a desired group of findings in a consistent position every time. Forms enable quick entry of positive and negative findings, as well as Entry Details field data such as value or results.

The Vitals Signs form is a good example. You could enter vitals on the Encounter Px tab by locating and clicking on individual findings on the Px tab, then repositioning your mouse at the bottom of the screen, then entering the value and unit of measurement for each vital sign. This would obviously be a time-consuming way to do it. As you have already experienced, vitals are much easier to enter using the Vitals form on which all the necessary findings are arranged with the value fields ready for data entry and the unit of measurement fields preset.

The Vitals form is only a very small example of what can be done with forms. Complete multipage forms can be created that make it fast and easy to document standard types of assessments.

Comparison of Lists and Forms

The value of lists is that they are dynamic and expand as necessary. A side effect of this is that sometimes findings do not appear on the screen, because they are in the nonexpanded portion of the tree, or the user must scroll the List to find them.

Forms, however, are static. Findings have a fixed position on the form and will remain in that location every time the form is used.

Lists arrange findings in the appropriate tab (Sx, Hx, Px, Tx, Dx, and Rx), but this means that nurses must change tabs as they work through the encounter. This is not a limitation with forms. The form designer is free to put any finding anywhere on the form. This allows each form to be designed to allow the quickest entry of data for a particular type of encounter. For example, if a nurse routinely enters the Chief complaint and records the client's symptoms at the same time she or he takes the vital signs, these could all be placed on one page of the form, even though the findings will appear in three different sections of the note.

Forms offer many additional features. These include check boxes, drop-down lists, and most of the fields in the Entry Details section. Free-text boxes in a form can be preassigned to a finding; therefore, they do not require the user to locate a free-text finding to record comments.

Forms may include the necessary fields required to meet regulatory requirements and the forms designer has the option to require entry of data for certain findings before the form can be closed.

Initial Intake Form for an Adult

The intake form used in the following exercise provides an example of different designs and features that are possible with forms. These include the unique ability to record two types of history at once, the Auto Negative feature, and other features you will explore during the exercise.

Figure 5-19 is an example of a form that might be found in any medical facility that uses paper medical records. You have probably been asked to fill out a similar form sometime in the past. As you complete the following exercise, notice the similarities

Memorial Hospital
Anytown, USA

Patient Name: _____
Date of Birth:
☐ Male   ☐ Female

Date: _____

Race: _____

What is the reason you are here today?

_____
_____

Please check any of the following conditions which you have had

General
☐ Serious Infections
   (e.g. pneumonia)
☐ Diabetes Mellitus
☐ Rheumatic fever
☐ HIV Infection
☐ Cancer

Cardiovascular
☐ High Blood Pressure
☐ Congestive Heart failure
☐ Heart Murmur
☐ Heart Valve Disease
☐ Angina
☐ Heart Attack
☐ High Cholesterol
☐ Abnormal Heart Rhythm
☐ Blood Clot in Veins
☐ Blocked Arteries in Neck
☐ Blocked Arteries in Legs

HEENT
☐ Glaucoma
☐ Allergies "hay fever"
☐ Frequent Ear Infections
☐ Frequent Sinus Infections

Respiratory
☐ Asthma
☐ Emphysema
☐ Blood Clot in Lungs
☐ Sleep Apnea

Musculoskeletal /
Extremities
☐ Osteoporosis
☐ Rheumatoid Arthritis
☐ Degenerative Joint Disease
☐ Fibromyalgia
☐ Neck Pain (herniated disk)
☐ Back Pain (herniated disc)

GI/GU
☐ Stomach Ulcers
☐ Ulcerative Colitis
☐ Crohns Disease
☐ Bleeding from Intestines
☐ Diverticulitis
☐ Colon Polyps
☐ Irritable Bowel Disease
☐ Hepatitis
☐ Cirrhosis of the liver
☐ Liver Failure
☐ Pancreatitis
☐ Gallstones
☐ Kidney Stones
☐ Kidney Failure
☐ Prostate Disease
☐ Endometriosis
☐ Sex Transmitted Infection

Lymphatic / Hematologic
☐ Thyroid Goiter
☐ Over Active Thyroid
☐ Under Active Thyroid
☐ Transfusions
☐ Anemia

Skin / Breast
☐ Acne
☐ Eczema
☐ Psoriasis
☐ Fibrocystic Breast Disease

Neurological / Psychiatric
☐ Chronic Vertigo (Meniere's)
☐ Peripheral Nerve Disease
☐ Migraine Headaches
☐ Stroke
☐ Multiple Sclerosis
☐ Depression
☐ Anxiety

Please check any of the following major illnesses in your family members:

☐ Tuberculosis
☐ Emphysema
☐ Heart Disease
☐ High Blood Pressure
☐ Osteoporosis

☐ Diabetes Mellitus
☐ Thyroid Disease
☐ Anemia
☐ Hemophilia
☐ Other _____

☐ Kidney Disease
☐ Epilepsy
☐ Neurological Disorder
☐ Liver Disease
☐ Other _____

☐ Breast Cancer
☐ Ovarian Cancer
☐ Colon Cancer
☐ Prostate Cancer
☐ Other _____

If you have had surgery please indicate the year:

Year	Surgery	Year	Surgery	Year	Surgery	Year	Surgery
____	Angioplasty	____	Colonoscopy	____	Neurosurgery	____	Tubal ligation
____	Appendectomy	____	Coronary Bypass	____	Sinus Surgery	____	C-Section
____	Back or Neck Surgery	____	Ear Surgery	____	Stomach Surgery	____	Hysterectomy
____	Bladder Surgery	____	Gallbladder	____	Thyroid Surgery	____	Ovary Removed
____	Carotid Artery Surgery	____	Hip Surgery	____	Tonsillectomy	____	Breast Surgery
____	Carpal Tunnel Surgery	____	Inguinal Hernia	____	Trauma Related Surgery	____	Thyroid Surgery
____	Chest/lung Surgery	____	Knee Surgery	____	Vascular Surgery	____	Other

Please indicate when you had the following preventative services:

Date	Immunizations	Date	Tests	Date	Tests / Exams	Date	Tests / Exams
____	Flu Vaccine	____	Chest X-ray	____	Colon Cancer Stool Test	____	Breast Exam
____	Hepatitis Vaccine	____	EKG	____	Flexible Sigmoidoscopy,	____	Mammogram
____	Pneumonia Vaccine	____	Echocardiogram	____	Rectal Exam	____	Pap Smear
____	Tetanus Booster	____	Stress Test	____	Barium Enema	____	Bone Density Test
____	Other	____	Cardiac	____	Prostate Cancer Blood	____	Date of last Physical
			Angiogram		Test		Exam

Personal Habits

Tobacco
☐ Never
☐ Previous user
☐ Current user
packs per day _____

Alcohol
☐ Never
☐ Previous user
☐ Current user
drinks per day _____

Caffeine
☐ Never
☐ Previous user
☐ Current user
cups per day _____

Illicit Drugs
☐ Never
☐ Previous user
☐ Current user

▶ **Figure 5-19 Sample Intake Form from a paper chart.**

between this paper form and the EHR form. Electronic forms are one of the easiest ways to use an EHR.

Guided Exercise 35: Using Forms

In this exercise, you will use an EHR form to record symptoms, history, and a physical exam. The EHR form, in this case, has been abridged to shorten the time it takes a student to complete the exercise; a full version of the form as it is used in a medical facility would have much more detail. A short intake form might be used by a nurse for prescreening.

Case Study

Terry Chun is a 31- year-old female complaining of an excruciating headache lasting greater than one week. She is being admitted for status migrainosus.

Step 1

If you have not already done so, start the Student Edition software.

Click Select on the Menu bar, and then click Patient.

In the Patient Selection window, locate and click on **Terry Chun** as shown in Figure 5-20.

Step 2

Click Select on the Menu bar again, and then click New Encounter.

Use the current date and time. Select the reason **Headaches** from the drop-down list. Click on the OK button.

Step 3

Enter the Chief complaint by locating the button in the Toolbar labeled "Chief" and clicking on it.

In the dialog window that opens, type "**Severe headaches**."

Compare your screen to Figure 5-21 before clicking on the button labeled "Close the note form."

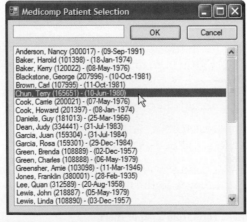

▶ **Figure 5-20 Selecting Terry Chun from the Patient Selection window.**

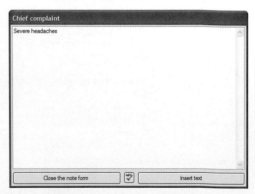

▶ **Figure 5-21 Chief complaint "Severe headaches."**

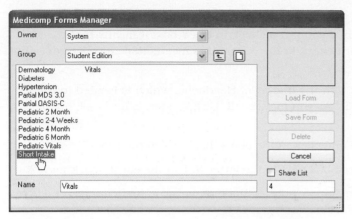

▶ **Figure 5-22 Select Short Intake in Forms Manager window.**

Step 4

Click on the Forms button in the Toolbar at the top of the screen.

In the Forms Manager window, select the Form labeled "Short Intake," as shown in Figure 5-22. The Short Intake form shown in Figure 5-23 will be displayed.

Step 5

Compare your screen to Figure 5-23. Take a few minutes to study the form on your screen.

Note that at the top of the form there are tabs labeled "Review of Systems," "Medical History," "Physical Examination," and "Outline View." This form has three pages on which you may enter data. In subsequent steps, you will use each of these pages to explore the features of this form.

▶ **Figure 5-23 Short Intake Form—Review of Symptoms tab.**

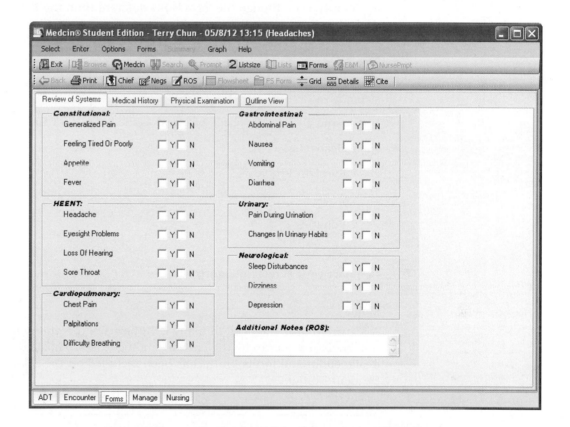

Probably what you first noticed are columns of check boxes with Y and N next to them. This is very similar to a paper form and very intuitive. With almost no training, people understand Y means yes and N means no.

Check boxes work very simply, here is how:

✓ If you click your mouse on an empty box, a check mark appears. The finding will be recorded.

✓ If you change your mind and click in the opposite box, the check mark moves to the box you just clicked.

✓ If you do not want either box checked, click on whichever box already has the check mark and you will be asked to confirm that you want the finding removed (as shown in Figure 5-24).

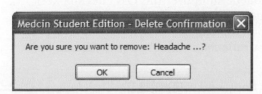

▶ **Figure 5-24 Confirmation that you want to remove a finding.**

Step 6

On the Review of Symptoms tab, if you put a check in the Y box, it means that the client has that symptom. If you put check in the N box, this means that the client does not have that symptom.

Practice using the check boxes with the finding of Headache, which is located in the section of the form labeled "HEENT." As you may recall, HEENT stands for head, eyes, ears, nose and throat.

Locate the finding of Headache and click in the check box next to the letter **Y**.

Now click the mouse in the check box next to the letter **N**. Did the check mark move?

Although you cannot see the encounter note at this moment, you just changed the note from the "headache" to "No headache."

Click the mouse again in the same box that already has the check mark in it; this should be next to the letter **N**. The confirmation message shown in Figure 5-24 should appear. Click on the OK button. Both check boxes should now be empty.

Remember, even though the form looks different than the Encounter tab, you really are adding and removing findings on the encounter note when you work with the form.

Step 7

Terry reports that she has headaches, vision problems, nausea, vomiting, and trouble sleeping.

Locate and click in the check box next to the letter **Y** for the following findings:

✓ **Y** Headache

✓ **Y** Eyesight Problems

✓ **Y** Nausea

✓ **Y** Vomiting

✓ **Y** Sleep Disturbances

Compare your screen to Figure 5-25.

Step 8

A feature that is included in many EHR forms is the ability to see where in the nomenclature hierarchy the current finding exists. This feature is not necessarily designed into all forms, but it has been included on the Short Intake form for the Student Edition.

> **Note** — **Left and Right Mouse Buttons**   A computer mouse typically has at least two buttons—we will refer to these as the "left-click" and "right-click" buttons. In this step, you will use the right-click button.

Position the mouse pointer over the word "Headache" (not over the Y/N check boxes). The finding will become highlighted in white and the mouse pointer will change shape to include a question mark. When your mouse pointer looks like the one circled in red in Figure 5-26, click the **right-click button** on your mouse. A small pane of Medcin findings will open in the middle of the form.

The Nomenclature pane shows the highlighted finding in context of the Medcin tree structure. When the Nomenclature pane is displayed, you can expand the tree structure as well as select additional or different findings.

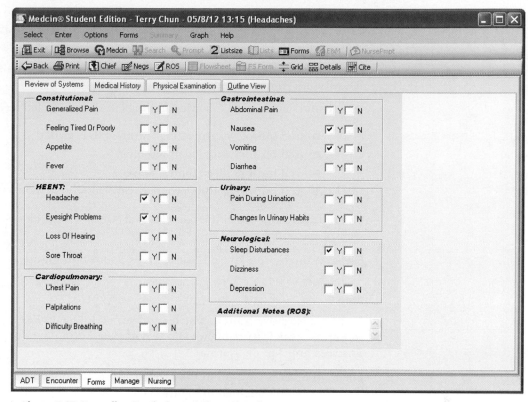

▶ **Figure 5-25 Recording Headache and Sleep Disturbances.**

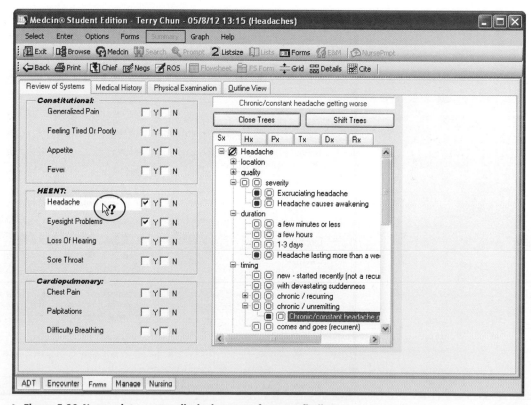

▶ **Figure 5-26 Nomenclature pane displaying tree of current finding.**

One reason for invoking the Medcin tree is to locate a more specific finding. In the previous step, you recorded the finding "Headache," but the client elaborates further.

Expand the tree for "Headache" by clicking on the small plus signs next to "Severity," "Duration," "Timing," and "Chronic/Unremitting."

Locate and click on the following findings in the expanded tree:

- (red button) excruciating - worse I've ever had
- (red button) causing awakening
- (red button) more than a week
- (red button) getting progressively worse

The button at the top of the pane labeled "Close Trees" closes the pane to restore your view of the entire form.

Click on the button labeled "Close Trees" (shown in Figure 5-26 outlined in orange).

Step 9

The Auto Negative button, which you learned to use in Exercise 33, also can be enabled in Forms. This feature allows you to complete Form pages quickly whenever most of the answers are "No" or "Normal."

Locate the "Negs" button in the Toolbar at the top of your form. Click your mouse on the Negs button (highlighted in Figure 5-27).

Compare your screen to Figure 5-27. Note what happened. Note that Auto Negative does not alter findings that are already recorded, such as "Headache," "Eyesight Problems," and "Sleep Disturbances."

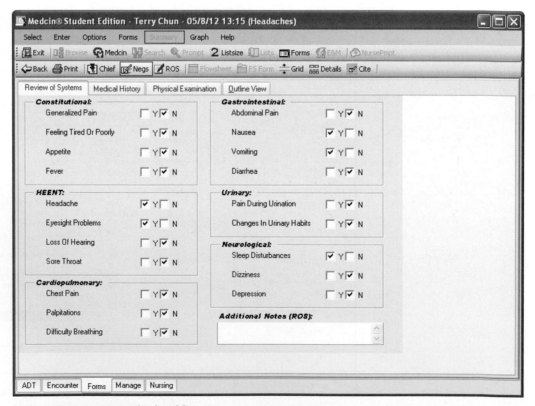

▶ **Figure 5-27 Auto Negative in a form.**

Step 10

Forms also can allow entry of free-text notes right on the form. This saves the nurse the time it takes to add notes to Entry Details, or open free-text findings. In this step, add a clinical impression to the ROS findings.

In the box at the bottom of your screen labeled "Additional Notes ROS," type the following text: **Patient denies depression but seems very sad**.

Compare your screen to Figure 5-28 before proceeding.

▶ **Figure 5-28 Free-text clinical impressions in a form.**

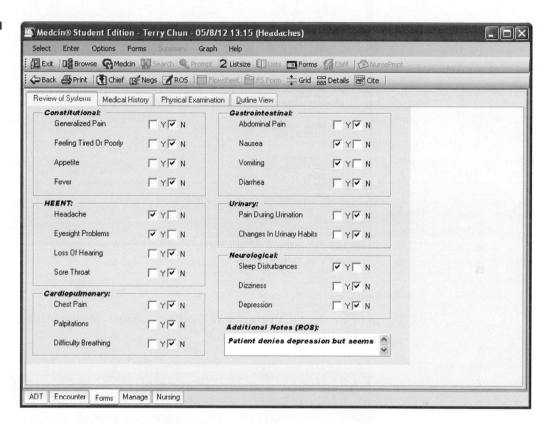

Step 11

During the course of this exercise, you have been recording findings in the encounter note with every click of your mouse on the form, but you cannot see them as you can on the Encounter tab.

In Forms, the Outline View tab allows you to take a quick look at the findings you have selected for the encounter note. Before entering data in the rest of the form, take a moment to look at what has been entered so far.

Locate and click on the tab labeled "Outline View" at the top of your form (circled in red in Figure 5-29).

The Outline View shows small folders for each section of the encounter. The small folder icons are the Finding Group titles you normally see in the encounter note.

Click the small plus sign next to the folder icons to expand them to show the findings.

Compare your screen to Figure 5-29. The Outline View uses blue text when the findings are negative or normal and red text when they are positive or abnormal. Notice under "Headache" the additional findings that you entered from the tree view.

Scroll the outline downward to locate the "Review of Systems" folder. Notice the free-text note you added in the previous step.

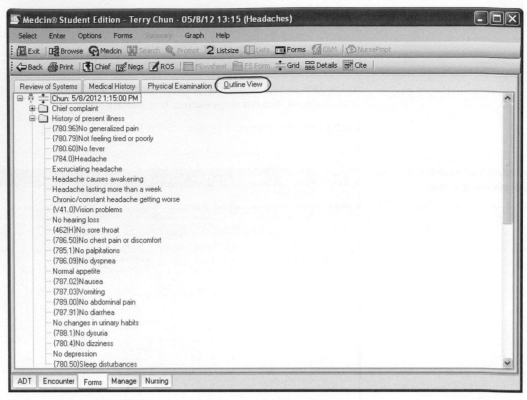

▶ **Figure 5-29 Outline View.**

Step 12

Locate the tab at the top of the form labeled "Medical History" (circled in red in Figure 5-30), and click on it.

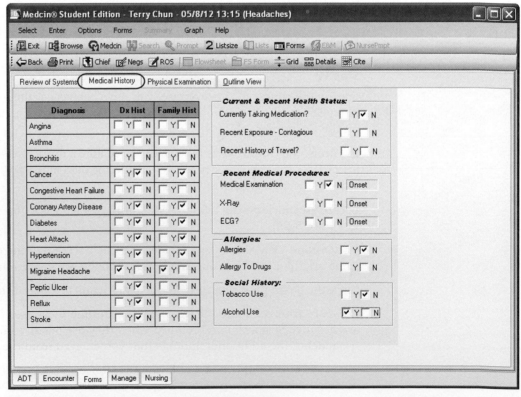

▶ **Figure 5-30 Medical History page of Short Intake Form.**

This page illustrates another advantage of forms. Normally, when you do an intake history for a client, you go through many items twice: "Have you ever had a heart attack? Has anyone in your family ever had a heart attack?" On this page, the form has been designed to save the nurse time, by making it easy to record answers to either personal, family history, or both types of history questions in two columns. Compare the information on this tab of the EHR form with the paper form in Figure 5-19.

Step 13

Sometimes clients do not know the medical history of other family members; therefore, you will only record findings the client is sure about. As the nurse asks Ms. Chun the history questions, she will only know the answer to some of them.

Enter the Dx History and Family History only for the following items:

Diagnosis	Dx Hist	Family History
Cancer	✓ N	✓ N
Coronary Artery Disease	✓ N	✓ N
Diabetes	✓ N	✓ N
Heart Attack	✓ N	✓ N
Hypertension	✓ N	✓ N
Migraine	✓ Y	✓ Y
Peptic Ulcer	✓ N	
Reflux	✓ N	
Stroke	✓ N	

Complete the rest of her medical history in the right side of the form by locating and clicking on the check boxes as follows:

Currently Taking Medication	✓ N
Recent Medical Examination	✓ N
Allergies	✓ N
Tobacco	✓ N
Alcohol	✓ Y

Carefully compare your screen to Figure 5-30 before proceeding.

Step 14

Locate the tab at the top of the form labeled "Physical Examination" (circled in red in Figure 5-31), and click on it.

The first thing you will notice about this page is that it includes the Vital Signs (in the upper left corner of the page). Recording vital signs as part of the intake physical saves the time it would take to load the Vitals form separately. This page illustrates how forms can combine many different elements to make data entry more convenient.

▶ **Figure 5-31 Physical Exam page of Short Intake Form.**

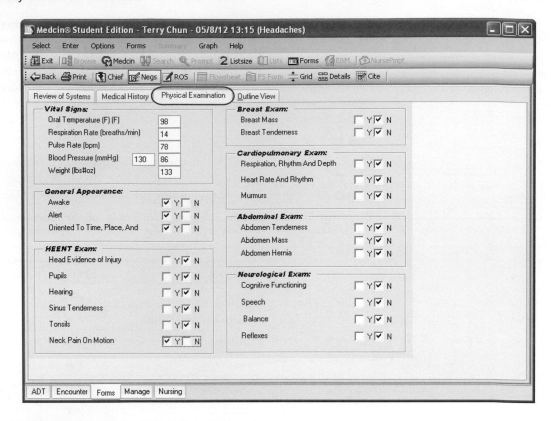

Enter the following vital signs for Terry Chun:

Temperature:	**98**
Respiration:	**14**
Pulse:	**78**
BP:	**130/86**
Weight:	**133**

Step 15

During the physical, the nurse observes the client has neck pain elicited by motion. Locate the finding **Neck pain on motion** and click the check box for **Y**.

Everything else is normal. Click on the button labeled "Negs" on the Toolbar at the top of your screen (highlighted in Figure 5-31).

Remember you can use the "Negs" button to quickly document "normals" on Symptoms and Physical Exam findings.

Compare your screen to Figure 5-31.

Did you see that the findings in the General Appearance group were checked Y instead of N by the Auto Negative feature? That is because for some findings such as these, the normal state is to be awake, alert, and oriented. If these were checked No, the condition would be abnormal. The Auto Negative feature is really an Auto Normal feature.

Step 16

Click on the Encounter tab at the bottom of your screen, to view the full text of the encounter note that was completed from within the form.

Click on the Dx tab in the left pane and enter an admitting diagnosis.

Locate and expand the tree for "Neurologic Disorders," "Headache Syndromes," and "History of migraine headache."

Locate and highlight the finding "status migrainosus."

Locate and click on the down arrow button in the Entry Details Prefix field and select "Admission diagnosis of"; the description should change to "Admission diagnosis of status migrainosus."

Compare your screen to Figure 5-32. Scroll the right pane upward so that you can view the entire contents of the note.

This exercise was intended to demonstrate how forms can be used to speed through pages of routine questions and provide the convenience of free-text or Entry Details fields as part of the form. Although the exercise does not create a medically complete intake history and assessment, you have successfully completed the goals of this exercise.

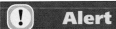 **Alert**

> *Do not close or exit the encounter until you have a printed copy in your hand.* **You will lose your work if you exit before printing.**

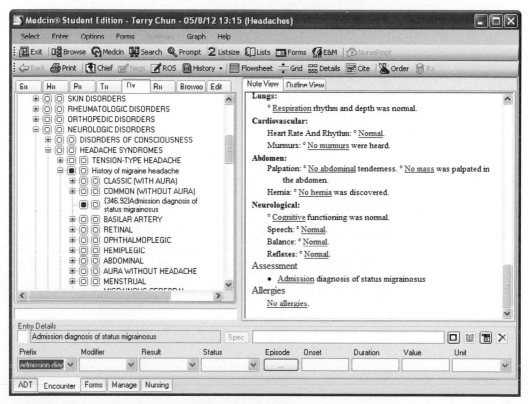

▶ **Figure 5-32 Encounter (in right pane) entered using a form.**

Step 17

Click on the Print button on the Toolbar at the top of your screen to invoke the Print Data window.

Be certain there is a check mark in the box next to "Current Encounter" and then click on the appropriate button to either print or export a file, as directed by your instructor.

Student: *your name or id here*
Patient: Terry Chun: F: 6/10/1980: 5/08/2012 01:15PM
Chief complaint
The Chief Complaint is: Severe headaches.
History of present illness
     Terry Chun is a 31 year old female.
     She reported: Headache is excruciating - 'worst I ever had', causing
     awakening, lasting for more than a week, and chronic/unremitting getting
     progressively worse. Vision problems.
     Normal appetite. Nausea and vomiting. No abdominal pain and no diarrhea.
     No depression. Sleep disturbances.
     No generalized pain, not feeling tired or poorly, and no fever. No hearing
     loss and no sore throat. No chest pain or discomfort and no palpitations.
     No dyspnea. No changes in urinary habits and no dysuria. No dizziness.
Past medical/surgical history
Reported History:
     Medical: No recent medical examination.
     Medications: Not taking medication.
Diagnosis History:
     No coronary artery disease
     No acute myocardial infarction.
     No hypertension.
     No esophageal reflux
     No peptic ulcer.
     No diabetes mellitus.
     Migraine headache.
     No stroke syndrome.
     No cancer
Personal history
     Behavioral: No tobacco use.
     Alcohol: Alcohol use.
Family history
     No coronary artery disease
     No acute myocardial infarction
     No hypertension
     No diabetes mellitus
     Migraine headache
     No cancer.
Review of systems
Patient denies depression but seems very sad.
Physical findings
Vital Signs:

Vital Signs/Measurements	Value	Normal Range
Oral temperature	98 F	97.6 - 99.6
RR	14 breaths/min	18 - 26
PR	78 bpm	50 - 100
Blood pressure	130/86 mmHg	100 - 120/56 - 80
Weight	133 lbs	98 - 183

General Appearance:
     °~Awake. °~Alert. °~Oriented to time, place, and person.
Head:
     Injuries: °~No evidence of a head injury.
Neck:
     Maneuvers: •~Neck pain was elicited by motion.
Eyes:
     General/bilateral:
     Pupils: °~Normal.

Continued on the following page…

▶ **Figure 5-33a Printout of encounter note for Terry Chun created using a form (Page 1 of 2).**

Terry Chun   Page 2 of 2

Ears:
     General/bilateral:
     Hearing: °~No hearing abnormalities.
Nose:
     General/bilateral:
     Sinus Tenderness: °~No sinus tenderness.
Pharynx:
     Oropharynx: °~Tonsils showed no abnormalities.
Breasts:
     General/bilateral:
     °~No breast mass was found. °~No tenderness of the breast.
Lungs:
      °~Respiration rhythm and depth was normal.
Cardiovascular:
      Heart Rate And Rhythm: °~Normal.
      Murmurs: ° No murmurs were heard.
Abdomen:
     Palpation: °~No abdominal tenderness. °~No mass was palpated in the abdomen.
     Hernia: °~No hernia was discovered.
Neurological:
     °~Cognitive functioning was normal.
     Speech: °~Normal.
     Balance: °~Normal.
     Reflexes: °~Normal.
Assessment
     •~Admission diagnosis of status migrainosus
Allergies
     No allergies.

▶ **Figure 5-33b Printout of encounter note for Terry Chun created using a form (Page 2 of 2).**

Compare your printout or file output to Figure 5-33. (Note your computer will print out two pages; the page breaks vary by printer and may not be in the same place as the figure in the book. However, the contents should be the same except for the encounter date and client's age.) If your work is correct, hand it in to your instructor. If there are any differences, review the previous steps in the exercise and find your error.

Customized Forms

Forms are not limited to the pages used in this exercise. Forms, as discussed earlier, also allow you to organize questions in the order you would ask them, regardless of where the findings may be grouped in the Medcin Nomenclature hierarchy.

Forms can be designed to include pages for any of the findings expected to be needed for a particular type of client encounter. For example, a therapy page is an excellent means of having quick access to standard treatments for specific conditions.

Medical facilities that have a large number of forms customized for their providers succeed very well in implementing an EHR. Form Design tools are a part of almost every EHR system on the market. Forms take longer for the designer to create than Lists, but if well constructed, make it significantly easier to document in real-time. Figure 5-34 shows an actual form created and used daily at an obstetrics and gynecology practice.

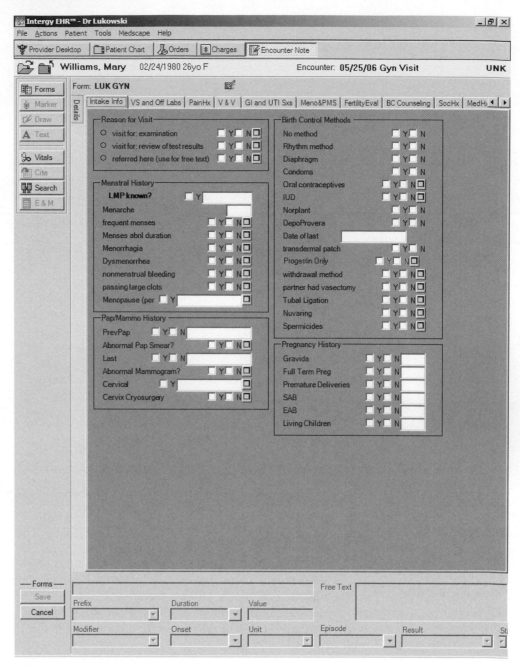

▶ **Figure 5-34 Intake tab of gynecology form.**

By Jayne Deal, RN

I work at a busy pediatrics practice. Our six pediatricians and two nurse practitioners see about 30 to 35 clients per day per provider. We have had our EHR system for a couple of years, but we finally went completely paperless about five months ago. Now all of our client visits are documented using EHR forms.

We have several different forms for well checks based on the child's age. We also have different forms for sick visits, attention deficit hyperactivity disorder (ADHD), and several other specialized forms for things like trauma that we don't have to use very often. On the well checks each of them are different; the ones we use for babies are different from one we would use for a 6- or 12-year-old.

I think using a form is very easy. On each form there are multiple tabs for symptoms, history, feeding questions, developmental milestones, and vitals. I complete those and then the doctor completes the exam tab.

One feature I like is that when I type free text in the comments area on some of our forms, the check box gets automatically checked on its own. As an example, instead of checking the yes box for current medications and then typing the medication in the form, when I just type the medication name, the Yes box is automatically checked.

Our practice administrator knows how to modify our forms as we identify additional questions or features we would like to have on the form. It is helpful that she can do it for us because we are still in the process of tweaking some of the forms to make the data entry more streamlined.

Obviously, with well check visits, immunizations are important. Immunization schedules in our EHR allow us to compare what vaccines the child has had to the CDC-recommended immunization schedule. We haven't loaded all our past client records on the EHR, so for older children we have to check the Florida Shots system and our old records. That process is slowing us down right now, but for children born since we went totally on the EHR, all the information is in there already.

Once the provider sees what vaccines that the child needs, there is a place on the form to check off the vaccines that will be given. So, we can order what is required right from the form by going to the immunizations section and ordering the vaccines—then we can administer them.

I also have spent some time at a large teaching hospital that uses a different EHR. In their system security settings prevent the nurse from entering orders. In our practice nurses have more autonomy and I can enter the pediatrician's orders for the vaccines, speeding the process and streamlining the visit for the child.

We can also generate growth charts from the EHR to give the parents. It is a great tool for showing them their child's development, and the computer takes the human error out of plotting the graph. We are also using the EHR to graph the child's body mass index, and we give that to the parents as well.

Critical Thinking Exercise 36: Using a Form and a List

In this exercise, you will use both the form and the list from the previous exercises. Using what you have learned so far, document Mr. Green's hospital admission.

Case Study

Charles Green is a 33-year-old male with a complaint of a new-onset, frequent cough that is progressively worse, especially at night. His chest hurts when he coughs and sometimes he vomits because of the coughing. Mr. Green was previously seen at his doctor's office and diagnosed with acute sinusitis. His condition has deteriorated. He is being admitted to the hospital for acute bronchitis.

Step 1

If you have not already done so, start the Student Edition software.

Click Select on the Menu bar, and then click Patient.

In the Patient Selection window, locate and click on Charles Green.

Step 2

Click Select on the Menu bar, and then click New Encounter.

Select the reason **Hospital Inpatient** from the drop-down list.

Make sure you have selected the reason correctly. You may use the current date for this exercise.

Step 3

Enter the Chief complaint by locating the button in the Toolbar labeled "Chief" and clicking on it.

In the dialog window that will open, type "**Recurrent cough and dyspnea**."

Click on the button labeled "Close the note form."

Step 4

Click on the Forms button in the Toolbar at the top of the screen.

In the Forms Manager window, select the Form labeled "Short Intake."

Step 5

The client reports that he is feeling poorly, and has a fever, headaches, chest pain, difficulty breathing, and trouble sleeping.

On the tab labeled "Review of Symptoms," locate and click in the check box next to the letter **Y** for the following findings:

✓ **Y** Feeling Tired or Poorly

✓ **Y** Fever

✓ **Y** Headache

✓ **Y** Chest Pain

✓ **Y** Difficulty Breathing

✓ **Y** Vomiting

✓ **Y** Sleep Disturbance

Step 6

Locate and click on the "Negs" button in the Toolbar at the top of your form.

All items on the Review of Symptoms tab should now have a check in either the Y or N boxes.

Step 7

Locate the tab at the top of the form labeled "Medical History."

Locate the finding "**Currently Taking Medication**" and click in the check box next to the letter **Y**.

Position the mouse pointer over the finding description "Currently Taking Medication" (not over the Y/N check boxes) and click the **right-click button** on your mouse.

Scroll the list of Medcin findings that opened on the left of the form, to locate and click on the plus sign next to "over-the-counter medications." Click on the following finding:

● (red button) for colds

Click on the button labeled "Close Trees" at the top of the pane.

Step 8

Locate the finding "Allergies" and click in the check box next to the letter **N**.

Locate the finding "Tobacco use" and click in the check box next to the letter **Y**.

Step 9

Enter the Dx History and Family History only for the following items:

Diagnosis	Dx Hist	Family Hist
Cancer	✓ N	✓ N
Coronary Artery Disease	✓ N	✓ N
Diabetes	✓ N	✓ N
Heart Attack	✓ N	✓ N
Hypertension	✓ N	
Migraine	✓ N	
Peptic Ulcer	✓ N	
Reflux	✓ N	
Stroke	✓ N	

Step 10

Locate the tab at the top of the form labeled "Physical Examination."

Enter Mr. Green's vital signs in the corresponding fields as follows:

Temperature:	**101**
Respiration:	**26**
Pulse:	**88**
BP:	**130/86**
Weight:	**170**

Step 11

On the Physical Examination tab, locate and click in the check box next to the letter **Y** for the following findings:

✓ **Y** Sinus Tenderness

✓ **Y** Neck Pain On Motion

✓ **Y** Respiration Rhythm And Depth

Locate and click on the "Negs" button in the Toolbar at the top of your form.

All items on the Physical Examination tab should now have data.

Step 12

Locate and click on the Encounter tab at the bottom of your screen to return to the encounter view.

Locate and click on the Lists button in the Toolbar at the top of your screen. The List Manager window will be invoked.

Locate and highlight the list named Adult URI. Click your mouse on the button labeled "Load List."

Step 13

You can verify that the list has been loaded because the first line of the Sx tab in the left pane should read "Templates (Symptoms)" and there should be an HPI button next to each symptom finding.

Locate and click on the following symptom findings:

- (red button) sinus pain
- (red button) cough
- (red button) coughing up sputum

Locate and click the small plus sign next to "Cough."

Locate and click the findings:

- (red button) worse at night
- (red button) causing awakening from sleep

Step 14

Locate and click on the ROS button in the Toolbar at the top of your form. Verify that the ROS button is orange.

Locate and click on the Negs button in the Toolbar at the top of your form.

Step 15

Click on the Hx tab. Locate and click on the following History findings:

- (red button) Recent upper respiratory infection (URI)
- (red button) current smoker

In the Value field at the bottom of your screen, type the number **20**.

Step 16

Click on the Dx tab to document a history of Sinusitis.

Locate and highlight **Sinusitis Acute**.

Locate and click on the down arrow button in the Prefix field. Select "**Recurrent history of**" from the drop-down list.

Step 17

Click on the Px tab to document the physical exam.

Locate and click on the following Physical Exam findings:

- (red button) Wheezing
- (red button) Rhonchi

Locate and click on the small plus sign next to "Respiratory movements" to expand the tree.

Locate and click on the following Physical Exam finding:

- (red button) Exaggerated Use Of Accessory Muscles For Inspiration

Locate and click on the Negs button in the Toolbar at the top of your form.

Step 18

Click on the Dx tab and then locate and highlight the finding **acute bronchitis**.

Locate the Entry Details Prefix field, click on the down arrow button and select "Admission diagnosis of" as you have in previous exercises. This will record the encounter note assessment.

Step 19

Click on the Rx tab.

Scroll down to Nursing Care and then locate and click on the following nursing interventions and nursing actions:

- (red button) RNRx Oxygen therapy care
- (red button) RNRx Pulmonary care
- (red button) RNOx Assess respiratory status
- (red button) RNOx Monitor lung sounds
- (red button) RNOx Assess sputum appearance
- (red button) RNOx Monitor Oxygen saturation
- (red button) RNOx Titrate O2 to maintain saturation value
- (red button) RNOx Provide oxygen therapy
- (red button) RNOx Teach inhaler instruction
- (red button) RNOx Collaborate with respiratory therapist

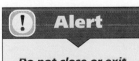
Alert

Do not close or exit the encounter until you have a printed copy in your hand. You will lose your work if you exit before printing.

Step 20

Click on the Print button on the Toolbar at the top of your screen to invoke the Print Data window.

Be certain there is a check mark in the box next to "Current Encounter" and then click on the appropriate button to either print or export a file, as directed by your instructor.

Compare your printout or file output to Figure 5-35. (Note your computer will print out two pages; the page breaks vary by printer and may not be in the same place as the figure in the book. However, the contents should be the same except for the encounter date and client's age.) If your work is correct, hand it in to your instructor. If there are any differences, review the previous steps in the exercise and find your error.

Charles Green   Page 1 of 2

Student: *your name or id here*
Patient: Charles Green: M: 5/06/1979: 5/08/2012 01:45PM
Chief complaint
The Chief Complaint is: Recurrent cough and dyspnea.
History of present illness
      Charles Green is a 33 year old male.
      He reported: No generalized pain. Feeling tired or poorly and fever.
      Headache and sinus pain.
      Chest pain or discomfort. No palpitations.
      Dyspnea, cough worse at night, causing awakening from sleep, and coughing
      up sputum.
      Normal appetite and no nausea. Vomiting. No abdominal pain and no
      diarrhea.
      No depression. Sleep disturbances.
      No vision problems. No hearing loss and no sore throat. No changes in
      urinary habits and no dysuria. No dizziness.
Past medical/surgical history
Reported:
      Medical: A recent URI.
      Medications: Taking over-the-counter cold medication.
Diagnoses:
      Recurrent history of acute sinusitis.
      No coronary artery disease
      No acute myocardial infarction.
      No hypertension.
      No esophageal reflux
      No peptic ulcer.
      No diabetes mellitus.
      No migraine headache
      No stroke syndrome.
      No cancer
Personal history
Behavioral: Current smoker was 20 years.
Family history
      No coronary artery disease
      No acute myocardial infarction
      No diabetes mellitus
      No cancer.
Review of systems
Systemic: No chills.
Neck: No swollen glands in the neck.
Otolaryngeal: No earache, no discharge from the ears, no nasal discharge, and no
nasal passage blockage.
Pulmonary: No hemoptysis.
Musculoskeletal: No muscle aches.
Physical findings
Vital Signs:

Vital Signs/Measurements	Value	Normal Range
Oral temperature	101 F	97.6 - 99.6
RR	26 breaths/min	18 - 26
PR	88 bpm	50 - 100
Blood pressure	130/86 mmHg	100-120/60-80
Weight	170 lbs	125 - 225

General Appearance:
      ° Awake. ° Alert. ° Oriented to time, place, and person.
Head:
      Injuries: ° No evidence of a head injury.

Continued on the following page…

▶ **Figure 5-35a Printed encounter note for Charles Green's hospital intake (page 1 of 2).**

Neck:
  Maneuvers: • Neck pain was elicited by motion.
Eyes:
  General/bilateral:
  Pupils: ° Normal.
Ears:
  General/bilateral:
  Hearing: ° No hearing abnormalities.
Nose:
  General/bilateral:
  Discharge: ° No nasal discharge seen.
  Cavity: ° Nasal septum normal. ° Nasal turbinate not swollen.
  Sinus Tenderness: • Tenderness of sinuses.
Pharynx:
  Oropharynx: ° Tonsils showed no abnormalities.
  Mucosal: ° Pharynx was not inflamed.
Lymph Nodes:
  ° Normal.
Breasts:
  General/bilateral:
  ° No breast mass was found. ° No tenderness of the breast.
Lungs:
  • Respiration rhythm and depth was abnormal. • Exaggerated use of accessory
  muscles for inspiration was observed. • Wheezing was heard. • Rhonchi were
  heard. ° Chest was normal to percussion. ° No rales/crackles were heard.
Cardiovascular:
  Heart Rate And Rhythm: ° Normal.
  Murmurs: ° No murmurs were heard.
Abdomen:
  Palpation: ° No abdominal tenderness. ° No mass was palpated in the abdomen.
  Hernia: ° No hernia was discovered.
Neurological:
  ° Cognitive functioning was normal.
  Speech: ° Normal.
  Balance: ° Normal.
  Reflexes: ° Normal.
Assessment
  • Admission diagnosis of acute bronchitis
Therapy
  • Oxygen therapy care
  • Pulmonary care
  • Respiratory status assessment performed
  • Lung sounds monitoring performed
  • Sputum appearance assessment performed
  • Oxygen saturation monitoring performed
  • O2 titration to maintain saturation value performed
  • Oxygen therapy provision performed
  • Teaching of inhaler instructions performed
  • Collaboration with respiratory therapist performed
Allergies
  No allergies.

▶ **Figure 5-35b Printed encounter note for Charles Green's hospital intake (page 2 of 2).**

Chapter Five Summary

In this chapter, you used to use Lists and Forms. Lists are selected from the List Manager window. Forms are selected from the Form Manager window. Both windows are invoked by clicking buttons on the Toolbar.

Forms   Invokes the Forms Manager window from which you may select and load a form as you have in previous chapters.

List   Invokes the List Manager window from which you may select and load a list.

List Size   Increases or decreases the number of findings in the displayed list. List Sizes are 1 to 3.

Lists allow the nurse to use a subset of the nomenclature that will typically be needed to document a particular condition. A List usually contains findings in every tab.

Because shorter lists mean less scrolling, Lists are a sure way to speed up data entry of routine or typical cases. Over time, medical facilities build a library of Lists covering the medical conditions that are frequently observed in their clients.

A List is accessed by clicking on the button labeled Lists in the Toolbar at the top of the screen and then selecting it from the List Manager window.

Forms display a desired group of findings in a presentation that allows for quick entry of not only positive and negative findings but of any Entry Details fields such as value or results as well. Forms also provide other features that lists cannot, for example:

1. Forms are static; findings have a fixed position on Forms, and will consistently remain in that position, every time the form is used.

2. Findings from multiple sections of the nomenclature can be mixed on the same page of the form in any way that will enable the quickest data entry.

3. Forms may include check boxes, drop-down lists, the fields in the Entry Details section, the onset date, and free-text boxes to record comments.

4. Forms can control which findings are required and which are optional; every question on a Form does not have to be answered for every visit.

The Outline View allows you to see the findings that have been selected without leaving the Forms tab.

A form is accessed by clicking the Forms button on the Toolbar and then selecting it from the Forms Manager window.

In addition to the List and Forms buttons, you learned to use the following new buttons:

Negs   Auto Negative button will automatically click set all the findings (that are not already set) to "normal" when you are on the Sx or Px tab.

ROS   On/Off button: when On (orange), symptoms are recorded in the Review of Systems section; when Off (blue), the same symptoms would be recorded in the History of Present Illness section.

After completing this chapter, you should be comfortable with the general process of locating findings and expanding the tree to view additional findings, using Lists and Forms to create encounter notes. If you are having difficulty with any area, it is suggested that you repeat Exercises 33 and 35 before proceeding further in the book.

Task	Exercise		Page No.
Load and use a list	33		146
How the ROS button works	33		150
HPI/ROS button on individual findings	33		150
Auto Negs button	33		150
Setting the Modifier field	33	(step 10)	152
Load and use Forms	35		166
How to access the nomenclature while in a form	35		166

Reference

Jackson Healthcare. (2010). *Hospital Nurses Study 2010 summary of findings.* Alpharetta, GA: Author.

Test Your Knowledge

You may run the Medcin Student Edition software and use your mouse on the screen to answer the following questions:

1. How do you select a List?

2. How do you select Forms?

3. List three features Forms have that Lists do not.

4. Describe what the ROS button on the Toolbar does.

Write the meaning of each of the following medical abbreviations (as they were used in this chapter):

5. ROS _____

6. HPI _____

7. HEENT _____

8. URI _____

9. How do you access the nomenclature without closing the form?

10. How do you close the Nomenclature pane when it is opened on the form?

11. Auto Negative (the Negs button) functions on what two tabs?

12. An extra icon appears next to Sx findings while using a List. Describe the function of this special button.

13. What Entry Details field was used with a finding to indicate the client's fever was "mild"?

14. How do you change the numbers on the List Size button and what do the numbers do?

15. You should have produced four narrative documents of client encounters, which you printed. If you have not already done so, hand these in to your instructor with this test. The printed encounter notes will count as a portion of your grade.

Ask your instructor for answers to Test Your Knowledge

nursing.pearsonhighered.com

Prepare for success with animated examples, practice questions, challenge tests, and interactive assignments.

Electronic Nursing Care Plans

Learning Outcomes

After completing this chapter, you should be able to:

1. Create and use nursing care plans in an EHR

2. Describe the six steps of the nursing process

3. Understand the Clinical Care Classification (CCC) System

4. Document the nursing process using the CCC System

5. Explain the difference between standardized, individualized, and interactive plans of care

6. Create an individualized nursing plan of care

7. Use an interactive nursing plan of care

8. Modify a plan of care

9. Document outcomes of nursing interventions and nursing actions

Nursing Care Plans

This chapter will discuss three types of nursing care plans: standardized plan of care, individualized plan of care, and interactive plans of care.

▶ Many healthcare facilities use standardized plans of care that are defined for a specific disease or medical condition. These predefine the nursing diagnosis with time-specific interventions. They may also be incorporated into interdisciplinary plans often referred to as "critical pathways" and may define a standard set of expected outcomes. Standardized plans of care are often based on expert content documents such as textbooks, evidenced-based research, or clinical guidelines of from professional nursing organizations. When a client has multiple diagnoses, the nurse may need to work with more than one standardized care plan to adequately address the variety of that client's needs.

▶ Individualized plans of care are tailored to meet the needs of a specific client with a specific medical condition, needs that are not met by a standard plan of care such as a client with comorbidities. The nurse enters the various nursing diagnoses and appropriate planned interventions to address the client's needs. These follow the traditional plan format, complementing the medical plan of care, and are based on the body of knowledge of nursing practice.

▶ Interactive plans of care allow for individualized adaptation for a client's specific conditions. This type of online care planning system allows the nurse to select the nursing diagnoses, appropriate outcomes, and interventions based on the specific client's conditions. An interactive care planning system, based on the CCC System, is designed to use branching logic to include evidence-based nursing guidelines and knowledge of nursing clinical practice. Interactive care plans may be based on a standardized plan of care, but are easily modified based on outcomes.

Bringing the EHR to Nursing

Unfortunately, EHR systems in many healthcare facilities were originally developed without consideration of the nursing process or the workflow necessary to facilitate nursing documentation at the point of care. As hospitals and clinics have selected EHR systems, decisions about those systems have generally been driven by administrative and revenue-generating departments. Also, most EHR systems were developed following the medical model, which may not adequately support documentation of the nursing process. The evaluation of EHR systems for the facility were often conducted by management with little or no input from the nursing personnel. Typically, nurses were too actively engaged in work to schedule time for participation or were turned away from being involved in the system selection or development process. Because of a professional focus on care delivery and lack of favorable computer experience, many nurses were not interested in computer systems that perceived nursing workflow as the scheduling of independent jobs on a computer. Nursing data collection was more than discrete facts stored in a computer system database. Nurses ignored the potential impacts of computerized nursing applications and their needs were not addressed by available computer programs. System selection often included the vision of how it could support the medical staff's need for information and were designed to support activities such as registration, billing, and diagnostics. Although nursing departments had printed policy and procedure manuals with documentation standards, preprinted care plans, and clinical pathways that direct nursing documentation and care of clients, implementation of the nursing workflow was usually omitted from core organizational requirements in the search for the EHR system. Most plans of care were written or printed. The preprinted versions were developed by the nursing department and were therefore unique to each facility.

Two major initiatives have raised the awareness of the need for codified electronic nursing documentation. The national attention on computerized provider order entry (CPOE) has raised an awareness of the need for electronic nursing records to confirm completion and measure the outcome of the physician's electronic orders. New quality initiatives by CMS require hospitals and other healthcare facilities to provide evidence of compliance to national patient safety, core quality, and outcome measures. These have created a critical need for electronic codified data from nursing about client care.

To provide that data, EHR systems must include a codified nursing language capable of allowing nurses to electronically document the nursing process at the point of care. The CCC System provides standardized codified terminologies specifically created for the practice of nursing that can be incorporated into the EHR.

CCC System

Based on studies of actual nursing practice, the CCC System was developed by nurses for nurses. It offers a definitive foundation for the design of codified computer applications that support computer-based expert systems, protocols, care plans, care paths, and nursing decision support for nurses. The CCC System is comprised of two inter-related, classified terminologies: the CCC of Nursing Interventions and Actions, and the CCC of Nursing Diagnoses and Outcomes. By linking standardized nursing diagnosis, interventions, and outcomes together, the CCC System follows the six steps of the nursing process and facilitates the creation of comparable nursing data for analysis and reporting (Saba, 2007). It also provides an evidence-based approach to guide electronic documentation that follows the nursing process.

You may already be familiar with the nursing process steps from another nursing course. Figure 6-1 illustrates the six steps of nursing as defined in the Standards of Care and Standards of Professional Performance in the Standards of Clinical Nursing

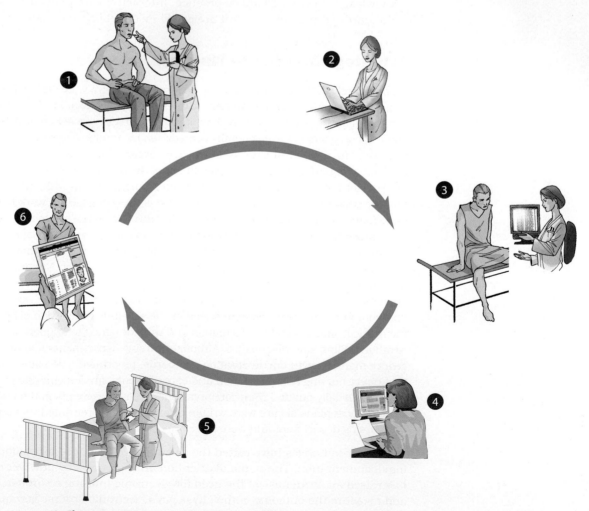

▶ **Figure 6-1 The six steps of the nursing process.**

Practice from the American Nurses Association. The six steps of the nursing process encompass the science and art of nursing, providing the basis for clinical decisions and provision of competent nursing care.

The CCC model follows the six steps of the Nursing Process Standard of Care (adapted from American Nurses Association, 1998):

1 Assessment—collect the client's health data

2 Diagnose by analysis of the assessment data, determining diagnosis

3 Identify expected outcome, individualized to the client

4 Plan—develop a plan of care that prescribes interventions to attain the expected outcomes

5 Implementation of the interventions/actions identified in the plan of care

6 Evaluate the client's progress toward attainment of outcome

Of course the nursing process is a flow where the sixth step, evaluation, leads back to the first, assess, to *reassess* the signs and symptoms and further modify the plan of care as the client's condition changes. The circular arrows in Figure 6-1 indicate the six steps of the nursing process model are a continuous flow. Note that the national licensure examination (NCLEX) and some texts define the nursing process in five steps by combining step 3 (identification of expected outcome) into either step 2 or 4.

The CCC System offers a codified and standardized approach to documenting the nursing care processes and workflow in an EHR. Twenty-one Care Components provide a structure that interrelates the 182 Nursing Diagnoses, 198 Nursing Interventions, 3 Nursing Outcomes, and 4 Nursing Intervention Actions Types. The correlation of the six steps of the nursing process to the CCC System framework is easily seen by comparing the left and right columns of the table in Figure 6-2.

ANA Standards of Clinical Nursing Steps of Nursing Process	CCC Documentation Steps
Assessment	Care Components (21)
Diagnosis	Nursing Diagnosis (182)
Outcome Identification	Expected Outcomes (3)
Planning	Nursing Interventions (198)
Implementation	Action Types (4)
Evaluation	Actual Outcomes (3)

▶ **Figure 6-2 Comparison of the six steps of nursing process and CCC System framework for nursing documentation.**

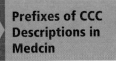

Prefixes of CCC Descriptions in Medcin

RNDx nursing diagnosis
RNRx nursing intervention
RNOx nursing order
(nursing action)

To put it simply, the nurse uses the assessment of the client's signs and symptoms to form the Nursing Diagnosis. The Nursing Diagnosis *drives* the selection of the appropriate interventions to accomplish the desired outcomes and justifies nursing actions, which are then evaluated.

Perhaps the easiest way to understand this is to examine a nursing plan of care created using the CCC codes. As we discussed in Chapter 2, CCC codes have been integrated into SNOMED-CT, LOINC, the Unified Medical Language System of the National Library of Medicine, and MEDCIN. This is helpful to the nursing student because the Medcin nomenclature used in this course already includes the CCC codes that we will be using in this chapter.

Guided Exercise 37: Reviewing a Nursing Plan of Care

In this exercise, you are going to learn to use a new tab in the Student Edition software, the ADT tab. ADT stands for Admission, Discharge and Transfer, and usually refers to the hospital registration computer. The ADT tab lists inpatients who are currently admitted to the hospital in the unit in which you work. In this software it is used to simulate the inpatient census of a particular nursing unit.

A variety of cases with diverse medical conditions are listed. In a real healthcare facility, these inpatients might have been on different floors or in different units. In the student software they are in the same unit only to simplify access for these exercises.

Case Study

Irene Smith is an 83-year-old female with right leg pain that started after a recent visit to her daughters, which included a prolonged cross-country airline flight. She stated that her leg hurts when she stands on it and aches so much at night that it is disturbing her sleep. She tried Tylenol® to relieve the pain, but it didn't help. She has erythema and edema of the right calf, which is warm to the touch. She has been admitted to the hospital with a diagnosis of DTV. You documented her admission in Chapter 4.

Step 1

Start the Student Edition software, and log in.

Locate the tab labeled **ADT** at the bottom of your screen and click on it.

Compare your screen to Figure 6-3.

Step 2

Locate and click on **Irene Smith** in the ADT list. This will highlight the row with her name as shown in Figure 6-3.

Locate and click on the button labeled "**Review Plan of Care**" (circled in Figure 6-3).

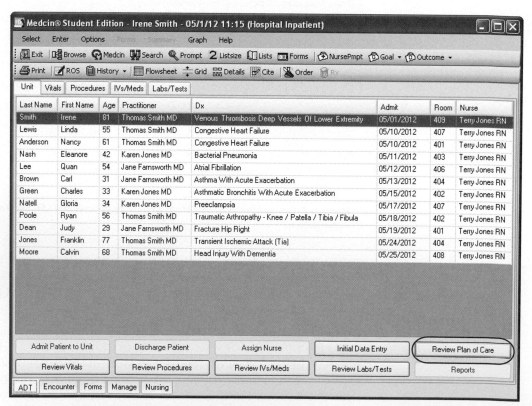

▶ **Figure 6-3 Selecting Irene Smith from the ADT tab.**

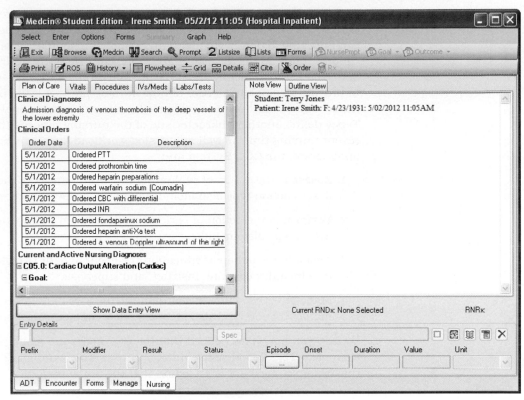

▶ **Figure 6-4 Client's Plan of Care showing the clinical orders.**

Step 3

The Plan of Care will display in the left pane. Compare your screen to Figure 6-4.

The first section of the Plan of Care contains the Clinical Diagnosis and Clinical Orders.

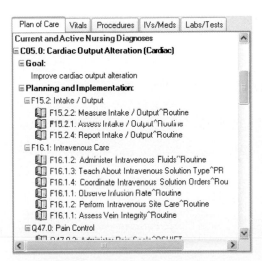

▶ **Figure 6-5 Nursing Plan of Care created using the CCC model.**

Step 4

Scroll the left pane downward until Active Nursing Diagnoses is at the top of the pane and you can see the portion of Plan of Care as shown in Figure 6-5. Review the Nursing Plan of Care on the screen as you read the following information.

Locate **Cardiac Output Alteration**. This is one of the 182 Nursing Diagnoses in the CCC System. It is defined as "change in or modification in the pumping action of the heart." In the Plan of Care it serves to identify the client problem being treated and needing care by nurses or other healthcare providers. This Plan of Care has a second CCC Nursing Diagnosis, Cardiovascular Alteration, which we will analyze in a moment.

Locate the **Goal** "Improve cardiac output alteration" below the nursing diagnosis. This is the expected outcome for this nursing diagnosis. The goal is typically identified before selecting the nursing interventions. The expected outcome is created by using one of the three CCC System qualifiers as the expected outcome or goal to provide a method to evaluate the care process. There are three Medcin goals to select from when creating the nursing plan of care: improve, stabilize, or support. In Medcin, the goal "Support" is defined as the CCC expected outcome of "support deterioration."

Locate **Intake/Output**, **Intravenous Care**, and **Pain Control** (listed under Cardiac Output Alteration). These are three of the 198 possible nurse interventions. Nurse interventions are designed to achieve a specific result for each diagnostic condition or client-assessed problem requiring therapeutic nursing care.

Listed under each of the Medcin Nursing Interventions there are a number of specific actions that the nurse will take to carry out the nursing intervention. Notice that each nursing action begins with an action verb such as "Assess," "Teach," "Perform," "Report," and "Manage." These are representative of the four CCC Action Type qualifiers that serve to modify the nursing interventions into "essence of care" actions used to provide a complete picture of how nursing process influences client outcomes, identify resources, and provide evidence for clinical decision making. The four CCC Action Types define another characteristic of the nursing process that can be used to represent nursing time as well as nursing workload and care cost. The four Action Type qualifiers in the CCC System are:

1. **Assess** is the action of evaluating the health status of the client's condition. The assess action type also includes monitor, observe, and evaluate.

2. **Perform** is the action of performing (hands-on) therapeutic client care. The perform action type also includes care, provide, and assist.

3. **Teach** is the action of education the client and/or caregiver. The teach action type also includes educate, instruct, and supervise.

4. **Manage** is the action of coordinating the care of the client and/or caregiver. The manage action type also includes refer, contact, coordinate, report, and notify.

By now you may have noticed that the CCC codes are displayed in the Plan of Care. For example, F15.2.2 is Measure Intake/Output. The last digit, 2, tells us the action type. In this example, measure is an action that the nurse *performs*.

> **Note**
>
> Note that the display of the CCC code is a pedagogical feature of the Student Edition software to help you visualize the code structure. Commercial EHRs using the Medcin/CCC nomenclature may elect to not display the codes.

Compare the Nursing Actions displayed in the right pane to the table in Figure 6-6 to identify the four CCC Action Types.

CCC	Nursing Action	Action Type
F15.2.**1**:	Assess Intake/Output	1. Assess
F15.2.**2**:	Measure Intake/Output	2. Perform
F15.2.**4**:	Report Intake/Output	4. Manage
F16.1.**1**:	Observe Infusion Rate	1. Assess
F16.1.**1**:	Assess Vein Integrity	1. Assess
F16.1.**2**:	Administer Intravenous Fluids	2. Perform
F16.1.**2**:	Perform Intravenous Site Care	2. Perform
F16.1.**3**:	Teach About Intravenous Solution Type	3. Teach
F16.1.**4**:	Coordinate Intravenous Solution Orders	4. Manage

▶ **Figure 6-6 Nursing Action Types.**

Step 5

Scroll the left pane downward until the nurse intervention "Pain Control" is at the top of the pane, as shown in Figure 6-7.

Using what you have learned in the previous step, identify the action type for each nursing action listed under Pain Control and Clinical Measurements. Write your answers on a sheet of paper and give it to your instructor.

Nurse Action	Action Type
Assess Pain Control	
Evaluate Effectiveness of Pain Control Measures	
Administer Pain Scale	
Administer Prescribed Pain Medication	
Teach Purpose of Pain Medication	
Teach Side Effects of Pain Medication	
Assess Breathing Status	
Notify Provider of Patient Status	
Measure Calf Circumference	
Teach Purpose of Clinical Measurement	
Assess Peripheral Pulses	
Mark Site of Peripheral Pulses	

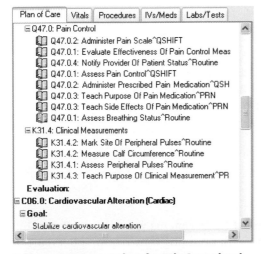

▶ **Figure 6-7 Nurse actions for Pain Control and Clinical Measurements.**

Step 6

Although the nursing interventions Pain Control and Clinical Measurements are still displayed in the left pane, notice that nursing actions in the Plan of Care also include a frequency at which the action is to be repeated.

In this Plan of Care the nurses are going to:

Assess Pain Control every shift

Evaluate Effectiveness of Pain Control Measures as needed

Administer Pain Scale every shift

Administer Prescribed Pain Medication every shift

Teach Purpose of Pain Medication as needed

Teach Side Effects of Pain Medication as needed

Assess Breathing Status routinely

Notify Provider of Patient Status routinely

Measure Calf Circumference routinely

Teach Purpose of Clinical Measurement as needed

Assess Peripheral Pulses routinely

Mark Site of Peripheral Pulses routinely

Step 7

The final item on the Plan of Care for this nursing diagnosis is evaluation. This is the step six in the nursing process described in Figure 6-1. The heading "Evaluation" is located in this Plan of Care beneath the nursing action "Teach Purpose of Clinical Measurement ^PRN."

When the plan of care was created, a goal was defined for each nursing diagnosis. This was the *expected outcome.* When the nursing diagnosis is resolved, the client is evaluated and the *actual outcome* is recorded. The CCC System defines three outcomes:

▶ Improved—the client's condition or problem improved.

▶ Stabilized—the client's condition or problem was stabilized.

▶ Supported—the client who is experiencing a deterioration of the condition was provided support.

Notice that these terms parallel the three goals described earlier.

Step 8

This completes this exercise. You may exit without printing. If you have not already done so, give your instructor the answers that you recorded in step 5.

Effectiveness of EHR Nursing Plans of Care Using CCC

In 2004, Veronica D. Feeg and colleagues conducted a study with student nurses to develop and test a bedside personal computer program designed to incorporate standardized CCC System terminologies into all aspects of the nursing process. Using randomized study design, the students' electronic charting was evaluated comparing two different methodologies for recording the nursing plan of care. One group of students used a laptop with an interactive CCC System. The control group of students used a text-based narrative software version of the CCC System to document the plan of care. The findings of the study supported the efficacy of a computer-based application using a standardized CCC System for documenting the plan of care while using the nursing process. However, the analysis of the students who charted using narrative documentation found the care plans were variable and nonstandardized (Feeg, Saba, & Feeg, 2004).

Standard Nursing Plans of Care

At healthcare facilities where the EHR lacks a codified interactive planning structure, the adequacy of the care planning process may vary greatly, like the control group in the Feeg study. Some of the reasons variances occur even with experienced nurses using an EHR include:

▶ Computer application deficiencies

▶ Varying levels of nursing experience and knowledge

▶ Time limitations allocated for care planning

▶ The assigned nursing caseload

As discussed in the beginning of this chapter, most EHR systems were not developed to support the nursing process. In an effort to reduce the nursing time required to create the plan of care and to reduce the variability, standard care plans are often adopted. The style and content may be based on a particular theorist, standards of practice established by a professional organization, best practice guidelines or care paths related to specific medical diseases, the programmed set in the software or to meet other specific institutional requirements. Regardless of the reference source, standard care plans were developed out a need to provide consistent plans of care for clients with like diagnoses. Standard care plans do not easily accommodate individualized needs of the client's plan of care. In addition, the needs of a client with multiple diagnoses may require the nurse to use multiple standardized plans of care documents.

Care Pathway

Another type of standard plan of care is sometimes referred to as a "critical pathway" or a "care pathway." This type of plan for the client may be generated from a CPOE standardized order set in an EHR system or be included in a paper version. As with the standard plan of care, the care pathway is also driven by the clinical diagnosis, but a care pathway creates orders for test and treatments by a variety of clinical staff. It may also include predefined nursing interventions and clinical orders. It usually is based on a best practice standard for each discipline involved for the diagnosis. This differs from standard care plans discussed earlier in that the pathway also defines the expected client outcomes for each day of the expected hospital stay. However, a care pathway is a prescriptive plan of care designed to address a single diagnosis. This type of plan is problematic when clients have multiple diagnoses or the client "falls off the path" by failing to meet the prescribed outcome each day.

Guided Exercise 38: Comparing Care Pathway and EHR Plan of Care

In this exercise you will learn how print the plan of care for review from the Nursing tab. You will use the printout to compare the EHR plan of care to a paper-based care pathway.

Case Study

Linda Lewis is a 53-year-old female. In an earlier exercise she was in the cath lab for a cardiac catheterization following an episode of chest pain and shortness of breath. She had evidence of mild coronary heart disease with ECG changes and known hypercholesterolemia; she has seen a cardiologist, but is now under follow-up care only with her primary physician. Her history includes parents and older bother with a history of cardiovascular disease, diabetes, and hypertension. She quit smoking 5 years ago.

In this exercise, it is a week later and she is being admitted as an inpatient with congestive heart failure. The nursing plan of care has been created using a heart failure care pathway, based upon best practice standards to generate a standardized plan of care. The clinical orders in the plan of care were entered by the attending physician using CPOE. These correspond to the interdisciplinary pathway standard predefined for 3 days of care.

Step 1

Start the Student Edition software, and log in.

Step 2

Locate the tab labeled **ADT** at the bottom of your screen and click on it.

Locate and click on **Linda Lewis** in the ADT list. This will highlight the row with her name, as shown in Figure 6-8.

▶ **Figure 6-8 Selecting Linda Lewis from the ADT tab.**

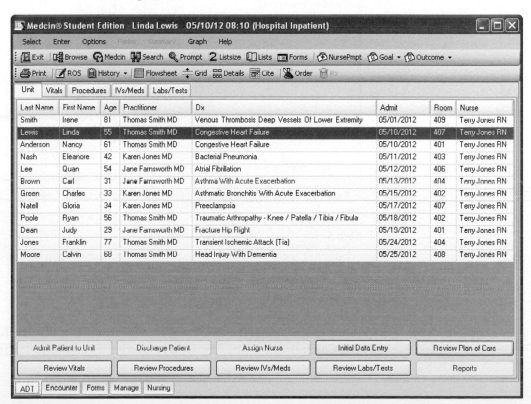

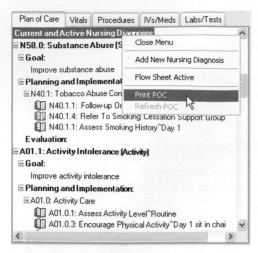

▶ **Figure 6-9 Selecting Print POC from the Plan of Care menu.**

Locate and click on the button labeled "**Review Plan of Care**" (circled in Figure 6-3).

Step 3

Scroll the left pane downward to locate the heading "Current and Active Nursing Diagnosis," just below Clinical Orders, and right-click on it.

Locate and click on "Print POC" in the drop-down menu, as shown in Figure 6-9.

Step 4

The Print Data window shown in Figure 6-10 will be displayed. Locate and click on the check box for Nursing Plan of Care in the left column.

At the bottom of the window, locate and click on the button labeled "Print and Close" (even if you normally export files for your instructor). This will produce a printed document you will use for step 6.

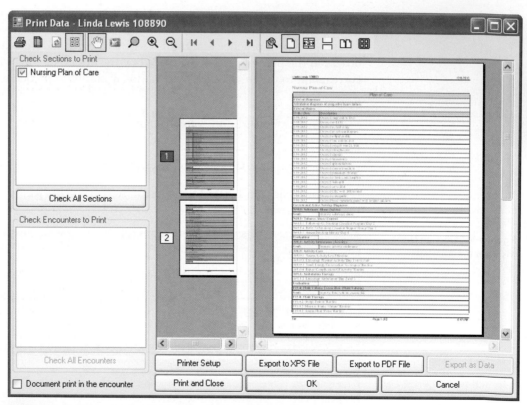

▶ **Figure 6-10 Select Nursing Plan of Care in the Print Data window.**

Step 5

When you have your printed plan of care in hand, you may exit the Student Edition software.

Step 6

Compare the clinical orders on your printed plan of care to those listed in the Paper Clinical Pathway Orders for Heart Failure (HF) shown in Figure 6-11.

Memorial Hospital Anywhere City **HEART FAILURE Care Pathway**	**Patient Label** Lewis, Linda ID: 108890 DOB: 12/3/1957

Admit to inpatient
Diagnosis: Acute Systolic CHF
Consult Dr. Hart
Vital Signs Q4H × 1st 24 hrs, then
    per unit standard,
Activity: Per Care Path
I&O, Weight on admission and daily
Diet: 2 gm NA, Low Chol
CXR: PA and Lateral if not done in ER
    re Pulmonary Edema
EKG ASAP if not done in ER and repeat
    on day 2 evaluation re CHF
Echocardiogram re edema S.O.B.
    hypertension if not done in last 6 months
Oxygen NC 2L/min Maintain O2 Sat 92%
Nursing Pathway Order Set
PT/OT Evaluate and Treat on Day 2
	Labs today not done in ER:
	    CBC with diff, BMP, MG, PT, PTT,
	    Fasting Lipid Panel in AM
	Pro BNP
	BMP and Mg daily × 2
	Order ACE or ARB if on at home:
	    Lisinopril 2.5 mg Daily
	Order Beta-blocker if on at home:
	    Carvedilol 3.125 mg PO BID
	Lasix 40 mg IV then PO BID
	KCl 20 meq po BID
	Spironolactone 25mg PO Daily
	Digoxin 0.125 mg PO Daily
	DVT Prophylaxis: Lovenox 40 mg
	    sq Daily
	Colace 100 mg PO Daily
	Case Management Referral for home
	    Health follow-up re HF monitoring

	Physician Signature: *Thomas Smith, MD* Date and time: *5/10/2012*

▶ **Figure 6-11 Standard CPOE order set for heart failure care pathway (Paper Version).**

Step 7

After reviewing the clinical orders, compare the nursing orders on your printed plan of care to Figure 6-12.

Identify the 5 Nursing Diagnoses and their Expected Outcomes (goals).

> Notice that the plan of care includes Tobacco Abuse, smoking cessation interventions (despite the fact that the Linda does not smoke) because it is a standard component of the CHF critical pathway.

Review the Interventions located directly below each Nursing Diagnosis.

Identify the type of action of each nursing order.

Identify the timing intervals on each nursing action, and note those that are planned to occur on specific days of the hospitalization.

Step 8

In this exercise you have learned about plans of care based on care pathways. Your instructor may want you to prepare a report on the items in step 7. Ask your instructor.

You have also learned how to print a nursing plan of care from the Student Edition software. You will need to print the plan of care in future exercises; refer back to this exercise if you need help.

Memorial Hospital Anywhere City **HEART FAILURE Care Pathway Guideline for Care**		**Patient Label** Lewis, Linda ID: 108890 DOB: 12/3/1957
ADMIT - DAY 1	**DAY 2**	**DAY 3**
Evaluate Tobacco Use	Tobacco Cessation Referral	Tobacco Cessation Program
Bedrest with BRP, HOB elevated if dyspnea	Up in chair BID, Walk in hallway 35 feet and evaluate dyspnea	Activity as tol, Walk 50 feet and eval dyspnea
PT/OT Evaluation	PT/OT Treat per evaluation	PT/OT Treat prn
Case Manager Assessment home situation – initiate Home Health Care Referral for HF Follow-up	Case Manager arrange Home Monitoring Program	Case Manager enroll patient in CMAP as needed for medication purchase support
Weight Saline loc or IV access Telemetry per standard I&O Monitor Fluid Status Oxygen Therapy at level to maintain oxygen saturation at or above 92%	Weight Saline loc Telemetry per standard I&O Monitor Fluid Status Wean Oxygen Therapy at level to maintain oxygen saturation at or above 92% If Foley in place – discontinue	Weight Saline loc I&O Monitor Fluid Status IV meds changed to oral schedule
Assess Respiratory Status Assess Circulation Q4H Assess Pain Control Q shift Report complication of activity level	Assess Respiratory Status Assess Circulation Q4H Assess Pain Control Q shift Report complication of activity level	Assess Respiratory Status Assess Circulation Q4H Assess Pain Control Q shift Report complication of activity level
Give HF Book Teach Cardiac Care and Diagnostic Tests	Review HF Book Teach Smoking Cessation Teach Energy Conservation Discuss Daily Weight Log Explore Emotional Response to illness	Continue HF education per standard Medication Teaching per prescribed meds Education re post discharge care
Outcome Goal: Stabilize Alteration of Cardiac Output Improve Fluid Volume Excess Stabilize Activity Intolerance	Outcome Goal: Stabilize Alteration of Cardiac Output Improve Fluid Volume Excess Stabilize Activity Intolerance	Outcome Goal: Stabilize Alteration of Cardiac Output Improve Fluid Volume Excess Stabilize Activity Intolerance

▶ **Figure 6-12 Paper version of heart failure care pathway document.**

Real-Life Story

Creating Care Plans the Hard Way

By David Robbins, RN, BSN

David Robbins is a registered nurse, currently working in a private hospital. Here he recalls his experiences developing nursing plans of care for clients at a large hospital.

After graduating from an accelerated bachelor of nursing program, my first job was at a large hospital where I worked for about two years. The first year I worked in acute care, med/surg, and oncology; the second year I worked on the long-term care floor, which included geriatric rehab and an eight-bed palliative care unit; a small nursing home was on that floor as well.

The nurses had to create an interim plan of care within 8 hours of a client's admission. It could take up to 4 hours to do the initial assessment; we were busy all the time there and very tightly staffed.

The interim plan of care was good for up to one week. We would start with the admission assessment and create all the required documentation. In the Computerized Patient Record System (CPRS), this process required three separate modules.

First was basic information about the client: addresses and phone numbers; whether the client has a living will or other advanced directives, a health surrogate, or a power of attorney for healthcare decision making; and some past medical history. Second was primarily physical assessment of essentially all the systems. The third was determining the client's level of education and preferences, such as what time the client likes to be wakened, what time the client likes to take meals, how the client learns best, and how the client likes to be taught.

Once those three portions were complete, we would go to another computer to enter the plan of care. This part of the process used software different from CPRS and once the plan of care was created in this system, we would then transfer it into CPRS.

Creating the plan of care required that we address nine specific areas—additional areas were available, but all plans of care included these nine at a minimum. These included admission diagnosis, code status, skin integrity, pain, fall risk, nutritional status, activities of daily living (ADL), social activity, and discharge plan.

For me, creating this interim plan of care was one of the most nerve-wracking aspects of the job, partly because of the 8-hour deadline, by which time it must be completed. So if it took you 4 hours to get through an initial assessment, and you had some other clients or duties, then you felt pressure to get the current client's plan done. Also, because the systems were separate, you couldn't make use of the assessment work you had already

done—you had to re-enter it into the plan of care system, save the plan, and get it imported back into the CPRS, within the required time frame.

If we had been in the same system, or able to take what we had already entered in CPRS and brought it into this system, it would have been easier. But no—I had to re-enter the data, consult my notes, or even go back and pull up the client's record in CPRS to check something.

The first thing we would enter would be the problem. Once that was done, there were two ways we could proceed. We could write our own interventions and goals, or we could select from some that had been pre-setup in the system. These didn't automatically populate the screens, but we could choose a list of standard interventions for the problem we had entered. If we took this approach, and there were multiple interventions, they would all come into the plan, and we then would erase the ones we didn't want or need. The process for writing the goals was similar.

The format of the plan was called an "I care plan." It was written as though the client was speaking: "I want to not be awakened before 6:00 AM." If there were components of the nursing plan that were not actually in the client's words, then we would write them as though they were. For example, if a client was on oxygen therapy and the nursing order was to titrate the oxygen saturation to 95 percent, the statement might be written as "I want the nurse to keep my oxygen adjusted so that I don't feel any shortness of breath." Similarly, goals might be stated as "My skin shall remain free of pressure ulcers throughout the duration of my stay."

In terms of care pathway standards to assist us, there were printed reference books on the shelves above the plan of care computers and there were some standard plans of care online in the computer, but I think mostly the system relied on the education and experience of the nurses to write the plan of care for the client.

When the plan of care was finished, we would copy the result into a document that could be cut and pasted into the CPRS system.

If the client's condition improved, degraded, or the doctors added new orders, then ideally the plan would have been updated or modified. However, this was the interim plan of care and was only intended to encompass the first week of long-term care. During that week, a nurse whose full-time responsibility was writing plans of care would develop the primary plan of care. So, in actuality, we didn't alter the interim plan—we would just make changes during nursing report, then the CPRS orders would change, and we would adjust accordingly.

One other difficulty with the plan of care system we used was that we were not able to create it while we were with the client. Because it was on a separate system, we could not do it at bedside. To have been able to create it while we were doing the initial assessment, would have been a vast improvement.

Individualized Plans of Care

In the previous exercise, the paper version of the care pathway reflected a best practice standard for the care of a client with the diagnosis of congestive heart failure, but should have been modified to meet the individual needs of the client. However, free-text plans of care are not the answer. The Feeg study, cited earlier, found the quality of plans for clients with similar diagnoses and problems can be variable, without some standardized framework to serve as the foundation for planning.

Individualized plans of care are entered into the EHR in real time for a client with a specific medical condition or for a client with comorbidities. The CCC System offers an interrelated, codified standardized framework for creating the plan of care. As you will see in the next exercise, using the CCC System offers nursing diagnoses related specifically to the medical diagnosis, but follows the nursing process to lead to an individualized plan of care.

The nurse enters the various nursing diagnoses and appropriate planned interventions to address the client's needs. These follow the traditional plan format, complementing the medical plan of care, and are based on the body of knowledge of nursing practice. The ability for a nurse to place nursing orders into a CPOE application permits the selection of electronic nursing orders related to the client's condition and problems. This facilitates a plan of care capable of addressing the individualized need of a client with comorbid diagnoses or problems, unlike standardized plans of care.

Guided Exercise 39: Creating an Individualized Nursing Plan of Care

In this exercise you will document the first four steps of the nursing process, which will culminate in an EHR plan of care based on the CCC System. Although you would normally document a full nursing assessment, this exercise has been shortened to allow you to focus your efforts on selecting the necessary items to create her initial plan of care. You will chart only a focused problem assessment of her acute symptoms.

Case Study

Eleanore Nash is a 42-year-old female admitted for bacterial pneumonia. She reported that she has had a "cold" for the past 2 weeks, but now she is experiencing shortness of breath with exertion, dyspnea when lying down, fever, and pain in her right chest when she coughs. She has a harsh, nonproductive cough and is experiencing extreme fatigue, and seems anxious. She has been admitted with an admission diagnosis of bacterial pneumonia and Dr. Karen Jones has entered the clinical orders.

Part 1: Document the RN Assessment

Before creating a plan of care, you will first need to chart the findings of your nursing assessment, which are recorded as Physical Findings.

Step 1

If you have not already done so, start the Student Edition software.

Click on the ADT tab at the bottom of your screen.

Locate and click on **Eleanore Nash** to highlight her name.

Locate and click on the button labeled "Initial Data Entry," circled in red in Figure 6-13.

▶ **Figure 6-13 Select patient Eleanore Nash.**

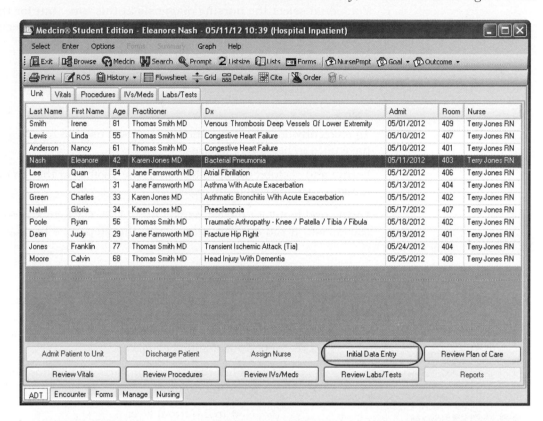

▶ **Figure 6-14 Initial assessment for client with bacterial pneumonia.**

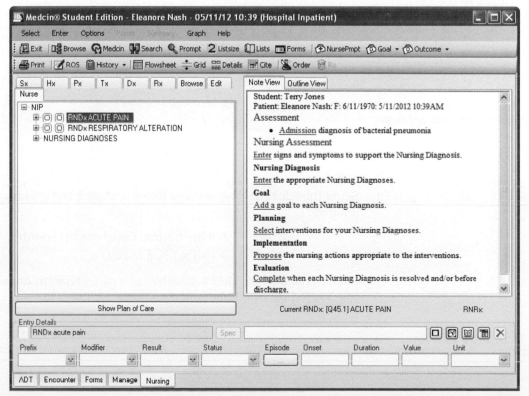

Step 2

The tab at the bottom of the screen will automatically change to the Nursing tab. Take a moment to study the screen shown in Figure 6-14). The right pane shows the clinical assessment (admission diagnosis) and a list of suggested steps for the nurse to take next. The left pane shows two Nursing Diagnoses that are associated with the clinical diagnosis "bacterial pneumonia."

You could select the nursing diagnosis at this time, but for this exercise you will follow the nursing process steps listed in the right pane, beginning with the nursing assessment.

Locate and click on the Sx tab.

Step 3

To efficiently document the findings, you will use the Adult Upper Respiratory list you have used in previous exercises.

Locate and click on the Lists button in the Toolbar at the top of your screen. The List Manager window will be invoked.

Locate and highlight the list named Adult URI. Click your mouse on the button labeled "Load List." If you need assistance with this step, refer to Chapter 5, Figure 5-4.

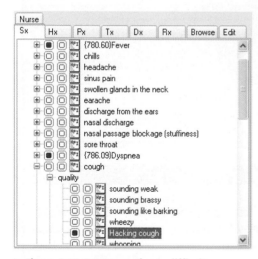

► **Figure 6-15 Symptoms: fever, difficulty breathing (dyspnea), and cough.**

Step 4

During your exam, Eleanore had indicated she had a fever, was feeling short of breath, and was coughing frequently, but she didn't expectorate any sputum. The muscles in her chest, back, and abdomen had become sore from so much coughing.

Record her reported symptoms by clicking the buttons indicated for the following findings:

- (red button) fever
- (red button) difficulty breathing (dyspnea)

Expand the list by clicking the small plus signs next to "Cough" and "Quality."

Locate and click on the following symptom finding:

- (red button) Hacking

Compare your left pane to Figure 6-15.

Step 5

Scroll the left pane downward to locate and click the buttons indicated for the following findings:

- (blue button) Coughing up sputum
- (red button) Muscle aches

Click in the free-text field below the right pane, type "**in chest, back and abdomen is aggravated by coughing**" and then press the Enter key on your keyboard.

Compare your screen to Figure 6-16.

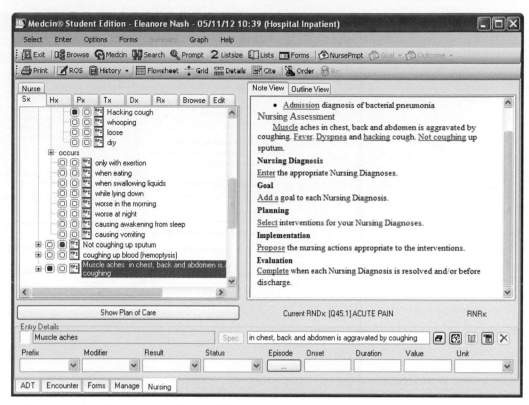

▶ **Figure 6-16 Muscle aches caused by coughing.**

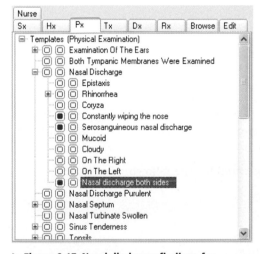

▶ **Figure 6-17 Nasal discharge findings for Eleanore Nash.**

Step 6

During the respiratory exam, Eleanore wiped her nose continuously. You observed bilateral serosanguineous nasal drainage, diminished respiratory effort, and shallow lung sounds with rhonchi heard more prominently in the right upper and mid-chest. She rated her pain as 7. You observed her hugging her sides and abdomen during the coughing spell.

Click on the Px tab to record your objective findings.

Locate and click on the small plus sign next to "Nasal Discharge."

Locate and click on the following findings:

- (red button) Constantly wiping the nose
- (red button) Serosanguineous
- (red button) Bilaterally

Compare your left pane to Figure 6-17.

Step 7

To continue documenting your respiratory exam, scroll the left pane downward to locate and click on the small plus signs next to "Respiratory Movements" and "Diminished Respiratory Excursion."

Locate and click on the following findings:

- (red button) Bilaterally
- (red button) Splinting

Click in the free-text field below the right pane, type "**when coughing**," and then press the Enter key on your keyboard.

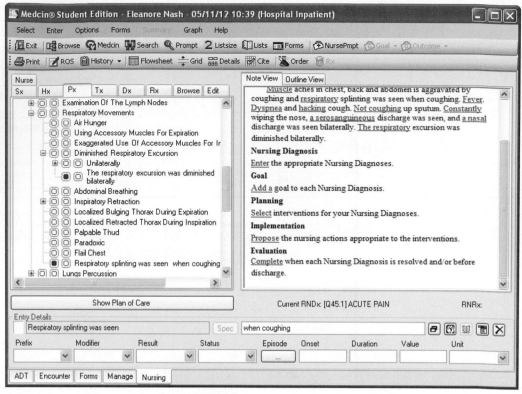

▶ **Figure 6-18 Respiratory movement findings.**

Compare your screen to Figure 6-18.

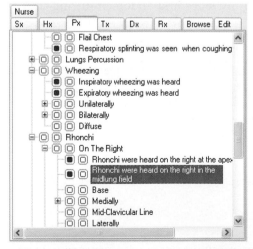

▶ **Figure 6-19 Lung sounds.**

Step 8

Record observed lung sounds. Scroll the left pane downward to locate and click the small plus signs next to "Wheezing," "Rhonchi," and "on Right" (as shown in Figure 6-19).

Locate and click the buttons indicated for the following findings:

- ● (red button) Inspiratory
- ● (red button) Expiratory
- ● (red button) Apex
- ● (red button) Midlung Field

Compare your left pane to Figure 6-19.

To keep this exercise short we will omit vital signs, history taking and other findings a nurse would normally record as part of the initial assessment.

Part 2: Document the Nursing Diagnosis

Now that you have your focused nursing assessment documented, you are ready to document the second step in the nursing process, defining your nursing diagnosis. The etiology of Eleanore's symptoms is related to her diagnosis of bacterial pneumonia. Because Medcin links the CCC nursing diagnosis to the medical diagnosis as part of its index structure, the Nurse tab already contains a short list of appropriate Nursing Diagnoses associated with Eleanore's clinical diagnosis.

Step 9

Locate and click on the tab at the top of the left pane labeled "Nurse."

Although there are 182 Nursing Diagnoses defined in the CCC System, the Nursing Diagnoses most commonly associated with bacterial pneumonia are already listed in the left pane. You will recall that in step 2 these were automatically identified by the software. Note the left pane may not display the tree of RNDx findings expanded as shown in Figure 6-20; it is not necessary to expand the tree in this step.

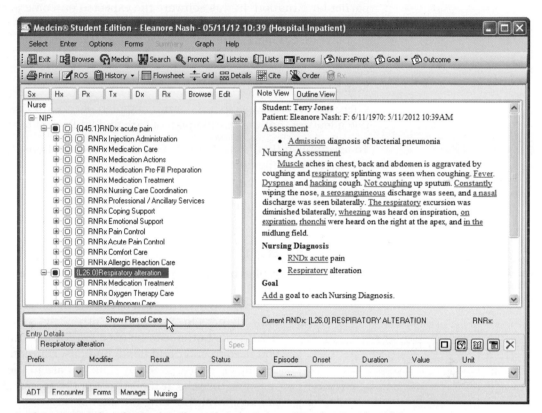

▶ **Figure 6-20 Select the Nursing Diagnosis Acute Pain and Respiratory Alteration.**

Locate and click the red button for the following RNDx findings:

- (red button) RNDx Acute Pain
- (red button) RNDx Respiratory Alteration

Although it would be possible to also select interventions from this pane, in this exercise we are going to follow the nursing process steps listed in the right pane. Scroll your right pane all the way upward and compare your screen to Figure 6-20.

You should now be able to see in the right pane the complete note created thus far. Under Assessment, the admission diagnosis is listed. This is sometimes also referred to as the "clinical diagnosis." Below that is Nursing Assessment, which includes the symptoms and physical exam findings observed by the nurse. Below that are the two nursing diagnoses we have just selected. At the bottom of the right pane is the next step in the workflow, add a goal for each nursing diagnosis.

Part 3: Identify the Expected Outcomes

The third phase of the nursing process requires the identification of an expected outcome for each nursing diagnosis in the plan of care, individualized to your client's particular situation. In this software the expected outcome is referred to as the "Goal." As discussed earlier, the CCC System defines three expected outcomes: Improve, Stabilize, or Support deterioration.

Step 10

There are several ways to build a nursing plan of care. In this exercise, we are going to use a feature that creates the plan of care and let us add to it dynamically.

To accomplish this, you will use a new button located beneath the left pane when you are on the Nursing tab.

Locate and click on the button labeled "Show Plan of Care" under the left pane. It is outlined in orange in Figure 6-20.

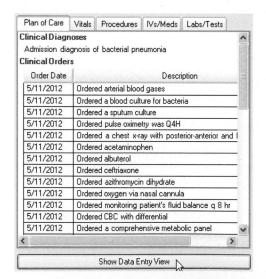

▶ **Figure 6-21 Plan of Care—clinical assessment and clinical orders.**

Step 11

A plan of care is created and replaces the nomenclature in the left pane. This is the Plan of Care View that you have used in the two previous exercises. When the Plan of Care is displayed, the button below the left pane changes to "Show Data Entry View" (outlined in orange in Figure 6-21). This button can be used to redisplay the Nomenclature pane, if you need to enter additional findings. Caution: you can change tabs at the top of the left pane any time you are in the Data Entry View, but do not click the tabs at the bottom of the screen (ADT, Encounter, Forms, or Manage) while building the plan of care.

Compare your left pane to Figure 6-21. You will recall from previous exercises that the first thing displayed in the Plan of Care is the clinical assessment and clinical orders.

Step 12

In the Plan of Care View there are many useful features that allow you to quickly build a nursing plan of care. Most of them are accessed by using the right-click button on the mouse. In this step we are going to set the expected outcome goals.

Scroll the left pane downward until you can see the Nursing Diagnoses that were added in step 9.

Position your mouse pointer over the description "Acute Pain," and click the right-click mouse button. A drop-down menu will appear. Move your mouse pointer down the items in the menu until you reach "Add a Goal for This Diagnosis." When your mouse is on this item, slide it to the right and click on the goal **"Improve"** from the list of three goals that will be displayed (as shown in Figure 6-22).

▶ **Figure 6-22 Right-click on Acute Pain; select the Goal "Improve" from the drop-down menu.**

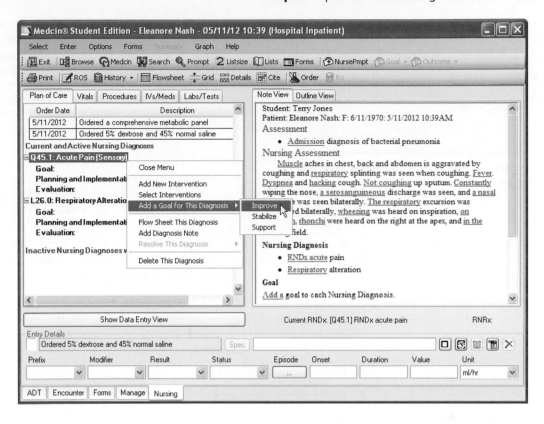

Step 13

The "Goal: Improve RNDx acute pain" has been added to the plan (circled in red in Figure 6-23).

Using what you have learned in step 12, set the goal for respiratory alteration, by right-clicking on the nursing diagnosis. Locate "Add a Goal for This Diagnosis" and click on **Stabilize** from the drop-down (as shown in Figure 6-23).

The "Goal: stabilize respiratory alteration" will be added to the Plan of Care in the left pane.

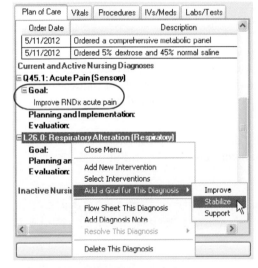

▶ **Figure 6-23 Right-click on Respiratory Alteration; select the Goal "Stabilize."**

Part 4: Planning

The next step is to add nursing interventions appropriate to the nursing diagnosis. There are several ways to add nursing interventions. In earlier chapters, you documented performed interventions by locating them in the nomenclature and clicking the red button. However, when developing the plan of care, we haven't necessarily performed that intervention; we just want to add it to the plan. Fortunately, the right-click menu has an option that will let us add interventions to the plan of care quickly and efficiently.

In addition to identifying nursing diagnoses related to the clinical diagnosis, the software also helps you select appropriate nursing interventions for each nursing diagnosis based on proven standards of care. This design enables you to efficiently create a plan of care based on best nursing practices individualized to meet needs of the client.

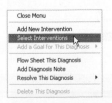

▶ **Figure 6-24 Right-click menu; Select Interventions.**

Step 14

Position the mouse pointer over the Nursing Diagnosis "Acute Pain" and click the right-click mouse button. The menu shown in Figure 6-24 will be displayed.

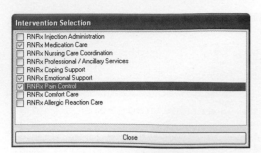

▶ **Figure 6-25 Intervention Selection window for Acute Pain.**

Notice the menu has two items related to interventions. The first, "Add New Intervention," adds interventions one at a time. It is generally used to add an intervention after the plan of care has already been created. The second, "Select Interventions," allows you to select multiple interventions by clicking on check boxes.

Locate and click the menu item **Select Interventions** (as shown in Figure 6-24). A small window, shown in Figure 6-25, will be displayed.

Step 15

The check boxes in the Intervention Selection window work like the check boxes you have used with Forms in Chapter 5; that is, if you click a check box, a check mark appears and you have selected the intervention. If you click a box that already has a check mark, the intervention will be unselected. When you have selected all the desired interventions, clicking the button labeled "Close" will add them to the plan. If you have not selected any interventions, the button labeled "Cancel" will close the window without adding interventions.

Eleanore seemed very apprehensive when she arrived on the unit and rated her pain at 7; and her doctor has ordered medications. By selecting interventions from this list, you will create a plan of care individualized for Eleanore Nash. Locate and click on the check boxes for the following acute pain interventions:

✓ RNRx Medication Care

✓ RNRx Emotional Support

✓ RNRx Pain Control

Compare your selected interventions to Figure 6-25. When everything matches, click on the button labeled "Close."

Step 16

The left pane should now display three nursing interventions for acute pain, under the heading "Planning and Implementation." These can be seen on the left in Figure 6-26. Using a process very similar to the previous step, we are going to add Nursing Actions for each of the three interventions.

Locate and right-click on Medication Care. In the drop-down menu, click on Select Nursing Actions as shown in Figure 6-26. A small window, shown in Figure 6-27, will be displayed.

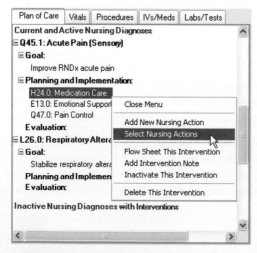

▶ **Figure 6-26 Right-click on Intervention to display menu; select Nursing Actions.**

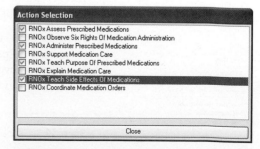

▶ **Figure 6-27 Nursing Action Selection window.**

Locate and click on the check boxes for the following nursing actions:

✓ Assess Prescribed Medications

✓ Administer Prescribed Medications

✓ Teach Purpose of Prescribed Medications

✓ Teach Side Effects of Medications

Compare your Action Selection window to Figure 6-27. When everything is correct, click on the button labeled "Close" and the nursing actions will be displayed in the left pane under the Medication Care intervention.

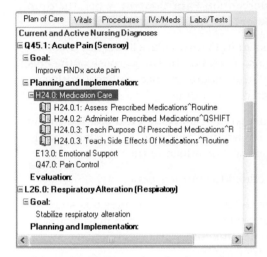

▶ **Figure 6-28 Nursing Actions for the nursing intervention Medication Care.**

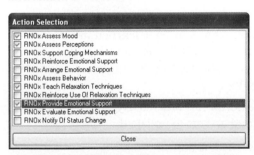

▶ **Figure 6-29 Nursing Actions for the nursing intervention Emotional Support.**

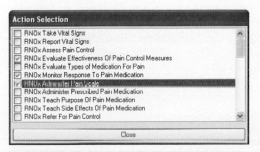

▶ **Figure 6-30 Nursing Actions for the nursing intervention Pain Control.**

Step 17

Compare your left pane to Figure 6-28. Notice that for each nursing action there is an interval or frequency at which the nursing actions are expected to occur such as QShift, Routine, or PRN.

As you selected the nursing actions, default intervals were automatically assigned. These time intervals can be modified if necessary after the nursing actions have been added to the plan. You do not need to modify the time intervals for any of Eleanore's plan.

Step 18

Using what you have learned in the previous step, right-click on the nursing intervention Emotional Support, in the drop-down menu click Select Nursing Actions.

When the Nurse Action Selection window is displayed, click the check boxes for the following nursing actions:

✓ Assess Mood

✓ Assess Perceptions

✓ Teach Relaxation Techniques

✓ Provide Emotional Support

Compare your Action Selection window to Figure 6-29. When everything is correct, click on the button labeled "Close."

Step 19

Locate and right-click on the nursing intervention Pain Control. In the drop-down menu, click Select Nursing Actions.

When the Nurse Action Selection window is displayed, click the check boxes for the following nursing actions:

✓ Evaluate Effectiveness Of Pain Control Measures

✓ Monitor Response To Pain Medication

✓ Administer Pain Scale

Compare your Action Selection window to Figure 6-30. When everything is correct click on the button labeled "Close."

Step 20

When you are done, your nursing plan of care for Acute Pain should resemble Figure 6-31. Scroll your left pane slightly upward, so that you can see the RNDx Acute Pain, its goal, the three interventions, and all

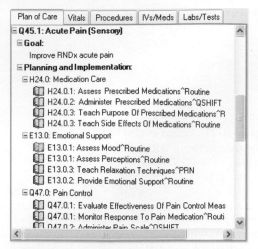

▶ **Figure 6-31 Completed plan of care for RNDx Acute Pain.**

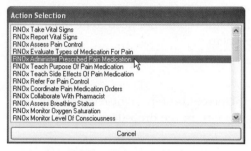

▶ **Figure 6-32 Action Selection window after initial actions have been added.**

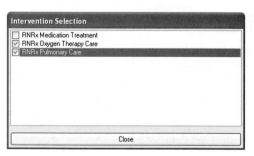

▶ **Figure 6-33 Intervention Selection window for Respiratory Alteration.**

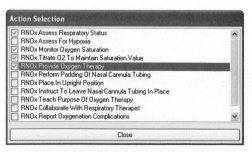

▶ **Figure 6-34 Action Selection window for oxygen therapy care.**

of the actions you have selected. Compare your screen to Figure 6-31. If anything is missing, perform step 21 before trying to correct it.

Step 21

In this step you will learn how to add something to plan after you have closed the selection window. This information applies to both the select interventions and the select actions windows.

The nurse wishes to add the action of "administer pain medication" to the plan.

Locate and right-click on the intervention **Pain Control**. When the drop-down menu appears, click on **Select Actions**.

The Action Selection window shown in Figure 6-32 will display a list of actions, but this time there are no check boxes. The purpose of the check boxes was to allow you to add all the actions at once. Subsequently actions (or interventions) are added one at a time.

Locate and double-click on **Administer Prescribed Pain Medication** in the Action Selection window as shown in Figure 6-32. The window will close automatically and the action will be added to the plan.

Verify that the action has been added to your left pane.

When you compared your screen to Figure 6-31 in the previous step, if there were any items missing, use what you have learned in this step to correct your plan, by adding the missing interventions or actions one at a time using the appropriate selection window.

Step 22

Once you have the plan for acute pain correct, use what you have learned in this exercise to add the interventions and then the actions for the RNDx Respiratory Alteration. Because the nursing actions are a subset of an intervention, we add the interventions first, then the actions.

Because Eleanore is acutely ill, the doctor has ordered oxygen. The nurse will add related nursing interventions and actions to update the plan of care.

Locate "Respiratory Alteration" in the left pane.

Right-click your mouse on the description; a drop-down menu will be displayed. Click on **Select Interventions**. The window shown in Figure 6-33 will be displayed.

Locate and click on the check boxes for the following nursing interventions:

✓ Oxygen Therapy Care

✓ Pulmonary Care

Compare your window to Figure 6-33. When everything is correct, click on the button labeled "Close." Verify the two interventions have been added to the left pane.

Step 23

Add the actions to the oxygen therapy intervention.

Locate and right-click your mouse on its description; a drop-down menu will be displayed. Click on **Select Nursing Actions**. The window shown in Figure 6-34 will be displayed.

Locate and click on the check boxes for the following nursing actions:

✓ Assess Respiratory Status

✓ Monitor Oxygen Saturation

✓ Titrate O2 To Maintain Saturation Value

✓ Provide Oxygen Therapy

Compare your window to Figure 6-34. When everything is correct, click on the button labeled "Close." Verify the four actions have been added below oxygen therapy care.

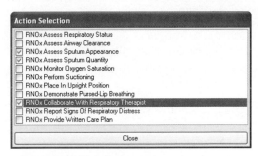

▶ **Figure 6-35 Action Selection window for pulmonary care.**

Step 24

Next add the nursing actions for the pulmonary care intervention.

Locate the intervention Pulmonary Care and right-click your mouse on its description; a drop-down menu will be displayed. Click on **Select Nursing Actions**. The window shown in Figure 6-35 will be displayed.

Locate and click on the check boxes for the following nursing actions:

✓ Assess Sputum Appearance

✓ Assess Sputum Quantity

✓ Collaborate With Respiratory Therapist

Compare your select action window to Figure 6-35. When everything is correct, click on the button labeled "Close." Verify the three interventions have been added below pulmonary care.

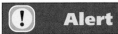

> ⓘ **Alert** ▶   *Do not leave the Nursing tab until you have a printed copy in your hand.* **You could lose your plan of care if you change tabs or exit before printing.**

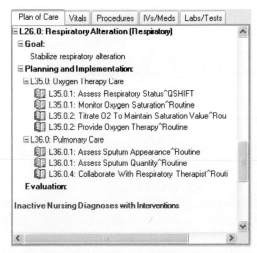

▶ **Figure 6-36 Plan of care for RNDx Respiratory Alteration.**

Step 25

Compare you left pane to Figure 6-36, if anything is missing, use the procedure you learned in step 21 to correct your plan. When everything is correct, remain on the nursing tab while you locate and click the Print button on the Toolbar at the top of your screen to invoke the Print Data window.

Locate and click the check boxes in the left column for *both* Current Encounter *and* Nursing Plan of Care, and then click on the appropriate button to either print or export a file, as directed by your instructor.

Compare your printout or file output to Figure 6-37. If it is correct, hand it in to your instructor. Note your printer will produce two pages, but the pagination will be different from Figure 6-37. If there are any differences (other than the pagination), review the previous steps in the exercise to find and correct your error.

Eleanore Nash   Page 1 of 2

Student: *your name or id here*
Patient: Eleanore Nash: F: 6/11/1970: 5/11/2012 10:39AM
Assessment
  • Admission diagnosis of bacterial pneumonia
Nursing Assessment
Muscle aches in chest, back and abdomen is aggravated by coughing and respiratory
splinting was seen when coughing. Fever. Dyspnea and hacking cough. Not coughing
up sputum. Constantly wiping the nose, a serosanguineous discharge was seen, and
a nasal discharge was seen bilaterally. The respiratory excursion was diminished
bilaterally, wheezing was heard on inspiration, on expiration, rhonchi were
heard on the right at the apex, and in the midlung field.
Nursing Diagnosis
  • RNDx acute pain
  • Respiratory alteration
Goal
  • Goal: Improve RNDx acute pain
  • Goal: Stabilize respiratory alteration
Planning
  • Medication care
  • Emotional support
  • Pain control
  • Oxygen therapy care
  • Pulmonary care
Implementation
  • Propose evaluation of effectiveness of pain control measures
  • Propose monitoring of response to pain medication
  • Propose pain scale administration
  • Propose prescribed pain medication administration
  • Propose respiratory status assessment
  • Propose sputum appearance assessment
  • Propose sputum quantity assessment
  • Propose oxygen saturation monitoring
  • Propose O2 titration to maintain saturation value
  • Propose oxygen therapy provision
  • Propose collaboration with respiratory therapist
  • Propose mood assessment
  • Propose perceptions assessment
  • Propose teaching of relaxation techniques
  • Propose assessment of prescribed medications
  • Propose administration of prescribed medications
  • Propose teaching purpose of prescribed medications
  • Propose teaching of side effects of medications
  • Propose provision of emotional support
Evaluation
Complete when each Nursing Diagnosis is resolved and/or before discharge.

▶ **Figure 6-37a Printed Encounter for Eleanore Nash (page 1 of 2).**

Plan of Care	
Clinical Diagnoses	
Admission diagnosis of bacterial pneumonia	
Clinical Orders	

Order Date	**Description**
5/11/2012	Ordered arterial blood gases
5/11/2012	Ordered a blood culture for bacteria
5/11/2012	Ordered a sputum culture
5/11/2012	Ordered pulse oximetry was Q4H
5/11/2012	Ordered a chest x-ray with posterior-anterior and lateral views
5/11/2012	Ordered acetaminophen
5/11/2012	Ordered albuterol
5/11/2012	Ordered ceftriaxone
5/11/2012	Ordered azithromycin dihydrate
5/11/2012	Ordered oxygen via nasal cannula
5/11/2012	Ordered monitoring patient's fluid balance q 8 hr
5/11/2012	Ordered CBC with differential
5/11/2012	Ordered a comprehensive metabolic panel
5/11/2012	Ordered 5% dextrose and 45% normal saline

Current and Active Nursing Diagnoses	
Q45.1: Acute Pain (Sensory)	
Goal:	Improve RNDx acute pain
H24.0: Medication Care	
H24.0.1: Assess Prescribed Medications^Routine	
H24.0.2: Administer Prescribed Medications^QSHIFT	
H24.0.3: Teach Purpose Of Prescribed Medications^Routine	
H24.0.3: Teach Side Effects Of Medications^Routine	
E13.0: Emotional Support	
E13.0.1: Assess Mood^Routine	
E13.0.1: Assess Perceptions^Routine	
E13.0.3: Teach Relaxation Techniques^PRN	
E13.0.2: Provide Emotional Support^Routine	
Q47.0: Pain Control	
Q47.0.1: Evaluate Effectiveness Of Pain Control Measures^PRN	
Q47.0.1: Monitor Response To Pain Medication^Routine	
Q47.0.2: Administer Pain Scale^QSHIFT	
Q47.0.2: Administer Prescribed Pain Medication^QSHIFT	
Evaluation:	
L26.0: Respiratory Alteration (Respiratory)	
Goal:	Stabilize respiratory alteration
L35.0: Oxygen Therapy Care	
L35.0.1: Assess Respiratory Status^QSHIFT	
L35.0.1: Monitor Oxygen Saturation^Routine	
L35.0.2: Titrate 02 To Maintain Saturation Value^Routine	
L35.0.2: Provide Oxygen Therapy^Routine	
L36.0: Pulmonary Care	
L36.0.1: Assess Sputum Appearance^Routine	
L36.0.1: Assess Sputum Quantity^Routine	
L36.0.4: Collaborate With Respiratory Therapist^Routine	
Evaluation:	
Inactive Nursing Diagnoses with Interventions	

▶ **Figure 6-37b Printed plan of care for Eleanore Nash (page 2 of 2).**

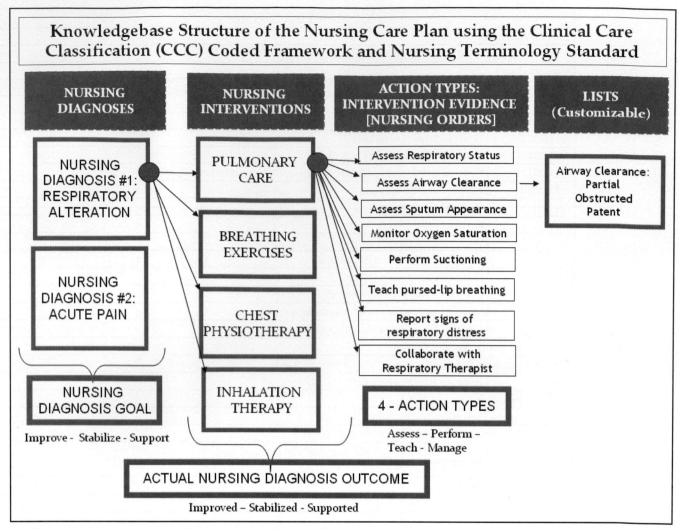

Knowledgebase Structure of the Nursing Care Plan using the Clinical Care Classification (CCC) Coded Framework and Nursing Terminology Standard

Courtesy of Medicomp Systems, Inc.
▶ Figure 6-38 The CCC Model.

Flow of the CCC Model

The CCC model provides an interactive plan of care interrelated with the continuous feedback of the six phases of the nursing process. Figure 6-38 illustrates the interrelationship between the CCC Nursing Diagnoses and Outcomes and the CCC Nursing Interventions and Actions. The figure illustrates the case of a client with an upper respiratory problem different from Eleanore Nash's.

The first column shows the selection of two relevant Nursing Diagnoses interrelated with the possible Expected Outcomes to create the planned goals. The second column shows the selected interventions related the nursing diagnosis. The third column shows nursing orders and the four types of related nursing actions. The fourth column further clarifies a nursing action for this particular client's condition.

Having created plan of care individualized to the specific needs and goals of the client, the plan can then guide the care and relevant documentation. Following the implementation of the interventions, the effectiveness of the planned interventions is evaluated against the planned goal to determine the actual outcome of the nursing diagnosis, as illustrated at the bottom of the columns.

The actual outcome of the therapeutic care or nursing interventions is the nurse's evaluation of whether the plan goal was met or not. The CCC Actual Outcomes correspond directly to the Expected Outcomes used to create the goal, as illustrated at the bottom of Figure 6-38.

The Interactive Nursing Plan of Care

In the previous exercise you followed the CCC System through four steps of the nursing process to create an individualize plan of care for Eleanore Nash.

1. You used the initial data entry button to chart the initial assessment.

2. You identified the appropriate Nursing Diagnosis related to the clinical diagnosis.

3. You used the Add Goals menu to identify an Expected Outcome for each of the Nursing Diagnoses.

4. You selected nursing interventions and nursing actions to create an individualize plan of care.

In the next exercise you will use a different case to learn how to interact with a CCC-based plan of care to complete the remaining steps of the nursing process:

5. Implement the interventions/actions in the plan of care and document them in the chart.

6. Evaluate the outcomes and document them in the chart.

As you learned earlier in Figure 6-1, after completing the sixth step the nursing process then returns to step 1, in which the nurse reassesses the client and modifies the plan of care accordingly. In the next exercise you will learn how to cite nursing interventions/ actions in the EHR as they are performed; how to record the actual outcome; and how to modify a plan of care in a system that is truly interactive.

Guided Exercise 40: Using an Interactive Nursing Plan of Care

In this exercise the client has been hospitalized for several days, another nurse performed the initial assessment, and nurses on other shifts have provided care for her. You will review her plan of care, her current progress, document nursing interventions/actions that have been performed, evaluate the client, and record the actual outcome.

Case Study

Nancy Anderson is a 61-year-old female who was admitted from the ER 3 days ago for congestive heart failure. She had 2+ pitting edema in her lower legs and feet with 1+ edema in both hands. She was experiencing shortness of breath and complaining of chest pain when she was seen in the ER. She has known mitral valve disease for the past 10 years, etiology unknown, but she has been stable until recently. She has been mildly hypertensive for the past 2 months, but is not on any antihypertensive medications at this time. She has no other significant medical history. Her father died of heart disease and her older brother has survived a recent myocardial infarction. She has been taking Lasix 20 mg oral BID, Lanoxin 0.125 mg oral daily, K-Dur 10mg oral BID before admission.

Her physician, Dr. Smith, recorded her medical history and home medications into her current record and entered his admitting orders through CPOE. Her initial orders were started in ER before she arrived on the nursing unit and the nurse on duty completed the initial assessment and plan of care.

You have reviewed her chart and the nursing notes from other shifts, which included the following observations: She had pitting edema and a fluid imbalance associated with her heart failure and was experiencing pain and dyspnea with all activity and diaphoresis with almost any exertion, orthopnea, pulmonary rales throughout her lungs with audible wheezing, and jugular vein distension.

She has been hospitalized for 3 days. She has IV fluids infusing and is wearing telemetry. She was painful when she arrived on the nursing unit, but denies pain at this time. She has been on bedrest with her head elevated and is receiving oxygen per nasal cannula.

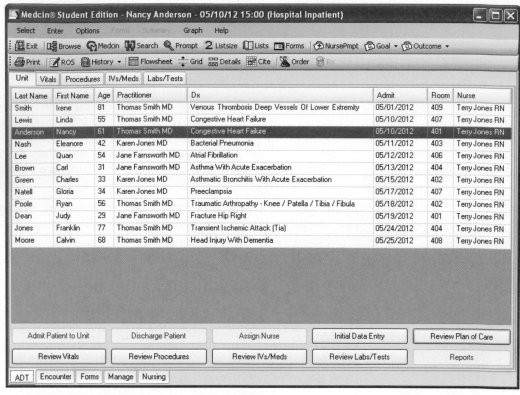

▶ Figure 6-39 Select Nancy Anderson on the ADT tab.

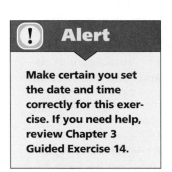

Alert

Make certain you set the date and time correctly for this exercise. If you need help, review Chapter 3 Guided Exercise 14.

Step 1

If you have not already done so, start the Student Edition software, and log in.

Locate the tab labeled "ADT" at the bottom of your screen and click on it.

Locate **Nancy Anderson** in the ADT list, and click on her name as shown in Figure 6-39.

Locate and click the button labeled "Review Plan of Care" (circled in red in Figure 6-3).

This will open Nancy Anderson's chart and automatically change to the Nursing tab.

Step 2

Locate and click Select on the Menu bar, and then click New Encounter from the drop-down menu.

Select the date **May 12, 2012**, the time **7:30 AM**, and the reason **Hospital Inpatient**.

Compare your screen to Figure 6-40. Make certain that the date and time match before clicking on the OK button.

Step 3

In this exercise you will learn to use several new buttons, but first take a moment to familiarize yourself with Nancy's clinical orders and nursing plan of care, scrolling the left pane as necessary.

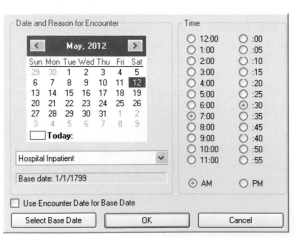

▶ Figure 6-40 Set encounter date to May 12, 2012 7:30 AM.

Nancy is on a care path standard for congestive heart failure. Her individualized plan includes edema control and oxygen therapy. She has a running IV and is receiving medications to treat the heart failure. Her fluid intake and output are being measured and she has had several cardiac and diagnostic tests. The swelling in her hands and feet has improved and she is no longer experiencing shortness of breath.

When you are sufficiently familiar with her plan of care, locate and click the button below the left pane labeled "Show Data Entry View."

Locate and click on the Px tab at the top of the left pane.

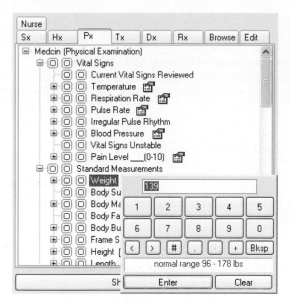

▶ **Figure 6-41 Entering the client's weight in the Nomenclature pane.**

Locate and click on the button labeled "Medcin" in the Toolbar at the top of your screen. This button is used to restore the full nomenclature to the left pane when the number of findings displayed has been limited by a list or other template.

Step 4

Because the treatment for congestive heart failure involves medications to help Nancy reduce the edema, she is weighed every morning.

Expand the tree by clicking the small plus signs next to "Vital Signs" and "Standard Measurements."

Notice that there is a special button in the left pane following the description of findings such as temperature, respiration, pulse, pain scale, and weight. This is a special feature of the Nursing tab that allows the nurse to enter numerical findings while remaining on the Nomenclature pane.

Locate and click the special button next to Weight. A small data entry window as shown in Figure 6-41 will open next to the description. Type **139** in the field.

Compare your screen to Figure 6-41 and then click on the button labeled "Enter." The text "Weight was 139 lbs." should display the right pane.

Step 5

For each of the vital signs listed below, click the small icon button next to the description, type the value indicated, and then click the button labeled "Enter" or press the Enter key on your keyboard.

🖻 Temperature **98.8**

🖻 Respiration **24**

🖻 Pulse **68**

🖻 Pain Level **2**

Compare your right pane to Figure 6-42.

▶ **Figure 6-42 Vital signs entered using the icon buttons (circled in red) on the Nomenclature pane.**

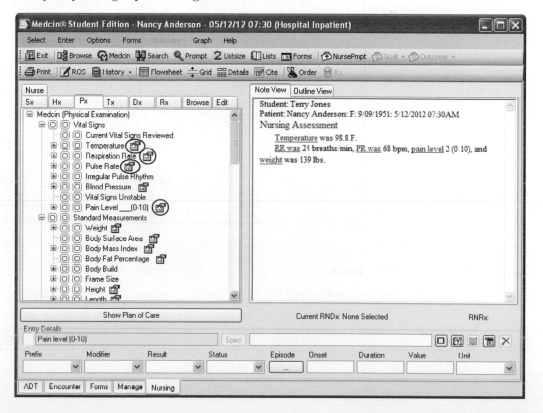

Step 6

Locate and click the small plus sign next to "Blood Pressure."

Locate and click the small icon buttons, type the value indicated, and then click the Enter button (or press the Enter key) for the systolic and diastolic readings:

☞ Systolic: **148**

☞ Diastolic: **92**

Verify that "Blood Pressure: 148/92" was added to your encounter note.

Step 7

Nancy is no longer experiencing shortness of breath and her oxygen saturation seems good. Pressing on her nails has a normal response.

Scroll the left pane downward to locate and click on the small plus sign next to "Nails."

Scroll the expanded list downward to locate and click the blue button for the following finding:

● (blue button) Prolonged capillary filling

Compare your screen to Figure 6-43.

▶ **Figure 6-43 No prolonged capillary filling of fingernails.**

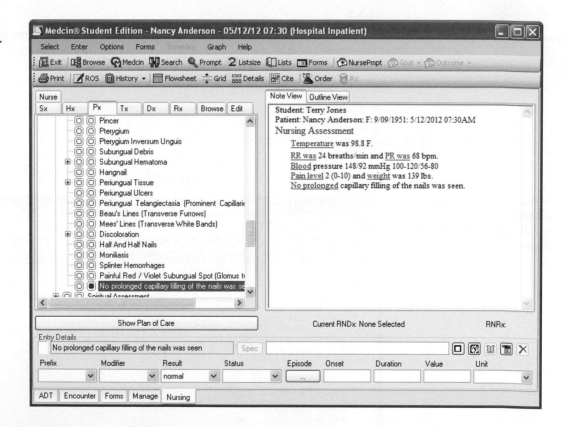

Step 8

Click on the Tx tab.

Locate and click on the small plus signs next to "Blood Analysis" and "Blood Gas Analyses."

Locate and click the small icon button next to the description, type the indicated value, and then click the Enter button for the following finding:

☞ Oxygen Saturation: **97**

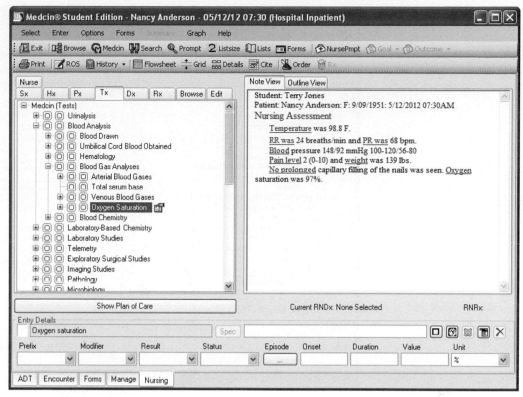

▶ **Figure 6-44 Arterial blood gas saturation 97%.**

Compare your screen to Figure 6-44.

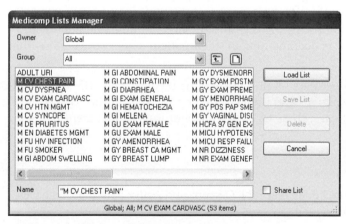

▶ **Figure 6-45 Select M CV Chest Pain list.**

Step 9

Click on the Px tab.

Locate and click the Lists button on the Toolbar to invoke the List Manager window.

Highlight the list named "M CV Chest Pain," as shown in Figure 6-45, and then click on the button labeled "Load List."

Step 10

Locate and click the blue buttons for the following findings:

- (blue button) Rales/crackles
- (blue button) jugular vein distension increased
- (blue button) edema
- (blue button) diaphoresis

Compare your screen to Figure 6-46. When everything is correct, locate and click on the button below the left pane labeled "Show Plan of Care."

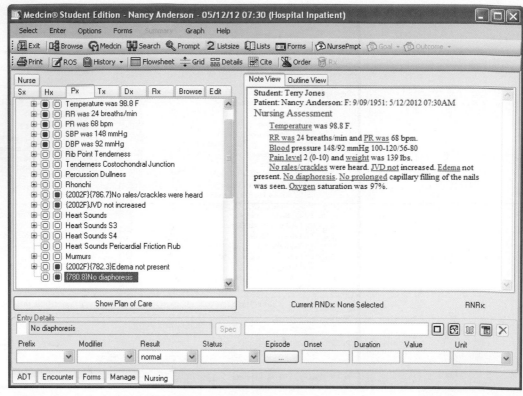

▶ Figure 6-46 Selected Px findings for Nancy Anderson.

Part 5: Implementation

As mentioned earlier, this exercise will continue with the fifth and sixth steps of the nursing process. While doing so, you will also learn several additional features of the EHR software. The fifth step is implementing the nursing interventions and actions in the care plan. Equally important is documenting in the inpatient's chart the actions that the nurse has taken.

In previous chapters you have documented nursing actions by expanding the tree, locating a finding that described the action, and then clicking on the red button. However, once you have defined a plan of care, there is a more efficient way to document using an interactive plan of care.

Step 11

Scroll the left pane downward until you can see the Current and Active Nursing Diagnoses, as shown in the left pane of Figure 6-47.

Locate and click on the button labeled "Cite" in the Toolbar at the top of your screen. The button icon resembles a teal check mark over a grid. Whenever Cite mode is enabled, the Cite button will change color, as shown in Figure 6-47. When the Cite button is off, it will be blue.

Verify your Cite button is on (orange).

Cite is used to bring information forward from previous encounters into the current one. You can also cite from the Plan of Care into the current encounter. The findings can be edited after they are in the current encounter, without affecting the previous entries in the chart.

In this step you are going to document nursing actions you have performed. Having discussed her improved status with the physician, Nancy's activity level is being advanced

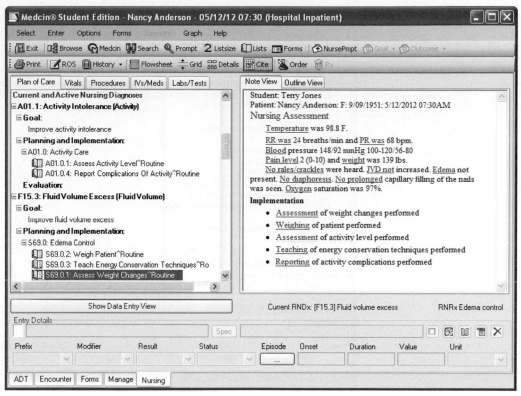

▶ Figure 6-47 Cite findings from nursing plan of care into encounter when Cite button is on.

and you have begun teaching Nancy about energy conservation. You have weighed her, assessed her activity level, and assessed her weight changes.

Locate the intervention Activity Care in the left pane and click your mouse on each of the following nursing actions:

A01.0.1: Assess Activity Level

A01.0.4: Report Complications Of Activity

Locate the intervention Edema Control and click your mouse on each of the following nursing actions:

S69.0.1: Assess Weight Changes

S69.0.2: Weigh Patient

S69.0.3: Teach Energy Conservation Techniques

Compare your right pane to the right pane of Figure 6-47. Each of the nursing actions has been recorded as performed. You will see how quickly you were able to document the nursing actions that were performed.

Click the Cite button on your Toolbar to turn Cite mode off. Verify the button has turned blue.

Part 6: Evaluation

The sixth and final step in the nursing process is to evaluate the outcome of the nursing interventions and actions and document it in the chart. During the nursing assessment, the nurse has noted that Nancy's oxygen saturation is much improved; therefore, she will no longer require oxygen therapy.

▶ **Figure 6-48 Oxygen Therapy no longer required.**

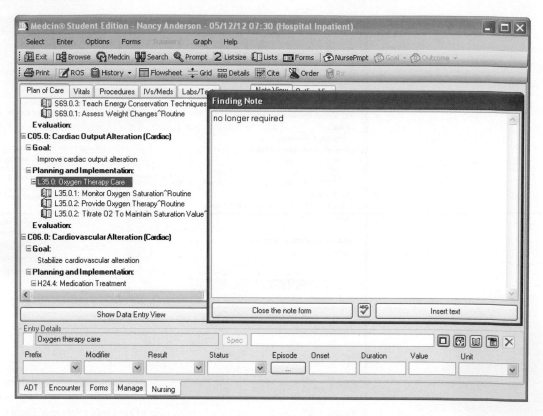

Step 12

In this example, we are going to begin by making a note in the chart. Scroll the left pane downward. Locate and highlight the intervention **Oxygen Therapy Care** in the plan.

Locate and click on the note button under the right pane. When the Finding Note window is displayed, type "**no longer required**."

Compare your screen to Figure 6-48 and then click on the button labeled "Close the note form."

▶ **Figure 6-49 Resolving Cardiac Output Alteration.**

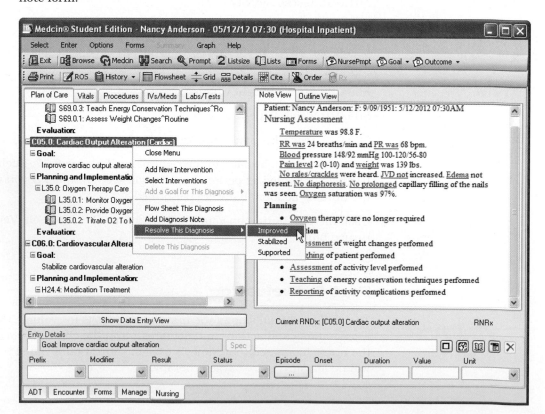

"Oxygen therapy care not longer required" will be added to the encounter note.

Step 13

We can record the evaluation of this nursing diagnosis and make it inactive (within the plan) in one step.

Right-click on **Cardiac Output Alteration**. Position your mouse pointer on "Resolve This Diagnosis" in the drop-down menu and then click on "Improved," as shown in Figure 6-49.

Note that the CCC outcomes parallel the CCC goals, but in the past tense.

Scroll your left pane all the way downward to locate Inactive Nursing Diagnoses and Interventions.

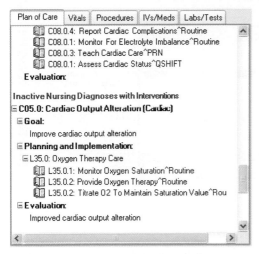

► **Figure 6-50 Inactive nursing diagnosis Cardiac Output Alteration with outcome Evaluation.**

Compare your screen Figure 6-50. Notice that the diagnosis has been moved to the inactive group and that the evaluation has been recorded.

Step 14

It is not necessary to set a nursing diagnosis to inactive to record an evaluation outcome.

It is also possible to make a nursing intervention or nursing action inactive without making the whole nursing diagnosis inactive by right-clicking on an intervention or action and selecting the corresponding menu option "Inactivate this Intervention" or "Inactivate this Action."

Scroll your left pane upward to locate and click on the nursing diagnosis of Fluid Volume Excess to highlight it.

Locate and click on the button labeled "Outcome" on the Toolbar at the top of your screen. This will display a drop-down list of the three possible CCC outcomes.

Click on "Improved." The evaluation will be added to your encounter note (as shown in Figure 6-51) but will not alter the plan of care or inactivate the diagnosis.

► **Figure 6-51 Recording outcome evaluation in the encounter using Toolbar button.**

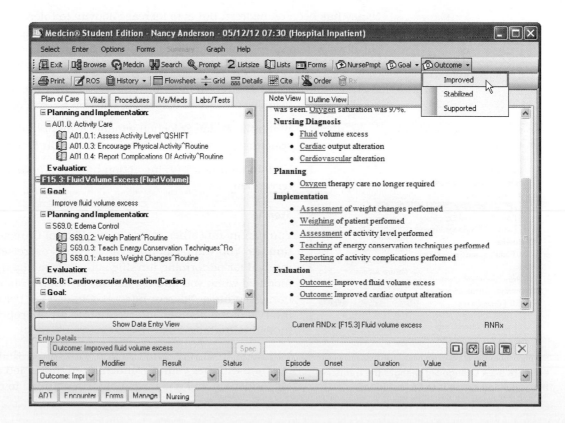

Reassess and Modify Plan

In Figure 6-1, once the last step has been reached, the nursing process circles back to the beginning. We assess the client's response to treatment and modify the plan of care accordingly. In the next steps you will learn a few examples of how to modify an interactive plan of care.

▶ **Figure 6-52 Modifying the nursing plan of care.**

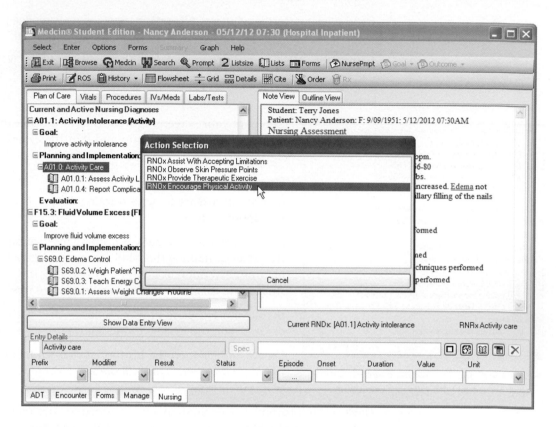

Step 15

Nancy has been on bedrest, but is to increase activity to tolerance beginning on your shift. Her cardiac monitor has been changed to telemetry, permitting mobility and increased activity. Therefore, we wish to add to her plan of care. The procedure is very similar to Exercise 39, Step 22, in which you learned to add an action while creating a plan.

Position your mouse pointer on the intervention Activity Care and right-click. When the dropdown menu is displayed, click on Select Nursing Actions.

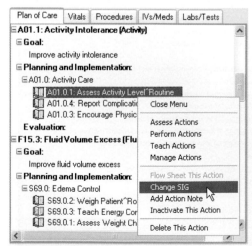

When the Action Selection window is displayed, locate and click on "Encourage Physical Activity," as shown in Figure 6-52.

Verify that a new nursing action has been added to the Activity Care intervention.

Step 16

You can modify other things in the Plan of Care such as the interval timings. You will recall from the previous exercise that the frequency or interval for performing nursing actions is set by default. These can be modified when you add the action, or when a change in Nancy's condition warrants a different interval. Change Sig is used to adjust the timing interval of the planned intervention to an appropriate frequency for her individualized need.

▶ **Figure 6-53 Change Sig changes the frequency that a nursing action is to be performed.**

You know from your conversation with Nancy that she enjoys spending time with her young grandchildren, has a job outside the home, and Mr. Anderson and she have a big trip planned to celebrate their 35th anniversary this year. Nancy's biggest priority is to be able to enjoy her active lifestyle. Because we are encouraging activity, we want to reassess her activity level on every shift to make sure she builds up gradually.

Highlight the nursing action Assess Activity Level and right-click your mouse. When the drop-down menu appears, click on **Change Sig**, as shown in Figure 6-53.

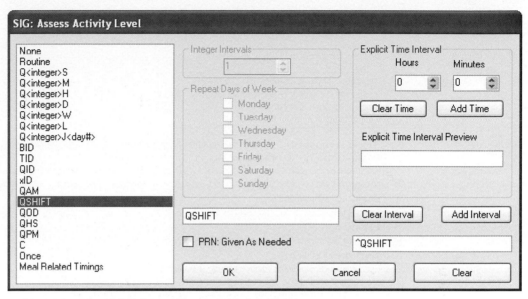

▶ **Figure 6-54 Select QShift interval for Access Activity Level.**

⊘ **Alert** **Do not close; exit the Encounter or change tabs. You will lose your work if you do.**

Step 17

The Change Sig window appears with the name of the action you are modifying displayed in the title bar.

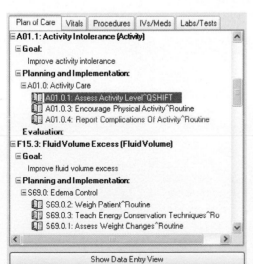

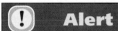

▶ **Figure 6-55 Assess Activity Level modified to QShift and new action Encourage Physical Activity.**

Locate and click on the button labeled "Clear Interval" to remove the old Sig.

The left column displays a number of standard intervals. Locate and click on the interval **QSHIFT** as shown in Figure 6-54).

Locate and click the OK button to close the window and modify the nursing action.

Compare your left pane to Figure 6-55. In the figure you can see the new interval has been set for Assess Activity Level and below it the new nursing action you added in step 15.

Step 18

Remain on the Nursing tab. You are going to print the encounter note and the modified plan of care.

Click on the Print button on the Toolbar at the top of your screen to invoke the Print Data window. Be certain there is a check mark in the boxes next to *both* Current Encounter *and* Nursing Plan of Care, and then click on the appropriate button to either print or export a file, as directed by your instructor.

Compare your printout or file output to Figure 6-56 and Figure 6-57. If it is correct, hand it in to your instructor. Note your printer will produce two to three pages and the pagination will be different from Figure 6-56 and 6-57. If there are any differences (other than the pagination), review the previous steps in the exercise to find and correct your error.

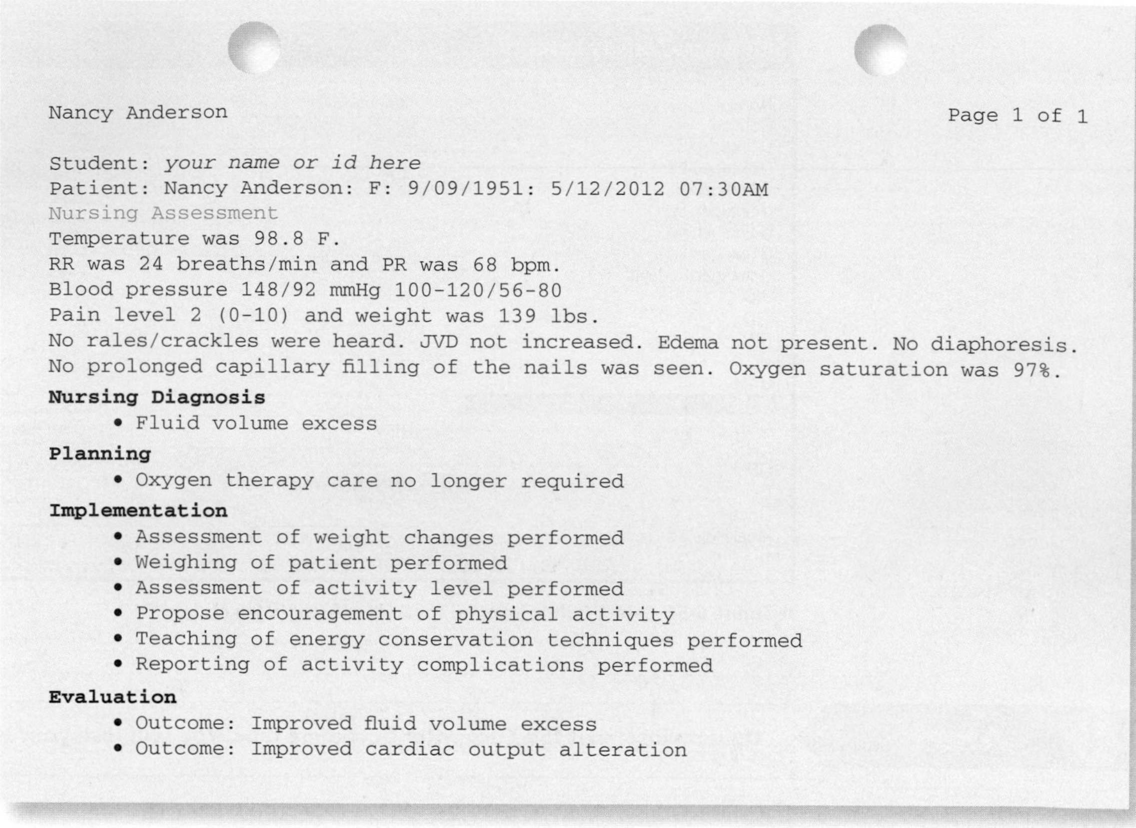

```
Nancy Anderson                                           Page 1 of 1

Student: your name or id here
Patient: Nancy Anderson: F: 9/09/1951: 5/12/2012 07:30AM
Nursing Assessment
Temperature was 98.8 F.
RR was 24 breaths/min and PR was 68 bpm.
Blood pressure 148/92 mmHg 100-120/56-80
Pain level 2 (0-10) and weight was 139 lbs.
No rales/crackles were heard. JVD not increased. Edema not present. No diaphoresis.
No prolonged capillary filling of the nails was seen. Oxygen saturation was 97%.
Nursing Diagnosis
    • Fluid volume excess
Planning
    • Oxygen therapy care no longer required
Implementation
    • Assessment of weight changes performed
    • Weighing of patient performed
    • Assessment of activity level performed
    • Propose encouragement of physical activity
    • Teaching of energy conservation techniques performed
    • Reporting of activity complications performed
Evaluation
    • Outcome: Improved fluid volume excess
    • Outcome: Improved cardiac output alteration
```

▶ **Figure 6-56 Printed encounter note for Nancy Anderson.**

Plan of Care	
Clinical Diagnoses	
Admission diagnosis of congestive heart failure	

Clinical Orders	
Order Date	**Description**
5/10/2012	Ordered a chest x-ray
5/10/2012	Ordered an echocardiogram
5/10/2012	Ordered a lipid profile
5/10/2012	Ordered low sodium diet
5/10/2012	Ordered oxygen was 2L/min
5/10/2012	Ordered aspirin
5/10/2012	Ordered metoprolol
5/10/2012	Ordered digoxin
5/10/2012	Ordered furosemide
5/10/2012	Ordered spironolactone
5/10/2012	Ordered docusate sodium
5/10/2012	Ordered heparin preparations
5/10/2012	Ordered potassium chloride
5/10/2012	Ordered lisinopril
5/10/2012	Ordered CBC with differential
5/10/2012	Ordered coagulation studies PT and PTT

Current and Active Nursing Diagnoses	
A01.1: Activity Intolerance (Activity)	
Goal:	Improve activity intolerance
A01.0: Activity Care	
A01.0.1: Assess Activity Level^QSHIFT	
A01.0.3: Encourage Physical Activity^Routine	
A01.0.4: Report Complications Of Activity^Routine	
Evaluation:	
F15.3: Fluid Volume Excess (Fluid Volume)	
Goal:	Improve fluid volume excess
S69.0: Edema Control	
S69.0.1: Assess Weight Changes^Routine	
S69.0.2: Weigh Patient^Routine	
S69.0.3: Teach Energy Conservation Techniques^Routine	
Evaluation:	
C06.0: Cardiovascular Alteration (Cardiac)	
Goal:	Stabilize cardiovascular alteration
H24.4: Medication Treatment	
H24.4.1: Monitor Medication Treatment^Routine	
H24.4.2: Administer Medication Treatment^Routine	
H24.4.3: Reinforce Home Medication Schedule^Routine	
F15.2: Intake / Output	
F15.2.1: Assess Fluid Status^Routine	
F15.2.1: Assess Intake / Output^Routine	
F15.2.1: Evaluate Urinary Output^Routine	

▶ **Figure 6-57a Printed plan of care for Nancy Anderson (page 1 of 2).**

F15.2.2: Measure Intake / Output^Routine	
F15.2.3: Teach Fluid Management Goals^PRN	
F15.2.4: Report Intake / Output^Routine	
F16.1: Intravenous Care	
F16.1.1: Assess Intravenous Access^Routine	
F16.1.1: Observe Infusion Rate^Routine	
F16.1.1: Assess Vein Integrity^Routine	
F16.1.2: Administer Intravenous Fluids^Routine	
F16.1.2: Perform Intravenous Site Care^Routine	
F16.1.3: Teach About Intravenous Solution Type^PRN	
F16.1.4: Coordinate Intravenous Solution Orders^Routine	
C08.0: Cardiac Care	
C08.0.1: Monitor Vital Signs^Routine	
C08.0.1: Assess Pain Control^QSHIFT	
C08.0.1: Monitor Response To Pain Medication^Routine	
C08.0.1: Assess Respiratory Status^QSHIFT	
C08.0.1: Observe Physical Appearance^Routine	
C08.0.1: Monitor For Electrolyte Imbalance^Routine	
C08.0.1: Assess Circulation^Routine	
C08.0.1: Assess Cardiac Status^QSHIFT	
C08.0.3: Explain Diagnostic Tests^PRN	
C08.0.3: Explain Cardiac Tests^PRN	
C08.0.3: Teach Cardiac Care^PRN	
C08.0.3: Review Symptoms To Report With Patient^Routine	
C08.0.4: Report Cardiac Complications^Routine	
Evaluation:	
Inactive Nursing Diagnoses with Interventions	
C05.0: Cardiac Output Alteration (Cardiac)	
Goal:	Improve cardiac output alteration
L35.0: Oxygen Therapy Care	
L35.0.1: Monitor Oxygen Saturation^Routine	
L35.0.2: Titrate 02 To Maintain Saturation Value^Routine	
L35.0.2: Provide Oxygen Therapy^Routine	
Evaluation:	Improved cardiac output alteration

▶ **Figure 6-57b Printed plan of care for Nancy Anderson (page 2 of 2).**

Guided Exercise 41: Reviewing an Inpatient Chart

In this exercise you will learn how to retrieve a previous encounter.

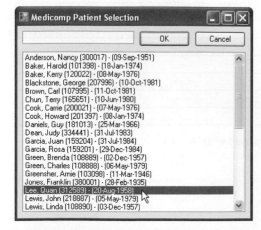

▶ **Figure 6-58 Select patient Quan Lee from Patient Selection.**

Case Study

Quan Lee is a 53-year-old female who presented at the emergency department with sudden onset of palpitations, feeling her heart was racing. The ER triage nurse recorded Ms. Lee's medical history, and she was admitted as an inpatient by the ER doctor, Jane Farnsworth, who diagnosed her with atrial fibrillation. You are about to start your nursing assessment, but before doing so you will review her chart.

Step 1

If you have not already done so, start the Student Edition software.

Click Select on the Menu bar, and then click Patient.

In the Patient Selection window, locate and click on **Quan Lee**, as shown in Figure 6-58.

▶ **Figure 6-59 Select the existing encounter for May 12, 2012.**

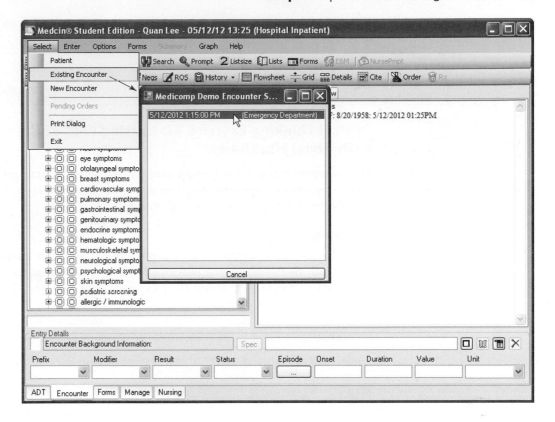

Step 2

In this exercise you will use a new feature you have not used before; you are going to retrieve and work with an encounter already in progress.

Click Select on the Menu bar, and then click **Existing Encounter**.

A small window of previous encounters will be displayed. Position your mouse pointer on the first encounter in the list, dated **5/12/2012 1:15 PM** (as shown in Figure 6-59), and click on it.

Step 3

Review the encounter, scrolling the right pane as necessary.

Quan Lee is a 53-year-old female seen in the emergency department for sudden onset of palpitations, feeling that her heart was racing. She reported this has happened before, but it was over so quickly that she didn't think it was important. She denies any pain.

She has no prior cardiac history and is not on medications at home except a daily vitamin. She reported that she had read about aspirin being taken during a heart attack could save your life and had taken 2 aspirin tablets before coming to the ER. She has no history of hypertension and has never smoked.

Scroll the right pane downward as necessary. She reported that both of her parents and one living brother have cardiovascular disease and hypertension. Her mother and sister have diabetes.

She was found to have an irregular heart rate with variation in her peripheral pulses and the electrocardiogram confirmed premature beats and persistent atrial fibrillation.

Scroll the right pane downward as necessary. While in the ER her oxygen saturation level was normal and she had a blood profile drawn with no significant findings.

Dr. Jane Farnsworth has diagnosed her with atrial fibrillation, admitted her as an inpatient. Her admitting orders entered into CPOE include daily laboratory studies PT, PTT and INR. Telemetry is ordered and she is to receive Lovenox 40 mg subcutaneously daily and Warfarin 2.5 mg by mouth every evening.

Step 4

If time permits, you may continue with Exercise 42, otherwise you may exit without printing.

Critical Thinking Exercise 42: Nursing Plan of Care for an Inpatient with Atrial Fibrillation

This exercise will provide an opportunity to practice what you have learned in this chapter while documenting Ms. Lee's hospital admission. Do not begin the exercise unless there is sufficient time remaining to complete it.

Case Study

Quan Lee is a 53-year-old female admitted from the ER for atrial fibrillation. She was very emotionally distraught at the time of admission, verbalizing fear of a heart attack. She remains very apprehensive about the diagnostic tests and what is happening with her heart.

Step 1

If you have not already done so, start the Student Edition software and log in.

Locate the tab labeled "**ADT**" at the bottom of your screen and click on it.

Step 2

Locate and click on **Quan Lee** in the ADT list. This will highlight the row with her name.

Locate and click on the button labeled "Initial Data Entry." This should automatically take you to the Nursing tab and create a new encounter for May 12, 2012, which includes her admitting diagnosis.

If you are continuing from the previous exercise, you may receive a warning that the previous encounter has not been printed. Click on the OK button to close the warning.

Step 3

Verify that the tab at the top of the left pane is the Nurse tab. It should be pre-populated with potential Nursing Diagnoses. Because we know her admitting diagnosis is atrial fibrillation, we already know at least one Nursing Diagnosis that will be needed.

Locate and click the red button for the following nursing diagnosis:

● (red button) RNDx Cardiac Output Alteration

Step 4

As you have seen from the previous exercise, the ER triage nurse has already taken her medical history, so begin by clicking on the Px tab to chart the findings of your assessment.

Locate and click the Medcin button on the Toolbar at the top of your screen.

During your nursing assessment, you found Quan Lee to be alert and oriented with a normal neurological, respiratory, gastrointestinal, renal urinary, and musculoskeletal findings; her skin assessment revealed no wounds, bruises, or rashes.

Scroll the left pane as necessary to locate and click the buttons indicated for each of the following findings:

● (blue button) Lungs
● (blue button) Urinary system
● (blue button) Musculoskeletal
● (blue button) Neurological
● (blue button) Skin

Step 5

Enter her vital signs except for the pulse. She is having varying pulse information; therefore, you will enter multiple pulse data in a moment.

Scroll your left pane upward to locate and click the small plus signs next to "Vital Signs" and "Blood Pressure."

Locate and click the small icon buttons next to each of the following findings, type the value indicated, and then click the Enter button or press the Enter key on your keyboard.

☞ Temperature: **97**

☞ Respiration: **20**

☞ Systolic: **130**

☞ Diastolic: **86**

Locate and click the button indicated for each of the following finding:

● (red button) Pulse Rhythm Irregular

A check of her peripheral pulses found pedal pulses diminished in strength but equal to her radial pulses. Her apical pulse was a regularly irregular rate.

Locate and click the small plus sign next to "Pulse."

Scroll the left pane slightly downward if necessary to locate and click the small icon buttons next to each of the following pulse findings, type the value indicated, and then click the Enter button (or press the Enter key):

☞ Apical: **108**

☞ Radial: **88**

☞ Dorsalis Pedis: **88**

Step 6

Quan Lee has expressed to you her fear of her present condition and the meaning of the diagnostic tests.

Locate and click on the Sx tab.

Locate and click the small plus signs next to "Psychological," "Mood," and "Fear."

Locate and click the button indicated for the following finding:

● (red button) of present medical condition

Step 7

After charting her assessment, you wish to add another nursing diagnosis.

Locate and click on the button below the left pane labeled "Show Plan of Care."

Locate and right-click on "Current and Active Nursing Diagnoses"; a drop-down menu will appear.

Click "Add Nursing New Diagnosis." A list of Nursing Diagnoses will display in the left pane.

Locate and click the small plus sign next to "Self-Concept."

Locate and click the red button for the following Nursing Diagnosis:

● (red button) RNDx Anxiety

Locate and click on the long button below the left pane labeled "Show Plan of Care."

Step 8

Now that the Nursing Diagnoses have been identified, the next phase in the nursing process is to identify an Expected Outcome.

Locate and right-click on "Cardiac Output Alteration."

In the drop-down menu, locate "Add a Goal for this Diagnosis," and click on the goal **Stabilize**.

Step 9

Next, identify the interventions to achieve this goal.

Right-click on "Cardiac Output Alteration" again.

In the drop-down menu, click on "Select Interventions" and a small window will be displayed. Locate and click on the check boxes for the following interventions:

✓ Intake/Output

✓ Intravenous Care

✓ Cardiac Care

Click on the Close button.

Step 10

Now, for each of the interventions, add the actions.

Right-click on the intervention "Intake/Output."

In the drop-down menu, click on "Select Nursing Actions" and a small window will be displayed. Locate and click on the check boxes for the following nursing actions:

✓ Assess Fluid Status

✓ Measure Intake/Output

✓ Explain Intended Effects of Medical Regimen

Click on the Close button.

Step 11

Right-click on the intervention "Intravenous Care."

In the drop-down menu, click on "Select Nursing Actions" and a small window will be displayed. Locate and click on the check boxes for the following nursing actions:

✓ Observe Infusion Site

✓ Observe Infusion Rate

✓ Perform Intravenous Site Care

✓ Coordinate Intravenous Solution Orders

Click on the Close button.

Step 12

Right-click on the intervention "Cardiac Care."

In the drop-down menu click on "Select Nursing Actions" and a small window will be displayed. Locate and click on the check boxes for the following nursing actions:

✓ Monitor Vital Signs

✓ Assess Pain Control

✓ Weigh Patient

✓ Monitor Arrhythmias

✓ Assess Cardiac Status

✓ Teach Cardiac Care

✓ Report Cardiac Complications

✓ Review Symptoms to Report with Patient

Click on the Close button.

Step 13

The doctor would like the client weighed every morning. Modify the frequency interval for that nursing action.

Locate and right-click on the nursing action "Weight Patient ^Routine."

In the drop-down menu click on "Change Sig" and the interval window will open.

Locate and click on the button labeled "Clear Interval."

In the left column locate and click on the interval **QAM** (which means every morning).

Click on the OK button to close the window. Verify that the interval has changed.

Step 14

Following the same sequence you used in step 12, complete the plan of care for the nursing diagnosis "Anxiety."

Add the Goal: **Improve**.

Select Intervention:

✓ Emotional Support

Select Nursing Actions:

✓ Assess Mood

✓ Assess Perceptions

✓ Teach Relaxation Techniques

✓ Provide Emotional Support

Step 15

You have determined that some of her anxiety is from a knowledge deficit about the cardiac and diagnostic tests.

Add nursing actions to an existing intervention.

Locate and right-click on the intervention Emotional Support.

In the drop-down menu click on **Add Nursing Action** (*not* select nursing actions); the left pane will change to the Nurse tab and display the findings for Nursing Orders.

Locate and click on the small plus sign next to "Specimens."

Scroll the expanded tree downward to locate and click the red buttons for the following findings:

● (red button) Explain Diagnostic Tests
● (red button) Explain Cardiac Tests

Locate and click on the button below the left pane labeled "Show Plan of Care."

Step 16

While implementing the plan of care, you used the "teach back method" to teach Ms. Lee a relaxation technique, and you want to add this to the measured outcome for the Anxiety diagnosis. After explaining the diagnostic tests and teaching the relaxation technique, you will record the evaluation outcome.

Locate and highlight the nursing diagnosis "Anxiety (self-concept)."

Locate and click the button labeled "Outcomes" on the Toolbar at the top of your screen. Select **Improved** from the drop-down list.

With the diagnosis still highlighted, type "**decreased, confirmed relaxation technique in teach back process**" in the Entry Details free-text field below the right pane. Press the enter key on your keyboard.

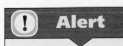

Alert

Do not close, exit the Encounter, or change tabs. You will lose your work if you do.

Step 17

Remain on the Nursing tab while you print the encounter note and the plan of care.

Click on the Print button on the Toolbar at the top of your screen to invoke the Print Data window. Be certain there is a check mark in the boxes next to *both* Current Encounter *and* Nursing Plan of Care, and then click on the appropriate button to either print or export a file, as directed by your instructor.

```
Quan Lee                                                    Page 1 of 2


Student: your name or id here
Patient: Quan Lee: F: 8/20/1958: 5/12/2012 01:25PM
Assessment
     • Admission diagnosis of atrial fibrillation
Nursing Assessment
Fear of present medical condition. Temperature was 97 F.
RR was 20 breaths/min.
Apical pulse rate was 108 bpm, radial was 88 bpm, dorsalis pedis was 88 bpm, and
the pulse rhythm was irregular.
Blood pressure 130/86 mmHg 100-120/56-80
Lungs: normal. Urinary system: normal. Musculoskeletal system: normal.
Neurological system: normal.
Skin: normal.
Nursing Diagnosis
     • Anxiety
     • Cardiac output alteration
Goal
     • Goal: Improve anxiety
     • Goal: Stabilize cardiac output alteration
Planning
     • Emotional support
     • Intake/output
     • Intravenous care
     • Cardiac care
Implementation
     • Propose vital signs monitoring
     • Propose pain control assessment
     • Propose assessment of fluid status
     • Propose infusion site observation
     • Propose infusion rate observation
     • Propose I/O measurement
     • Propose IV site care
     • Propose coordination of IV solution orders
     • Propose mood assessment
     • Propose perceptions assessment
     • Propose teaching of relaxation techniques
     • Propose weighing of patient
     • Propose explanation of diagnostic tests
     • Propose explanation of cardiac tests
     • Propose provision of emotional support
     • Propose arrhythmia monitoring
     • Propose assessment of cardiac status
     • Propose cardiac care teaching
     • Propose reporting of cardiac complications
     • Propose review of symptoms to report with patient
     • Propose explanation of intended effects of medical regimen
Evaluation
     • Outcome: Improved anxiety decreased, confirmed relaxation technique in
       teach back process
```

▶ **Figure 6-60a Printed encounter note and plan of care for Quan Lee (page 1 of 2).**

Compare your printout or file output to Figure 6-60. If it is correct, hand it in to your instructor. Note your printer will produce 2 pages, but the pagination will be different from Figure 6-60. If there are any differences (other than the pagination), review the previous steps in the exercise to find and correct your error.

Plan of Care	
Clinical Diagnoses	
Family history of diabetes mellitus	
Atrial fibrillation	
No history of hypertension	
Clinical Orders	
Order Date	**Description**
5/12/2012	Ordered PTT
5/12/2012	Ordered prothrombin time
5/12/2012	Ordered warfarin sodium (Coumadin)
5/12/2012	Ordered INR
5/12/2012	Ordered enoxaparin
5/12/2012	Ordered telemetry
Current and Active Nursing Diagnoses	
C05.0: Cardiac Output Alteration (Cardiac)	
Goal:	Stabilize cardiac output alteration
F15.2: Intake / Output	
F15.2.1: Assess Fluid Status^Routine	
F15.2.2: Measure Intake / Output^Routine	
F15.2.3: Explain Intended Effects Of Medical Regimen^Routine	
F16.1: Intravenous Care	
F16.1.1: Observe Infusion Site^Routine	
F16.1.1: Observe Infusion Rate^Routine	
F16.1.2: Perform Intravenous Site Care^Routine	
F16.1.4: Coordinate Intravenous Solution Orders^Routine	
C08.0: Cardiac Care	
C08.0.1: Assess Cardiac Status^QSHIFT	
C08.0.1: Assess Pain Control^QSHIFT	
C08.0.1: Monitor Arrhythmias^Routine	
C08.0.1: Monitor Vital Signs^Routine	
C08.0.2: Weigh Patient^QAM	
C08.0.3: Review Symptoms To Report With Patient^Routine	
C08.0.3: Teach Cardiac Care^PRN	
C08.0.4: Report Cardiac Complications^Routine	
Evaluation:	
P40.0: Anxiety (Self Concept)	
Goal:	Improve anxiety
E13.0: Emotional Support	
E13.0.1: Assess Mood^Routine	
E13.0.1: Assess Perceptions^Routine	
E13.0.3: Teach Relaxation Techniques^PRN	
E13.0.2: Provide Emotional Support^Routine	
E13.0.3: Explain Diagnostic Tests^PRN	
E13.0.3: Explain Cardiac Tests^PRN	
Evaluation:	
Inactive Nursing Diagnoses with Interventions	

▶ **Figure 6-60b** Printed plan of care for Quan Lee (page 2 of 2).

Chapter Six Summary

In this chapter you have had an opportunity to explore how to use the software to create a plan of care for a variety of clients. You have used many features specifically designed only for the professional nurse, who is responsible for creating, coordinating, and maintaining a plan of care. A quality plan of care for the client must not only meet standards of best nursing practice but also be individualized to the client's specific needs. You have learned how the CCC-codified structure facilitates meeting both of these care-planning requirements.

Two major national initiatives have fostered the growing awareness of the need for codified electronic nursing documentation. The national attention on computerized provider order entry (CPOE) has resulted in the need for electronic nursing records to confirm order completion and to measure the client outcome of ordered care. New quality initiatives by CMS require hospitals and other healthcare facilities to provide evidence of compliance to national patient safety goals, core quality indicators, and outcome measures. These have created a critical need for electronic codified data from nursing about client care that can be quantified and electronically communicated. To provide that data, EHR systems must include a codified nursing language capable of allowing nurses to electronically document the nursing process at the point of care.

The Clinical Care Classification (CCC) system provides standardized codified research-based terminologies specifically addressing the practice of nursing. The CCC terminologies offer a common nursing codified language that can support electronic data sharing with nationally required reporting databases and best practice standards of care.

It also can provide an interrelated structure of codified terminologies to support documentation that flows with the nursing process. The six steps of the nursing process are assessment, diagnosis, establishing expected outcomes, planning, implementation, and evaluation. In this chapter, we have used the CCC System to follow the nursing process and discussed several types of nursing plans of care:

- **Standardized** plans of care are defined for a specific disease or medical condition which use predefined nursing diagnoses and time-specific interventions. These plans often lack individualization or are difficult to adapt to comorbid conditions.

- **Individualized** plans of care work well for specific medical condition or for a client with comorbidities permitting a variety of nursing diagnoses and appropriate planned interventions to address the client's problems.

- **Interactive** plans of care allow for individualized adaptation for a client's specific conditions, while enabling the nurse to select the nursing diagnoses, appropriate outcomes, and interventions. As the client's condition changes, the outcomes of nursing interventions are evaluated and the interactive plan can be modified to meet the changing client needs.

In this chapter you learned to use the ADT and Nursing tabs. You learned to create nursing care plans and to retrieve an existing encounter. You also learned new buttons on the Toolbar:

Medcin   Restores the full Medcin nomenclature when the left pane has been limited by a List or other type of template.

Cite   Records a finding from a previous encounter or plan of care into the current encounter.

Outcome   Allows you to record an evaluation outcome in the encounter without resolving the nursing diagnosis.

As you continue through the course, you can refer to the Guided Exercises in this chapter when you need to remember how to perform a particular task that you learned in this chapter.

Task	Guided Exercise(s)	Page No.
Selecting Patients from the ADT tab	37	192
Printing a plan of care	38	197
Creating an individualized plan of care	39	203
Modifying a plan of care		
Adding a new nursing action	39, step 21	212
Adding free text to a nursing intervention	40, step 12	223
Setting a nursing diagnosis inactive	40, step 13	223
Setting an outcome using the Toolbar button	40, step 14	225
Changing the interval of a nursing order	40, step 16	226
Retrieve a previous encounter	41	227

References

American Nurses Association. (2010). *Nursing: Scope and standards of nursing practice* (2nd ed.). Silver Spring, MD: Author.

Feeg, V. D., Saba, V. K., & Feeg, A. (2004). Development and testing of a bedside personal computer (PC) Clinical Care Classification System (CCCS) for nursing students using Microsoft Access. *Computers in Nursing.*

Saba, V. (2007). *Clinical Care Classification (CCC) System manual: A guide to nursing documentation.* New York: Springer Publishing Company.

Test Your Knowledge

1. What are the three Expected Outcomes of the CCC System terminologies?
2. Name the two related CCC terminologies that comprise the CCC System.
3. What is the first step of the nursing process?
4. Why does nursing need a codified standardized documentation system?
5. Name one of the national initiatives that raised awareness for improvement in EHR nursing documentation.
6. What are the three phases of the nurse process that result in the creation of a plan of care?
7. Name the four nursing actions types in the CCC terminologies.
8. Name the three Actual Outcomes in the CCC System.
9. What is a standard plan of care?
10. Describe an individualized plan of care.
11. What button on the Toolbar allows you to record an evaluation in the encounter?

The following prefixes precede descriptions of CCC findings. Write the meaning of each:

12. RNOx _____
13. RNDx _____
14. RNRx _____
15. You should have printed two narrative documents of client encounters and two plans of care. If you have not already done so, hand these in to your instructor with this test. These will count as a portion of your grade.

Ask your instructor for answers to Test Your Knowledge

nursing.pearsonhighered.com

Prepare for success with animated examples, practice questions, challenge tests, and interactive assignments.

Comprehensive Evaluation of Chapters 1–6

This comprehensive evaluation will enable you and your instructor to determine your understanding of the material covered so far. Complete both the written test and the two exercises provided below. Depending on the time provided, it may be necessary to do this in two separate sessions. Your instructor will advise you. Do not begin the hands-on exercise if there will not be enough class time to complete it.

Part I—Written Exam

You may run the Student Edition software and use your mouse on the screen to answer the following questions. You will also need access to the Internet to answer some of the questions.

Give a brief description of the purpose of each of the following coding systems:

1. Medcin _____
2. CCC _____
3. Explain the difference between an EHR nomenclature and a billing code set.
4. Which screen do you use to set the reason for the visit?
5. How do you load a form?
6. How do you load a list?

Write the meaning of each of the following acronyms:

7. ROS _____
8. Hx _____
9. HPI _____
10. Dx _____
11. HEENT _____
12. URI _____
13. How does the HITECH Act influence EHR adoption?
14. What Entry Details field is used with a finding to indicate an "admission" diagnosis?
15. Name the two related CCC terminologies that are used in the CCC System.
16. List the six steps of the nursing process, in order.
17. Compare the advantages of codified EHR data over scanned document data.
18. Name at least three things that are checked by a DUR alert system.
19. What is a care pathway?
20. Name the four nursing actions in the CCC terminologies.
21. Name the three Actual Outcomes in the CCC System.

Describe the purpose of the following buttons on the Medcin Toolbar:

22. Negs   _____

23. ROS   _____

24. Outcome   _____

25. Medcin   _____

Part II—Online Student Exercise Questions

Use the document image simulation program on the Online Student Resources web site to answer the next five questions.

Case Study

Raj Patel is an 80-year-old male who arrives in the emergency department accompanied by his daughter. His daughter informs the triage nurse that Mr. Patel was previously an inpatient at this hospital.

Using what you have learned in Guided Exercise 5, find the information that the triage nurse needs about Mr. Patel's previous stay.

Step 1

Start your web browser, go to the Online Student Resources web site and log in. Select Exercises and Activities from the drop down list and click on Evaluation 1–6 in the left menu.

Locate and click the link "Document/Image System program."

Step 2

Select patient **Raj Patel**.

Step 3

Locate and click on the catalog entry for his Admission Face Sheet.

26. What was the date of admission?

27. What was the date of discharge?

28. What was the admitting diagnosis?

29. What was the name of the attending physician?

Step 4

Locate and click on the catalog entry for his Discharge report.

30. Where was the client discharged to?

Part III—Hands-on Exercise

The following exercise will use features of the software with which you have become familiar. Complete each step in sequential order using the instructions and other information provided.

When you have finished the complete exercise, print out the encounter note and plan of care. Give them to your instructor. Do not begin the hands-on exercise if there will not be enough class time to complete it.

Critical Thinking Exercise 43: Admission of an Inpatient with Asthma

In this exercise, you use the skills you have acquired to document this exam.

Case Study

Carl Brown is a 30-year-old male who comes to the hospital complaining of awakening in the night short of breath. Carl does not smoke, but he is exposed to second-hand smoke and has pets in the house. His admitting doctor has diagnosed his condition as asthma with acute exacerbation and has entered orders for oxygen, pain medication, and respiratory medications.

Step 1

If you have not already done so, start the Student Edition software.

Click Select on the Menu bar, and then click Patient.

In the Patient Selection window, locate and click on **Carl Brown**.

Step 2

Click Select on the Menu bar, and then click New Encounter.

Select the date **May 13, 2012**, the time **4:45 PM**, and the reason **Hospital Inpatient**.

Make certain that you set the date and reason correctly. Compare your screen to the date, time, and reason printed in bold type before clicking on the OK button.

Step 3

Before beginning your assessment, you provided care to help make the client comfortable and need to document the care provided.

Locate and click on the Nursing tab at the bottom of your screen.

Click on the Px tab at the top of the left pane.

Locate and click the small plus sign next to "Vital Signs."

Locate and click the small icon button, type the value indicated, and then click the Enter button (or press the Enter key) for the following:

☞ Pain Level: **6**

Step 4

Click on the Rx tab at the top of the left pane.

Locate and click the small plus signs next to "Nursing care" and "Nursing Interventions."

Scroll the pane downward to locate and click the small plus sign next to "Sensory."

Locate and click the button indicated for the following intervention:

● (red button) RNRx Pain Control

Scroll the pane downward to locate and click the small plus signs next to "Nursing Orders" and "RNOx Vital Signs."

Scroll further downward to locate and click the small plus sign next to "RNOx Pain."

Locate and click the buttons indicated for the following nursing orders:

● (red button) RNOx Administer Pain Scale
● (red button) RNOx Administer Prescribed Pain Medication

Step 5

You have also performed the ordered pulmonary care.

Locate and click on the Lists button in the Toolbar at the top of your screen. The List Manager window will be invoked.

Two fields at the top of the List Manager window organize the display of List names, filtering them by Owner and Group. The Student Edition has two groups.

Click on the down arrow in the Group field and select the Group "Student Edition."

Locate and highlight the list named **Asthma**. Click your mouse on the button labeled "Load List."

Verify that you are still on the Rx tab.

Locate and click the buttons indicated for the following nursing intervention and orders:

- (red button) RNRx Inhalation Therapy
- (red button) RNOx Provide Oxygen Therapy
- (red button) RNOx Provide Nebulizer Therapy
- (red button) RNOx Instruct to Leave Nasal Cannula Tubing in Place
- (red button) RNOx Teach Inhaler Instructions
- (red button) RNOx Teach Purpose of Nebulizer

Step 6

Locate and click on the description **RNOx Titrate O2 to Maintain Saturation Value**, but do not click the red or blue button.

Locate and click in the Entry Details field "Value." Type **92%** and press the Enter key on your keyboard.

Step 7

After Carl was more comfortable, you were able to continue your nursing assessment.

Click on the Sx tab and the title of first line should be "Templates (Symptoms)."

Locate and click on the following symptom findings:

- (red button) feeling tired or poorly
- (red button) headache
- (red button) recurrent episodes of acute difficulty breathing

The description will change to Episodic dyspnea.

- (red button) awakening at night short of breath

The description will change to Paroxysmal nocturnal dyspnea.

Step 8

Locate and click the small plus signs next to "cough" and "quality."

Scroll the pane downward as necessary to locate and click on the buttons indicated for the following findings:

- (red button) sounding like barking
- (red button) wheezy
- (red button) hacking
- (red button) worse at night
- (red button) causing awakening from sleep

Step 9

Locate and click the small plus sign next to "wheezing."

Scroll the pane downward as necessary to locate and click on the buttons indicated for the following findings:

- (red button) only when breathing in
- (blue button) responding to bronchodilators

Step 10

Click on the Hx tab.

Locate and click on the buttons indicated for the following findings:

- (red button) previous hospitalization for a pulmonary problem
- (red button) exposure to secondhand smoke
- (red button) exposure to animal dander
- (blue button) current smoker
- (red button) never a smoker

Step 11

Click on the Px tab to document the physical exam.

Locate and click the small plus sign next to "Respiratory Movements."

Locate and click on the buttons indicated for the following findings:

- (red button) Exaggerated Use of Accessory Muscles for Inspiration
- (red button) Inspiratory Retraction
- (red button) Wheezing
- (red button) Auscultation Prolonged Expiratory Time
- (red button) Rales/Crackles

Step 12

Locate and highlight the finding **Wheezing was heard**.

Locate the Status field in the Entry Details section at the bottom of the screen. Click your mouse on the down arrow button in the status field. A drop-down list of status phrases will appear.

Position your mouse pointer on the status "inadequately controlled" and click the mouse button.

The description should change to "Wheezing was heard which is inadequately controlled."

Step 13

Click on the Dx tab.

Locate and highlight the diagnosis **Asthma with Acute Exacerbation**.

Locate the Prefix field in the Entry Details section and click your mouse on the down arrow button. Locate **Admission diagnosis of** in the drop-down list and click on it.

Step 14

Enter the Chief complaint by locating and clicking on the button labeled "Chief" in the Toolbar at the top of your screen.

In the dialog window that will open, type "**Client reports waking at night short of breath.**"

When you have finished typing, click on the button labeled "Close the note form."

Step 15

Click on the Forms tab at the bottom of your screen.

Record Carl's medical history and vital signs using the Short Intake form.

Locate and click on the button labeled "Forms" in the Toolbar at the top of your screen.

Select the **Short Intake** form in the Forms Manager window.

When the Short Intake form is displayed, locate and click on the check box next to:

✓ **Y** Sleep disturbances

Locate and click on the ROS button in the Toolbar at the top of your screen. Verify that it has turned orange and then locate and click the Negs button in the Toolbar at the top of your screen.

Again, locate and click on the ROS button in the Toolbar at the top of your screen. Verify that it is no longer orange.

Step 16

Locate and click on the tab labeled "Medical History" at the top of the form.

Enter the Dx History and Family History by clicking on the Y (yes) check box or the N (no) check box for the following items:

Diagnosis	Dx Hist	Family Hist
Angina	✓ N	✓ N
Asthma	✓ Y	✓ Y
Bronchitis	✓ Y	✓ N
Cancer	✓ N	✓ N
Congestive Heart Failure	✓ N	✓ N
Coronary Artery Disease	✓ N	✓ N
Diabetes	✓ N	✓ N
Heart Attack	✓ N	✓ N
Hypertension	✓ N	✓ N
Migraine Headache	✓ N	✓ N
Peptic Ulcer	✓ N	✓ N
Reflux	✓ N	✓ N
Stroke	✓ N	✓ N

Complete the rest of his medical history on the right side of the form by locating and clicking on the check boxes as follows:

Currently Taking Medication	✓ N
Recent Exposure (Contagious Disease)	✓ N
Recent History of Travel	✓ N
Recent Medical Examination	✓ Y
Recent X-Ray	✓ N
Allergies	✓ Y
Allergy to Drugs	✓ N

Step 17

Locate and click on the tab at the top of the form labeled "Physical Examination."

Enter Carl's vital signs in the corresponding fields on the form as follows:

Temperature:	**98.8**
Respiration:	**26**
Pulse:	**78**
BP:	**120/80**
Weight:	**165**

Alert

Do not continue with
Step 19 until you
have a printed copy
in your hand. You
will lose your work
if you exit before
printing.

Locate and click on the Negs button in the Toolbar at the top of your screen. The physical exam findings should now have a check mark.

Locate and click on the Encounter tab at the bottom of the screen.

Step 18

Before proceeding to the nursing plan of care, you are going to print your encounter.

Click on the Print button on the Toolbar at the top of your screen to invoke the Print Data window.

Be certain there is a check mark in the box next to "Current Encounter" and then click on the appropriate button to either print or export a file, as directed by your instructor. Your print out or file should consist of 2–3 pages.

Do not close or exit the Student Edition; continue with Step 19.

Step 19

Once you have your printed encounter in hand, you will create an individualized nursing plan of care for Mr. Brown.

Locate and click on the ADT tab at the bottom of your screen.

Locate and click on **Carl Brown** to highlight his name.

Locate and click on the button labeled "Initial Data Entry." The tab at the bottom of the screen will automatically change to the Nursing tab.

Step 20

Locate and click the red buttons for the following nursing diagnoses:

- (red button) RNDx Acute Pain
- (red button) RNDx Respiratory Alteration

Locate and click on the button below the left pane labeled "Show Plan of Care."

Step 21

Now that the nursing diagnoses have been identified, the next phase in the nursing process is to identify the expected outcomes, interventions, and actions.

Locate and right-click on "Respiratory Alteration (Respiratory)."

In the drop-down menu, locate "Add a Goal for this Diagnosis," and click on the goal **Stabilize**.

Right-click on "Respiratory Alteration (Respiratory)" again.

In the drop-down menu click on "Select Interventions" and a small window will be displayed. Locate and click on the check box for the following interventions:

✓ Medication Treatment

✓ Oxygen Therapy Care

✓ Pulmonary Care

Once the interventions are added, right-click on "Medication Treatment" and then click "Select Nursing Actions" in the drop-down menu.

In the Action Selection window locate and click on the check boxes for the following nursing actions:

✓ Monitor Medication Treatment

✓ Administer Medication Treatment

Step 22

Right-click on "Oxygen Therapy Care" and then click "Select Nursing Actions" in the drop-down menu.

In the Action Selection window, locate and then click on the check boxes for the following nursing actions:

✓ Assess Respiratory Status

✓ Monitor Oxygen Saturation

✓ Titrate O2 To Maintain Saturation Value

✓ Provide Oxygen Therapy

✓ Collaborate With Respiratory Therapist

Step 23

Right-click on "Pulmonary Care" and then click "Select Nursing Actions" in the drop-down menu.

In the Action Selection window, locate and click the check boxes for the following nursing actions:

✓ Assess Airway Clearance

✓ Assess Sputum Appearance

✓ Assess Sputum Quantity

✓ Demonstrate Pursed-Lip Breathing

✓ Report Signs of Respiratory Distress

Step 24

Following the same sequence you used in Steps 21 and 22, complete the plan of care for the nursing diagnosis "Acute Pain (Sensory)."

Add the Goal: **Improve**.

Select Intervention:

✓ Pain Control

Select Nursing Actions for Pain Control:

✓ Assess Pain Control

✓ Administer Pain Scale

✓ Administer Prescribed Pain Medication

Because you will only administer pain medication if the client needs it, modify the frequency interval for that nursing action.

Locate and right-click on the nursing action "Administer Prescribed Pain Medication ^QSHIFT."

In the drop-down menu click on "Change Sig" and the interval window will open.

Locate and click on the button labeled "Clear Interval."

Locate and click on the check box for the interval:

✓ **PRN (Given as needed)**.

Click on the OK button to close the window. Verify that the interval has changed.

Step 25

Scroll the left pane upward to locate and right-click on "Current and Active Nursing Diagnoses"; a drop-down menu will appear. Click on "Print POC."

When the Print Data window opens, be certain there is a check mark in the box next to "Plan of Care" and then click on the appropriate button to either print or export a file, as directed by your instructor. Your plan of care should consist of one page.

Give your encounter and plan of care printout or output files from this exercise to your instructor.

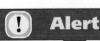

① Alert

Do not change tabs, close, or exit the encounter until you have the printed plan of care in your hand. You will lose your work if you exit before printing.

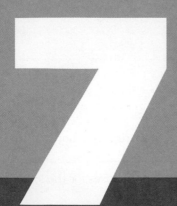

Chapter

7 Understanding Electronic Orders

Learning Outcomes

After completing this chapter, you should be able to:

1. Discuss the importance of electronic orders and results
2. Compare paper and electronic workflow of orders and results
3. Search for a finding using the Search button
4. Understand and use the Prompt feature
5. Record orders for tests
6. Order tests to confirm or rule out a diagnosis
7. Describe the workflow of radiology orders and reports
8. Discuss Closed Loop Safe Medication Administration
9. Name the ten rights of medication administration
10. Use a CPOE to write a prescription
11. Order medications using a quick-pick list
12. Compare ICD-9-CM codes and ICD-10 codes
13. Use a diagnosis to find protocols

The Importance of Electronic Orders and Results

All types of treatments and care events are the result of provider orders. Examples include labs, x-rays, other diagnostic tests, medications, oxygen, diet, therapy, and even home medical devices such as a walker or wheelchair.

As you learned in Chapter 1, computerized provider order entry, or CPOE, is viewed by IOM, Leapfrog, and others as one of the key features of an EHR that can improve quality of care, patient safety, and clinician efficiency. The IOM report suggests, when care is ordered electronically, the care is expedited and the workflow process is improved to the benefit of the client. According to an IOM report (Dick & Steen, 2000), CPOE systems can improve workflow processes by:

▶ Preventing lost orders

▶ Eliminating ambiguities caused by illegible handwriting

▶ Reduce the medication errors of dose and frequency, drug–allergy, and drug–drug interactions

▶ Monitoring for duplicate orders

▶ Reducing the time to fill orders

▶ Automatically generating related orders

▶ Improve clinician productivity

Computerized results improve workflow processes because:

▶ They can be accessed more easily than paper reports by the provider at the time and place they are needed.

▶ They reduce lag time, allowing for quicker recognition and treatment of medical problems.

▶ Automated display of previous test results makes it possible to reduce redundant and additional testing.

▶ They allow for better interpretation and for easier detection of abnormalities, thereby ensuring appropriate follow-up.

▶ Access to electronic consults and patient consents can establish critical linkages and improve care coordination among multiple providers, as well as between provider and patient.

To help visualize these important points, we will compare workflows of paper versus electronic orders and results. We will then discuss laboratory and radiology orders and you will learn to record them in the EHR. While recording orders, you will learn to use the search, prompt, and order features of the software. Next, we will discuss medication orders and closed loop administration of medications, and will use an electronic prescription writer in several exercises. The chapter concludes with an explanation of diagnosis codes and order protocols based on diagnosis, and you will write orders using a protocol list.

Recording Orders in the Student Edition

CPOE is used by many types of healthcare providers. Some examples include physicians, licensed nurse practitioners, physician assistants, registered nurses, pharmacists, and others, within the scope of their license or role in the healthcare team. Although you may not yet be a nurse who writes orders, there are a number of reasons we include orders in this course:

1. Orders are an essential component of any chart and a key objective for the IOM, Leapfrog, HITECH Act, and CMS "meaningful use" criteria.

2. Charts that include electronic orders and results offer the student a more realistic view of the complete EHR workflow.

3. Nurses often enter verbal orders into an EHR on behalf of the ordering clinician.

4. Nurses or other allied health professionals may enter their own orders directly in the EHR within their particular scope of practice. (You have already entered nursing orders while creating the nursing plan of care in Chapter 6.)

5. Nurse practitioners and physician assistants in nearly all states are licensed to write prescriptions and thus will use an electronic prescription writer. Nurse practitioners order laboratory, radiology, and other diagnostic tests with the same authority as their physician counterparts.

6. In some critical care units, a nurse will act as a scribe for the *code* team, documenting the emergency care as it is being delivered, including the ordering of stat tests and meds.

Exercises in this textbook simulate the process of ordering and tracking lab results on a computer and simulate writing prescriptions electronically. However, the Student Edition software does not write or send actual orders to a lab, nor can it write or send actual prescriptions to a pharmacy. These capabilities would be inappropriate in a student edition. Even though it would not be the role of a student nurse to write orders for tests or prescriptions, the exercises help the student experientially understand CPOE processes.

Lab Orders and Reports

Laboratory and other diagnostic tests are ordered to determine the health status of the client, to confirm, or to rule out, a suspected diagnosis. In most healthcare settings these tests and the associated results are referred to simply as lab tests or lab results and will be designated with this more common name throughout this chapter.

Laboratory services consist of nine sciences:

▶ Hematology

▶ Chemistry

▶ Immunology

▶ Blood bank (donor and transfusion)

▶ Pathology

▶ Surgical pathology

▶ Cytology

▶ Microbiology

▶ Flow cytometry

Early in the process the order is assigned a unique ID called a *requisition or accession* number, which is used to track the order in both the CPOE and the Laboratory Information System (LIS).

Many laboratory tests use automated instruments to analyze blood and other samples. These instruments typically have an electronic interface to the LIS. This enables automated test equipment to transfer test results directly to the LIS database. Test results are first stored in the LIS and then transferred to the EHR or printed on a paper lab result report.

Some lab tests cannot be performed by automated equipment. For example, some pathology tests are performed by growing cultures and examining them, or examining tissue samples through a microscope. There are three areas of pathology:

▶ Clinical pathology uses chemistry, microbiology, hematology, and molecular pathology to analyze blood, urine, and other body fluids.

▶ Anatomic pathology performs gross, microscopic, and molecular examination of organs and tissues and autopsies of whole bodies.

▶ Surgical pathology performs gross and microscopic examination of tissue removed from a patient by surgery or biopsy.

Hospitals and some medical practices have a laboratory in the medical facility. There are also outside testing facilities called *reference laboratories*. These labs process tests for facilities that do not have their own labs and perform esoteric tests that are beyond the capability of the hospital laboratory.

There are also medical tests that do not have to be performed in a laboratory. Certain tests may be performed by handheld instruments at the client's bedside or even the client's home. This is called *point-of-care testing*. One example of such an instrument is a *glucose monitor*. The glucose monitor measures the amount of a type of sugar in a client's blood. The results of this test can be electronically transferred from the glucose monitor device to the EHR. In a hospital, the data may be transferred via the LIS or entered manually in the chart by the nurse or other caregiver.

The fluid or tissue to be examined is called the *specimen*. The specimen may be collected from the client at the medical facility and then transported to the laboratory, or the client may be sent to the laboratory to have his or her blood drawn there.

Whether blood is drawn at a medical office, laboratory, or in a hospital at the client's bedside, a phlebotomist or nurse will collect a specified amount of blood in one or more vials.

A physician usually only collects the specimen when it is part of the exam or procedure—for example, taking a swab for a throat culture, or removing a mole that is to be sent to pathology.

If a test requires a urine sample or stool specimen, this might be obtained from the client at the medical facility or might be brought by an outpatient to his or her appointment.

Here are examples of the various ways a sample for a blood test might be obtained from the client and given to the laboratory:

▶ A nurse in the emergency department may draw blood from a client, but a different person may carry the sample to the hospital laboratory.

▶ A laboratory at an inpatient hospital may send a phlebotomist to the client's room to draw the blood required for ordered tests.

▶ Someone scheduled for surgery may be directed to the hospital laboratory during preadmission, where a phlebotomist or laboratory technician may draw the sample before the client is admitted.

▶ A physician's office may have a small laboratory where certain tests can be performed in the office.

▶ A physician's office may draw the blood but send the specimen to an outside reference lab. In this case a courier will collect the specimens from the medical office and transport them to the lab.

▶ A physician's office may give a written lab requisition to the client and send that person to the outside reference lab. When the client arrives at the lab, a phlebotomist employed by the lab company will draw the blood.

Certain tests may not be covered by the client's insurance and the client must sign an acknowledgment that he or she has been advised that the test will not be paid by insurance. This is called an Advance Beneficiary Notice, or ABN. An example of an ABN form is shown in Chapter 2, Figure 2-23.

If the clinician's diagnosis or plan of treatment is dependent on the outcome of the test, then timeliness is important. In such a case, the client cannot be treated until the provider receives and reviews the results. Although many of the steps are the same, electronic lab orders enable the provider to begin treatment sooner because the provider is aware of the results sooner.

Similarly, tissue samples need to be examined for certain surgical pathologies and the results made available to the surgeon during the surgery.

The results of tests that are performed by automated equipment are communicated to the LIS, which assigns codes and records values for each component of the test. The LIS then compiles the results into a report that includes the information from the original requisition, test codes, codes for each component of the test, as well as standard reference ranges for each associated with the actual value measured with the component. Additional notes, such as whether the value is considered outside the reference range (high or low) and whether the results were verified by repeat testing, also are merged into the report data.

When the report is complete, it is sent to the ordering clinician. The clinician will review the results of the test and take appropriate action. Often in the hospital or clinic setting the lab results are previewed by the nurse and critical values are called to the physician's attention.

From the beginning of the order to completion of the review by the clinician, the status of the order is important. If too much time lapses between when the client needs the test and a treatment is given based on that test's results, the client's condition could deteriorate.

To determine how much time has elapsed, the medical staff must know which clients have tests pending results and when they were ordered. This knowledge enables the nurse to follow up on the test by calling the lab or the client.

Orders are tracked in an EHR from the moment they are entered in the system. If an outpatient or presurgical client fails to show up for a test, the lab can inform the medical staff because the lab received the requisition electronically and is expecting the client.

In the EHR system, all orders have a status. Lab orders that have been sent but have no results are "pending." A report of pending orders is always available.

Labs may sometimes send "preliminary" results to give the clinician an early indication of the test and then send "final" results once the test has been repeated for verification. For example, a bacterial culture's preliminary results may appear after 24 hours, but the culture may be monitored for 72 hours before the final results.

EHR systems may connect to the lab system frequently as new orders are written or at predefined intervals throughout the day. Whenever a connection is established between the two systems, all available results for all of the facility's clients are downloaded to the EHR. When lab results are received, most systems merge the data instantly into the chart. Software matches each result to the original requisition order.

The status will then be preliminary, final, or corrected, as designated by the lab.

With an electronic order system, the lab results are usually available the same day or the next morning. The ordering clinician is electronically notified as soon as results are ready. The clinician may order follow-up tests, a follow-up visit, send a "task" to have the client called, add comments or annotations to the test, and compare the results to previous similar tests results. The EHR system also keeps track of which results have not yet been reviewed by the clinician.

An important tool that clinicians use to care for their clients is "trending," which is comparing the change of certain test components or vital signs over a period of time. In a paper chart, the trend is observed by paging through past tests, locating the desired component on each report, and making a mental comparison. However, when the lab results are stored as fielded, coded data in the EHR, the computer can instantly create trending reports and graphs of any finding with a numerical value. Chapter 2, Figures 2-19 and 2-20 showed examples of trending computerized lab result data.

The benefit of electronic lab results is that the codified data is merged into the EHR. Most medical facilities cannot afford the personnel to have paper lab results keyed into the computer. Without an electronic laboratory interface, the provider and the client both miss the advantages that codified lab data provides.

Electronic lab orders and results benefit both the client and the practice. Waiting for the results of an important test is stressful to clients. Electronic laboratory interfaces help expedite the process, ensuring the provider knows about the results as soon as they are ready at the lab. Whether the client is subsequently contacted by the phone or has access to lab results via the web, the waiting time (and accompanying anxiety) is reduced.

Comparison of Orders and Results Workflows

Chapter 1 compared the workflow of an office using paper charts with an office that fully uses an EHR. In this chapter Figure 7-1 and Figure 7-2 allow us to compare the workflow of an outpatient clinic that writes orders on paper with one that uses electronic orders and results.

In this scenario, the clinician wants additional information about the client's health that can be obtained by analyzing the client's blood. The provider "orders" a blood test.

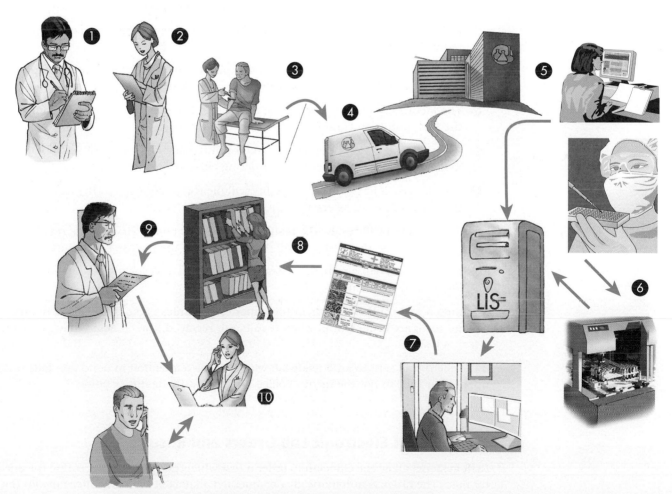

▶ **Figure 7-1 Workflow of paper-based lab orders and results.**

Implied within the order is a request for a nurse, phlebotomist, or other medical personnel to draw a sample of the client's blood.

Workflow of Paper Lab Orders and Results

Figure 7-1 illustrates the workflow of paper-based lab orders and results in an outpatient clinic. Follow the workflow as you read the following:

❶ The workflow begins when the clinician decides a lab test will be useful and writes an order. In a facility that uses paper orders, this may be a verbal order to the nurse, who will obtain and complete the paper requisition form. The test order may be noted in the handwritten paper chart or mentioned in the clinician's dictation.

❷ A paper requisition form supplied by the reference laboratory is filled out. The client's demographic and insurance information is copied by hand, onto the form, with inherent risks of a mistake while copying by hand.

Certain tests may not be covered by the client's insurance and the client must sign an ABN. Whether an ABN will be required for a particular test relies on either a call to the lab, a call to the insurance plan, or the nurse's memory.

❸ The specimen of the client's blood is drawn.

The paper form is accompanied by uniquely numbered labels. The nurse will write the client name and ID on the labels and attach them to the specimen vial or container.

❹ If the blood is drawn at the clinic, the sample is picked up by a courier and transported to the lab. The paper requisition will accompany the specimen.

If the client is going to have the blood drawn at the lab, the client will bring the requisition form.

❺ The paper requisition is keyed into the lab system computer by a lab employee. There is an inherent risk of a typing error or a loss of the paper requisition.

❻ The laboratory performs the tests, assigns codes and values for each component of the test, and then compiles the results into a report.

❼ A pathologist reviews the results and a printed copy of the results will be faxed, mailed, or sent by courier to the ordering clinic or facility.

❽ A staff person at the medical facility will file the paper copy in the client's chart and make the clinician aware that the report has arrived.

❾ The clinician will review the results in the paper chart. To compare results with any previous tests, the clinician will thumb through the pages of the chart.

❿ The clinician will handwrite notes, or leave voice mail for his staff, who will call the client with the results.

Although a copy of the order is in the paper chart, unless a separate list is maintained of what tests are ordered and when results are received, the clinician may never know if a test is lost.

If the client was sent to an outside lab with a paper requisition in hand and fails to show up, neither the lab nor the medical office knows that the test is pending.

Workflow of Electronic Lab Orders and Results

EHR systems allow the clinician to order a test while the clinician is creating the encounter note. The order is automatically documented as part of the encounter note (in the Plan section). You will see this in Guided Exercise 44.

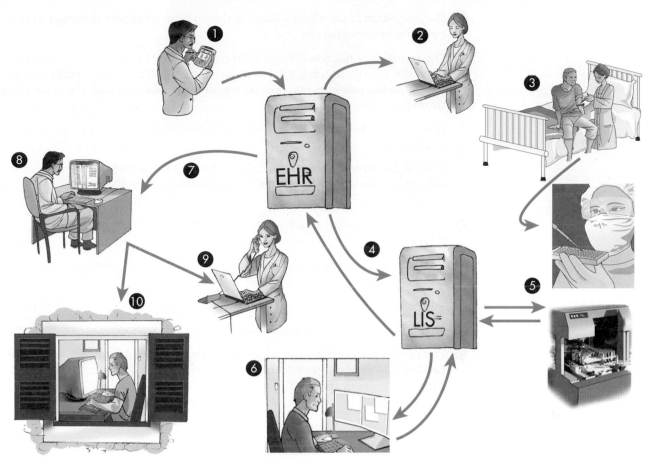

▶ **Figure 7-2 Workflow of electronic lab orders and results.**

Figure 7-2 illustrates the workflow of electronic lab orders and results in an outpatient setting. Follow the workflow as you read the following:

❶ The workflow begins when the provider orders a lab test. Using an EHR at the point of care, the provider can create the order from within the EHR.

The electronic order system compares the test codes on the order to coverage rules for the client's insurance and automatically alerts the user if a signed ABN is required.

CPOE systems also display a list of recent and pending orders for the client. This serves two purposes. First it can prevent unintentional duplicate orders as the clinician is aware if another provider has already ordered the same or similar test. Second, the clinician is made aware of regular preventative or health maintenance tests for which the client is due.

❷ In CPOE systems, the provider does not complete the actual requisition form. The lab order initiates a "task" for a nurse or phlebotomist to act on. The task involves at least two actions: completing the requisition and obtaining a specimen.

A nurse, phlebotomist, or other staff person will complete the electronic requisition in a computer. The client's demographic and insurance information is populated automatically, eliminating mistakes caused by retyping.

Uniquely numbered labels are automatically printed as part of the electronic requisition process.

❸ The specimen of the client's blood is drawn. The labels are attached to the specimen vial or container.

❹ The requisition is transmitted electronically to the lab system computer and contains the information required to process the test. Electronic orders are transmitted to the lab either in real time as each requisition is completed or in batches throughout the day.

Specimens obtained by the nurse are transported to the lab one or more times a day.

Note, if the client is sent to the lab for the blood to be drawn there, the requisition will already be waiting in the lab system when the client arrives because it was sent electronically.

❺ The lab performs the requested tests and communicates the results through the LIS.

❻ As soon as any results are ready at the lab, they are reviewed by the pathologist and made available to the medical facility's EHR.

❼ The results are returned electronically and merged into the client's EHR.

The EHR can alert the clinician that the results are ready.

❽ The clinician will review the results on screen. Access to other components of the EHR allows easy comparison of current results with previous tests and allows the clinician to graph trends. The clinician can then order the treatments and follow-up tests, send messages to the staff or the client, and do it all from the EHR.

❾ In an outpatient setting, a nurse or other staff member receives an electronic "task" to call the client.

❿ Alternatively, some facilities allow the client to view the test results online via a secure web site.

Electronic lab orders are assigned a status the moment they are created. This makes it easy for a clinician to see that a test has already been ordered by another provider. It also means that the order is not buried in some paper chart, but electronically tracked so the clinic is alert to missing or overdue results.

Learning to Use the Search and Prompt Features

In preparation for learning to place electronic orders, you will find it helpful to learn to use the search and prompt features. As you learned in Chapter 2, medical nomenclatures such as SNOMED-CT and Medcin have hundreds of thousands of findings. The challenges with large clinical vocabularies include:

▶ How can you locate a finding among hundreds of thousands?

▶ Does the nomenclature use the same term for the finding as you do?

▶ Where are other related findings?

The Search feature provides a quick way for the nurse to locate a desired finding in the nomenclature. This feature is helpful for locating and documenting any finding, including but not limited to orders. Search produces a list of the findings almost instantly. Medcin addresses semantic differences in medical terms in several ways:

1. Search performs automatic word completion; if you search for "knee" but the finding is for "knees," it will still find it.

2. Medcin includes an extensive list of synonyms that are used in an alternate word search. For example, if you search for knee injury, the search results will also include findings for knee burns, knee trauma, and fractured patella, among others.

3. Search identifies related findings in other tabs so that when you search for a word or phrase in a particular tab, related findings are automatically available in the other tabs. This means that when you are using Search while documenting an encounter, as you proceed, the other tabs may already have related findings that you will use.

How Search Works

Search is not designed to find every instance that contains the words being searched because the search results would often have too many findings. Instead, search uses the Medcin hierarchy (the tree view you have expanded in previous exercises). It finds and shows the highest level match and does not list all the expanded findings below it.

For example, in Chapter 5 you did an exercise with Headache during which you expanded the tree to show many types of headache. If you searched for Headache, the search results would display the finding "Headache" with a small plus sign next to it. If you wanted to peruse the various types of headaches, you would click on the plus sign to expand the next level of the tree. If, however, you were searching for "migraine headache," the search results would have expanded the tree for Headache to show migraine.

Search always begins in the tab you are currently in when you start the search. If there are search results in another tab but none in the current tab, the software will automatically change tabs to the first one with results. The order of the tabs you see on the screen is the same order in which search will display the results. For example, if you are on the Tx tab when you search and there are no results but there are results for the other tabs, it will automatically change the left pane to the Dx tab to display those results because Dx is the next tab in order.

Guided Exercise 44: Using Search and Prompt

When there are referrals for diagnosis or follow-up care, a battery of diagnostic tests may be ordered to be done before the scheduled appointment so the results can be available when the clinician sees the client. This is especially true of tests that require more time for results or require the capabilities of an outside lab or radiology center.

Having the results ready when the clinician sees the client allows the results to be considered during the exam, used in the current assessment, and used to educate and counsel the client.

In this exercise, you will learn to use the Search and Prompt features as well as several new buttons on the Toolbar. The exercise minimizes the nursing assessment portion of the encounter to focus on learning the new features.

Case Study

The client, Gary Yamamoto, has been referred the hospital's cardiology clinic with suspected angina. Gary did not seem in any immediate danger when he was seen by his family physician at the time of the referral and has been given an appointment at the clinic later this week. In the meantime, we are going to enter orders for some tests to be done before the scheduled appointment so the results will be available at the scheduled clinic visit.

Step 1

If you have not already done so, start the Student Edition software.

Click Select on the Menu bar, and then click Patient.

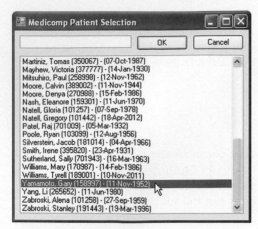

▶ **Figure 7-3 Selecting Gary Yamamoto from the Patient Selection menu.**

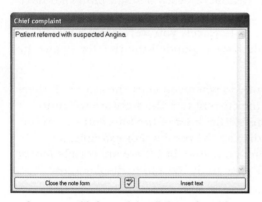

▶ **Figure 7-4 Chief complaint dialog referral for suspected angina.**

In the Patient Selection window, locate and click on **Gary Yamamoto**, as shown in Figure 7-3.

Step 2

Click Select on the Menu bar again, and then click New Encounter.

You may use the current the date and time for this exercise.

Select the reason **Pre-visit Workup** from the drop-down list. Click on the OK button.

In the next two steps, the nurse enters the Chief complaint and Vital Signs.

Step 3

Enter the Chief complaint by locating the button in the Toolbar labeled "Chief" and clicking on it.

In the dialog window that will open, type "**Patient referred with suspected Angina.**"

Compare your screen to Figure 7-4 before clicking on the button labeled "Close the note form."

Step 4

Enter Mr. Yamamoto's vital signs using the Vitals Form.

Locate and click on the button labeled "Forms" in the Toolbar at the top of your screen.

Select the form labeled "Vitals" from the list in the Form Manager window.

Enter Gary Yamamoto's vital signs in the corresponding fields as follows:

Temperature:	**98.6**
Respiration:	**20**
Pulse:	**70**
BP:	**130/86**
Height:	**65**
Weight:	**138**

When you have finished, compare your screen to Figure 7-5. If it is correct, click on the tab labeled "Encounter" at the bottom of the window.

Step 5

Rather than navigate the entire Medcin nomenclature, you can start with a known symptom or disease and work forward. To quickly locate the desired findings, we will use the Search function.

Locate the Search button on the Toolbar near the top of the screen. The search icon resembles a small pair of binoculars. It is highlighted orange in Figure 7-6.

Click your mouse on it to invoke the "Search String" window. Position your mouse in the Search String field and enter the medical term "**angina pectoris.**" Verify that you have spelled this correctly, and then click the button in the search window that says "Search."

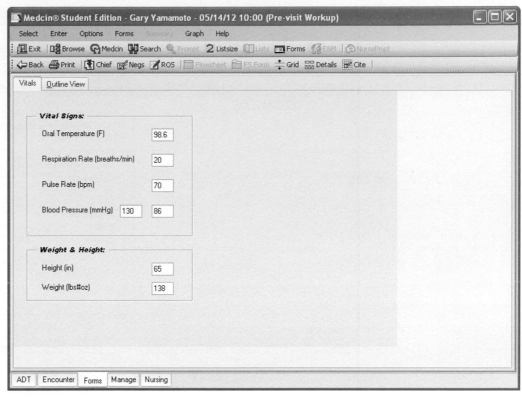

▶ **Figure 7-5 Vital Signs form for Gary Yamamoto.**

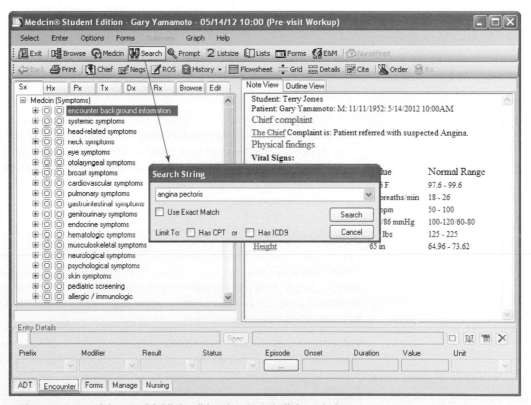

▶ **Figure 7-6 Search button (highlighted) invokes Search dialog window.**

▶ **Figure 7-7 Search results (Prompt button highlighted).**

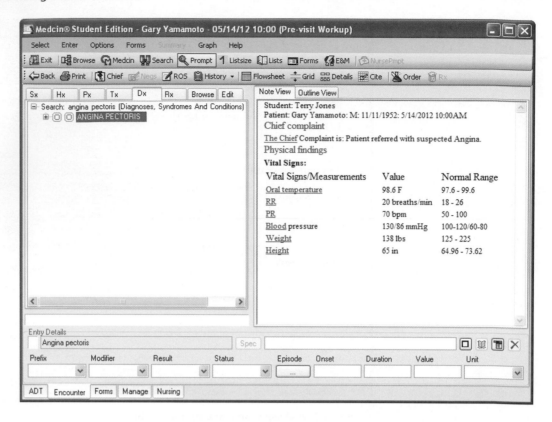

Step 6

Compare your screen to Figure 7-7, which shows the search has succeeded. Notice that you started the search on the Sx tab but the screen is now on the Dx tab. This is because the search was for a very specific pair of words that did not exist in the other tabs.

As discussed earlier in this section, the Search result displays in the current tab if there are any findings that match the search string; otherwise, it displays in the first tab with findings that match. Had the search simply been for angina, History of Angina would have been found and the Hx tab would have been displayed.

Note

No Results?

If your screen does not match Figure 7-7, or you received the message "nothing found to match search," repeat step 5 and verify that you have spelled the medical terms correctly. In this exercise you are searching for a very specific match, and a spelling error will alter the search results.

Step 7

Locate the Prompt button on the Toolbar near the top of the screen. The Prompt icon resembles a small magnifying glass. It is highlighted orange in Figure 7-7. The full name of the feature is "Prompt with current finding." This feature generates a list of findings that are clinically related to the finding currently highlighted. For this step, Angina Pectoris should be highlighted in blue on your screen.

Once the list is displayed, you can use it just like you have been using Lists in previous exercises. That is, you can record findings by clicking on the red or blue buttons next to the findings. You also can change tabs; however, the findings displayed in the other tabs will be limited to those that are clinically related to the finding that was highlighted when you clicked the Prompt button.

Click your mouse on the Prompt button at this time.

Step 8

Locate the button labeled "Listsize" on the Toolbar near the top of the screen. You have used this button in Chapter 5. As with other lists, the List Size controls the number of findings that will be displayed in a "prompt list."

For this step, set the List Size to **1**. If the List Size is currently greater than 1, click your mouse on the List Size button repeatedly until it displays a **1**.

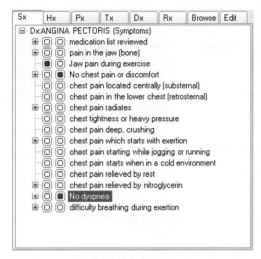

▶ **Figure 7-8 Sx tab displaying findings related to angina (shown after findings selected).**

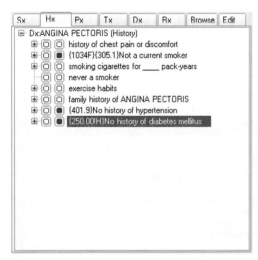

▶ **Figure 7-9 Hx tab displaying findings related to angina.**

Step 9

The left pane should have automatically changed to the Sx tab; if it did not, click on the tab labeled "Sx."

Compare the list in the left pane of your screen to Figure 7-8, ignoring the red and blue buttons for the moment. Note that the list of findings is much shorter than is normally displayed in the Sx tab.

The first line in the left pane usually includes the name or source of the list. Heretofore, this was just the name of the tab, for example, Medcin (Symptoms); now, however, the first line reads "Dx: ANGINA PECTORIS (Symptoms)." This indicates that the list is limited to findings that are clinically related to the diagnosis of angina pectoris.

Proceed with the exercise by locating and clicking on the following symptoms reported by the client:

- (red button) jaw pain during exercise (myocardial)
- (blue button) chest pain or discomfort
- (blue button) difficulty breathing (dyspnea)

Compare your left pane to the selected red and blue buttons in Figure 7-8 before proceeding.

Step 10

The client does not smoke, and denies any history of high blood pressure or diabetes. Click on the Hx tab and enter the client's history information by locating and clicking on the following history findings:

- (blue button) current smoker
- (blue button) history of HYPERTENSION (Systemic)
- (blue button) history of DIABETES MELLITUS

Compare your screen to Figure 7-9.

Step 11

The first test to be ordered is an electrocardiogram (ECG). Although some tests, such as electrocardiograms, are performed in the clinic, most lab tests and many radiology procedures are "ordered" at the clinic, but the test is performed elsewhere.

The ECG was performed today at the clinic.

Verify the List Size displays the numeral **1**.

Click on the Tx tab, which will display a list of tests that might be ordered for angina pectoris.

You can indicate that the test was performed at the clinic by clicking on the red button next to its name. Locate and click on the following finding:

- (red button) Electrocardiogram

► Figure 7-10 Recording the finding "An ECG was performed."

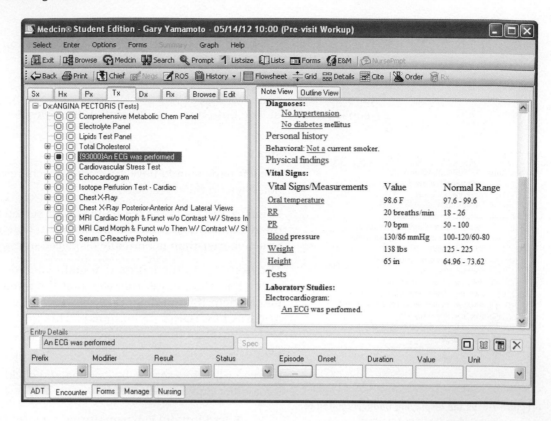

The encounter note should now read, "An ECG was performed," as shown in Figure 7-10 under the heading "Tests."

Do not exit the program until you have completed the following exercise.

► Figure 7-11 Drop-down list of the Prefix field used for electrolyte panel.

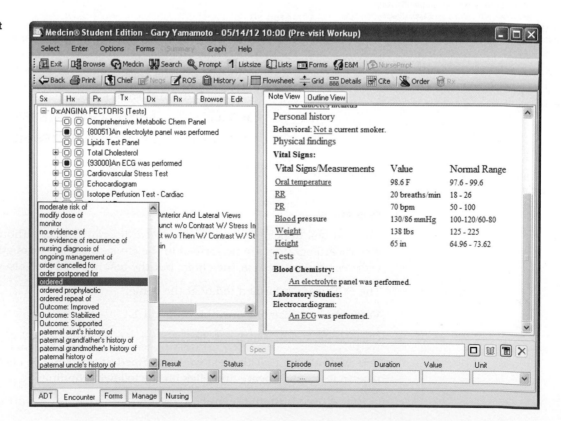

Guided Exercise 45: Ordering Diagnostic Tests

Continuing with Mr. Yamamoto's visit, this exercise will explore several methods of recording tests and orders.

In this exercise, you will order several lab tests. There are two ways to do this: by using the Entry Details Prefix field or by using the Order button on the Toolbar. In step 12, you are going to use a prefix.

Step 12

Locate and click on the following test:

- (red button) Electrolyte panel

Note that the electrolyte panel appears in the encounter note under Tests; "An Electrolyte Panel was performed." However, your clinic did not really perform the Electrolyte panel test; the clinician just wanted to order it.

With the finding of "Electrolyte panel was performed" still highlighted, click on the Prefix field in the bottom of the screen. A drop-down list will appear, as shown in Figure 7-11. Locate and click on the word "Ordered" in the list of prefixes.

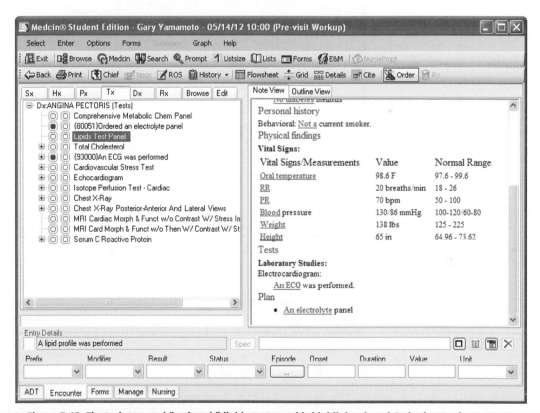

▶ **Figure 7-12** Electrolyte panel "ordered," lipids test panel is highlighted, and Order button is orange.

Step 13

Compare your right pane to the right pane in Figure 7-12. Notice that when you added the prefix "Ordered" to the finding Electrolyte Panel, it not only changed the meaning in the encounter note but also moved the test to a different category in the encounter notes. Medcin assigns a test that was performed or has a result status to the category of test procedures, but assigns a test that is ordered to the category "Plan."

Now that you are familiar with one method of ordering, you can see that it requires several steps, clicking the finding, clicking the down arrow button in the Prefix field, and then locating and clicking the prefix. However, all of these actions can be accomplished in a single step by using the "Order" button on the Toolbar. To order a test using the Order button, you only need to highlight the finding and click the Order button. You do not have to click either the red or blue button for the finding.

Locate and click on the description "Lipids Test Panel" to highlight it (as shown in Figure 7-12).

Locate and click on the button labeled "Order" in the Toolbar at the top of your screen. The Order icon resembles a lab beaker and test tube. It is highlighted orange in Figure 7-12.

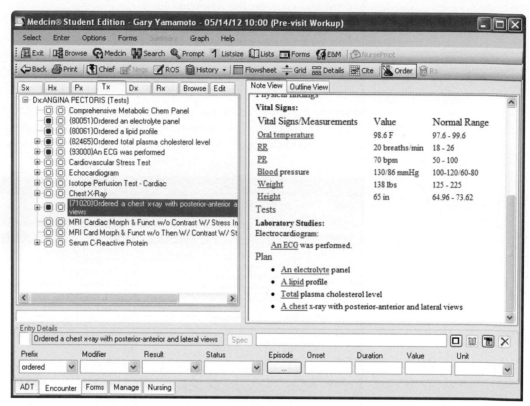

▶ **Figure 7-13 Tests and x-rays ordered using the Order button.**

Step 14

Using what you have learned in the previous step, order an additional test and an x-ray. Highlight each of the following findings and then click on the Order button. Do not click on the red or blue buttons beside these findings. The Order button will set them once they are ordered.

- 🧪 Total Cholesterol

- 🧪 Chest X-Ray Posterior-Anterior and Lateral Views

Compare your screen to Figure 7-13. From this exercise, you can see the advantage of using Toolbar buttons for orders. A different button is used for ordering medications, as you will learn in subsequent exercises.

> **Note**

> ## Electronic Lab Orders
>
> **Most commercial EHR systems offer sophisticated laboratory interface systems that electronically send orders, receive results, and automatically populate the EHR with lab data. In an EHR, a button similar to the lab orders button shown here will typically invoke a window in which you create the actual electronic lab order and send it to the lab.**

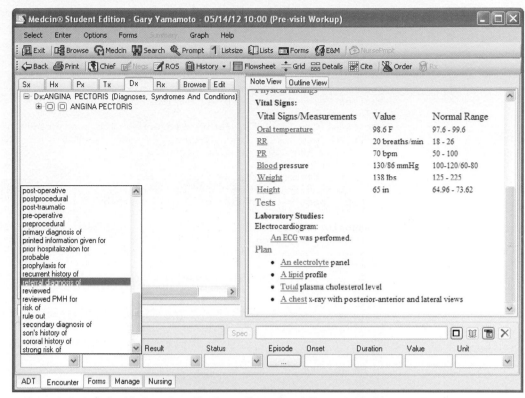

▶ **Figure 7-14 Dx tab with drop-down list for Prefix—referral diagnosis Angina Pectoris.**

Step 15

The clinician will determine the final assessment after the complete workup later this week however the lab requires a diagnosis for the orders. Therefore, the diagnosis at this time will be the referral diagnosis of angina pectoris.

Click on the Dx tab and record the assessment.

Locate and highlight Angina Pectoris.

Locate the Prefix field in the Entry Details section. Click the mouse on the button with the down arrow in the Prefix field.

Scroll the drop-down list to locate and click on the words **Referral diagnosis of**, as shown in Figure 7-14.

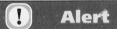 **Alert**

> *Do not close or exit the encounter until you have a printed copy in your hand.* **You will lose your work if you exit before printing.**

Step 16

This completes Mr. Yamamoto's previsit workup. Print your completed encounter note. Click on the Print button on the Toolbar at the top of your screen to invoke the Print Data window.

Be certain there is a check mark in the box next to "Current Encounter" and then click on the appropriate button to either print or export a file, as directed by your instructor.

Compare your printout or file output to Figure 7-15. If it is correct, hand it in to your instructor. If there are any differences (other than date or the client's age), review the previous steps in the exercise and find your error.

```
Gary Yamamoto                                              Page 1 of 1

Student: your name or id here
Patient: Gary Yamamoto: M: 11/11/1952: 5/14/2012 10:00AM
Chief complaint
The Chief Complaint is: Patient referred with suspected Angina.
Referred here
Referral diagnosis of angina pectoris.
History of present illness
     Gary Yamamoto is a 59 year old male.
     He reported: Jaw pain during exercise.
     No chest pain or discomfort. No dyspnea.
Past medical/surgical history
Diagnosis History:
     No hypertension.
     No diabetes mellitus
Personal history
Behavioral: Not a current smoker.
Physical findings
Vital Signs:
Vital Signs/Measurements        Value              Normal Range
Oral temperature                98.6 F             97.6 - 99.6
RR                              20 breaths/min      18 - 26
PR                              70 bpm              50 - 100
Blood pressure                 130/86 mmHg          100 - 120/60 - 80
Weight                         138 lbs             125 - 225
Height                          65 in              64.96 - 73.62
Tests
Laboratory Studies:
     Electrocardiogram:
     An ECG was performed.
Plan
     • An electrolyte panel
     • A lipid profile
     • Total plasma cholesterol level
     • A chest x-ray with posterior-anterior and lateral views
```

▶ **Figure 7-15 Printed encounter note with angina orders for Gary Yamamoto.**

Radiology Orders and Reports

Most acute care hospitals have radiology departments. Radiology departments typically have a radiology information system (RIS), a picture archiving and communication system (PACS) for storing diagnostic images, and a dictation/transcription or voice recognition system for reports. (These were discussed in Chapter 1 and Chapter 2.)

When diagnostic information is needed, the provider may order an x-ray or other radiology study. CPOE Systems in a hospital may create an electronic requisition for the required study or send orders directly to the radiology department RIS system. Radiology orders may also be handwritten or verbal orders. Most medical offices do not yet send electronic radiology orders unless the x-ray or other device is located in the same facility as the ordering provider. Whatever the original form of the order, virtually all radiology department orders are entered into the RIS, where they become electronic orders for the remainder of the process.

Many of the diagnostic imaging devices used in the radiology department are capable of receiving order and client data electronically from the RIS system. Client data is then incorporated in the image data. Once the image is captured, it will transfer electronically into the PACS.

Traditional x-rays used to be taken on photographic film. To be stored in a PAC system, the film then had to be digitized using a scanner. Today, x-ray systems can record the image on a special plate that captures the image digitally, eliminating the steps of developing the film and then scanning it. Another advantage of this technology is that the radiologist can enlarge specific portions of the digital image for further analysis without requiring an additional "view" to be taken. This reduces the client's exposure to radiation.

In addition to x-rays, other types of diagnostic images studied by radiologists include:

▶ Computerized axial tomography (CAT) systems use x-rays to see into the body and capture thousands of digital images. Using computer software, it then constructs a view of cross sections of the body from the digital images. In some facilities this is also referred to as CT or computed tomography.

▶ Magnetic resonance imaging (MRI) uses magnetic fields and pulses of energy to create images of organs and structures inside the body that cannot be seen by x-ray or CAT scan.

▶ Positron emission tomography (PET) combines CT and nuclear scanning using a radioactive substance called a *tracer*, which is injected into a vein. A computer records the tracer as it collects in certain organs, then converts the data into three-dimensional images of the organ. PET can be used to detect or evaluate cancer.

A set of related images interpreted by the radiologist is called a *study*; a *hanging protocol* refers to the number of images that simultaneously display on the radiologist's monitor.

Once the x-ray, CAT scan, or other study images have been captured, a radiologist interprets the results. Increasingly, these images are stored and read in a digital format. The radiologist uses a computer monitor with much higher resolution than standard computer screens to view the images. Special software not only displays the image but also allows the radiologist to manipulate it, zooming in and out, changing the contrast, reversing the image colors, and offering many other capabilities that help the radiologist.

While looking at the image, radiologists dictate a report; describe what they see, its size, location, and any other comments. Because the radiologists are using the computer controls to manipulate and control the image, their observations are seldom keyed into an EHR program. It is standard practice for a radiologist's report to be dictated and then typed by a medical transcriber. However, some radiology departments use speech recognition software, which converts the human voice into typed reports. This was discussed in Chapter 1.

When the report is complete and reviewed by the radiologist, it is sent to the ordering provider. Radiology reports are almost always originated in an electronic text format in the radiology department, but are often sent on paper as a letter or fax, especially to a provider outside the hospital.

Radiology reports are seldom available as a codified EHR record, but some medical facilities may scan the paper reports as document images as you did in Chapter 2. Radiological observations that are codified are those related to the size and stage of tumors.

Additionally, within most hospital systems and from some radiologist's offices, electronic text files of the reports may be available. Copies of the images studied by the radiologist also are sometimes sent to the ordering provider. These images are usually in an electronic format, although x-rays may be sent as film. Electronic transmission of images uses a national standard called DICOM, which stands for Digital Imaging and Communications in Medicine. Electronic orders, results, and other data may be communicated between the hospital systems using another standard, called HL7. Both DICOM and HL7 were discussed in Chapter 2.

Critical Thinking Exercise 46: Ordering an X-Ray

Case Study

Patient Juan Garcia has injured his knee and is examined by a nurse practitioner, who will order an x-ray.

Using what you have learned in this chapter, document Juan Garcia's visit and the nurse practitioner's orders.

Step 1

Click Select on the Menu bar, and then click Patient.

In the Patient Selection window, locate and click on **Juan Garcia**.

Step 2

Click Select on the Menu bar, and then click New Encounter.

You may use the current the date and time for this exercise.

Select the reason **Office Visit** from the drop-down list. Click on the OK button.

Step 3

Enter the Chief complaint by locating the button in the Toolbar labeled "Chief" and clicking on it.

In the dialog window that will open, type "**Twisted his knee.**"

Click on the button labeled "Close the note form."

Step 4

Locate and click on the Search button on the Toolbar near the top of the screen. (The Search button was highlighted in Figure 7-6.)

Click your mouse in the Search String field and enter the medical term "**knee sprain.**" Verify that you have spelled this correctly, and then click the button in the box labeled "Search."

If you see the message "nothing found to match search," repeat step 4 and verify that you have spelled the medical term correctly.

Step 5

If Knee Sprain is not automatically highlighted, click on the description "Knee Sprain" to highlight it.

Locate and click on the Prompt button on the Toolbar near the top of the screen. (The Prompt button was highlighted in Figure 7-7.)

Step 6

If the left pane is not automatically on the Symptoms tab, click the Sx tab. List Size should be 1.

Locate and click on the following findings:

- (red button) joint pain localized in the knee
- (red button) joint swelling of the lateral left knee

Step 7

Click the Hx tab.

Click on the small plus sign next to "Reported trauma to the knee."

Locate and click on the following finding:

- (red button) due to twisting

Step 8

Click the Px tab.

Click on the small plus sign next to "Knee swelling."

Locate and click on the following findings:

- (red button) Left

Scroll the list and then click on the small plus sign next to "Knee tenderness on palpitation."

Locate and click on the following findings:

- ● (red button) On the left

Step 9

Click the Dx tab.

Locate and click on the following finding:

- ● (red button) Knee sprain

Step 10

Click the Tx tab.

Locate and highlight the following finding. When the finding is highlighted, locate and click the Order button on the Toolbar:

- 🧪 (order button) X-Ray Knee Views W/oblique(s), 3 or more views

Step 11

Click the Rx tab.

Locate the List Size button on the Toolbar and click on it. It should change to size **2**.

Locate and click on the following findings:

- ● (red button) ordered knee brace
- ● (red button) ordered pain management by immobilization

Step 12

Click on the Print button on the Toolbar at the top of your screen to invoke the Print Data window.

Alert

Do not close or exit the encounter until you have a printed copy in your hand. You will lose your work if you exit before printing.

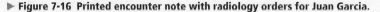

```
Juan Garcia                                                    Page 1 of 1


Student: your name or id here
Patient: Juan Garcia: M: 7/31/1984: 5/14/2012 02:30PM
Chief complaint
The Chief Complaint is: Twisted his knee.
History of present illness
Juan Garcia is a 27 year old male.
He reported: Knee joint pain and knee joint swelling on the left laterally.
Past medical/surgical history
Reported History:
Physical Trauma: Trauma to the knee due to twisting.
Physical findings
Musculoskeletal System:
Knee:
Left Knee:
     • Swelling. • Tenderness on palpation.
Assessment
     • Knee sprain
Plan
     • X-rays of the knee with oblique(s), three or more views
     • Knee brace
     • Pain management by immobilization
```

▶ **Figure 7-16 Printed encounter note with radiology orders for Juan Garcia.**

Be certain there is a check mark in the box next to "Current Encounter" and then click on the appropriate button to either print or export a file, as directed by your instructor.

Compare your printout or file output to Figure 7-16. If it is correct, hand it in to your instructor. If there are any differences (other than date or the client's age), review the previous steps in the exercise and find your error.

Medication Orders

The most common type of order is for medication. Ever since the IOM report revealed that high numbers of deaths have occurred because of preventable medical errors, hospitals have increased their expenditures on systems that are designed to protect client safety. Hospitals' efforts have included CPOE, computerizing pharmacy systems, and using positive identification systems to correctly match the medication with the client, thus ensuring the right client receives the right medication. In ambulatory settings, electronic prescription writers have been incorporated into EHR software and include drug utilization review and formulary checking functions (described in Chapter 2 and below). The HITECH Act and CMS incentive requirements discussed in Chapter 1 require electronic prescribing.

Written Prescriptions

At an inpatient facility using paper charts, the order is written on a Doctor Order sheet and a copy is sent to the hospital pharmacy. The clerk or nurse transcribes the medication order onto a medication administration record or fluid infusion form in the chart. On subsequent hospital days, the pharmacy system may generate an electronically produced medication record that is printed on paper, but this requires the nurse to double-check these records against the physician orders to ensure the printed copy has the most current orders and to manually correct the forms as the new orders are updated.

In an outpatient facility using a paper system, drug prescriptions are written by hand on a prescription pad and given to the client to have filled at a pharmacy. Information about the medication is recorded in the chart by hand or the prescription is copied and filed in the paper chart. Alternatively, a member of the clinic staff may phone the prescription to the pharmacy or the clinician may give the client samples of drugs provided by pharmaceutical companies.

When an outpatient goes to the pharmacy to have the prescription filled, the pharmacist will enter the information in the pharmacy computer system. The client's insurance may require that a generic or less costly drug be substituted for a brand-name drug on the prescription. Unless the provider has indicated DAW (Dispense As Written) on the prescription, it is very likely that the pharmacist will substitute a medically equivalent drug for the one prescribed by the provider.

The pharmacy computer system is also likely to perform two other functions: "formulary compliance checking" and "drug utilization review," or "DUR."

DUR and formulary compliance were discussed earlier in Chapter 2 as an example of decision support. Formulary lists are usually per insurance plan, and because there are so many different plans, the pharmacy system usually checks the formulary by electronically communicating with an intermediary company called a *pharmacy benefit manager*.

If either the formulary checking or the DUR indicates any problem with the handwritten prescription, the pharmacist must contact the prescribing provider. Often the call from the pharmacist comes when the provider is with another client, so a message is left and the call is returned at a later time. This creates a delay for the client and pharmacist and consumes extra time for the provider, who has to return the phone calls. Also when the pharmacy performs the DUR check, its system may not factor in prescriptions filled at other pharmacies or drugs dispensed directly to the client by the clinic.

Electronic Prescriptions

Writing prescriptions electronically has several advantages over the paper chart method. First, the provider issues the prescription and records it in the chart in one step. Second, the prescription can be transmitted electronically from the provider's computer system to the pharmacy, saving time for the client, eliminating the need for the provider's staff to call in the prescription, and reducing errors caused by handwritten prescriptions. Also, the prescription is not lost by the client before arriving at the pharmacy. Finally, the DUR and formulary compliance checking can be performed by the clinician's computer at the time the prescription is written. This allows any problems with the prescription to be corrected before sending it to the pharmacy. This drastically reduces phone calls back to the prescribing provider from the pharmacy, saving everyone time. Figure 2-21 and Figure 2-22 in Chapter 2 show examples of DUR and formulary compliance screens in an electronic prescription system.

DUR is a very important feature that reduces the client's risk of adverse drug reactions. DUR works best when all of the known drugs and allergy information is available and current. Therefore, an EHR should record not only prescriptions issued by the provider's system but also medications prescribed elsewhere. These are usually reported by the client during the nurse's interview or during the exam. The current medications list should be updated each visit before the provider issues any prescriptions.

The electronic prescription component of an EHR can provide additional benefits to both the clinician and the client. Because each medication is automatically recorded in the medications list as the prescription is created, a current and recent medications list is available to the clinician when writing the prescription. Also, the EHR contains a list of medication allergies that the client has experienced. The provider receives a warning if the chosen medication is contraindicated. This reduces prescribing errors.

EHR systems also shorten the time it takes to write a prescription by maintaining a list of prescriptions that the clinician writes frequently. This speeds up the writing of prescriptions for common ailments seen at the practice. Clients with chronic diseases frequently require renewals for existing prescriptions; with EHR systems, this task can be performed with a few clicks of the mouse. Additional time is saved because all FDA-approved drugs are listed in the computer, eliminating the need to use a drug reference book to find less frequently prescribed drugs. An example of an EHR prescription writer will be used in Exercise 47.

Closing the Loop on Safe Medication Administration

Hospital EHR systems help protect clients by closing the loop on medication administration. This safety initiative starts with electronic medication prescription from CPOE to the pharmacy computer system, where the order is checked and approved by the pharmacist for dispensing to the nurse. The nurse can then use an electronic documentation process to ensure the ten rights of medication administration safety. Before administering the medication, a handheld scanner device is used to read a barcode on the client's armband to ensure the medication is being given to the right person. Next, the nurse scans the barcodes on each medication or intravenous solution, and the computer program checks the electronic orders and warns the nurse of any discrepancies. If the medication dose, route, and time match the order for the client, the nurse can then administer the medication. In some electronic systems a repeat scan of the client armband or the scan of the nurse's identification badge completes the documentation, confirming that the medication has been administered.

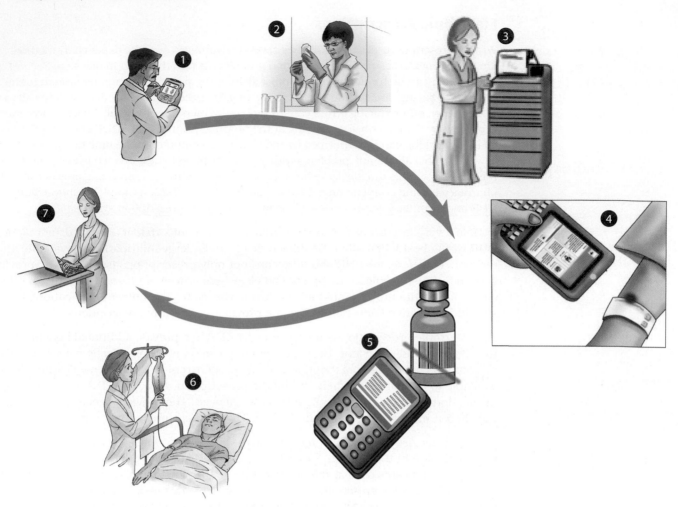

▶ **Figure 7-17 Medication safety—the closed loop process.**

Follow the numbers in Figure 7-17 as you read the following:

❶ The clinician writes prescription using CPOE.

❷ The prescription is checked and approved by the pharmacist.

❸ The nurse receives order electronically and removes vial from medication-dispensing system.

❹ A handheld scanner device is used to read a barcode on the client's armband to ensure the medication is being given to the right person and the nurse verifies the correct name is displayed on the computer.

❺ The nurse scans the barcodes on each medication or intravenous solution and the computer program checks the electronic order and warns the nurse of any discrepancies.

❻ The nurse explains the medication and administers it to the client.

❼ The nurse documents in the chart that the medication was administered. (In some hospital systems a repeat scan of the client's armband or the scan of the nurse's identification badge completes the chart documentation, without manual entry.)

> ### Medication Administration—The Ten Rights
>
> 1. Right client
> 2. Right time and frequency
> 3. Right medication
> 4. Right dose
> 5. Right route of administration
>
> 6. Right documentation
> 7. Right client education
> 8. Right of client to refuse
> 9. Right assessment
> 10. Right response

Guided Exercise 47: Writing Prescriptions in an EHR

In this exercise you will learn to use the Student Edition prescription writer to enter orders that a nurse has received by phone from the doctor. It is necessary for the nurse to enter the prescription, because the hospital's closed loop medication safety policy prevents the automated medication system from dispensing drugs without an order and the doctor does not have remote access to his EHR to write the prescription himself.

Case Study

You will recall from the previous chapter that Eleanore Nash is a 42-year-old female admitted for bacterial pneumonia. She is unable to sleep and informs the nurse that she is in pain from too much coughing. The nurse administers the pain scale and determines the client is at level 7. The nurse contacts Eleanore's physician, who orders Tylenol No. 3 and Ambien. The nurse will write the prescription and the doctor will cosign the order later, usually within 24 hours or in accordance with the facility policies.

► **Figure 7-18 Select patient Eleanore Nash on ADT tab.**

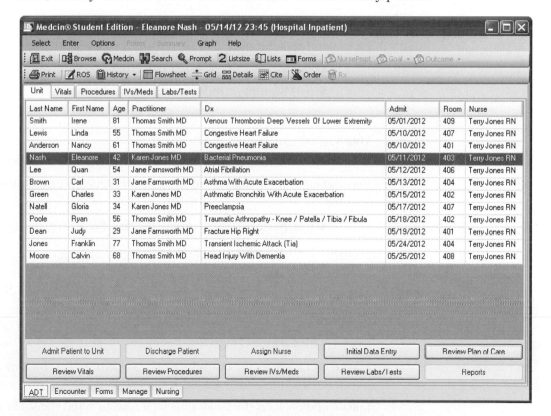

Step 1

If you have not already done so, start the Student Edition software.

Click on the ADT tab at the bottom of your screen, and then locate and click on **Eleanore Nash**, as shown in Figure 7-18.

Locate and click on the button labeled "Review Plan of Care."

Step 2

The nurse reviews the clinical orders in the plan of care as shown in Figure 7-19 to determine if pain medication has been ordered. Notice that a stronger pain medication is not listed in the clinical orders.

Locate the button labeled "Show Data Entry View" below the left pane, and click on it.

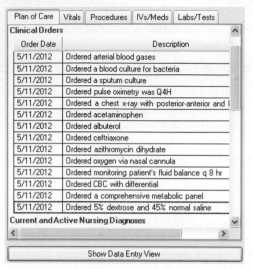

▶ **Figure 7-19 Clinical orders for Eleanore Nash.**

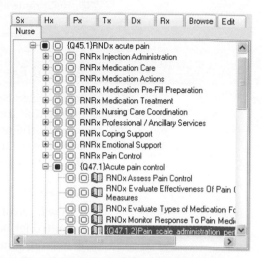

▶ **Figure 7-20 Nursing diagnosis acute pain selected with intervention and action.**

Step 3

Locate and click on the following findings:

- (red button) RNDx Acute Pain
- (red button) RNRx Acute Pain Control

Step 4

Locate and click on the small plus sign next to "Acute pain control."

Scroll the left pane downward to locate and click on the following finding:

- (red button) RNOx Administer Pain Scale

Compare your left pane to Figure 7-20.

Step 5

The nurse next administers and records the pain scale.

Click on the Px tab.

Locate and click on the button labeled "Medcin" in the Toolbar at the top of your screen to restore the full nomenclature in the left pane.

Locate and click on the small plus sign next to "Vital Signs" to expand the list.

Locate and click the small icon button, type the value indicated, and then click the Enter button (or press the Enter key) for the following finding:

☞ Pain scale **7**

Compare your screen to Figure 7-21.

▶ **Figure 7-21 Pain level 7 recorded in chart.**

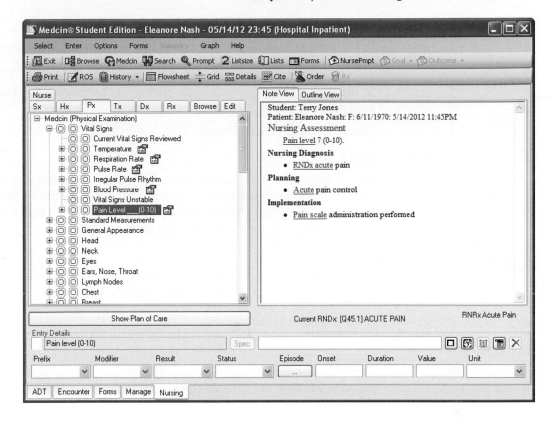

Step 6

At this point the nurse contacts the doctor and receives verbal orders that you will document in the next steps.

Click back on the tab at the top of the left pane labeled "Nurse."

Locate and click on the small plus sign next to "Acute pain control."

▶ **Figure 7-22 Coordination of pain medication orders with Dr. Thomas.**

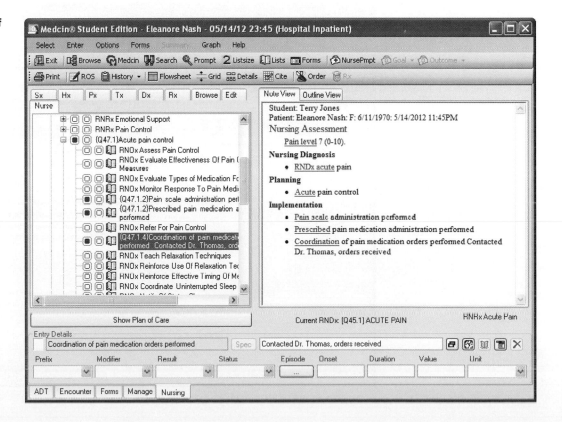

Locate and click on the following findings:

● (red button) RNOx Administer Prescribed Pain Medication

● (red button) RNOx Coordination of pain medication orders

In the free-text field below the right pane, type "**Contacted Dr. Thomas, orders received**."

Compare your screen to Figure 7-22.

Step 7

You will now enter the medication order using the prescription writer. Although clinicians usually have personal order sets that allow them to quickly pick from a list of frequently prescribed drugs, you do not have access to this doctor's list. Therefore you will use Search to locate the ordered drug.

Click on the Rx tab.

Locate and click on the Search button on the Toolbar to invoke the Search String window. Refer to Figure 7-6 if you need help locating the Search button.

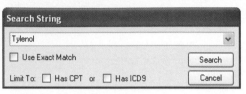

Type "**Tylenol**" in the Search dialog window and click on the button labeled "Search" as shown in Figure 7-23.

▶ **Figure 7-23 Search for Tylenol.**

Note that even when you type in a brand name, the search will automatically find the generic version of the drug for you. In this case, the generic name for Tylenol is "Acetaminophen."

Step 8

The prescription writer is invoked by clicking the Rx button in the Toolbar at the top of your screen. The button is shown highlighted orange in Figure 7-24. The icon resembles a small prescription bottle. In previous exercises the Rx button has been grayed out.

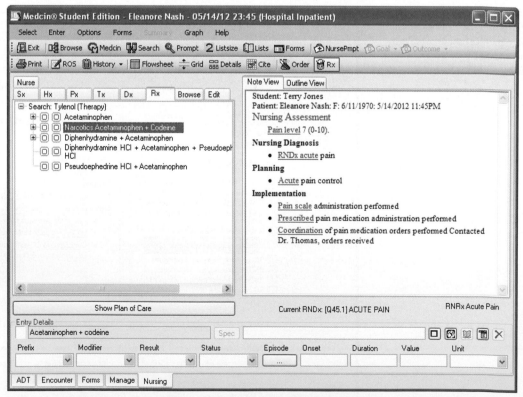

▶ **Figure 7-24 Rx button enabled when a medication finding is highlighted.**

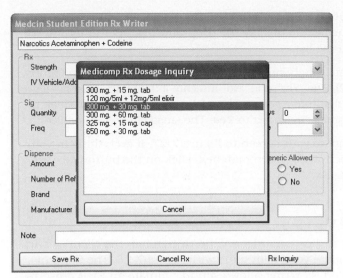

▶ **Figure 7-25 Prescription writer with Dosage window.**

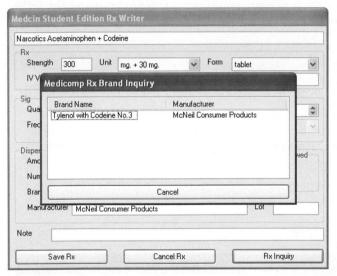

▶ **Figure 7-26 Prescription brand selection.**

This is because the Rx button is only available when you are on the Rx tab, and only when the currently selected or highlighted finding is a medication.

Locate and highlight "**Narcotics Acetaminophen + Codeine**," by clicking on its description (do not click on the red or blue button).

The Rx button on the Toolbar is now active. If you position the mouse pointer over it, it will change color (as shown in Figure 7-24).

With the finding "Narcotics Acetaminophen + Codeine" highlighted, locate and click on the Rx button in the Toolbar. A simple prescription writer window will be invoked, as shown in Figure 7-25.

Step 9

When you clicked on the prescription (Rx) button and invoked the prescription writing window, the drug was automatically selected from the finding. A list of available dosages is automatically displayed.

Locate and click your mouse on the dosage "**300 mg + 30 mg tab**," shown highlighted in Figure 7-25. This means one tablet contains 300 milligrams of acetaminophen and 30 milligrams of codeine.

As soon as you select the dosage, the next window displaying available brands (as shown in Figure 7-26) will be displayed automatically.

Step 10

Locate and click on the brand "**Tylenol with Codeine No. 3**," as shown in Figure 7-26. The brand selection window will close automatically; the dosage and the brand information will be displayed in the Rx Writer window.

Note: if you ever accidentally select the wrong dosage or brand, click on the button labeled "Rx Inquiry" in the Rx Writer window to invoke the Dosage and Brand windows again.

Step 11

The remaining fields on the prescription writer will be available for entry. In this step you will enter data to complete the "Sig" information that the pharmacist and nurse will need. Sig, from the Latin *signa*, was used in Chapter 6 to refer to the interval timing in nursing orders. In prescriptions, the Sig not only conveys the timing but also the dosage and administration instructions for the prescription. It consists of the quantity prescribed, the number of times per day, number (of tablets) to take each time, number of days to take the drug, the total quantity prescribed, the number of refills allowed, and any free-text instructions for the client.

Locate and click your mouse in the "Quantity" field, and then type **1**.

Locate the frequency field (labeled "Freq") and click on the down arrow in the field to display the drop-down list. Select **every 4 hours**, from the list.

Locate the field labeled "Per Day" and type the numeral **6**.

Locate the field labeled "When" and click on the down arrow in the field to display the drop-down list. Select **as needed**, from the list.

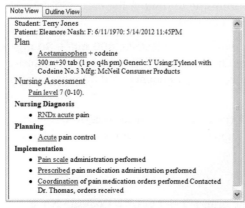

▶ **Figure 7-27 Prescription for Tylenol with Codeine No. 3 (generic circled in red).**

▶ **Figure 7-28 Right pane showing prescription in encounter note.**

▶ **Figure 7-29 Rx Writer dosage window for Hypnotics Zolpidem Tartate (highlighted in left pane).**

Locate the field labeled "Route" and click on the down arrow in the field to display the drop-down list. Select **by mouth**, from the list.

Locate the "Generic Allowed" fields (circled in red in Figure 7-27). The "Yes" and "No" indicate if the pharmacist is allowed to substitute a generic drug for a prescribed brand. Click in the small circle next to **Yes**. The small circle is then filled in.

Compare your screen to Figure 7-27. If everything in your prescription screen matches, click on the button labeled "Save Rx."

Step 12

The medication order will be written into the client's chart. Compare your right pane with Figure 7-28. The Student Edition Rx Writer allows you to simulate an EHR prescription system. In an actual CPOE system, at this point the prescription system would automatically transmit the order to the pharmacy.

Step 13

Using what you have learned in the previous steps, add the order for the second prescription.

Locate and click on the Search button on the Toolbar to invoke the Search String window. Type "**Ambien**" in the Search dialog window and click on the button labeled "Search."

The search function will locate and automatically highlight the generic form of the drug "Zolpidem Tartate."

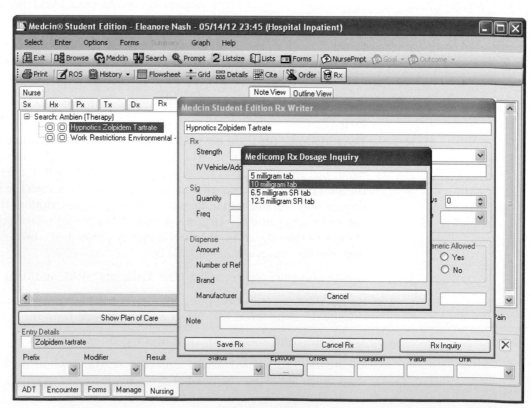

Step 14

Verify that "**Hypnotics Zolpidem Tartate**" is highlighted, as shown in Figure 7-29, and then click the Rx button on the Toolbar to invoke the prescription writer.

A list of available dosages is automatically displayed. Locate and click your mouse on the dosage "**10 milligram tab**" as shown in Figure 7-29.

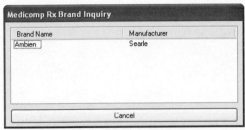

Step 15

When the list of available brands is displayed, locate and click your mouse on the brand "**Ambien**" as shown in Figure 7-30.

Step 16

Complete the medication order by entering the following information:

Locate and click your mouse in the "Quantity" field, and then type **1**.

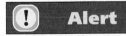
▶ **Figure 7-30 Select Ambien in Rx Brand window.**

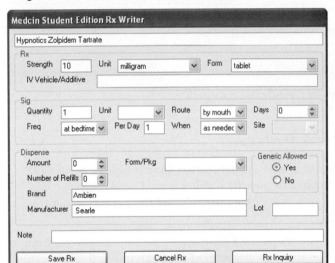

Locate the frequency field (labeled "Freq") and click on the down arrow in the field to display the drop-down list. Select **at bedtime**, from the list.

Locate the field labeled "Per Day" and type the numeral **1**.

Locate the field labeled "When" and click on the down arrow in the field to display the drop-down list. Select **as needed**, from the list.

Locate the field labeled "Route" and click on the down arrow in the field to display the drop-down list. Select **by mouth**, from the list.

Locate the "Generic Allowed" fields and click in the small circle next to **Yes**.

Compare your screen to Figure 7-31. When everything in your prescription screen matches, click on the button labeled "Save Rx."

▶ **Figure 7-31 Rx Writer with Sig information for Ambien order.**

(!) Alert

Do not close or exit the encounter until you have a printed copy in your hand. **You will lose your work if you exit before printing.**

Step 17

Click on the Print button on the Toolbar at the top of your screen to invoke the Print Data window.

Be certain there is a check mark in the box next to "Current Encounter" and then click on the appropriate button to either print or export a file, as directed by your instructor.

Compare your printout or file output to Figure 7-32. If your work is correct, hand it in to your instructor. If there are any differences except for the encounter date, review the previous steps in the exercise and find your error.

```
Eleanore Nash                                          Page 1 of 1

Student: your name or id here
Patient: Eleanore Nash: F: 6/11/1970: 5/14/2012 11:45PM
Plan
    • Acetaminophen + codeine
300 m+30 tab (1 po q4h prn) Generic:Y Using:Tylenol with Codeine No.3 Mfg:
    McNeil Consumer Products
    • Zolpidem tartrate
10 mg tab (1 po hs prn) Generic:Y Using:Ambien Mfg: Searle
Nursing Assessment
    Pain level 7 (0-10).
Nursing Diagnosis
    • RNDx acute pain
Planning
    • Acute pain control
Implementation
    • Pain scale administration performed
    • Prescribed pain medication administration performed
    • Coordination of pain medication orders performed Contacted Dr. Thomas,
      orders received
```

▶ **Figure 7-32 Printed encounter note with Rx orders for Eleanore Nash.**

Quick Access to Frequent Orders

In the previous exercise we mentioned a time-saving feature that is typical in all CPOE systems: a quick-pick list of a clinician's frequently used orders. These may take the form of diagnosis-based order sets, or a more generalized list of the prescriptions that the clinician writes most frequently.

With thousands of tests that could be ordered and thousands of drugs to choose from, a clinician does not have the time to go through a search of medications or tests to write a prescription or order a lab. Many clinicians find that they order a fairly narrow range of tests (appropriate to their specialty and client population) and write prescriptions for only a small group of medications.

It makes sense for clinicians to keep a list of the items that they most frequently use from which they can select when writing the order. Commercial EHR systems handle this in different ways; some automatically create the list by memorizing what the clinician has been ordering, whereas other systems allow the clinician (or a staff member) to build their own lists. Most EHR systems offer clinicians both methods of creating the order list.

The EHR system that you will use in a medical facility will most certainly have this type of feature. Making use of the feature is definitely a good way to speed up data entry at the point of care. Creating or customizing Rx and orders lists will certainly save time when the clinician is with the client.

The next exercise emulates this feature by allowing you to select from a small list of medications instead of searching for each drug. However, commercial EHR systems provide a much more robust application that allows the clinician to save the complete Sig information, which enables the clinician to write an entire prescription or lab order with a single click of the mouse.

Critical Thinking Exercise 48: Ordering Medications Using a Quick-Pick List

In this exercise you will learn to use a quick-pick list with the prescription writer to enter multiple medication orders that a nurse has received by phone from the doctor. In this exercise you will also experience a feature that is found in virtually all commercial

EHR prescription systems: the ability to store the Sig information for prescriptions that are frequently used. When the dosage is selected, the other fields in the Rx Writer are automatically set as well. This feature makes writing the prescription very fast.

Case Study

Nancy Anderson is a 61-year-old female who was admitted to the hospital for congestive heart failure. She is to be discharged today and is anxious to leave. Her doctor has called you with orders for her discharge medications. As you have in the previous exercise, you will enter medication orders on the doctor's behalf. The doctor has ordered Lasix 40 mg BID, Lanoxin 0.125 mg daily, Potassium chloride 20 mg BID, and Nitroglycerine sl PRN. The doctor will cosign the orders later.

Step 1

If you have not already done so, start the Student Edition software.

Click on the ADT tab at the bottom of your screen.

Locate and click on **Nancy Anderson**.

Locate and click on the button labeled "Review Plan of Care."

When the Plan of Care is displayed, locate the button labeled "Show Data Entry View" below the left pane, and click on it.

Step 2

Click Select on the Menu bar, and then click New Encounter.

Select the date **May 15, 2012**, the time **11:00 AM**, and the reason **Hospital Inpatient**.

Make certain that you set the date and reason correctly. Compare your screen to the date, time, and reason printed in bold type before clicking on the OK button.

Step 3

The nurse reviews with the client the symptoms she should report and gives her discharge instructions in a book provided by the hospital to clients with heart problems. Document the nursing intervention and action.

Click on the Nurse tab at the top of the left pane.

Scroll the list of nursing diagnoses downward until you can see "Cardiovascular Alteration."

Locate and click the red button for the following intervention:

- (red button) RNRx Cardiac Care

Locate and click on the small plus sign next to "Cardiac care" to expand the list.

Scroll the left pane downward to locate and click on the following nursing action:

- (red button) RNOx Review Symptoms to Report With Patient

In the free-text field below the right pane, type "**Gave patient heart book to take home.**"

Step 4

Next you will enter the orders for her medications. Because certain meds are routinely prescribed for heart clients, the hospital has a list that makes writing orders easier.

Click on the Rx tab.

Locate and click on the "List" button on the Toolbar at the top of your screen to invoke the List Manager window.

Scroll the List Manager window to the right until you see the list named "N CHF Discharge Meds." Highlight it (as shown in Figure 7-33) and then click the button labeled "Load List."

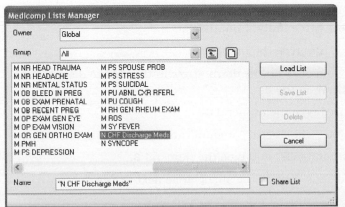

▶ **Figure 7-33 Load the list "N CHF Discharge Meds."**

The CHF Discharge Meds list displays medications typically prescribed to CHF clients when they are discharged.

Step 5

Locate and highlight the medication finding **ordered Anginal Preparations Nitroglycerine**, and then click on the Rx button on the Toolbar. This will invoke the prescription writer.

The dosage selection will automatically be displayed. Select the first dosage: **0.15 milligram tab 1 sl prn DSP 100**

When the brand window is displayed, click on the brand **Nitrostat.**

When the prescription is displayed, locate the "Generic Allowed" fields and click in the small circle next to **Yes**.

Click on the Save Rx button.

Step 6

Enter the next order by highlighting the medication finding **ordered Cardiac Glycosides Digoxin** and then click on the Rx button on the Toolbar.

When the dosage selection is displayed, select the first dosage on the list **0.125 milligram tab 1 po qd DSP: 100**.

When the brand window is displayed, click on the brand **Lanoxin.**

Locate the Generic Allowed fields and click in the small circle next to **Yes**.

Click on the Save Rx button.

Step 7

Locate and highlight the medication finding **ordered Diuretic Loop Acting Furosemide** and then click on the Rx button on the Toolbar.

When the dosage selection is displayed, select the second dosage on the list **40 milligram tab 1 po BID DSP: 100**.

When the brand window is displayed, click on the brand **Lasix.**

Locate the Generic Allowed fields and click in the small circle next to **Yes**.

Click on the Save Rx button.

Step 8

Enter the last order by highlighting the medication finding **ordered Potassium Chloride** and then click on the Rx button on the Toolbar.

When the dosage selection is displayed, select the last dosage on the list: **20 mEq tab**.

The brand will not be selected; click the button labeled "Cancel" in the brand window.

When the prescription is displayed, locate and click your mouse in the "Quantity" field, and then type **1**.

Locate the frequency field (labeled "Freq") and click on the down arrow in the field to display the drop-down list. Select **twice daily**, from the list.

Locate the field labeled "Per Day" and type the numeral **2**.

Locate the field labeled "Route" and click on the down arrow in the field to display the drop-down list. Select **by mouth**, from the list.

Locate the field labeled "Days" and type the numeral **30**.

In the Dispense section, locate the field labeled "Amount" and type the numeral **60**.

Locate the field labeled "Number of Refills" and type the numeral **3**.

Locate the Generic Allowed fields and click in the small circle next to **Yes**.

Click on the Save Rx button.

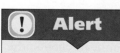

Alert

Do not close or exit the encounter until you have a printed copy in your hand. You will lose your work if you exit before printing.

By Marney Thompson, RN

Marney Thompson is a registered nurse working in the critical care unit of a large hospital.

When I was in nursing school I did a 17-week rotation in a critical care setting and I loved it. Since then I have always worked in medical intensive care or critical care units. I like the challenges of that type of nursing where you have an intensive care client with multiple needs and you are managing all the complications that come along with the acute phase—so you can get that client to the next phase, which is recovery. I feel a strong sense of purpose being part of the team who responds when there is a client who is coding.

I have been fortunate that all the hospitals I have worked in used electronic records. The client's vital signs, CVP (cerebral vascular pressure) monitoring, heart rate, oxygenation, blood pressure—all transfer directly into our charts electronically. Our hospital EHR also has CPOE, so all lab and medication orders are electronic. The lab results are also electronic, which means the intensivist and I can both be looking at a client's most recent results at the same time, even though the doctor might be in a different part of the hospital.

In addition, our hospital pharmacy is computerized, which means that when a situation is critical I can order meds on behalf of the doctor; the pharmacist can then review them and communicate with the Pyxsis Medstation in the nursing unit to dispense them. Here is a situation that happened recently.

This client was on BIPAP (bilevel positive airway pressure) and his respirations were agonal looking. He was not responsive—had not been responsive since coming to the unit—but he started to look like he was going downhill. I contacted the doctor (our intensivist), who ordered some stat lab tests: a BMP (basic metabolic panel), a CBC (complete blood count), and a magnesium level—pretty standard stuff for any client who is crashing. We drew the specimens and sent them to the lab stat. The BMP takes about 45 minutes to be processed. In the meantime, I noticed that his QRS intervals started to widen. I suspected that it was related to possible electrolyte imbalances because his urine output had significantly decreased despite fluid boluses. I got an EKG, which confirmed it. I, another nurse, and an RT (respiratory therapist) were in the room trying to get an ABG (arterial blood gas) from the femoral artery, when suddenly none of us could feel a pulse. Basically, he was in PEA (pulseless electrical activity). Of course at that point we called the code.

The code team arrived. We had started CPR (cardio-pulmonary resuscitation) and shortly after starting CPR we got a pulse back. We still had to intubate the client because of his respiratory status. While the CRNA (Certified Registered Nurse Anesthesiologist) was intubating, I was able to bring up his lab results so we could get a bigger picture. At that time his potassium was extremely high. The doctor was at the bedside assessing the client, assisting with intubation, and calling out orders. I was at the computer looking at the labs and entering orders.

The doctor said, "Let's go ahead and push an amp of D-50 (dextrose) and ten units of insulin. Then we'll push an amp of calcium chloride after that. His bi-carb is low—push 2 amps of bi-carb and put an order in for another ABG right away."

The doctor was ordering this in rapid succession, while I entered the orders and transmitted them to the pharmacist, who cleared them very quickly; my co-worker went to pull the meds from the Pyxsis machine. Literally in a matter of minutes, people were handing the drugs through the door, scanning and administering them. It was over and done, just that quick.

Our hospital policy supports the closed loop medication administration safety initiative that you will read about elsewhere in this chapter. Let me describe how that works. When the doctor was giving me verbal orders, I was entering them in the CPOE. The medication orders were automatically sent to the pharmacy. The pharmacist interacted with that order on the pharmacy system, validated that the orders were safe and ready to dispense, and sent an order to the dispensing system. When the nurse went to the drawer to pull it out of the machine, the order was in there and allowed her to get it. Then she gave it to the nurse in the room, who scanned the client's ID, scanned the medication, and then administered it. The system also documented it. There is no transcription error, no misinterpretation of the orders errors—it is all electronically one order moving through the systems. I love it. I feel like I am getting double-checked five times. The pharmacist is also getting double-checked because when the order goes to the Pyxsis machine it is also comes up on my order list screen, highlighted in yellow for the nurse to confirm this is in fact the correct order for the correct client. I know instantly what the pharmacist is dispensing. If there is any miscommunication, the nurse will have the ability to catch any error from the pharmacy.

When the crisis is over and the doctor has time to get into his own CPOE system, there is a button there labeled "cosign." He can click the cosign button and it will show him all the verbal orders that he given—that someone else has entered for him. He can select them and cosign them at that time. Also, each doctor has a work folder in the EHR, so if he does not cosign them at that time they will show up in his work folder as items he needs to attend to. Most of the intensivists on our unit cosign their orders before the end of their shift

Even when we are not in a code situation, there are times throughout the night when nurses are entering orders. For example, last night I had a client come in who was already on a dopamine drip at 20 micrograms. The client was tachycardic; blood pressure was 70 and 80 systolic. The doctor was at the bedside speaking with the surgeon when the anesthesiologist came to intubate. I said to the doctor, "Can I have Levophed?" and entered the order. I got the Levophed hanging, but the client's pressure was still dumping. Because the physicians were evaluating the client for septic versus cardiogenic shock, I asked, "How about some dobutamine?" The doctor told me to go ahead with the order.

Even with all three of those hanging, the client still was not improving, and the anesthesiologist was requesting a better BP before sedation for intubation. I asked, "What else do we want to hang to get some blood pressure—can I have some vasopressin?" The doctors preferred to have me enter the orders in the computer while they continued to confer about the client. Because I entered the orders at the bedside, pharmacy was able to get the drugs to me more quickly as well.

I enjoy working in the CCU. Nurses in this kind of unit are responsible for almost every aspect of their clients' care. They have to be an advocate for their client, and the type of person who can handle themselves in stressful situations and think quickly in crises.

```
Nancy Anderson                                          Page 1 of 1

Student: your name or id here
Patient: Nancy Anderson: F: 9/09/1951: 5/15/2012 11:00AM
Plan
    • Nitroglycerin
0.15 mg tab (1 sl prn) DISP:100 Refill:5 Generic:Y Using:Nitrostat Mfg:
    Parke Davis
    • Digoxin
0.125 mg tab (1 po qd) DISP:100 Refill:5 Generic:Y Using:Lanoxin Tablets Mfg:
    Burroughs Wellcome
    • Furosemide
40 mg tab (1 po bid) DISP:100 Refill:3 Generic:Y Using:Lasix Mfg: Hoechst
    • Potassium chloride
20 mEq SR tab (1 po bid 30) DISP:60 Refill:3 Generic:Y
Nursing Assessment
Planning
    • Cardiac care
Implementation
    • Review of symptoms to report with patient performed Gave patient heart
    book to take home
```

▶ **Figure 7-34 Printout of Nancy Anderson's discharge medication orders.**

Step 9

Click on the Print button on the Toolbar at the top of your screen to invoke the Print Data window.

Be certain there is a check mark in the box next to Current Encounter and then click on the appropriate button to either print or export a file, as directed by your instructor.

Compare your printout or file output to Figure 7-34. If your work is correct, hand it in to your instructor. If there are any differences, review the previous steps in the exercise and find your error.

Protocols Based on Diagnosis Codes

Disease-based protocols can help the clinician write the orders and document the encounter more quickly. Instead of searching through a list of a thousand prescription drugs, the clinician can access a short list of drugs that are regularly prescribed for a particular type of infection. These lists can be created for individual prescribing clinicians, for the practice as a whole, or by some recognized authority such as a medical association.

Similarly, the hospital or clinic can create a specific group of orders used to test for certain conditions. These may be groups of orders that are consistent with an identified best practice order sets or a clinical pathway. Once a suspected diagnosis is identified, the list can be quickly located and the clinician can order tests, consults, or radiological studies all at once.

Introducing Diagnosis Codes

Before we study diagnosis-based protocols, we are going to briefly discuss the international standard code set used for diagnoses. Then we will further study how the diagnosis aids the clinician in locating appropriate orders.

Each of the encounters you have documented in the previous exercises included an Assessment finding that was selected on the Dx tab of the software. As you are already aware, Dx is an acronym for "Diagnosis." Diagnoses are assigned codes using the ICD-9-CM code set (or ICD-10 after 2013).

ICD stands for International Classification of Diseases, which is a system of standardized codes developed collaboratively between the World Health Organization (WHO) and 10 international centers. The number "9" represents the ninth revision of the coding system; the number "10" represents the tenth revision.

People sometimes erroneously think of ICD-9-CM codes as "billing" codes, because reimbursement is tied to the diagnoses codes and they are required on health insurance claims. However, ICD-9-CM codes are important for reasons other than billing, including statistical studies of causes of death, disease, and injury. ICD-9-CM provides an internationally recognized system of codifying the client's condition.

Because ICD-9-CM standardized codes for diseases, those codes can be used for problem lists and associated with protocols and treatment plans. Many professional journals, associations, and practices create protocols for treating certain diseases. These may consist of specific regimens such as an oncologist might use to treat a particular form of cancer, or they might consist of a list of all possible antibiotics known to be effective for a certain type of infection. In either case, the protocol or plan of treatment can be easily communicated to other clinicians by linking it to the diagnoses for which it is effective.

Even without creating specific protocols, the diagnosis can be used to help locate orders and treatment plans. Guided Exercise 45, earlier in this chapter, demonstrated this with Gary Yamamoto's encounter. Once you found the diagnosis "Angina Pectoris," the Prompt feature was able to generate a list of appropriate test orders related to the condition. The ICD-9-CM code for angina pectoris is 413.9.

History of ICD-9-CM

Today's ICD coding system evolved from the International List of Causes of Death, which was used by physicians, medical examiners, and coroners to facilitate standardized mortality studies. The codes were revised about every 10 years from 1900 to 1979, incrementing the revision number each time. In 1948, WHO expanded and renamed the system to make it useful for coding medical conditions as well.

By the time the ninth revision was published, the U.S. National Center for Health Statistics began to modify the statistical study with clinical information. The letters "CM" stand for Clinical Modification. Clinical modifications provided a way to code the clinical information about the health of a client beyond that needed for statistical reports. With the addition of clinical modifications, the codes became useful for indexing medical records and medical case reviews, and communicating a client's condition more precisely.

ICD-9-CM is currently published in three volumes. The first two volumes provide a listing and an index of diagnosis codes; the third volume lists codes for hospital inpatient procedures. Figure 7-35 shows a sample list of codes from volumes 1 and 2.

▶ **Figure 7-35 Small sample of ICD-9-CM codes.**

ICD-9-CM Codes (Diagnosis)	
Code	**Description**
Diseases of Other Endocrine Glands	
250	Diabetes mellitus
250.0	Diabetes mellitus without mention of complication (NOS)
250.00	Diabetes mellitus type II, not stated as uncontrolled
250.01	Diabetes mellitus type I (juvenile) not stated as uncontrolled
250.02	Diabetes mellitus type II, uncontrolled
250.03	Diabetes mellitus type I, (juvenile) uncontrolled
250.1	Diabetes with ketoacidosis
250.2	Diabetes with hyperosomolarity
250.3	Diabetes with other coma
V Codes (Circumstances other than disease or injury)	
V22.0	Supervision of normal first pregnancy
V22.1	Supervision of other normal pregnancy
V70.0	Routine general medical examination (health check up)
V72.1	Examination of ears and hearing
V72.1	Encounter for hearing following a failed hearing screening
E Codes (Classification of external causes of injury or poisoning)	
E813.0	Driver in a motor vehicle accident involving collision with other vehicle
E813.1	Passenger in a motor vehicle accident involving collision with other vehicle
E813.3	Motorcyclist in a motor vehicle accident involving collision with other vehicle

The diagnosis codes are three characters, followed by a decimal point and up to two numerals. The first three characters of an ICD-9-CM code identify the primary diagnosis; the two digits to the right of the decimal point further refine the diagnosis specificity.

Insurance billing allows for the use of multiple ICD-9-CM codes for a single procedure, indicating one code as the primary diagnosis and additional codes as secondary conditions for which the treatment was done.

The historical intent of the ICD was to classify similar causes of mortality and disease conditions into statistical reportable data. When in 1989 ICD-9-CM codes became required by insurance carriers to process claims, the code set had to be further modified. The problem was that if an ICD-9-CM code was required for an insurance claim, but the client was perfectly healthy, what code should be used? To solve this problem, ICD-9-CM added a section of codes that start with the letter "V"; these V codes can be used to describe healthy clients. For example, children have regular pediatric checkups; these are coded as "V20.2 Well-Child."

Volume 1 also includes "E" codes (listed at the bottom of Figure 7-35). These are not used for diagnosis, but to classify the cause of an injury or poisoning. For example, the diagnosis code 823.0 indicates the client had a closed fracture of the tibia. The code E813.1 provides further detail that the broken leg is the result of a motor vehicle crash in which the client was a passenger.

Future Developments: ICD-10

ICD-10 is the latest revision to the International Classification of Diseases. It was released by WHO in 1992 and is used broadly in Europe and Canada. ICD-10 contains

Comparison of ICD-10 and ICD-9-CM Codes

ICD-10	Description	ICD-9-CM	Description
R31.0	Gross hematuria	599.7	Hematuria
R31.1	Benign essential microscopic hematuria	599.7	Hematuria
R31.2	Other microscopic hematuria	599.7	Hematuria
R31.9	Hematuria, unspecified	599.7	Hematuria
N36.41	Hypermobility of urethra	599.81	Urethral hypermobility
N36.42	Intrinsic sphincter deficiency	599.82	Intrinsic sphincter deficiency
N36.43	Combined hypermobility of urethra and intrinsic sphincter deficiency		
N364.4	Muscular disorders of urethra		
N36.8	Other specified disorders of urethra	599.83	Urethral instability
N36.8	Other specified disorders of urethra	599.84	Other specified disorders of urethra

▶ **Figure 7-36 A comparison of ICD-10 codes and ICD-9-CM codes.**

about twice as many categories as ICD-9 and uses more alphanumeric codes. Effective January 1, 1999, ICD-10 was officially implemented in the United States for reporting the cause of death on death certificates. It has not been implemented for billing, and should not be used in place of ICD-9-CM for reporting diagnoses on insurance claims. The U.S. Department of Health and Human Services (HHS) has proposed that the ICD-10 code sets be used for billing effective October 1, 2013.

Use Figure 7-36 to compare several ICD-9-CM and ICD-10 codes.

ICD-9-CM and EHR Nomenclatures

The ICD-9-CM is not an EHR nomenclature. However, most EHR systems contain a "cross-walk" or internal reference table that can produce ICD-9-CM codes automatically. The advantage of using an EHR with a codified nomenclature is that the ICD-9-CM codes will always be in sync with the encounter documentation produced. Another advantage is that the EHR allows the clinician to record nuances beyond the scope of ICD-9-CM such as "mild" or "improving." The EHR software will automatically translate the assessment to the correct diagnosis code.

Primary and Secondary Diagnoses

The concept of the primary diagnosis is also important. The primary diagnosis is the reason why the client came to the office or hospital. Other conditions addressed during the visit are listed as secondary diagnoses (also called *comorbidity*). In a hospital, secondary diagnoses are classified as POA, present on admission, or HAC, hospital acquired condition.

Any conditions that exist concurrently with the primary diagnosis should be reviewed, examined, or treated and documented. Often this is facilitated by a "problem list," which is a summary of ongoing or previous conditions. The problem list helps the clinician keep track of the client's needs beyond the scope of the chief complaint for today's visit. You will see an example of a problem list in Chapter 8.

Multiple Diagnoses

Multiple diagnoses occur mainly in clients with ongoing or chronic conditions requiring regular visits. It is correct and appropriate to continue to use diagnosis codes from past visits for as long as the client continues to have the illness or condition and that condition is clearly documented in the record. For example, a client with diabetes mellitus poorly controlled might be seen regularly. With this disease, on some visits the client will likely have other problems as well. Therefore, the diagnosis 250.2, "Diabetes Mellitus," should be included in every visit note and on insurance claims for those visits.

The Rule-Out Diagnosis

The ICD-9-CM code set has neither specific codes nor modifiers to use with diagnosis codes to communicate the concept of "ruling out" a disease or condition. One inconsistency in the ICD-9-CM guidelines is that services performed during inpatient settings support the concept of "rule-out," but guidelines for the outpatient setting does not.

The diagnosis for an outpatient may take more than one visit to be determined or confirmed, but the outpatient visit guidelines do not allow for "possible," "probable," "suspected," "rule-out," or similar diagnoses. Although the prefix "possible" may be appropriate and necessary in the encounter note, the insurance claim for an outpatient visit should not be coded with a diagnosis for the suspected disease.

This creates a dilemma when ordering diagnostic tests from outside facilities. Reference laboratories cannot bill for the test unless they have a diagnosis. Only the clinician ordering the test is allowed to assign the diagnosis; the reference lab cannot. Therefore, the labs require an order for a test to include a diagnosis code, even though the purpose of the test is only to determine if the client in fact has the disease.

Using Diagnosis to Find Orders and Treatments

In the next two exercises, you will learn to use multiple diagnoses and to create different sets of orders based on established plans associated with each diagnosis. You must complete both Exercise 49 and Exercise 50 in one session. **Do not begin this exercise unless there is enough class time remaining to complete both exercises.**

Guided Exercise 49: Orders Based on Diagnosis

Case Study

Alena Zabroski is a 53-year-old female who complains of jaw pain. She has been to her dentist, who has found nothing wrong. She has come to the clinic to be seen by a nurse practitioner. The nurse practitioner initially suspects angina and orders tests to confirm or rule out the diagnosis. However, Alena mentions that she has moved back to her childhood home and has been restoring it. Knowing that the client was born in 1959 and therefore her home is an old house, the nurse realizes there is a possibility that she is being exposed to lead-based paints. This fact alters the direction of inquiry and of the tests ordered.

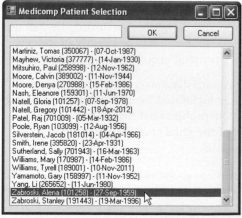

► Figure 7-37 Select patient Alena Zabroski.

Step 1

If you have not already done so, start the Student Edition software.

Click Select on the Menu bar, and then click Patient.

In the Patient Selection window, locate and click on **Alena Zabroski** as shown in Figure 7-37.

Step 2

Click Select on the Menu bar, and then click New Encounter.

Use the current date and time. Select the reason **Office Visit** from the drop-down list and click on the OK button.

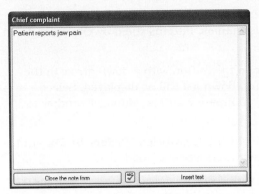

► **Figure 7-38 Chief complaint "Patient reports jaw pain."**

Step 3

In this exercise, the nurse will begin the visit by recording the chief complaint and taking Alena's vital signs.

Enter the chief complaint by locating the button in the Toolbar labeled "Chief" and clicking on it.

In the dialog window which will open, type: "**Patient reports jaw pain**."

Compare your screen to Figure 7-38 before clicking on the button labeled "Close the note form."

Step 4

Locate and click the Forms button on the Toolbar at the top of your screen. Select the form labeled "Vitals" from the Forms Manager (as you have done in previous exercises).

Enter Alena's vital signs in the corresponding fields on the form as follows:

Temperature:	**99**
Respiration:	**20**
Pulse:	**70**
BP:	**114/70**
Height:	**70**
Weight:	**150**

When you have finished, compare your screen to Figure 7-39 and, when it is correct, click on the Encounter tab at the bottom of the screen.

► **Figure 7-39 Vital Signs form for Alena Zabroski.**

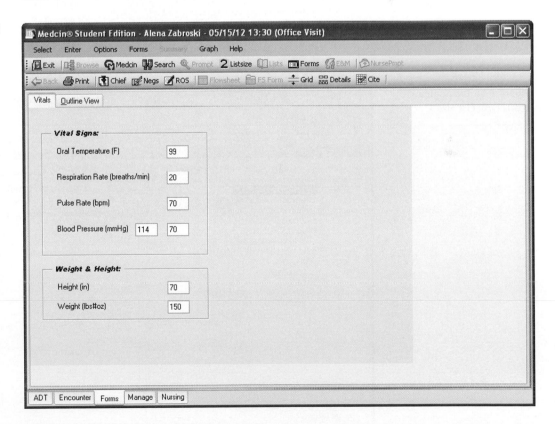

Step 5

Locate and click on the Lists button in the Toolbar at the top of your screen. The List Manager window will be invoked.

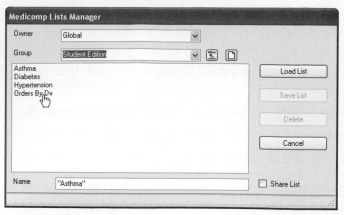

▶ **Figure 7-40 Load orders by Dx list.**

As you learned in Chapter 5, the List Manager organizes the display of List names, filtering them by Owner and Group.

Locate and click on the button with a down arrow in the Group field; a drop-down list will be displayed. Select Student Edition. Compare your List Manager window to Figure 7-40.

Locate and highlight the list labeled "**Orders By Dx**" and then click on the button labeled "Load List."

The Orders By Dx List has been especially created for this exercise. It demonstrates the use of protocols of orders and treatments by associating them with particular diseases. In this exercise there is one list for several diseases. In an actual medical clinic, there would likely be many separate lists.

Step 6

The list will load and automatically change to the Dx tab. If the left pane is not on the Dx tab, click on the tab labeled "Dx."

Locate the List Size button in the Toolbar at the top of your screen and click it until it is set to **2**.

Locate and click on the finding:

- (red button) ANGINA PECTORIS

Compare your screen to Figure 7-41.

Locate and click on the Prompt button in the Toolbar at the top of your screen.

▶ **Figure 7-41 Dx: Angina Pectoris with List Size 2.**

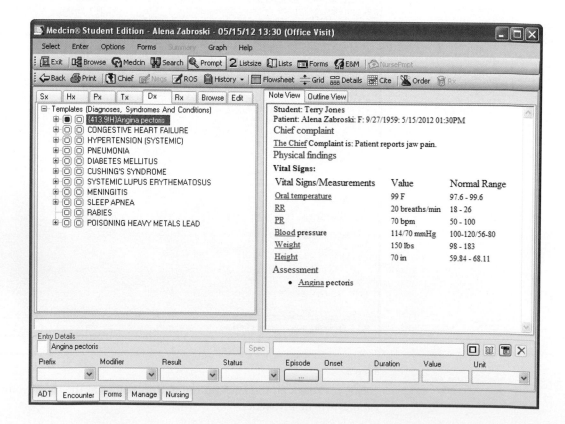

▶ **Figure 7-42 Sx tab with Dx: Angina Pectoris List Size 2 and ROS On.**

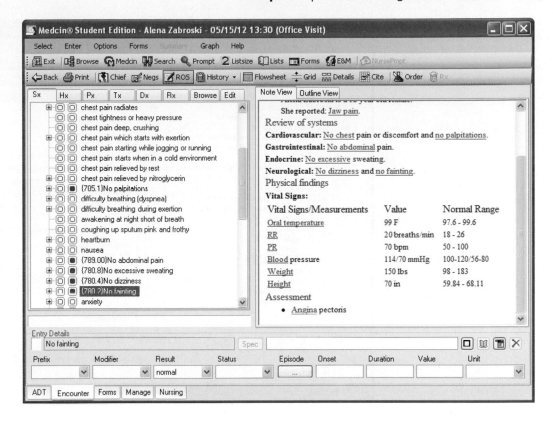

Step 7

Click on the Sx tab.

Locate and click on the following finding:

- (red button) jaw pain in jaw (bone)

Locate the ROS button in the Toolbar at the top of your screen and click it. It should change color (as shown in Figure 7-42).

Locate and click on the following findings (you will need to scroll the left pane to find them all):

- (blue button) chest pain or discomfort
- (blue button) palpitations
- (blue button) abdominal pain
- (blue button) excessive sweating
- (blue button) dizziness
- (blue button) fainting (syncope)

Step 8

Click on the Hx tab.

Locate and click on the following findings:

- (blue button) current smoker
- (red button) Family history of Angina Pectoris

Locate and expand the tree for "exercise habits."

Locate and click on the following finding:

- (red button) Sedentary

Compare your screen to Figure 7-43.

▶ **Figure 7-43 Hx tab with Dx: Angina Pectoris List Size 2.**

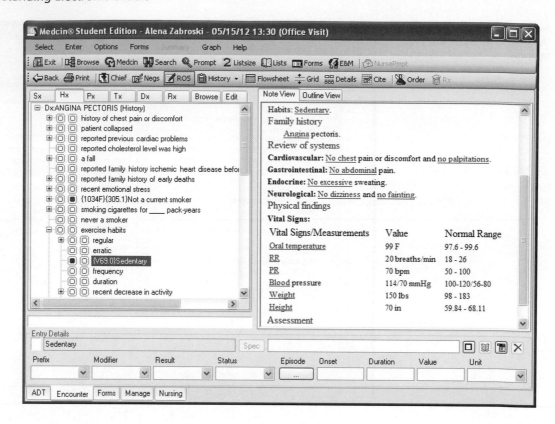

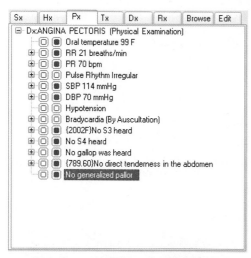

▶ **Figure 7-44 Px tab with Dx: Angina Pectoris List Size 2.**

Step 9

Click on the Px tab.

The nurse practitioner listens to the client's heart sounds and palpitates the abdomen.

Locate and click on the following findings:

- (blue button) Heart Sounds S3
- (blue button) Heart Sounds S4
- (blue button) Heart Sounds Gallop
- (blue button) Abdomen Tenderness Direct
- (blue button) Pallor, Generalized

Compare your screen to Figure 7-44.

Step 10

At this point, the nurse practitioner will order a number of tests.

Locate the List Size button in the Toolbar and click it until it is set to **1**.

Click on the Tx tab.

Locate the Order button in the Toolbar at the top of your screen (highlighted orange in Figure 7-45).

For each of the following findings, highlight the finding and then click on the Order button:

- (order) Comprehensive Metabolic Chem Panel
- (order) Lipids Test Panel
- (order) Electrocardiogram
- (order) Cardiovascular Stress Test

Compare your screen to Figure 7-45.

► **Figure 7-45 Tx tab with Dx: Angina Pectoris List Size 1.**

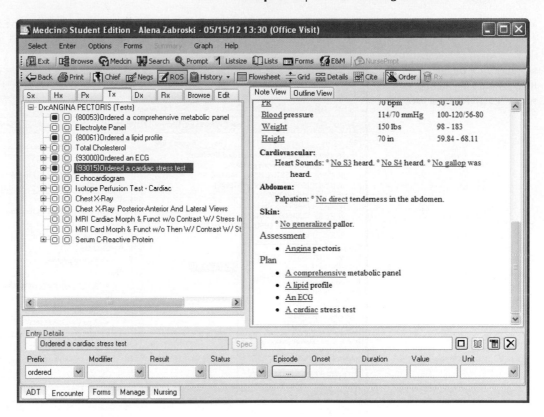

► **Figure 7-46 Rx tab with Dx: Angina Pectoris List Size 1.**

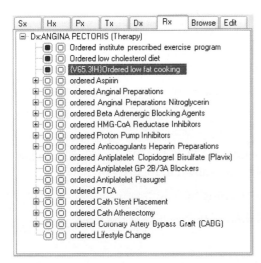

Step 11

The nurse counsels the client on diet and exercise.

Click on the Rx tab.

Locate and click on the following findings (you do not need to use the Order button):

- (red button) ordered Institute Prescribed Exercise Program
- (red button) ordered Low Cholesterol Diet
- (red button) ordered Patient Education Dietary Low Fat Cooking

Compare your left pane to Figure 7-46.

Continue with Guided Exercise 50. Do not exit the Student Edition software or you will lose your work.

Guided Exercise 50: Multiple Diagnoses

It is not unusual during the course of an office visit for a client to bring up additional problems or provide another piece of information that suddenly brings focus on another area of the client's health.

When Alena Zabroski mentions that she has been scraping a lot of old layers of paint off the walls of her childhood home, the nurse realizes that Alena was born in 1959 and there is a possibility that she is being exposed to lead-based paints.

Step 12

Locate the List button in the Toolbar at the top of your screen and click it to invoke the List Manager window.

Reload the List "Orders By Dx" by selecting it and clicking the button labeled "Load List." If you have difficulty, see Figure 7-40 and review step 5 above.

▶ **Figure 7-47 Dx tab with Heavy Metals highlighted— select "Possible" from list.**

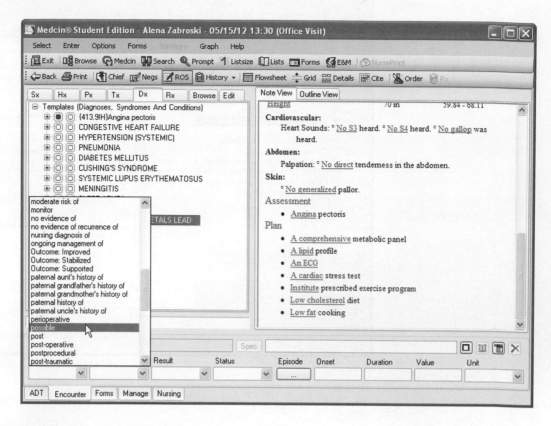

Step 13

The list will be reloaded and the Dx tab will be displayed.

Verify the List Size is 1. If it is not, then locate and click on the button labeled "List Size" in the Toolbar until it is set to 1.

Locate and highlight the finding "Poisoning Heavy Metals Lead."

Locate and click the down arrow in the Entry Details field labeled "Prefix." Scroll the list of prefixes. Locate and click on the term "Possible" as shown in Figure 7-47.

The text of the finding will change to "Possible poisoning by lead."

Locate and click on the Prompt button in the Toolbar at the top of your screen.

Step 14

The nurse is going to first record this new piece of information. Click on the Hx tab. Locate and click on the following finding:

● (red button) house has peeling paint which is lead based

Compare your left pane to Figure 7-48.

Step 15

Click on the Sx tab. Verify the ROS button in the Toolbar at the top of your screen is still orange. If it is not, then click it.

Locate and click on the following findings:

● (blue button) headache

● (blue button) nausea

● (blue button) vomiting

▶ **Figure 7-48 Hx tab with List from Dx: Poisoning Heavy Metals Lead.**

- (blue button) confusion
- (blue button) disorientation
- (blue button) convulsions, generalized

Compare your left pane to Figure 7-49.

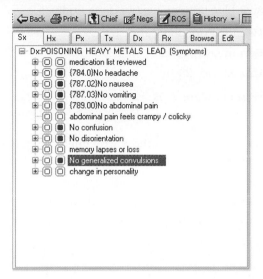

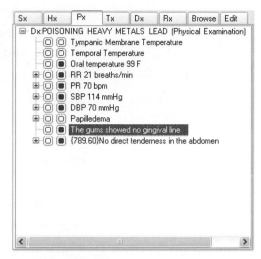

▶ **Figure 7-49 Sx tab with List from Dx: Poisoning Heavy Metals Lead.**

▶ **Figure 7-50 Px tab with List from Dx: Poisoning Heavy Metals Lead.**

Step 16

Click on the Px tab. Note some findings are already selected (from the previous exercise).

Locate and click on the following finding:

- (blue button) Gums Gingival Line

Compare your left pane to Figure 7-50.

▶ **Figure 7-51 Tx tab with list from Dx: Poisoning Heavy Metals Lead.**

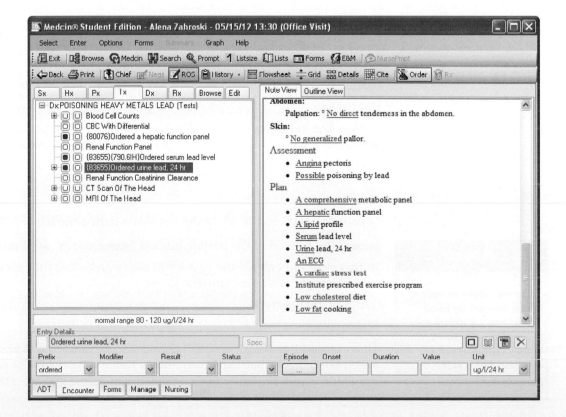

Step 17

Click on the Tx tab.

Locate the Order button in the Toolbar at the top of your screen.

Locate and highlight each of the following findings and then click on the Order button. Do not click on the red or blue buttons next to these findings.

     🏺 (order) Hepatic Function Panel

     🏺 (order) Serum Lead Level

     🏺 (order) Urine Lead, 24 hr

Compare your screen to Figure 7-51.

Step 18

The nurse is also concerned about others who might be in the home and will need to be screened for lead poisoning as well.

Click on the Rx tab.

Locate and click on the following finding (you do not need to use the Order button):

     ● (red button) Screen Family

Compare your left pane to Figure 7-52.

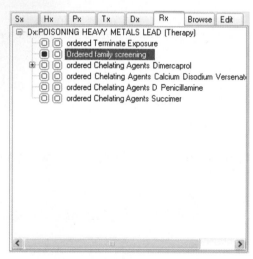

▶ **Figure 7-52 Rx tab with Dx: Poisoning Heavy Metals (List Size 1).**

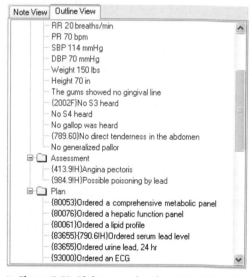

▶ **Figure 7-53 Right pane showing ICD-9-CM codes under Assessment heading.**

Step 19

Locate and click on the tab at the top of the right pane labeled "Outline."

Locate the section of the outline labeled "Assessment" as shown in Figure 7-53.

In this view you can see the ICD-9-CM codes preceding the description of each of the two diagnoses in this encounter:

413.9 Angina pectoris

984.9 poisoning by lead

This exercise has shown how a diagnosis can be used to find and display lists of orders and treatments for particular conditions. Using the possible or suspected diagnosis, we were able to quickly locate the most likely symptoms and tests that would be used to rule out the condition.

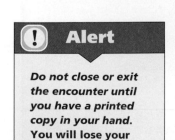

Alert

Do not close or exit the encounter until you have a printed copy in your hand. You will lose your work if you exit before printing.

```
Alena Zabroski                                              Page 1 of 1

Student: your name or id here
Patient: Alena Zabroski: F: 9/27/1959: 5/15/2012 01:30PM
Chief complaint
The Chief Complaint is: Patient reports jaw pain.
History of present illness
Alena Zabroski is a 52 year old female. She reported: Jaw pain.
Personal history
     Behavioral: Not a current smoker.
     Habits: Sedentary.
     Home Environment: Housing has peeling lead-based paint.
Family history
Angina pectoris.
Review of systems
     Head: No headache.
     Cardiovascular: No chest pain or discomfort and no palpitations.
     Gastrointestinal: No nausea, no vomiting, and no abdominal pain.
     Endocrine: No excessive sweating.
     Neurological: No dizziness, no fainting, no confusion, no disorientation,
and no generalized convulsions.
Physical findings
Vital Signs:
Vital Signs/Measurements         Value                Normal Range
Oral temperature                 99 F                 97.6 - 99.6
RR                               20 breaths/min       18 - 26
PR                               70 bpm               50 - 100
Blood pressure                   114/70 mmHg          100 - 120/56 - 80
Weight                           150 lbs              98 - 183
Height                           70 in                59.84 - 68.11
Oral Cavity:
Gums: ° Showed no gingival line.
Cardiovascular:
Heart Sounds: ° No S3 heard. ° No S4 heard. ° No gallop was heard.
Abdomen:
Palpation: ° No direct tenderness in the abdomen.
Skin:
° No generalized pallor.
Assessment
     • Angina pectoris
     • Possible poisoning by lead
Plan
     • A comprehensive metabolic panel
     • A hepatic function panel
     • A lipid profile
     • Serum lead level
     • Urine lead, 24 hr
     • An ECG
     • A cardiac stress test
     • Institute prescribed exercise program
     • Low cholesterol diet
     • Low fat cooking
     • Family screening
```

▶ **Figure 7-54 Printed encounter note for Alena Zabroski.**

Step 20

Click on the Print button on the Toolbar at the top of your screen to invoke the Print Data window.

Be certain there is a check mark in the box next to "Current Encounter" and then click on the appropriate button to either print or export a file, as directed by your instructor.

Compare your printout or file output to Figure 7-54. If your work is correct, hand it in to your instructor. If there are any differences (other than encounter date or client's age), review the previous steps in the exercise to find your error.

Chapter Seven Summary

This chapter introduced several new buttons on the Medcin Toolbar. In this chapter you learned to use the Search and Prompt features and one way of recording a clinician's order. You also learned to use Order and Rx buttons on the Medcin Toolbar.

Search provides a quick way to locate a desired finding in the nomenclature. Medcin addresses semantic differences in medical terms in three ways:

1. Search performs automatic word completion, so if you search for knee but the finding is for knees, it will still find it.

2. Medcin includes an extensive list of synonyms that are used in an alternate word search. For example, if you search for knee injury, the search results will also include findings for knee burns, knee trauma, and fractured patella, among others.

3. Search identifies related findings in other tabs so that when you search for a word or phrase in a particular tab, related findings are automatically available in the other tabs. This means that when you are using Search while documenting a client exam, as you continue through the exam, the other tabs may already have findings that you will use.

Search is not designed to find every instance that contains the words being searched because the search results will often have too many findings. Instead, Search finds and displays the highest level match but does not list all the expanded findings below it.

Prompt is short for "prompt with current finding." Prompt generates a list of findings that are clinically related to the finding currently highlighted.

The prompt list that is displayed is shorter than the full nomenclature, containing only relevant findings, making it easier to read and navigate. The list generated by the prompt feature populates all the tabs, creating shorter lists of any relevant findings in each tab (Sx, Hx, Px, Tx, Dx, and Rx).

The **Order** button orders a test. Clicking on the red button for a test records the test as performed. Highlighting the name of the test and clicking the Order button records the test as ordered.

The **Rx** button on the Toolbar is available only on the Rx tab and only when the highlighted finding is a drug or medication. Clicking the Rx button invokes the prescription writer.

ICD-9-CM codes are an international standard for coding diseases and death. A supplemental section of ICD-9-CM also provides codes for reasons that clients come to the doctor other than illness or injury. These codes are called "V Codes" and start with the letter "V." They are used for checkups, physicals, vaccinations, maternity care, screening for diabetes, and so on.

Another supplemental section of the ICD-9-CM codes is titled "External Causes of Injury and Poisoning." These codes begin with the letter "E." E codes cover injuries ranging from bee stings to war; other examples include falling and vehicle crash injuries. E codes are use in addition to the numeric ICD-9-CM codes, never alone. E codes are used to codify the cause of an injury or adverse event.

The ICD-9-CM codes are from three to five digits long. The fourth and fifth digits add specificity. Insurance billing rules require that clinicians code to the most specific level. EHR systems automatically reference ICD-9-CM codes at the fourth or fifth digit specificity. EHR systems based on Medcin can automatically resolve the assessment to the most specific level of diagnosis code.

ICD-9-CM codes also are used as a key to problems and protocols in healthcare. Examples of protocols might be a specific set of tests used to monitor a particular disease or a list of antibiotics known to be effective for a certain type of infection. Creating protocols and finding them based on the assessment can help the clinician write orders and document the exam quickly.

Multiple diagnoses codes can be assigned to a single encounter. This occurs mainly because clients with ongoing or chronic conditions require regular visits. It is correct and appropriate to continue to use diagnosis codes from past visits for as long as the client continues to have that illness or condition.

ICD-10 is the latest revision to the International Classification of Diseases. HHS has proposed that ICD-10 codes should begin being used in the United States effective October 2013.

As you continue through the course, you can refer to the Guided Exercises in this chapter when you need to remember how to perform a particular task.

Task	Exercise	Page No.
Search for a finding in the nomenclature	44	257
Prompt (locate findings related to highlighted finding)	44	257
Record orders (or change order status) using the drop-down list	45	263
Record orders using the order button	45	263
Use the prescription writer	47	273
Use a quick-pick list to write prescriptions	48	280
Order tests based on diagnosis	49 and 50	288 and 293

Reference

Dick, R. S., & Steen, E. B. (2000). *The computer-based patient record: An essential technology for health care*. Washington, DC: Institute of Medicine, National Academy Press. (Original work published 1991, revised 1997)

Test Your Knowledge

You may run the Medcin Student Edition software and use your mouse on the screen to answer the following questions:

1. Describe how to record a test that was ordered and describe how to record a test that was performed.

2. How do you indicate a "possible" diagnosis?

Describe the function of each of the following buttons on the Toolbar:

3. Search

4. Medcin

5. Order

6. Prompt

7. What does the acronym ICD stand for?

8. According to the textbook, what year is ICD-10 scheduled to replace ICD-9-CM?

9. Give an example of how a diagnosis-based protocol could be useful when writing orders.

10. When you click the Prompt button, what List will be generated?

11. Which button on the Toolbar invokes the prescription writer?

Answer True or False for the following statements:

12. Orders are an essential component of any medical chart.

     True   False

13. Nurses sometimes enter verbal orders into an EHR on behalf of the ordering clinician.

     True   False

14. The use of CPOE, in conjunction with an EHR, also improves clinician productivity.

     True   False

15. You should have produced five narrative documents of client encounters, which you printed. If you have not already done so, hand these in to your instructor with this test. The printed encounter notes will count as a portion of your grade.

Ask your instructor for answers to Test Your Knowledge

nursing.pearsonhighered.com

Prepare for success with animated examples, practice questions,
challenge tests, and interactive assignments.

Problem Lists, Results Management, and Trending

Learning Outcomes

After completing this chapter, you should be able to:

1. Understand and use Patient Management
2. Understand and use Problem Lists
3. Cite information from previous visits in a new encounter
4. View pending orders
5. Review lab test results
6. Create a graph of lab results
7. Create a graph of vital signs in the chart

Important Information about the Exercises in This Chapter

Many exercises thus far have permitted you to skip setting the encounter date and time. In the next few chapters, you will work with clients' longitudinal medical history using information from several previous encounters. In certain exercises it will be necessary to match the encounter date and time exactly as instructed in step 2 of the exercise in order to maintain the correct chronology of data in the exercise. If you need to review how to set the date and time when creating a new encounter, see Chapter 3, Guided Exercise 14.

Longitudinal Records to Manage Clients' Health

The majority of inpatient records typically concern a particular inpatient stay or episode of care. Although part of inpatient EHR will likely contain some longitudinal data such as problem history and allergies, the majority of the data will pertain only to the current visit. It will be easier to demonstrate the concept of longitudinal records by outpatient examples. In this chapter we shift from inpatient to outpatient facilities.

In addition to the traditional medical office, hospitals are increasingly operating specialty clinics focusing on problematic diagnoses—for example, diabetes, asthma, or hypertension. Regardless of the type of outpatient clinic or medical office, the EHR is a longitudinal record encompassing numerous encounters over an extended period of time.

In a medical office or outpatient clinic, clients are frequently seen by nurse practitioners instead of physicians. In this chapter, we use the term *clinician* or *provider* to represent equally a nurse practitioner or a physician.

Providers in a specialty clinic or primary care practice come to know their regular clients, helping to monitor and hopefully improve the client's health. To do so, the clinician must review the records from the client's past visits and recheck previous problems on every new encounter.

Providers also must keep track of what medications the client is currently taking, which tests have results, and any other orders that have been issued. A clinician will always check the medications list before writing a new prescription, as well as to renew chronic care prescriptions that are about to expire.

In an office using paper charts, this is done by flipping through the papers in the chart and reviewing the previous notes. In some offices, current medications and current problems are copied by hand to a list in the front of the paper chart. In other cases, the clinician simply remembers them while skimming the chart, keeping a mental list as he or she reads the chart.

In a codified electronic chart, the software itself can dynamically locate the necessary information and organize it for quick review. Additionally, the clinician can note the items reviewed, make updates to the problems, and then record them in the current encounter. The clinician does not have to search for findings in the system because the findings are already identified in the previous encounter notes.

The Student Edition software includes a Patient Management feature that will allow you to explore some of these concepts. Although commercial EHR vendors use national standard nomenclatures such as Medcin, they differentiate their software with unique visual styles. Software you will use in your workplace may have similar concepts and features of Patient Management, but the presentation of the information is likely to have a different appearance than the Student Edition.

Understanding Problem Lists

Nurses of all levels are trained to work with Problem Lists and depend on the information contained in the Problem Lists when providing care. Furthermore, maintaining a Problem List is a requirement for facility accreditation by organizations such as the Joint Commission.

Problem Lists are used to track both acute and chronic conditions related to the care of the client. Care team members should be able to easily see the active problems for a client and view the history of problems. Although chronic diseases that are poorly controlled or malignancies take precedence in clinical decision making over mild conditions that are not life threatening, the idea of a Problem List is to make sure everyone who cares for the client knows what conditions are present.

The relationship between diagnoses and problems is very close. In most EHR software, they are synonymous. Most clinical information recorded in the chart will be related to one or more problems. However, the concept of a primary diagnosis used for billing does not apply to a Problem List.

The concept of a "problem-oriented" view is to organize entries in a medical record by problem. The Problem List provides an up-to-date list of the diagnoses and conditions that affect that particular client's care. Typically, it links the data from all encounters, orders, and prescriptions to the respective problem. This problem-oriented view allows the clinician to quickly see the client's problems and what has been done thus far.

Problem Lists usually have an onset date, indicate Chronic or Acute, and show whether or not the problem is active. Problems are removed from the list or set inactive once the client is "cured" or the problem is "resolved." Some problems have a natural period of time in which they normally resolve themselves. These problems are called Acute Self-Limiting.

In some systems, Problem Lists can include findings that are not disease related but are, rather, wellness conditions. Wellness conditions are based on the age and sex of the client and used in health maintenance and preventative screening programs to keep healthy clients healthy. Both disease conditions and wellness conditions have preventive measures typically performed for clients with that condition. Here are some examples:

▶ an annual EKG for a person with congestive heart failure

▶ a quarterly blood sugar test for a client with diabetes

▶ a mammogram for a healthy woman over 35

▶ immunizations for a healthy infant

These recommendations can be driven by the data in the Problem List. An example of a health maintenance preventive screening program was discussed in Chapter 2.

In many EHR systems, a problem is added to the Problem List either manually or automatically from the assessment in the encounter note. Some clinicians prefer to add the problems manually so that diagnoses for "possible" and "rule-out" conditions do not appear on the Problem List until the diagnosis is confirmed. Manually adding a problem to the Problem List is especially useful when the problem is being treated by a specialist at another office, but the clinician wants to remain aware of the condition. It is also possible to manually add findings to the Problem List that would normally be in other sections of the narrative, such as Past Medical History or Symptoms.

Guided Exercise 51: Exploring the Manage Tab

The Manage tab in the Student Edition software is representative of a function found in many EHR used to manage a client's problems over time. The function, sometimes called Patient Management, presents a clinical summary view of the client's previous visits. The view presents historical data obtained from findings recorded in past encounters. The clinical summary can be updated from the current encounter or, conversely, the encounter note for the current visit can be created using data from the Manage tab.

In this exercise you are going to start a new encounter, but the system will automatically retrieve and display information from previous encounters. For the first exercise, you are just going to become familiar with the Patient Management features of the software. In the subsequent exercise you will learn to cite information from previous encounters into the current encounter note.

Case Study

Juan Garcia, an outpatient who has been treated previously, is returning for a follow-up visit.

Step 1

If you have not already done so, start the Student Edition software.

Click Select on the Menu bar, and then click Patient.

In the Patient Selection window, locate and click on **Juan Garcia** as shown in Figure 8-1.

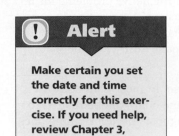

! **Alert**

Make certain you set the date and time correctly for this exercise. If you need help, review Chapter 3, Guided Exercise 14.

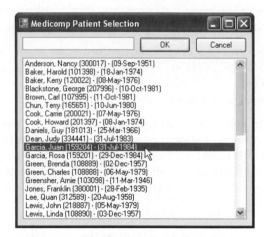

▶ **Figure 8-1 Selecting Juan Garcia from the Patient Selection window.**

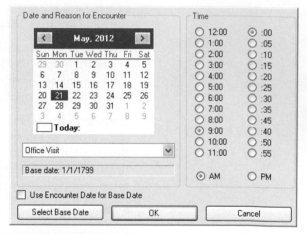

▶ **Figure 8-2 New encounter for an office visit, May 21, 2012 9:00 AM.**

Step 2

Click Select on the Menu bar, and then click New Encounter.

Select the date **May 21, 2012**, the time **9:00 AM**, and the reason **Office Visit**.

Compare your screen to Figure 8-2. Make certain the date and time match before clicking on the OK button.

Step 3

Enter the Chief complaint by locating the button in the Toolbar labeled "Chief" and clicking on it.

In the dialog window, type "**Knee injury follow-up**."

Compare your screen to Figure 8-3 before clicking on the button labeled "Close the note form."

Step 4

Locate and click on the tab labeled "Manage" at the bottom of your screen. It is circled in red in Figure 8-4.

▶ **Figure 8-3 Chief complaint dialog for knee injury follow-up.**

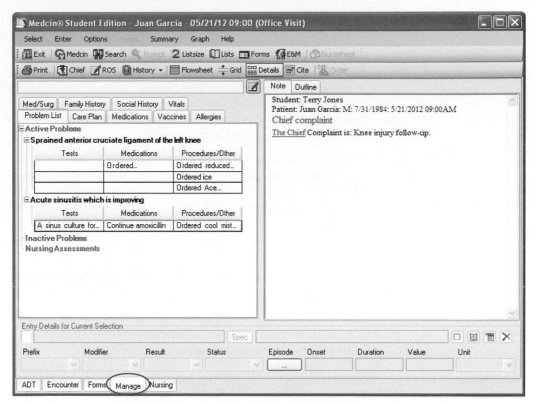

▶ Figure 8-4 Manage tab (circled in red) and Details button (highlighted orange).

Compare your screen to Figure 8-4. The Medcin Nomenclature normally displayed in the left pane of your screen has been replaced by an information window displaying information from previous encounters.

In this step we will learn a new button on the Toolbar. The button labeled "Details" allows you to see more of the information in the left pane by hiding the Entry Details section at the bottom of the screen. The Entry Details section can be restored whenever it is hidden by clicking the Details button again.

Locate and click on the button in the Toolbar labeled "Details." It is highlighted orange in Figure 8-4.

Look at the left pane of your screen. Note that the pane contains nine tabs:

▶ Problems (the Manage tab opens on the Problem List tab)

▶ Care Plan

▶ Medications

▶ Vaccines

▶ Allergies

▶ Past Medical/Surgical History (Med/Surg)

▶ Family History

▶ Social History

▶ Vitals

In the following steps, you will examine each tab.

Step 5

The Manage tab opens on the Problem List tab (circled in red in Figure 8-5). The Problem List includes a view of both active and inactive problems, as well as nursing assessments. This example has two active problems.

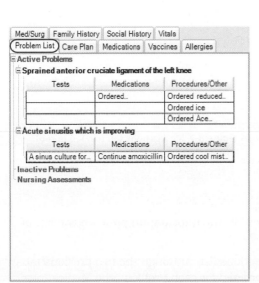

▶ Figure 8-5 Problem List tab (circled in red) with details hidden.

Compare your screen to Figure 8-5. Within the Problem List, there are three columns: Tests, Medications, and Procedures/Other. The most recent active findings (from the Tx and Rx sections of previous encounters) are listed in these columns for each problem.

If tests have been ordered, they appear in the first column. If a test has results, the name of the test is displayed in bold. Any medications prescribed for the problem appear in the second column. The last column lists any other orders or procedures from past encounters related to this problem.

The nurse also can focus on a particular problem by closing the others. A small plus or small minus sign next to a problem description allows you to open and close the details of the problem in the same way that you expand or contract the tree structure when browsing the Nomenclature List. You will work more with the Problem List in the next exercise.

Step 6

Locate and click on the tab labeled "Care Plan" in the information pane on the left of your screen.

The Care Plan tab displays each problem, followed by the date of each encounter that the client was seen for that problem. Small plus signs next to the encounter allow you to expand the encounter to display the Care Plan for that date.

Click on the plus sign beside each encounter date. Compare your screen with Figure 8-6.

Findings from the Plan section of the encounter note are displayed beneath the encounter date; however, findings from any group can be manually added to the Care Plan.

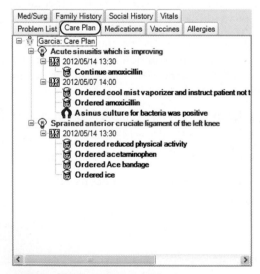

▶ **Figure 8-6 Care Plan tab (circled in red).**

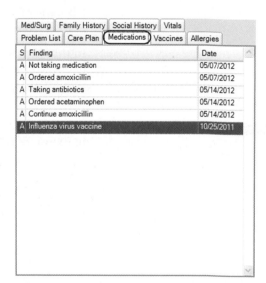

▶ **Figure 8-7 Medications tab (circled in red).**

Step 7

Locate and click on the tab labeled "Medications" in the information pane on the left of your screen. Compare your screen to Figure 8-7.

The Medications tab provides a traditional medications list. Although the two previous tabs (Problem and Care Plan) listed the medications ordered for each problem, the Medications tab displays all medications ordered by any clinician in the practice as well as those reported by the client.

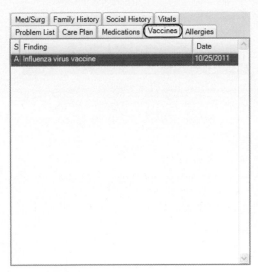

▶ **Figure 8-8 Vaccines tab (circled in red).**

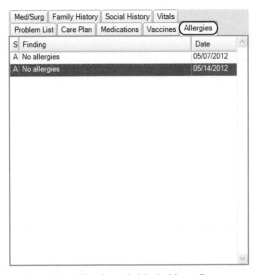

▶ **Figure 8-9 Allergies tab (circled in red).**

Step 8

Locate and click on the tab labeled "Vaccines" in the information pane on the left of your screen. Compare your screen to Figure 8-8.

The tab displays the client's history of vaccines. Note that vaccines also appear in the Medications list; these are not duplicate findings. The software deliberately shows vaccines in both lists.

Step 9

Locate and click on the tab labeled "Allergies" in the information pane on the left of your screen. Compare your screen to Figure 8-9.

The tab displays any allergy information from any of the previous encounters. In this case, the pertinent fact is that the client reported "No allergies."

Before writing a prescription, a nurse practitioner would check both the Medications and Allergies tabs. Most electronic prescription systems also check allergy data automatically at the time the prescription is written. Drug utilization review was discussed in Chapter 2 and Chapter 7.

Step 10

Locate and click on the tab labeled "Med/Surg" in the information pane on the left of your screen. Compare your screen to Figure 8-10. Note that the tabs in the left pane are arranged in two rows; when you click any tab in the upper row, the entire row moves down. The tab for the data currently displayed in the left pane is always in the (bottom) row of tabs closest to the grid.

The "Med/Surg" tab displays Medical and Surgical History findings that have been recorded in the Past History section of previous encounters. The date column displays the date the finding was recorded.

Step 11

Locate and click on the tab labeled "Family History" in the information pane on the left of your screen. Compare your screen to Figure 8-11.

The tab displays all findings that have been recorded in the Family History section of previous encounters. The date column displays the date that the finding was recorded.

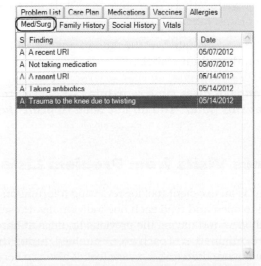

▶ **Figure 8-10 Past Medical and Surgical History tab.**

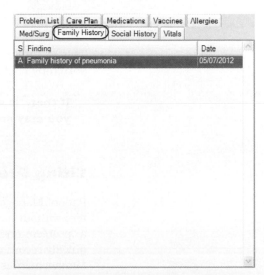

▶ **Figure 8-11 Family History tab (circled in red).**

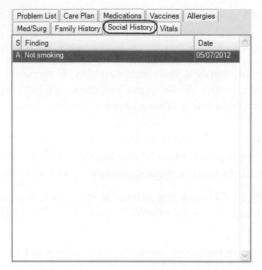

▶ **Figure 8-12 Social History tab (circled in red).**

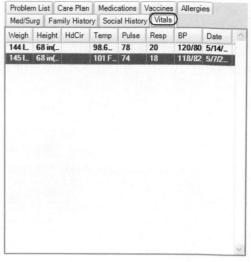

▶ **Figure 8-13 Vital Signs tab (circled in red).**

Step 12

Locate and click on the tab labeled "Social History" in the information pane on the left of your screen. Compare your screen to Figure 8-12.

The tab displays all findings that have been recorded in the Social History section of previous encounters. The date column displays the date that the finding was recorded.

Step 13

Locate and click on the tab labeled "Vitals" in the information pane on the left of your screen. Compare your screen to Figure 8-13.

The tab displays the Vital Signs findings that have been recorded in multiple encounters.

Step 14

In each of the tabs the data can be sorted. This is done by clicking on the labels over the columns of data. For example:

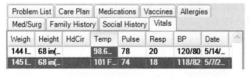

▶ **Figure 8-14 Vital signs sorted by temperature.**

Locate and click on the column labeled "Temp" within the Vitals tab. Compare the Vitals tab on your screen with Figure 8-14. You will notice that the rows of vital signs data changed places and the date that Juan had a temperature of 101°F is now the top row. When sorting, the entire row stays together. To restore the Vitals tab to its original order, click on the column labeled "Date."

This example used the Vitals tab, but the data in any tab of Patient Management can be sorted by clicking on the column labels.

> **If there is not enough class time remaining to complete the next exercise, you may stop at this point. You do not need to print the encounter.**

Citing Previous Visits from Problem Lists

Patient Management is an excellent tool for reviewing information from previous encounters without having to open and read each one individually. Presenting the information in a "problem-oriented" view and having the previous findings at hand enables the clinician to quickly record the reexamination of each area examined during the previous visits. Patient Management is much more than just a review tool; it also is a very efficient method of documenting a follow-up visit.

In Chapter 6 you learned to cite individual nursing actions using the Cite button on the Toolbar. On the Manage tab, you can cite whole sections of a previous encounter and update the finding to reflect changes in the client's condition—for example, as a follow-up to a previous visit.

Guided Exercise 52: Following Up on a Problem

You will recall from a previous chapter that the mouse typically has at least two buttons, a left button and a right-click button. In this exercise, when instructed, you are going to be using the right-click button on the mouse as well as the left button.

Case Study

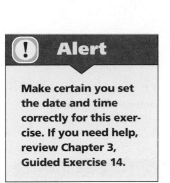

Alert

Make certain you set the date and time correctly for this exercise. If you need help, review Chapter 3, Guided Exercise 14.

Juan Garcia has returned for a follow-up on his previous knee injury. Using Patient Management, you will see how easy it is to document this type of visit.

Step 1

If you are continuing from the previous exercise, proceed to step 4.

Otherwise, start the Student Edition software.

From the Select Menu, click Patient, and from the Patient Selector window select **Juan Garcia** (see Figure 8-1).

Step 2

From the Select Menu, click New Encounter. Use the date **May 21, 2012**, the time **9:00 AM**, and the reason **Office Visit**.

Make certain the date and time match before clicking on the OK button (see Figure 8-2).

Step 3

Enter the Chief complaint by locating the button in the Toolbar labeled "Chief" and clicking on it.

In the dialog window, type "**Knee injury follow-up**."

When it is correct, click on the button labeled "Close the note form" (see Figure 8-3).

▶ **Figure 8-15 Vital Signs form for Juan Garcia.**

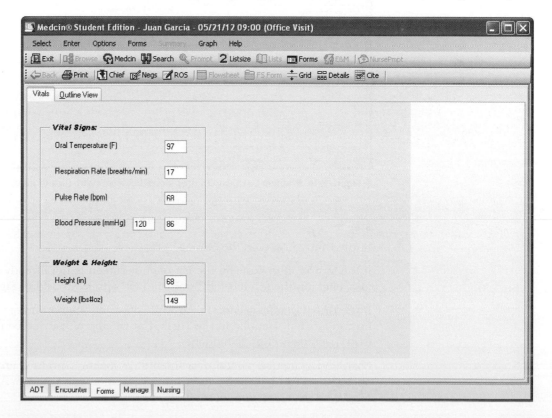

Step 4

Click the Forms button on the Toolbar and select "Vitals" from the Form Manager window. Enter Juan Garcia's vital signs on the Vitals Form in the corresponding fields as follows:

Temperature: **97**

Respiration: **17**

Pulse: **68**

BP: **120/86**

Height: **68**

Weight: **149**

When you have finished, compare your screen to Figure 8-15. If it is correct, click on the tab labeled "Manage" at the bottom of the window. (If you have difficulty locating Manage, refer to Figure 8-4).

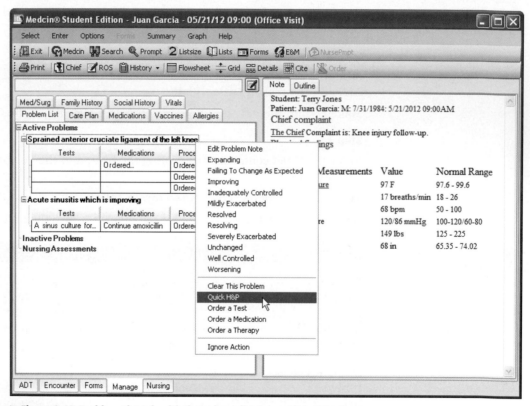

▶ **Figure 8-16 Problem List tab with drop-down list from right-click of mouse.**

Step 5

Verify that you are on the Manage tab.

If the information pane on the left of your screen is not already displaying the Problem List, click on the tab labeled "Problem List" (circled in red in Figure 8-5).

If the Entry Details section is currently covering the bottom of your screen, locate the button labeled "Details" in the Toolbar at the top of your screen and click it until the Entry Details section is hidden.

Position the mouse pointer over the first problem, "Sprained anterior cruciate ligament of the knee," and click the **right-click** button on your mouse. A drop-down list will be displayed, as shown in Figure 8-16.

If the drop-down list does not match the list shown in Figure 8-16, your mouse was not positioned correctly on the problem description. Reposition your mouse and click the **right-click** mouse button again.

Without clicking on any of the options, study the options on the drop-down list. Most of these options are used to cite updated findings into the new encounter. Do not select any option until directed to do so. The following is a brief explanation of each option in the drop-down list:

Edit Problem Note: Allows you to edit a free-text note that is attached to the problem.

The next 11 options are used to record the status of the problem. Selecting any of the following items from the drop-down list will add a new finding to today's encounter. The finding will have a status set with one of the following:

> **Expanding**
>
> **Failing to Change as Expected**
>
> **Improving**
>
> **Inadequately Controlled**
>
> **Mildly Exacerbated**
>
> **Resolved**
>
> **Resolving**
>
> **Severely Exacerbated**
>
> **Unchanged**
>
> **Well Controlled**
>
> **Worsening**

The remaining options allow the clinician to take multiple actions quickly. They are as follows:

Clear This Problem: Clears all test orders, discontinues medications related to the problem, clears therapy orders, and sets the problem as inactive.

Quick H&P: This option invokes a data entry window that lists symptoms, history, and physical findings as they appeared in the most recent encounter for this problem. The clinician can quickly review the last History and Physical (H&P) taken for this problem and update the new encounter with any findings in the Quick H&P window. The Quick H&P window will be shown in the next step.

Order a Test: This option is provided to allow the clinician to order a new test for this problem. When the option is selected, the right pane will temporarily display a list of tests you would normally see in Tx tab. When the Tx list is displayed, you can order directly from the list in the right pane.

Order a Medication: This option is provided to allow the clinician to order a new medication for this problem. When the option is selected, the right pane will temporarily display the Rx list of medications. When the Rx list is displayed, you can order directly from the list in the right pane. If the drug selected requires a prescription, the prescription writer will be invoked automatically.

Order a Therapy: This option is provided to allow the clinician to quickly order any type of therapy other than medications. As with the previous two options, a list of therapies will temporarily display in the right pane. You can order directly from the displayed list.

Ignore Action: This option cancels the drop-down list without recording anything. You also can cancel the drop-down list by clicking anywhere else on the screen.

▶ **Figure 8-17 Quick history and physical for knee injury.**

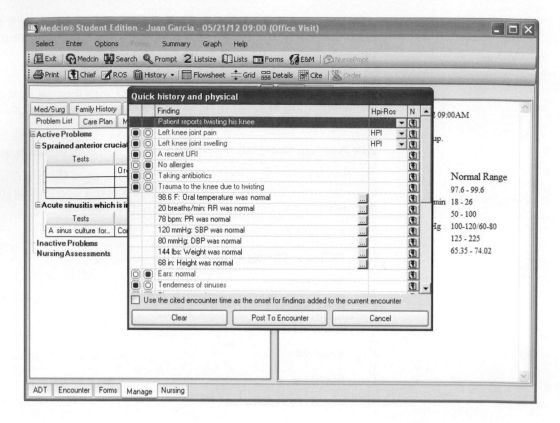

Step 6

Locate and click on the Quick H&P option in the drop-down list (shown highlighted in Figure 8-16). The Quick History and Physical window will be invoked.

Compare your screen to Figure 8-17. The window displays findings from the previous exam for this condition.

Using the findings in the list, the nurse practitioner can be certain to update anything that was observed in the previous visit. Items that have already been entered in today's encounter appear on the Quick H&P list in gray. Examples of today's findings that are gray in Figure 8-17 include Chief complaint and Vital Signs.

The patient reports that his knee is better. Locate and click on the following findings (you will need to scroll the window to get them all):

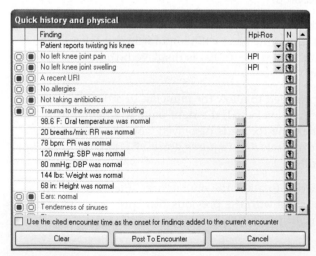

▶ **Figure 8-18 Knee injury findings set to normal, ready to post to encounter.**

- (blue button) Left knee joint pain

- (blue button) Left knee joint swelling

- (blue button) Taking antibiotics

- (blue button) Localized swelling of the left knee

- (blue button) Warmth of the left knee

- (blue button) Pain was elicited by motion of the left knee

Important—do not click every finding in the H&P list. Click only those indicated above.

Step 7

Compare your screen to Figure 8-18. Scroll the window and verify that you have selected only the items listed in step 6. If you find an error, click on the button labeled "Cancel," and repeat steps 5 and 6.

When all the findings have been selected correctly, click on the button labeled "Post To Encounter."

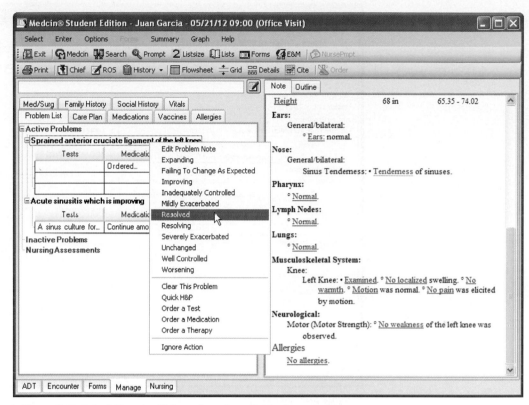

▶ **Figure 8-19 Select "Resolved" from drop-down list for knee problem.**

Step 8

The findings you selected in the Quick H&P window should now be displayed in the encounter note (as shown in the right pane of Figure 8-19).

The problem is resolved. To indicate this in today's encounter note, position the mouse over the first problem, "Sprained anterior cruciate ligament of the right knee," and click the **right-click** button on your mouse. Again, the drop-down list will be displayed, as shown in Figure 8-19.

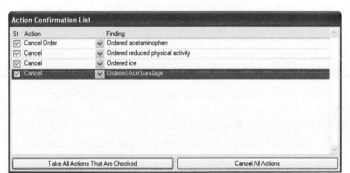

▶ **Figure 8-20 Resolving a problem—Action Confirmation List.**

Locate and click on the option labeled "Resolved." The window shown in Figure 8-20 will be invoked.

Step 9

When a problem is resolved, there are certain actions the clinician may want to take: canceling previous orders, discontinuing any medications, or setting the problem as inactive. The Resolved option invokes a window of all active orders related to the problem and sets appropriate default actions.

A check box next to each item indicates that you wish to take the action indicated. A drop-down list of possible actions is available for each order (shown later in Figure 8-22). You can use the list to select a different action or you can indicate that no action is to be taken by unchecking the box.

Do not make any changes to the default list. When you have reviewed the list, locate and click the button labeled "Take All Actions That Are Checked."

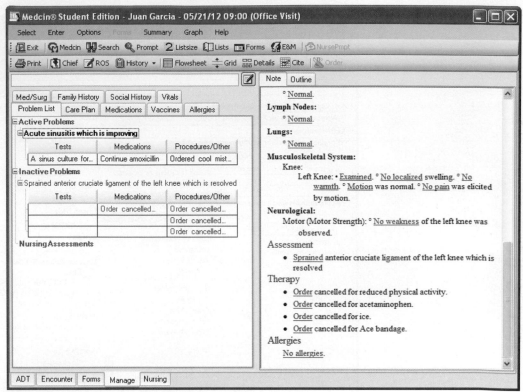

▶ **Figure 8-21 Inactive problem on Problem List.**

Step 10

The knee problem in the left pane has moved to the section labeled "Inactive Problems." If it is not currently displayed, locate and click the small plus sign next to "Inactive Problems."

Compare your screen with Figure 8-21. Note in the right pane that the previous therapy orders have been canceled.

Step 11

The Problem List also listed a second problem, acute sinusitis, for which the client was recently treated. Juan reports that his sinusitis has cleared up and that he has finished the prescribed course of antibiotics. Using what you have learned in the previous steps, resolve the acute sinusitis problem.

Position your mouse pointer on the active problem, "Acute sinusitis." Click the right-click button on the mouse and select Resolved from the options on the drop-down list. The Action Confirmation List window (shown in Figure 8-22) will be invoked.

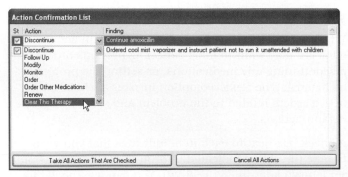

▶ **Figure 8-22 Resolve acute sinusitis Action Confirmation List.**

Step 12

Because Juan has reported taking all the amoxicillin, there is no reason to discontinue the order. Locate and click on the down arrow next to "Cancel" and select "Clear This Therapy" from the drop-down list as shown in Figure 8-22.

Click on the button labeled "Take All Actions That Are Checked."

When you have completed this step, you will notice that both problems are now in the inactive problem list.

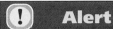

Do not close or exit the encounter until you have a printed copy in your hand. **You will lose your work if you exit before printing.**

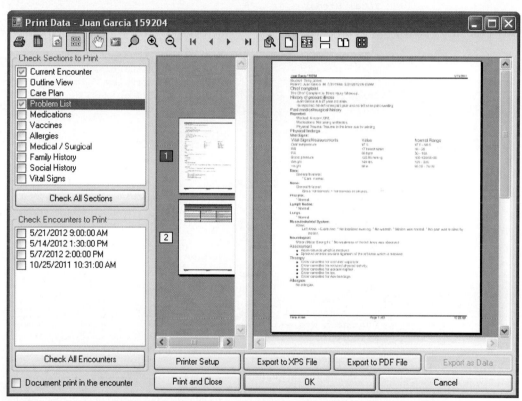

▶ **Figure 8-23 Check marks next to Current Encounter and Problem List in Print Data window.**

Step 13

Remain on the Manage tab. Click on the Print button on the Toolbar at the top of your screen to invoke the Print Data window.

Be certain to put a check mark in the boxes next to both "Current Encounter" and "Problem List" as shown in Figure 8-23.

Click on the appropriate button to either print or export a file, as directed by your instructor.

Compare your printout or file output to Figure 8-24a and 8-24b. If it is correct, hand it in to your instructor. If there are any differences, review the previous steps in the exercise and find your error.

Juan Garcia   Page 1 of 2

Student: *your name or id here*
Patient: Juan Garcia: M: 7/31/1984: 5/21/2012 09:00AM
Chief complaint
The Chief Complaint is: Knee injury follow-up.
History of present illness
       Juan Garcia is a 27 year old male.
       He reported: No left knee joint pain and no left knee joint swelling.
Past medical/surgical history
Reported History:
       Medical: A recent URI.
       Medications: Not taking antibiotics.
       Physical Trauma: Trauma to the knee due to twisting.
Physical findings
Vital Signs:

Vital Signs/Measurements	Value	Normal Range
Oral temperature	97 F	97.6 - 99.6
RR	17 breaths/min	18 - 26
PR	68 bpm	50 - 100
Blood pressure	120/86 mmHg	100 - 120/60 - 80
Weight	149 lbs	125 - 225
Height	68 in	65.35 - 74.02

Ears:
General/bilateral:
° Ears: normal.
Nose:
General/bilateral:
Sinus Tenderness:
       • Tenderness of sinuses.
Pharynx:
° Normal.
Lymph Nodes:
° Normal.
Lungs:
° Normal.
Musculoskeletal System:
Knee:
Left Knee:
       • Examined. ° No localized swelling. ° No warmth. ° Motion was normal.
° No pain was elicited by motion.
Neurological:
Motor (Motor Strength): ° No weakness of the left knee was observed.
Assessment
       • Acute sinusitis which is resolved
       • Sprained anterior cruciate ligament of the left knee which is resolved
Therapy
       • Order cancelled for cool mist vaporizer.
       • Order cancelled for reduced physical activity.
       • Order cancelled for acetaminophen.
       • Order cancelled for ice.
       • Order cancelled for Ace bandage.
Allergies
No allergies.

▶ **Figure 8-24a Printed encounter note for Juan Garcia (page 1 of 2).**

Problem List		
Tests	Medications	Procedures/Other
Inactive Problems		
Sprained anterior cruciate ligament of the left knee which is resolved		
	Order cancelled for acetaminophen 5/21/2012	Order cancelled for reduced physical activity 5/21/2012
		Order cancelled for ice 5/21/2012
		Order cancelled for Ace bandage 5/21/2012
Acute sinusitis which is resolved		
A sinus culture for bacteria was positive 5/7/2012		Order cancelled for cool mist vaporizer 5/21/2012

▶ **Figure 8-24b   Printed Problem List from Juan Garcia encounter (page 2 of 2).**

Orders and Results Management

You will recall from Chapter 1 that Results Management was one of the eight criteria for an EHR in the IOM report. Orders are tracked in an EHR from the moment they are entered in the system. In Chapter 7 we discussed one of the benefits of CPOE systems is that they keep track of what has been ordered for each client. Benefits of CPOE order tracking include:

▶ Preventing lost orders.

▶ Preventing duplicate orders.

▶ Detecting when a client sent to an outside lab has failed to show up.

Benefits of results tracking include:

▶ Notifying the provider as soon as "preliminary" results are available.

▶ Notifying the provider anytime results status are updated to "final" or "corrected."

▶ Keeping track of which results need to be reviewed by the clinician.

As you will see in subsequent exercises, the benefits of having test results available to the provider during the client encounter include the ability to graph or "trend" the results. Another benefit is the ability to review results online and to quickly order subsequent or additional tests when it is warranted.

The Student Edition software does not contain an electronic laboratory order and result system. It would be inappropriate to order tests from a classroom. Because the Student Edition does not contain the electronic lab interface, the following two exercises have been created solely to demonstrate how useful it is to have lab data at hand while seeing the client. The features you will find in commercial EHR software automate the lab order/result workflow differently and more elegantly than these simple exercises.

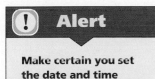

Alert

Make certain you set the date and time correctly for this exercise. If you need help, review Chapter 3, Guided Exercise 14.

Guided Exercise 53: Viewing Pending Orders and Lab Results

In Guided Exercises 50 this client's mother reported the possible exposure to lead-based paints while remodeling their older home. You will recall her treatment plan recommended screening other family members.

Case Study

Stanley Zabroski is a 16-year-old male living with his mother in a home built in 1959 that has peeling lead-based paint. During his mother's previous visit, lab tests were ordered to screen other family members for lead poisoning. Stanly has already visited the

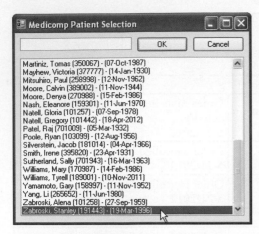

▶ **Figure 8-25 Selecting Stanley Zabroski from the Patient Selection window.**

lab before his appointment today. The purpose of his office visit is for an examination and to review the test results.

Step 1

If you have not already done so, start the Student Edition software.

Click Select on the Menu bar, and then click Patient.

In the Patient Selection window, locate and click on **Stanley Zabroski** as shown in Figure 8-25.

Step 2

Click Select on the Menu bar, and then click New Encounter.

Select the date **May 22, 2012**, the time **4:00 PM**, and the reason **Office Visit**.

Compare your screen to Figure 8-26. Make certain the date and time match before clicking on the OK button.

In the next two steps, the nurse enters the Chief complaint and Vital Signs.

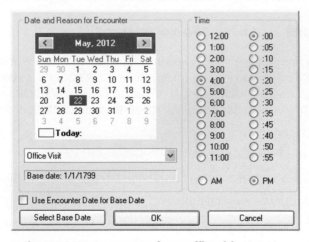

▶ **Figure 8-26 New encounter for an office visit, May 22, 2012 4:00 PM.**

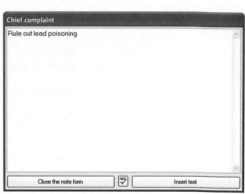

▶ **Figure 8-27 Chief complaint dialog for "Rule out lead poisoning."**

Step 3

Enter the Chief complaint by locating the button in the toolbar labeled "Chief" and clicking on it.

In the dialog window that will open, type "**Rule out lead poisoning**."

Compare your screen to Figure 8-27 before clicking on the button labeled "Close the note form."

Step 4

Enter the client's Vital Signs using the Vitals Form. Vital Signs for Stanley Zabroski are as follows:

Temperature: **98.6**

Respiration: **20**

Pulse: **76**

BP: **120/80**

Height: **73**

Weight: **155**

When you have finished, compare your screen to Figure 8-28. If it is correct, click on the tab labeled "Encounter" at the bottom of the window.

Step 5

Click on the Dx tab.

▶ **Figure 8-28 Vital Signs form for Stanley Zabroski.**

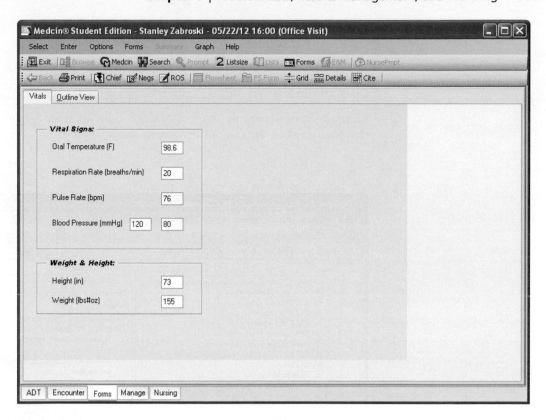

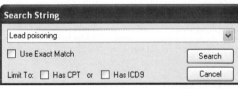

▶ **Figure 8-29 Search for Lead Poisoning.**

Click on the button labeled "Search" on the Toolbar near the top of the screen. (The Search button icon resembles a small pair of binoculars.) The Search String window will be invoked.

Enter the search string "Lead poisoning" and click on the button labeled "Search" in the window, as shown in Figure 8-29.

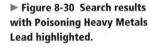

▶ **Figure 8-30 Search results with Poisoning Heavy Metals Lead highlighted.**

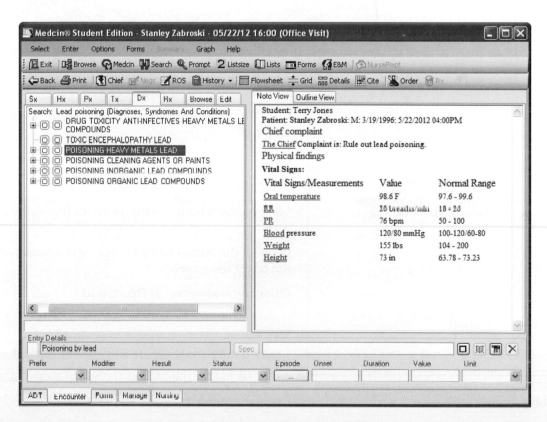

Step 6

Click on the Dx tab.

Locate and highlight the finding "POISONING HEAVY METALS LEAD."

Click on the List Size button until the list size is **1**.

Compare your screen to Figure 8-30, and then click on the button labeled "Prompt" on the Toolbar near the top of the screen.

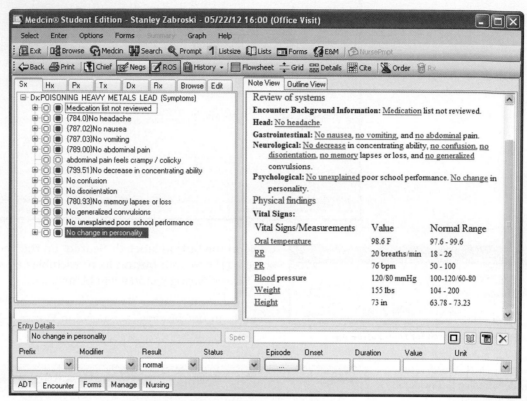

▶ **Figure 8-31 Symptoms for Heavy Metal Poisoning Lead.**

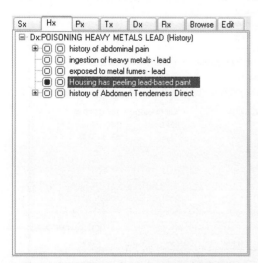

▶ **Figure 8-32 History for Heavy Metal Poisoning Lead.**

Step 7

Click on the Sx tab.

Verify that List Size is set to **1**.

Click on the button labeled "ROS" on the Toolbar near the top of the screen.

Click on the button labeled "Negs" (Auto Negative) on the Toolbar near the top of the screen.

Compare your screen to Figure 8-31.

Step 8

Click on the Hx tab. Locate and click on the following finding:

● (red button) house has peeling paint which is lead based

Compare your left pane to Figure 8-32.

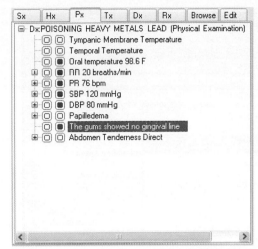

▶ **Figure 8-33 Physical Exam for Heavy Metal Poisoning Lead.**

▶ **Figure 8-34 Tx tab showing tests results with normal results.**

Step 9

Click on the Px tab. Locate and click on the following finding:

- (blue button) Gums gingival line

Compare your left pane to Figure 8-33.

Step 10

As discussed at the beginning of the exercise, Stanley has had several lab tests performed before the office visit. The results were within normal limits. The nurse practitioner will review results of the tests and document them in the encounter note.

Click on the Tx tab. Locate and click on the following finding:

- (blue button) CBC with differential
- (blue button) Serum Lead Level
- (blue button) Urine Lead, 24 hr

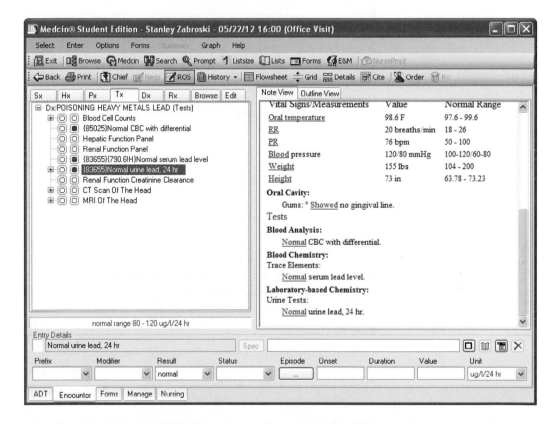

Compare your screen to Figure 8-34. If it is correct, click on the tab labeled "**Manage**" at the bottom of the window.

Step 11

Your screen should display the Problem List. If the information pane on the left of your screen is not already displaying the Problem List, click on the tab labeled "Problem List."

If the Entry Details pane is covering part of your list, locate and click on the button labeled "Details" in the Toolbar at the top of your screen.

Knowing which orders are still pending results is especially useful in offices in which multiple clinicians share clients, because it prevents duplicate orders. A nurse practitioner can see what orders are outstanding on a client, including those ordered by another provider.

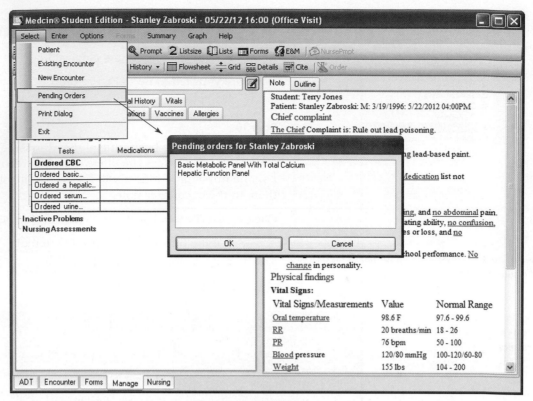

▶ **Figure 8-35 Patient Management—Pending Orders window.**

Click Select on the Menu bar, and then click **Pending Orders**. A window of pending orders will be displayed.

Compare the window in your screen labeled "Pending Orders for Stanley Zabroski" to Figure 8-35. This window contains a list of tests that have been ordered but for which results have not yet been entered.

Close the window by clicking on the Cancel button. Note: If you click OK by mistake, you will invoke a results entry window. Simply click the Cancel button in that window, and proceed to the next step.

Step 12

From the Manage tab, you also can see the results of any tests that have been entered. As we discussed earlier, EHR systems can receive results from the lab electronically and merge them directly into the client's chart. Typically, the ordering provider is notified that results are ready for review.

Look at the Problem List in the left pane of your screen, under the test column.

Test names that are in bold type in the list indicate those that have results in the system.

Position the mouse over the test labeled "Ordered CBC" and click the **right-click** button on your mouse. A drop-down list will be displayed.

If the drop-down list does not match the list shown in Figure 8-36, your mouse was not positioned correctly on the test. Reposition your mouse and click the right mouse button again.

Locate the option to Show Results and click the left mouse button. A window displaying the "Results for Ordered CBC" will be displayed, as shown in Figure 8-36.

The nurse can review the actual test results. Click the Cancel button to close the results window.

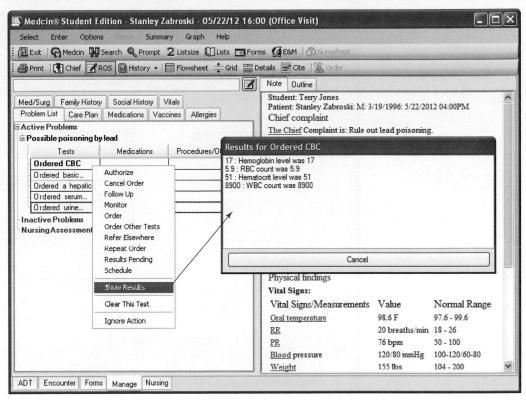

▶ Figure 8-36 Right-click menu: "Shows Results" invokes window of ordered CBC results.

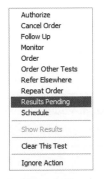

▶ Figure 8-37
Select option Results Pending
for basic metabolic panel.

Step 13

You will recall that tests displayed in the Pending Orders window (shown in Figure 8-35) did not yet have results. This fact can be easily noted in the encounter note using Patient Management.

Position the mouse over the test labeled "Ordered Basic Metabolic Panel" and click the **right-click** button on your mouse. A drop-down list will be displayed. Without clicking on any of the options, look at the list that is displayed. In addition to the "Show Results" option, used in the previous step, the drop-down list options include the ability to reorder a test, order additional follow-up tests, or enter the status of a test into the current encounter.

Locate and highlight the option "Results Pending" in the drop-down list (as shown in Figure 8-37) and click the left mouse button. This will record a finding into the exam narrative that the test results are pending.

Step 14

Locate and click on the **Encounter** tab at the bottom of your screen.

Click on the Dx tab (which has now returned to the full list of findings).

Again, click on the Search button in the Toolbar at the top of your screen.

The Search String window will be invoked and should still contain the words "**lead poisoning**." If it does not, type them again.

Click on the button in the window labeled "Search." (If you need help, refer to Figure 8-29.)

When the list of diagnoses is displayed, locate and highlight the finding "POISONING HEAVY METALS LEAD." (If you need help, refer to Figure 8-30.)

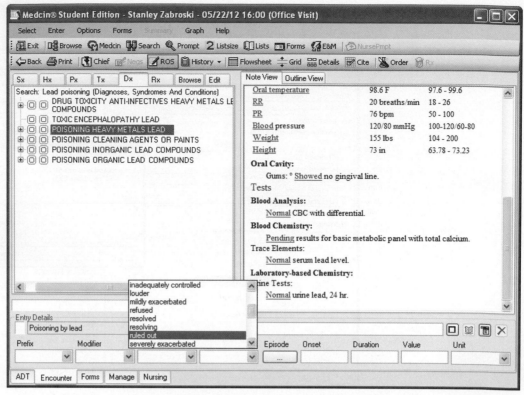

▶ **Figure 8-38 Dx tab—Select the status "Ruled out" for Poisoning Heavy Metals Lead.**

In the Entry Details section at the bottom of your screen, locate the Status Field and click on the down arrow button in it.

Scroll the drop-down list that is displayed to locate and click on "ruled out" as shown in Figure 8-38.

Alert

Do not close or exit the encounter until you have a printed copy in your hand. You will lose your work if you exit before printing.

Step 15

Click on the Print button on the Toolbar at the top of your screen to invoke the Print Data window.

Be certain there is a check mark in the box next to "Current Encounter" and then click on the appropriate button to either print or export a file, as directed by your instructor.

Compare your printout or file output to Figure 8-39. If it is correct, hand it in to your instructor. If there are any differences, review the previous steps in the exercise and find your error.

Stanley Zabroski   Page 1 of 1

Student: *your name or id here*
Patient: Stanley Zabroski: M: 3/19/1996: 5/22/2012 04:00PM
Chief complaint
The Chief Complaint is: Rule out lead poisoning.
Personal history
Home Environment: Housing has peeling lead-based paint.
Review of systems
Encounter Background Information: Medication list not reviewed.
Head: No headache.
Gastrointestinal: No nausea, no vomiting, and no abdominal pain.
Neurological: No decrease in concentrating ability, no confusion, no
       disorientation, no memory lapses or loss, and no generalized convulsions.
Psychological: No unexplained poor school performance. No change in personality.
Physical findings
Vital Signs:

Vital Signs/Measurements	Value	Normal Range
Oral temperature	98.6 F	97.6 - 99.6
RR	20 breaths/min	18 - 26
PR	76 bpm	50 - 100
Blood pressure	120/80 mmHg	100 - 120/56 - 80
Weight	155 lbs	83 - 176
Height	73 in	60.24 - 71.26

Oral Cavity:
Gums: ° Showed no gingival line.
Tests
Blood Analysis:
Normal CBC with differential.
Blood Chemistry:
Pending results for basic metabolic panel with total calcium.
Trace Elements:
Normal serum lead level.
Laboratory-based Chemistry:
Urine Tests:
Normal urine lead, 24 hr.
Assessment
      • Poisoning by lead which is ruled out

▶ **Figure 8-39   Printed encounter note for Stanley Zabroski.**

Real-Life Story

A Nurse Practitioner Talks about Her Profession

By Sharron Carr, ARNP-BC

Sharron Carr is a nurse practitioner affiliated with a large family practice medical group. During her nursing career, she has worked at every level of nursing from LPN to ARNP. She is currently working on her PhD.

A nurse practitioner is a provider of healthcare. We provide healthcare and prevention in different primary care settings as well as specialized offices. Our duties are very similar to those of a physician. We can prescribe medications; order, perform, and interpret different diagnostic tests; provide treatment plans; and perform minor office procedures—we essentially do the same job that the physician does with the exception of the prescription of controlled substances. There are currently five states that don't allow this, but that will change.

Each state governs the way a nurse practitioner can operate within the state and the scope of practice that is available to that nurse practitioner. The requirement in my state is that I have a collaborating physician with whom I am associated. I file with the board each year a letter of agreement between my collaborating physician and myself, but I can be a private practitioner; I do not need to practice under the care of a physician or in the same office. That is one of the main differences between the role of a nurse practitioner and a physician assistant. The nurse practitioner can practice independently; a physician assistant can never practice without the physician on the premises.

Educationally, the training for a nurse practitioner and physician assistant is very similar, but the program requirements are not. Most people who enter the physician assistant program have their bachelor's degree in some aspect of healthcare, but that is not mandatory. Then they progress on through their master's degree and graduate as a physician assistant. A nurse practitioner enters with a nursing degree (either an associate or bachelor degree in nursing) and the experience that goes along with that. We then advance into the master's degree level and graduate as a nurse practitioner.

Many types of nurse practitioner degrees are available and you can specialize within the practice as well. The Board of Nursing, the American Nursing Association, and the various societies are trying to adopt even higher levels of education and standards for nurse practitioners. In the future, a doctorate degree may be required in order to practice as a nurse practitioner.

There is also a clinical component to our training. Anytime you obtain a nursing degree, there is always a clinical component assigned to provide you the skills you will need to practice at that level. So for the nurse practitioner level, you are assigned within the type of care setting that you wish to work in when you leave school. For me, it was a primary care office. We had four different semesters during which we were required to do clinical rotations. The number of hours required differed each semester. We rotated through different clinical settings. We started out on campus at the health science center and then spread out into community as the semesters progressed. The settings depended on what our specialty was. If you were in pediatrics, you'd stay in the pediatric field; if you were into family medicine, you'd be exposed to both pediatric and adult practices.

Nursing in general is a field that has many avenues to explore and you can choose many paths. If one is not the right fit for you, you can choose another path. As a nurse practitioner, I feel like I have been able to make a difference in people's lives and promote healthcare and health in general to the population.

I started out in the world of nursing as an LPN, so I started out at the most basic level. As life allowed, I advanced my degree and moved through the ranks of nursing. I went from LPN to an associate degree RN, and from that I went back to school and earned my bachelor's and master's degrees. I am currently working on my doctorate.

As an RN, I worked in a hospital setting on a renal intensive care unit and did a little bit of management through that hospital. Subsequently, I began doing home infusion nursing, which I did for eight years. This is a very specialized, highly technological service for a registered nurse. I also assumed the director of nursing position and the director of professional services position within that company, giving me managerial experience as well.

My employer was eventually purchased by another company and was downsized. Although I was given a new job with the new company, after two years I decided I wanted to have more control over my working environment. I wanted to have responsibility for my own actions and to provide quality care. So I decided to go back to school and get my degree as a nurse practitioner. Now, by working on my doctorate, I hope to expand my knowledge and provide better care to my clients.

I am also involved in clinical trials research. My current family practice office participates in pharmaceutical clinical trials for new medications. I also continue my affiliation with a university, where a few times each year I participate in their clinical trials research.

I think what makes a nurse practitioner different from a physician is the component of prevention. We bring that provision to healthcare; we take a more holistic approach. I am concerned with how clients arrived at this point in their health when they present in front of me. What brought them to this level of illness? I look at environmental factors, their health behaviors, what their attitudes and beliefs are, and what their personal involvement is in their scheme of wellness. These are important

concepts in the disease process. We look at a whole person rather than just treat the symptom.

The more knowledge that I receive and the more that I am exposed to in the healthcare industry, the more eager I am to know. It is a continually evolving field that I'm practicing in and I try to keep up with the latest technological advances to provide even better care to the clients that I serve.

Trending

One important service that clinicians want to perform for their clients is "trending," which is comparing the change of certain test components or measurements over a period of time. In Chapter 1 the IOM identified this as one of the functional benefits derived from an EHR.

In a paper chart, the trend is observed by paging through past tests, locating the desired component on each report, and making a mental comparison. However, when the lab results or other measurements are stored as data in the EHR, the computer can instantly find all instances of any component that the clinician wishes to compare.

Additionally, with computerized data, graphs and charts can be easily created for any finding that has numerical results. This provides the clinician with a quick picture of the changes over time. Not only are graphs useful to the clinician, but they also provide an excellent means of clarification when counseling or for client education.

Using Graphs to View Trends of Lab Results

Chapter 2 discussed the advantages of EHR records with codified results as opposed to EHR records that are scanned images of printed reports. Nowhere is that more evident than with lab result reports.

An EHR system can graph any component of a lab test that has numerical values. However, to create a meaningful graph, the test must have been performed multiple times.

Guided Exercise 54: Graphing Lab Results

In the next exercise you will learn to graph a specific lab test by locating it using the search tool.

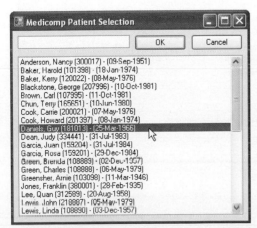

▶ **Figure 8-40 Selecting Guy Daniels from the Patient Selection window.**

Case Study

Guy Daniels has been seen at the clinic for several years. He has hypertension, Type II diabetes, and a weight problem. Several tests were ordered to be drawn before Mr. Daniels's scheduled visit to allow the results to be ready when the doctor or nurse practitioner sees him. He is scheduled for a clinic visit tomorrow and his lab results have been received from the lab. You have been asked to generate two graphs to be used for client education.

Step 1

If you have not already done so, start the Student Edition software.

Click Select on the Menu bar, and then click Patient.

In the Patient Selection window, locate and click on **Guy Daniels** as shown in Figure 8-40.

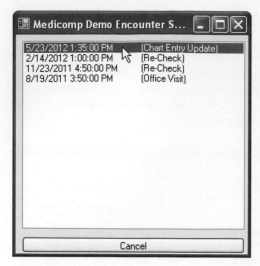

▶ **Figure 8-41 Select Existing Encounter for May 23, 2012 10:00 AM.**

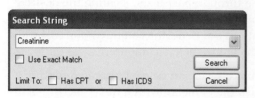

▶ **Figure 8-42 Search for Creatinine.**

Step 2

In this exercise you will retrieve an encounter already in progress.

Click Select on the Menu bar, and then click **Existing Encounter**.

A small window of previous encounters will be displayed. Compare your screen to the window in the center of Figure 8-41.

Position your mouse pointer on the first encounter in the list, dated **5/23/2012 1:35 PM** (as shown in Figure 8-41) and click on it.

The encounter will be displayed in the right pane of your screen; take a moment to review it. The record essentially consists of the results of his previsit lab tests. However, the encounter also contains a finding for blood pressure because while having his blood drawn, Mr. Daniels felt faint. The nurse took his blood pressure and recorded it in the chart.

Step 3

Click on the Tx tab.

Click on the button labeled "Search" on the Toolbar near the top of the screen. The Search String window will be invoked.

Type the search string "**Creatinine**" and click on the button in the window labeled "Search" as shown in Figure 8-42.

▶ **Figure 8-43 Select Graph Current Finding from the menu.**

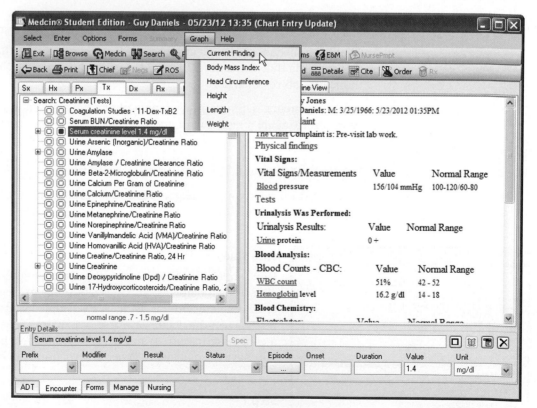

Step 4

Your left pane should automatically be on the Tx tab.

Locate and highlight the finding of Serum Creatinine (as shown in Figure 8-43).

Click Graph on the Menu bar, and then click "Current Finding" from the drop-down list. The Medcin Graph window will be invoked.

▶ **Figure 8-44 Graph of Guy Daniel's serum creatinine.**

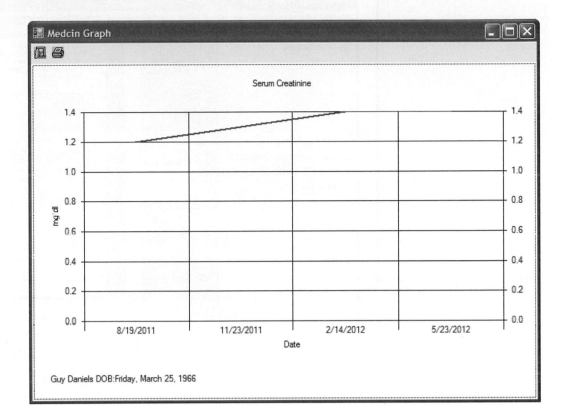

Step 5

The software will find and graph Mr. Daniels's creatinine over the last four tests.

Compare your screen to Figure 8-44.

This example shows the increase in creatinine level. Similar graphs could have been created for any of the lab results that have numeric values for their results.

Step 6

The Graph window has two buttons in the upper left corner that are identical in appearance and purpose to the corresponding buttons on the Student Edition Toolbar. The first button is Exit, which closes the graph window. The second button is the Print button, which prints your graph.

Locate and click on the Print button (circled in Figure 8-45) in the upper left corner of the graph window to invoke the Print Data window.

In the left column of the Print Data window where you normally see a check box for Current Encounter, you will see a check box with the name of the graph. Click your mouse in the check box next to Serum Creatinine and then click on the appropriate button to either print or export a file, as directed by your instructor.

When your graph has printed successfully, click on the Exit button in the window displaying the Serum Creatinine graph.

Do not close or exit the Student Edition software until you have completed the next exercise.

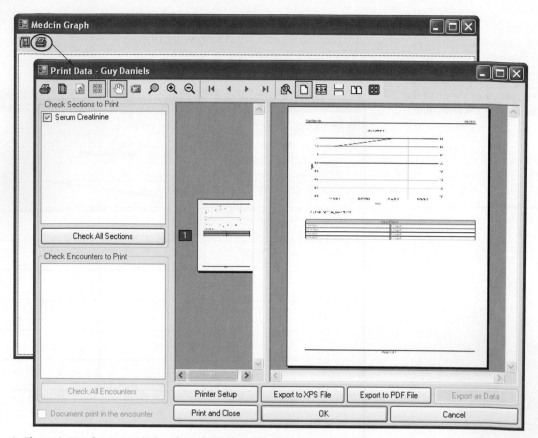

▶ **Figure 8-45 Print Data window for Graphs is invoked from Graph window Print icon.**

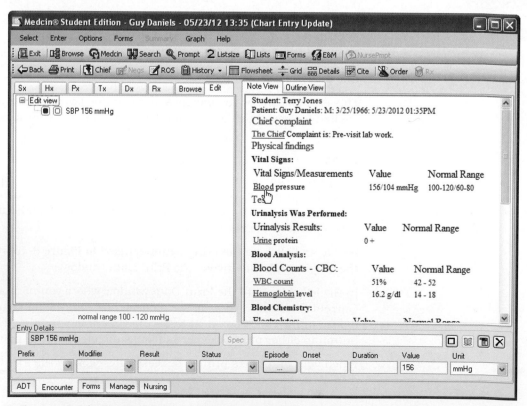

▶ **Figure 8-46 Selecting Guy Daniels's blood pressure from the encounter.**

Guided Exercise 55: Graphing Vital Signs in the Chart

As previously stated, any finding with a numeric value can be graphed. For example, vital signs are recorded at every encounter. A chart of the client's blood pressure and weight measurements could be used for client education and might stimulate the client to keep his own chart at home.

Step 7

In the right pane, the encounter note, locate and click on the vital sign **Blood Pressure** as shown in Figure 8-46.

Step 8

Click the word "Graph" on the Menu bar, and then click "Current Finding" on the list of menu options, as you did in the previous exercise.

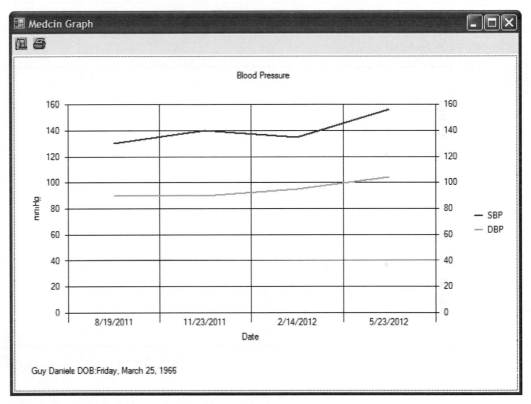

▶ **Figure 8-47 Blood pressure graph for Guy Daniels.**

Step 9

The software will find and graph Guy's blood pressure over the last four visits. Compare your screen to Figure 8-47. The blue line is his systolic blood pressure readings and the green line is his diastolic readings, as noted in the graph legend, SBP and DPB, respectively.

Locate and click on the Print button in the upper left corner of the graph window to invoke the Print Data window, as you did in the previous exercise.

Be certain there is a check in the box next to Blood Pressure and then click on the appropriate button to either print or export a file, as directed by your instructor.

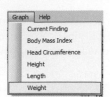

► **Figure 8-48**
Select Weight from the Graph menu.

When your graph has printed successfully, click on the Exit button in the window displaying the graph.

Step 10

For some vital signs it is not necessary to locate the finding to generate a graph. Several popular measurements are always available for graphing. In this example, the nurse wants to print a graph of the client's weight to use for weight counseling.

Click the word "Graph" on the Menu bar, and then click "Weight" on the list of menu options (as shown in Figure 8-48).

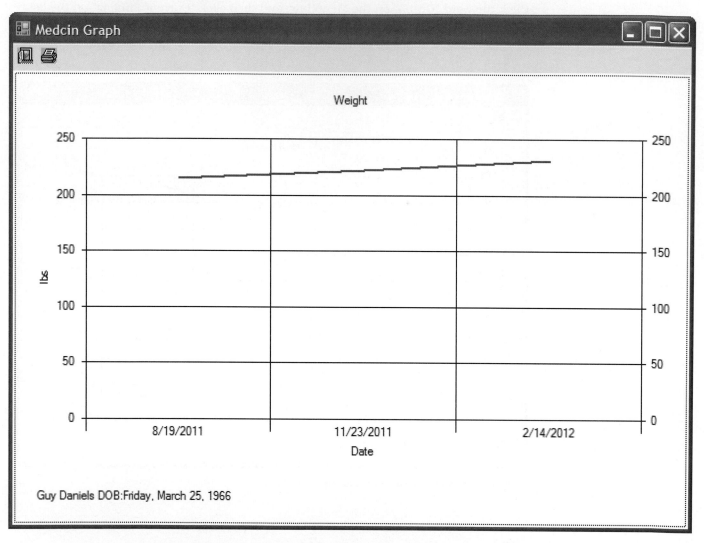

► **Figure 8-49 Graph of change in Guy Daniels's weight.**

Step 11

Compare your screen to Figure 8-49.

A graph of the client's weight measurements from previous visits is instantly displayed. You do not have to select a finding or even load an existing encounter. The graph menu allows the clinician to instantly create graphs of several key measurements without having to locate a specific finding.

Step 12

Locate and click on the Print button in the upper left corner of the graph window to invoke the Print Data window.

Locate the check box for Weight in the left column and click on it.

Locate and click on the appropriate button to either print or export a file, as directed by your instructor. When your graph has printed successfully, click on the Exit button in the window displaying the Weight graph. Give your graphs to your instructor.

Visual Aides to Engage Clients in Their Own Healthcare

Clients must become involved in their own healthcare to effectively manage and prevent diseases. A chart of the client's weight measurements and graphs of key indicators such as cholesterol and blood glucose levels can be effective visual aides for client education and may help to stimulate compliance with health regimens.

Critical Thinking Exercise 56: Graphing Total Cholesterol and Weight

Case Study

The clinic has been helping Sally Sutherland monitor her cholesterol by testing her at each annual exam. In this exercise, you are going to create a graph of Sally's total cholesterol and her weight. You will not enter any new data, but consider how these tools could aid the nurse to educate Sally about reducing her health risks.

Step 1

If you are continuing from the previous exercise, proceed to select the patient; otherwise start the Student Edition software.

Click Select on the Menu bar, and then click Patient.

In the Patient Selection window, locate and click on **Sally Sutherland**.

You do not have to set the date or time.

Step 2

Click the word "Graph" on the Menu bar, and then click "Weight" on the list of menu options.

Step 3

Locate and click on the Print button in the upper left corner of the graph window to invoke the Print Data window.

Locate the check box for Weight in the left column and click on it.

Locate and click on the appropriate button to either print or export a file, as directed by your instructor. When your graph has printed successfully, click on the Exit button in the window displaying the Weight graph.

Click on the Exit button in the window displaying the weight graph.

Step 4

Locate and click the button labeled "Search" on the Toolbar to invoke the Search String window. Type the words "**Total Cholesterol**" in the Search String window and click on the Search button.

Step 5

Verify you are on the Tx tab.

Locate and highlight the finding of Total Cholesterol.

Click Graph on the Menu bar, and then click "Current Finding" from the drop-down list.

The Graph window will be invoked, displaying a graph of Sally's Total Cholesterol test results over the last four years.

Step 6

Locate and click on the Print button in the upper left corner of the graph window to invoke the Print Data window.

Locate the check box for Total Cholesterol in the left column and click on it.

Locate and click on the appropriate button to either print or export a file, as directed by your instructor. When your graph has printed successfully, click on the Exit button in the window displaying the Total Cholesterol graph. Give your graphs to your instructor.

Chapter Eight Summary

This chapter explored the Patient Management feature to demonstrate the way an EHR can organize information from past encounters. Patient Management has the following tabs:

Problems—Problem lists and problem-oriented views of the chart organize the data by problem and encounter date.

Problem lists provide an up-to-date list of the diagnoses and conditions that affect that particular client's care. Problem lists track both acute and chronic conditions. Problems are removed from the list or set inactive once the client is "cured" or the problem is "resolved." Problems that normally resolve themselves over a short period of time are called "Acute Self-Limiting." The status of the problem is updated at each visit.

The following are typical of the types of status assigned to active problems:

> Resolved
>
> Resolving
>
> Improving
>
> Well controlled
>
> Unchanged
>
> Inadequately controlled
>
> Mildly exacerbated
>
> Failing to change as expected
>
> Expanding
>
> Worsening
>
> Severely exacerbated

Care Plan—Provides a quick review of the plan from each previous encounter. It is organized by problem and encounter date for which the client was seen for that problem. Clicking on the encounter reveals the findings recorded in the plan for that visit.

Medications—Keeps track of what medications the client is currently taking. The Medications list is reviewed before writing new prescriptions.

Vaccines—Lists the client's immunizations that have been administered at the clinic.

Allergies—Lists food, drug, and other allergies the client may have. This information is reviewed before writing a prescription.

Past Medical/Surgical History—Lists past history items recorded in the EHR during all previous encounters.

Family History—Lists family history items recorded in the EHR during all previous encounters.

Social History—Lists social and behavioral history items recorded in the EHR during all previous encounters.

Vitals—Displays key vital signs taken on previous visits in a column format.

Clicking the mouse on the label of a column within any tab of Patient Management will sort the rows in the tab by the values in the column that was clicked.

The Patient Management feature allows information from previous encounters to be updated and cited in the current encounter.

Citing means to bring a finding from a previous encounter note into the current encounter. Tests can be ordered, reordered, or the results can be viewed. Prescriptions can be renewed or discontinued as well.

You also learned to view pending lab orders. All lab orders have a status; these include:

Pending—Sent but have no results.

Preliminary—Results provide an early indication of the test but awaiting verification.

Final—Results have been verified and are ready for review.

Corrected—A change occurred as a result of repeat verification.

The ability for a clinician to see what tests are pending helps prevent duplicate orders.

The ability to graph weight, height, and test results can provide an excellent means of clarification when counseling clients or for the clinician to observe trends in the client's condition.

Any finding with a numerical value can be graphed. Several standard graphs—for example, height and weight—can be generated without locating the specific finding, simply by selecting them from the Graph menu.

As you continue through the course, you can refer to the Guided Exercises in this chapter when you need to remember how to perform a particular task.

Task	Exercise		Page No.
How to use Patient Management	51		303
How to use problem lists and cite findings	52		309
Viewing pending orders and lab results	53		317
How to graph lab results or any current finding	54		327
How to print a graph	54	Step 6	329
How to graph weight or height	55		330

Test Your Knowledge

1. What is a Problem List?

2. What is the idea of a Problem List?

3. Name at least two reasons why clinicians use a Problem List.

4. What is a reason that a "wellness" condition would appear on a Problem List?

5. Where does the data that appears in the Manage tab come from?

6. What does it mean to cite a finding?

7. Define trending of lab values.

8. Describe how to graph a client's weight.

9. What type of lab results can be graphed?

10. What is a pending order?

11. List the steps you would take to graph a lab value.

12. What type of data is on the Care Plan tab?

13. How do you sort the data display on the Vital Signs tab?

14. How do you set a problem as inactive?

15. You should have produced two narrative documents of client encounters and five graphs. If you have not already done so, hand these in to your instructor with this test. The printed encounter notes and graphs will count as a portion of your grade.

Ask your instructor for answers to Test Your Knowledge

nursing.pearsonhighered.com

Prepare for success with animated examples, practice questions, challenge tests, and interactive assignments.

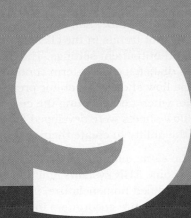

Chapter

9

Data Entry Using Flow Sheets and Anatomical Drawings

Learning Outcomes

After completing this chapter, you should be able to:

1. Describe flow sheets
2. Work with a flow sheet
3. Create a Form-based flow sheet
4. Create a Problem-based flow sheet
5. Create a flow sheet based on a nursing plan of care
6. Use an EHR drawing tool to annotate drawings in an encounter

Learning to Use Flow Sheets

Flow sheets present data from multiple encounters in column form. This format allows for a side-by-side comparison of findings over a period of time. Some nurses prefer to view a client chart this way because it is easier to spot trends in the client's health conditions. Flow sheets are used in both inpatient and outpatient settings. The flow sheet is ideal for chronic disease management such as diabetes or long-term conditions such as pregnancy. Nurses who work in OB offices use flow sheets to monitor pregnancy because it affords them a view of the previous visits when documenting the current one. Paper flow sheets have been in use long before flow sheets were developed for EHR systems. The difference is that EHR systems have the ability to create them dynamically.

Not all EHR systems implement flow sheets in the same manner, so flow sheets in your hospital or clinic may vary from these exercises. Some EHR systems limit flow sheets to lab results or vital signs. However, by using a codified nomenclature, it is possible to create clinical flow sheets that present findings from entire encounters in columns by encounter date. Additionally, there are several different ways for an EHR to create a flow sheet based on a list, a problem, a form, or nursing plan of care.

Guided Exercise 57: Working with a Flow Sheet

In previous exercises, you worked with multiple diagnoses for a single client. You also have learned that creating and using forms for specific diseases, conditions, or types of visits can speed up data entry because the form presents all of the findings likely to be needed by the clinician for a particular type of exam. This exercise will combine those two concepts and add a third concept, the flow sheet. In this exercise you will learn to use a flow sheet to document an encounter.

Clients with chronic diseases such as diabetes often develop additional chronic diseases—for example, hypertension, cardiovascular disease, macular degeneration, and a number of other diseases. Rather than try to develop complicated forms that cover different combinations of diseases, a clinic can simply develop one form for each disease. As you will see in this exercise, you can switch forms throughout the exam without reentering findings. Because the forms share the same nomenclature, a finding that is used on both forms automatically displays the entered data when either form is loaded.

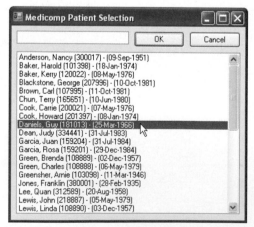

▶ **Figure 9-1 Selecting Guy Daniels from the Patient Selection window.**

Case Study

Guy Daniels is a client with hypertension and borderline diabetes who has been seen quarterly at the outpatient clinic to better manage his health. Mr. Daniels returns for a three-month checkup. Lab tests have been ordered and performed before his visit. The results were reviewed by the clinician when they arrived electronically earlier today.

Step 1

If you have not already done so, start the Student Edition software.

Click Select on the Menu bar, and then click Patient.

In the Patient Selection window, locate and click on **Guy Daniels** as shown in Figure 9-1.

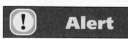

Make certain you set the date and time correctly for this exercise. If you need help, review Chapter 3, Guided Exercise 14.

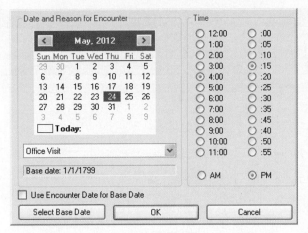

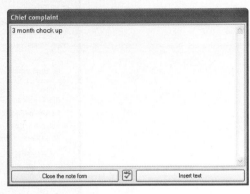

▶ **Figure 9-2 New encounter for an office visit, May 24, 2012 4:15 PM.**

▶ **Figure 9-3 Chief complaint dialog for three-month check-up.**

Step 2

Click Select on the Menu bar, and then click New Encounter.

Select the date **May 24, 2012**, the time **4:15 PM**, and the reason **Office Visit**.

Compare your screen to Figure 9-2. Make certain that the date and time match before clicking on the OK button.

Step 3

Enter the Chief complaint by locating the button in the Toolbar labeled "Chief" and clicking on it.

In the dialog window that will open, type "**3 month check up**."

Compare your screen to Figure 9-3 and then click on the button labeled "Close the note form."

Step 4

Locate and click on the Forms button in the Toolbar at the top of your screen, as you have done in previous exercises.

Select the form labeled "Hypertension" as shown in Figure 9-4.

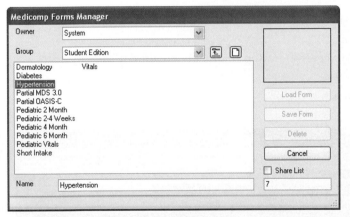

▶ **Figure 9-4 Select Hypertension Form.**

Step 5

Locate the Diagnosis of Hypertension at the top of the form.

Click the **Y** check box for Hypertension. A circle next to the finding will turn red.

To save time at the practice, the form designer has incorporated the Vital Signs fields into the first page of the form. Enter the following vital signs for Guy Daniels:

Temperature:	**98.2**
Respiration:	**20**
Pulse:	**68**
BP:	**125/85**
Weight:	**229**

Step 6

The nurse practitioner performs the Quick Screening exam.

▶ Figure 9-5 Hypertension
Form.

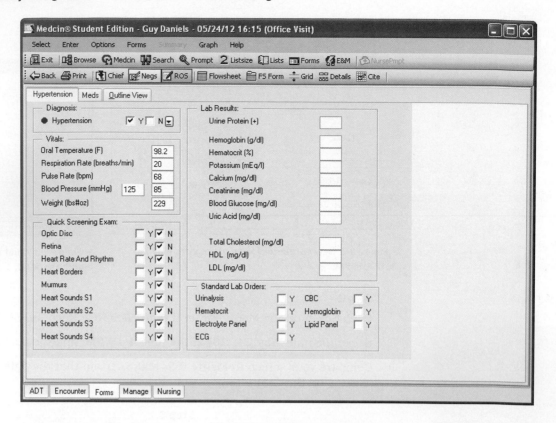

Locate and click on ROS button in the Toolbar near the top of your screen. The button should appear orange.

Locate and click the Negs (Auto Negative) button to quickly document the physical findings.

Compare your screen to Figure 9-5.

▶ Figure 9-6 Flow sheet based on Hypertension Form.

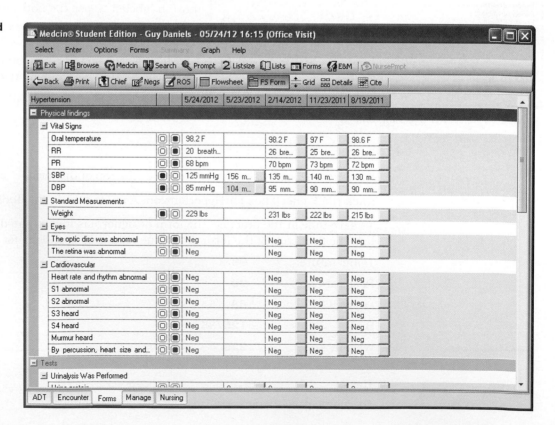

Step 7

You may have noticed previously that the Toolbar near the top of your screen has additional buttons when you are on the Forms tab. Two of the buttons are used for invoking the Flow Sheet view. One button creates a flow sheet based on a form and the other creates a flow sheet based on a problem or list. In this exercise, you will learn to create a flow sheet based on the form.

To invoke the Flow Sheet view of Guy Daniels's chart, follow these steps:

Click on the button labeled List Size until the list size is set to 1.

Locate and click on the button labeled "FS Form" in the Toolbar near the top of your screen. (The icon resembles a file folder with a grid pattern.)

The screen will change to the Flow Sheet view. The button should now be orange.

The FS Form button is used to view a flow sheet when you are in the Forms tab.

Compare your screen to Figure 9-6 as you read the following information.

About the Flow Sheet View

The Flow Sheet view resembles a spreadsheet similar to Microsoft Excel® or Lotus 1-2-3®; that is, it is made up of rows and columns of "cells." The first column displays descriptions as well as red and blue buttons for findings on the current form. The date of the current encounter is at the top of the column. The remaining columns to the right display encounter data from previous visits.

The flow sheet rows are grouped vertically into logical sections that match the sections you are accustomed to seeing in the encounter note. The title of each section is printed in blue on a teal background. For example, sections in Guy Daniels's flow sheet are titled "Physical Findings" and "Tests," "Assessment," and "Plan." A small plus or minus sign next to the section title allows you to hide or display the findings below it. Functionally, this is comparable to the ability to expand or collapse trees in the Nomenclature pane or to expand folders in the Outline view.

The list of findings in the first column and how they are displayed is determined by the way the flow sheet is invoked as follows:

FS Form—When a flow sheet is invoked from a form, the software uses the data elements on the form to populate the first column.

Problem—If the flow sheet were invoked instead from the Problem List on the Manage tab, the first column would be populated with findings pertinent to the problem selected on the Problem List.

List—A flow sheet can also be created from a list. When a list is used, the first column of the flow sheet is populated with findings in the list, findings that are within the tree view of the list, and findings of similar body systems.

Nursing Plan of Care—If the flow sheet were invoked instead from the Plan of Care on the Nursing tab, the first column would be populated with findings pertinent to the nursing diagnoses, nursing interventions, and nursing actions in the plan of care, as well as symptoms or physical findings in lists related to those nursing CCC codes.

Step 8

The columns on the right display the dates of previous visits. The cells within the column display the words POS (in red) or NEG (in blue), or a numerical value for the finding. A blank cell indicates no finding was recorded on that encounter date.

Each cell that has a finding recorded can display only one field of data. Where there is more data (for example, if entry detail fields have been used for a finding), the cell will contain a button with an ellipsis (three dots). Clicking on the ellipsis button will invoke a small window allowing you to view the additional details.

▶ **Figure 9-7 Data Details window invoked from ellipsis button for 02/14/2012 Respiration Rate.**

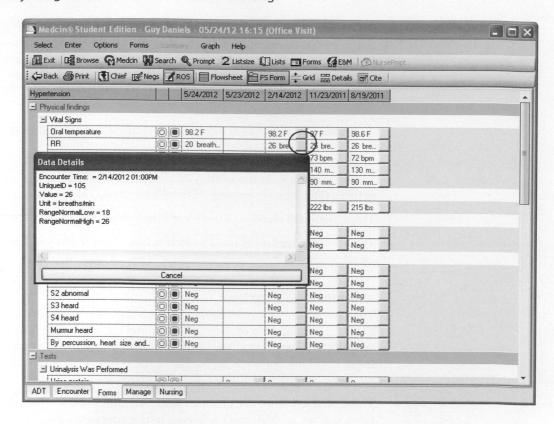

Try this yourself. Locate the row under vital signs labeled RR (respiration rate); next, locate the column dated 02/14/2012; now position your mouse on the gray ellipsis button in the cell containing the value "26 breaths." Click on the ellipsis button.

A Data Details window will be invoked, as shown in Figure 9-7. This cell has additional details showing the normal range.

▶ **Figure 9-8 Narrative window of previous encounter (02/14/2012).**

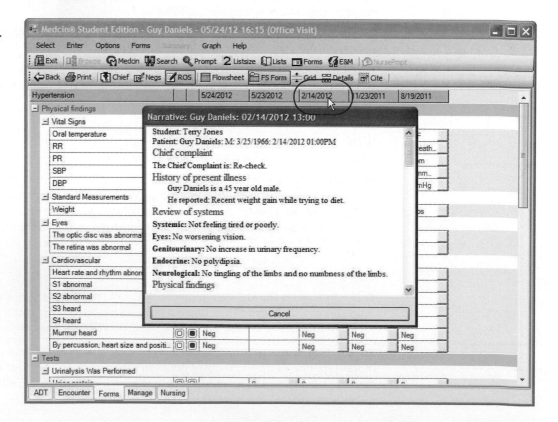

When you have finished looking at the data details, click on the button labeled "Cancel" to close the data details window.

Step 9

The full encounter note for any previous encounter can be viewed by positioning the mouse over the date at the top of any of the columns on the right and clicking the mouse on the date.

Locate and click on the column header date **02/14/2012**.

(Note that you must click on the date itself, not on the row or spaces adjoining it.)

A window displaying the full encounter note will be invoked. Compare your screen to Figure 9-8.

Click on the Cancel button to close the Narrative window for 2/14/2012.

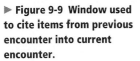

► Figure 9-9 Window used to cite items from previous encounter into current encounter.

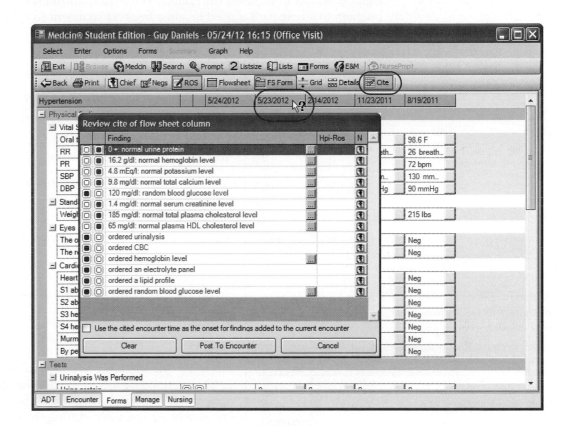

Step 10

Locate and click on the button labeled "Cite" in the Toolbar at the top of your screen. The Cite button will turn orange, as shown in Figure 9-9.

You have previously used the Cite function in Chapter 6 and Chapter 8. The Cite feature in a flow sheet does the same thing. It brings information forward from previous encounters into the current one. The information can be updated as it is brought forward, allowing you to bring the finding into the current note and edit it in one step.

Step 11

When the Cite button is on (orange), clicking on the date of a column header will invoke a different window. The "Review cite" window will list findings from that encounter instead of the encounter narrative. The Cite button changes which window is invoked. When the Cite button is on, a window of findings is invoked; when it is off, the Narrative window is invoked.

When the Cite button is on, the mouse pointer will change to resemble a large question mark whenever you move over the cells of the flow sheet. With the cite button **on**, position the mouse pointer on the column header date **05/23/2012**, as shown in Figure 9-9, and click the mouse. (Note that you must click on the date itself, not on the row or spaces adjoining it.)

A window of findings from the May 23, 2012, encounter will be invoked. Compare your screen to Figure 9-9.

The red and blue buttons for each finding are used to select the finding just as they are elsewhere in the software. The description of the finding will include any numerical values entered in the previous encounter. Two additional buttons appear on the right of each finding.

The first is the ellipsis button, which you used in step 7 to view results. However, when Cite mode is on, instead of displaying results, the ellipsis button allows you to modify any numerical data while citing the finding. The second button (whose icon resembles a red pushpin in a note pad) is used to add a free-text comment to a finding while citing it.

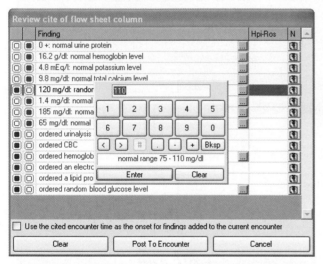

▶ **Figure 9-10 Modify numeric values of finding in Cite window with ellipsis button.**

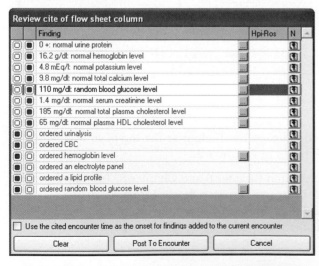

▶ **Figure 9-11 Random blood glucose level after modification.**

Step 12

A new glucose test has been performed.

In the "Review cite of flow sheet column" window, locate and highlight the finding for the "random blood glucose test" result.

Click on the ellipsis button for that finding. A small window resembling a calculator will appear.

Use your mouse to point to the numeric buttons and click on each number to update the cited test result from 120 to the current test result 110.

Click the number buttons **11** and **0**. (Note you can also type the numbers on a keyboard.)

Compare your screen to Figure 9-10, and then click on the button labeled "**Enter**." This will record your modification and close the number pad.

Step 13

From the Cite window you can also select or deselect the red or blue buttons for any of the findings listed. Although it may appear that you are editing a past encounter, you are not. You are simply selecting and editing the findings that will copy to the current encounter. Do not be concerned that this will change any of the findings in a previous encounter.

Compare your screen to Figure 9-11.

Click on the button labeled "Post To Encounter" to cite the findings.

Step 14

Individual findings can be cited without invoking the Cite Review window. When the Cite button is on, instead of positioning the mouse pointer on the date in the column header to invoke a window, you can position the mouse pointer on an individual cell of the flow sheet and click the mouse button. The data from that specific cell will be copied into the current encounter.

Scroll the flow sheet downward until you can see all the rows of the section labeled "Tests."

▶ **Figure 9-12 Cite the individual finding plasma LDL from the 02/14/2012 column.**

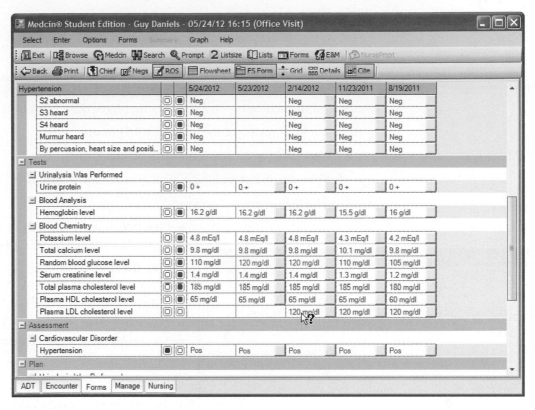

Locate the finding "Plasma LDL cholesterol" in the last row of that section.

Position your mouse pointer in that row, under the column dated 02/14/2012; click the mouse on the cell that reads "120 mg/dl," as shown in Figure 9-12.

This will cite a normal Plasma LDL in the column for the current encounter.

Locate and click on the button labeled "Cite" in the Toolbar at the top of your screen. This will turn Cite off.

▶ **Figure 9-13 Hypertension Form redisplayed with cited data.**

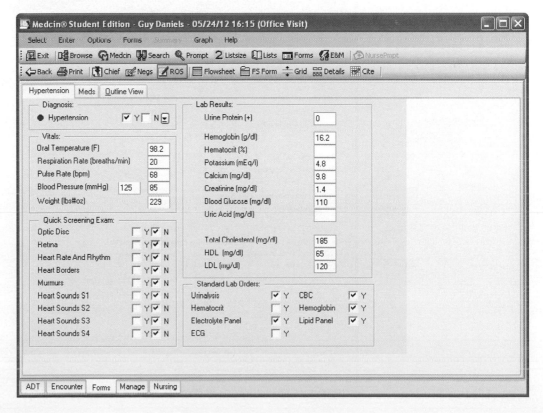

Step 15

As you learned earlier in this exercise, this FS form button acts like a toggle, shifting the screen between the Flow Sheet view and the Form view.

Locate and click on the button labeled "FS Form" in the Toolbar at the top of your screen. The form will redisplay. Compare your screen to Figure 9-13; notice the lab results in the center of the screen now have values that have been filled by using Cite.

Here is a brief review of the buttons FS Flow and Cite:

▶ **FS Flow Off** (button normal) displays the Form.

▶ **FS Flow On** (button orange) displays the Flow Sheet view.

When the flow sheet is displayed:

▶ **Cite Off** (button normal)—Clicking on a column header date invokes the narrative of that encounter.

▶ **Cite On** (button orange)—Clicking on a column header date invokes the findings from that encounter, which will be copied forward into today's encounter.

▶ **Cite On** (button orange)—Clicking on an individual cell will copy only the specific finding forward into today's encounter.

Step 16

To document the client's second problem, locate and click on the Forms button in the Toolbar at the top of your screen.

Select and load the form for diabetes (as shown in Figure 9-14).

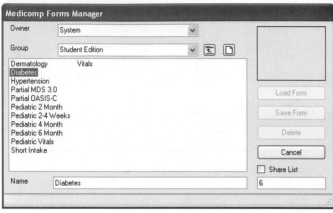

▶ **Figure 9-14 Selecting the Diabetes Form from the Form Manager window.**

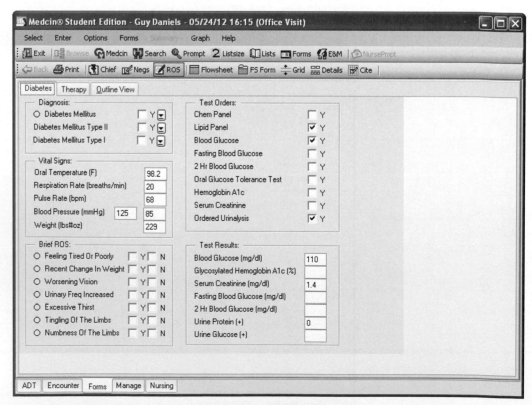

▶ **Figure 9-15 Diabetes Form shows data entered on Hypertension Form.**

Step 17

Compare your screen to Figure 9-15. Notice that vital signs and several of the fields on the diabetes form already contain data, because these findings were entered on the hypertension form. As mentioned earlier, any findings already in the current encounter will appear automatically as you change forms.

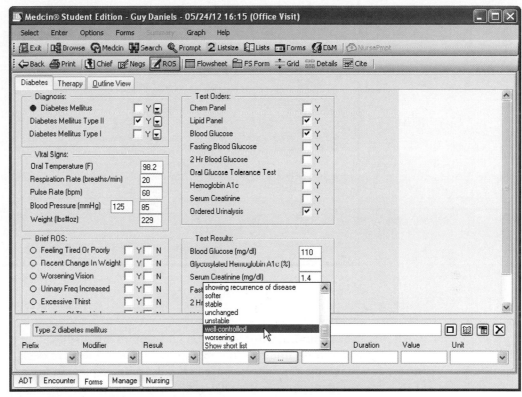

▶ **Figure 9-16 Setting the diagnosis diabetes mellitus well controlled.**

Step 18

Record the second diagnosis.

Locate the diagnosis Diabetes Mellitus Type II at the top of the form. Click on the check box next to the **Y**. A circle next to the finding will turn red.

Locate and click on the button labeled "Details" in the Toolbar at the top of your screen. This will open the Entry Details section over the bottom of the form.

In previous exercises, you have used the Details button to hide the details entry fields. In this step, we will display the fields so the status of the disease can be updated.

Locate the status field in the Entry Details section and click on the down arrow button in the field. Select the status "well controlled" from the drop-down list, as shown in Figure 9-16.

Click on the button labeled "Details" in the Toolbar at the top of your screen again, to hide the Entry Details section and to restore the full view of the form.

Step 19

Verify that the ROS button is still on, and then click on the button labeled "Negs" (Auto Negative) in the Toolbar near the top of your screen.

▶ **Figure 9-17 ROS Findings recorded with Auto Negative.**

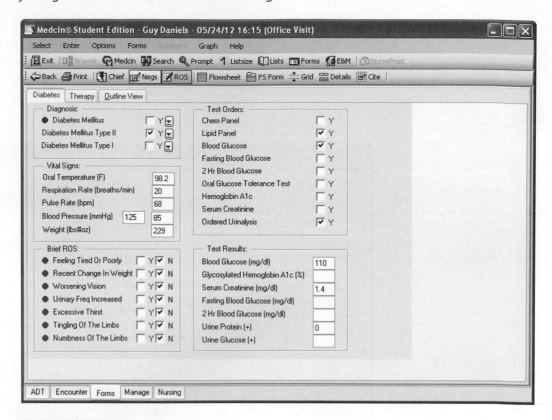

Compare your screen to Figure 9-17.

Step 20

Not all findings from previous encounters are displayed in a form-based flow sheet. Only those findings that match the items in the form design are listed in the columns. Similarly, flow sheets based on a list only display findings that match the list. This step will demonstrate the difference a form design makes in a flow sheet.

▶ **Figure 9-18 Flow Sheet view based on Diabetic Form.**

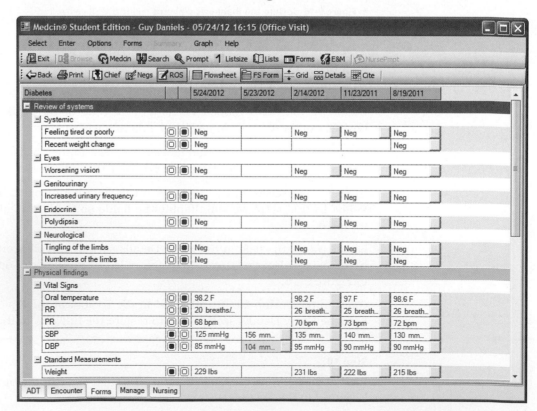

Verify that the List Size is still set to **1**; if it is not, then locate and click on the List Size button until it is **1**.

Locate and click on the button labeled "FS Form" in the Toolbar at the top of your screen. The diabetes flow sheet will be displayed. Your screen should resemble Figure 9-18.

Turn back in your book and compare your screen with the earlier flow sheet shown in Figure 9-6. Notice that the diabetes flow sheet has a review of system section, which the hypertension does not. There also are differences in the tests ordered for the two diseases. From this comparison, you can easily see how the flow sheets for diabetes and hypertension differ.

▶ **Figure 9-19 Cite of Therapy tab items.**

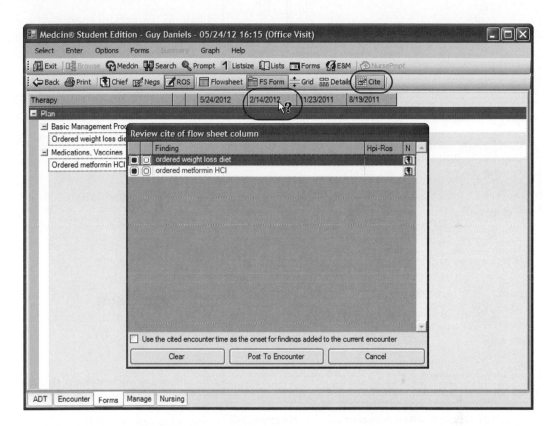

Step 21

Locate and click on the button labeled "FS Form" in the Toolbar at the top of your screen. The diabetes form will be redisplayed. Locate and click on the tab at the top of the diabetes form labeled "Therapy."

Locate and click on the button labeled "FS Form" in the Toolbar at the top of your screen. The flow sheet of the diabetes plan will be displayed.

Locate and click the Cite button on as you did early in this chapter (the button will appear orange).

Locate and click on the column header date **02/14/2012**.

A small window of findings from that encounter will appear. Compare your screen to the review cite findings window in Figure 9-19. Notice that because these findings do not have numerical values, the gray ellipsis button is not present.

There also are fewer findings to cite. This is partly because of the items on the form, but also because the Cite feature is intelligent. It omits findings already recorded in the current encounter during previous steps of the exercise.

After you have looked at the findings that are displayed, click the button labeled "Post To Encounter" to cite the findings.

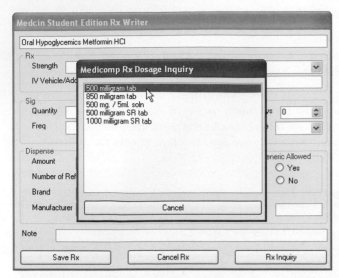

▶ **Figure 9-20 Select 500 mg Metformin HCl.**

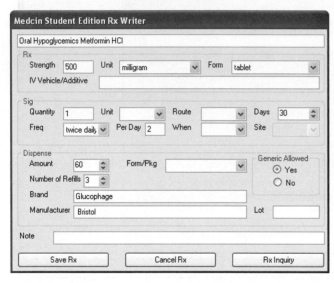

▶ **Figure 9-21 Writing Guy Daniels's prescription for Metformin HCl.**

Because one of the items in the list is a prescription, the prescription writer window will be invoked automatically.

Step 22

The prescription is for Metformin HCl. The prescription writer will display the Rx Dosage Inquiry window, as shown in Figure 9-20.

Locate and click on the Rx dosage **500 mg tab**; the window will next display a list of manufacturers.

Click on the default manufacturer when that window is displayed. (A figure of that window has been omitted.)

Step 23

Using what you have learned in Chapter 7, enter the following prescription information in the appropriate fields:

Sig

> Quantity: **1**
>
> Freq: **Twice daily**
>
> Per Day: **2**
>
> Days: **30**

Dispense

> Amount: **60**
>
> Refill: **3**

Generic

> Locate and click on the circle next to **Yes**.

Compare your screen to Figure 9-21. When everything is correct, click on the button labeled "Save Rx."

Step 24

Locate and click on the button labeled "Cite" in the Toolbar at the top of your screen to turn Cite off.

Locate and click on the button labeled "FS Form" in the Toolbar at the top of your screen to return to the view of the form. If the form is not on the Therapy tab, locate and click on the tab labeled "Therapy" (at the top of the form).

Locate the section labeled "Dietary Orders" in the upper right corner of the form. Note that Weight Loss should already have a check next to the Y. This box was checked by citing the findings in step 21.

Click the check box next to **Y** for the following findings:

✓ **Y** Diabetic (diet)

✓ **Y** Controlled Carbohydrate

Compare your screen to Figure 9-22.

Locate and click on the Encounter tab at the bottom of your screen.

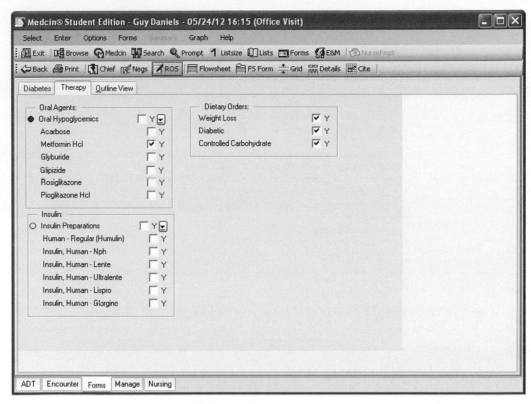

▶ **Figure 9-22 Diabetic Form—enter dietary orders.**

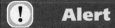 **Alert**

> *Do not close or exit the encounter until you have a printed copy in your hand.* **You will lose your work if you exit before printing.**

Step 25

Click on the Print button on the Toolbar at the top of your screen to invoke the Print Data window.

Be certain there is a check mark in the box next to "Current Encounter" and then click on the appropriate button to either print or export a file, as directed by your instructor.

Compare your printout or file output to Figure 9-23. If it is correct, hand it in to your instructor. If there are any differences, review the previous steps in the exercise and find your error.

> **You may stop at this point or, if time permits, you may continue with the next exercise without exiting.**

Guy Daniels   Page 1 of 1

Student: *your name or id here*
Patient: Guy Daniels: M: 3/25/1966: 5/24/2012 04:15PM
Chief complaint
The Chief Complaint is: 3 month check up.
Review of systems
Systemic: Not feeling tired or poorly and no recent weight change.
Eyes: No worsening vision.
Genitourinary: No increase in urinary frequency.
Endocrine: No polydipsia.
Neurological: No tingling of the limbs and no numbness of the limbs.
Physical findings
Vital Signs:

Vital Signs/Measurements	Value	Normal Range
Oral temperature	98.2 F	97.6 - 99.6
RR	20 breaths/min	18 - 26
PR	68 bpm	50 - 100
Blood pressure	125/85 mmHg	100 - 120/60 - 80
Weight	229 lbs	125 - 225

Eyes:
    General/bilateral:
    Optic Disc: ° Normal.
    Retina: ° Normal.
Cardiovascular:
    Heart Rate And Rhythm: ° Normal.
    Heart Sounds: ° S1 normal. ° S2 normal. ° No S3 heard. ° No S4 heard.
    Murmurs: ° No murmurs were heard.
    Heart Borders: ° By percussion, heart size and position were normal.
Tests
Urinalysis Was Performed:

Urinalysis Results:	Value	Normal Range
Urine protein	0 +	

Blood Analysis:

Blood Counts - CBC:	Value	Normal Range
Hemoglobin level	16.2 g/dl	14 - 18

Blood Chemistry:

Electrolytes:	Value	Normal Range
Potassium level	4.8 mEq/l	3.5 - 5.5
Total calcium level	9.8 mg/dl	8.5 - 10.5
Endocrine Laboratory Tests:	Value	Normal Range
Random blood glucose level	110 mg/dl	75 - 110
Metabolic Tests:	Value	Normal Range
Serum creatinine level	1.4 mg/dl	0.7 - 1.5
Total plasma cholesterol level	185 mg/dl	140 - 200
Plasma HDL cholesterol level	65 mg/dl	30 - 70
Plasma LDL cholesterol level	120 mg/dl	80 - 130

Assessment
    • Hypertension
    • Type 2 diabetes mellitus which is well-controlled
Plan
    • Urinalysis
    • CBC
    • Hemoglobin level
    • An electrolyte panel
    • A lipid profile
    • Random blood glucose level
    • Weight loss diet
    • Diabetic diet
    • Controlled carbohydrate diet
    • Metformin HCl
500 mg tab (1 bid 30) DISP:60 Refill:3 Generic:Y Using:Glucophage Mfg: Bristol

▶ **Figure 9-23 Printed encounter note for Guy Daniels.**

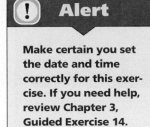

Alert

Make certain you set the date and time correctly for this exercise. If you need help, review Chapter 3, Guided Exercise 14.

Guided Exercise 58: Creating a Problem-Oriented Flow Sheet

In this exercise, you are going to view a flow sheet that is focused on a particular problem, rather than a form.

Step 1

If you are continuing from the previous exercise, proceed to step 3.

Otherwise, start the Student Edition software.

Click Select on the Menu bar, and then click Patient.

In the Patient Selection window, locate and click on **Guy Daniels**.

Step 2

Click Select on the Menu bar, and then click New Encounter.

Select the date **May 24, 2012**, the time **4:15 PM**, and the reason **Office Visit**.

Make certain you set the date, time, and reason correctly. If necessary, refer to Figure 9-2.

▶ **Figure 9-24 Problem List for Guy Daniels.**

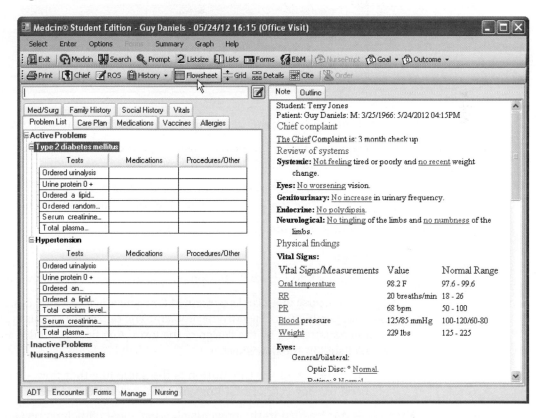

Step 3

Locate and click on the Manage tab at the bottom of your screen.

If the left pane of your screen is not currently displaying the Problem List, click on the tab labeled "Problem List."

(Note that the right pane of Figure 9-24 is showing the encounter note as if you were continuing from the previous exercise. If you are not, the right pane will contain less information; that is acceptable for this exercise.)

Step 4

Verify that the button labeled "List Size" in the Toolbar at the top of your screen is **1**. If it is not, click on it until the list size is 1.

▶ **Figure 9-25 Flow sheet from Problem List for Guy Daniels.**

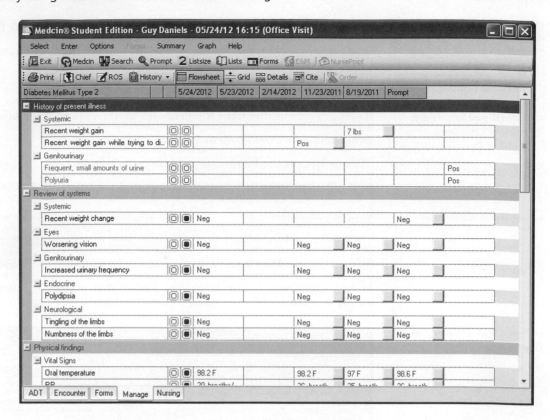

Locate and click the Details button on the Toolbar to hide the Details section.

Locate and click on the diagnosis **Type 2 diabetes mellitus** in the Problem List (left pane). This will highlight the diagnosis as shown in Figure 9-24.

Locate and click on the button labeled "Flowsheet" in the Toolbar at the top of your screen. (Note that this is not the FS Form button that you used in the previous exercise.)

A flow sheet similar to that in Figure 9-25 will be displayed.

Step 5

Turn back to Figure 9-18. Compare your screen to the flow sheet in that figure.

The purpose of a problem-oriented flow sheet is to provide a historical view of the client's data pertinent to the current problem. The difference in this type of flow sheet is that it is not constrained by the design of the form. Any finding related to the selected problem will be listed in the flow sheet.

The function of the Cite button is the same in either flow sheet. That is, Cite can be used to copy relevant findings into the current encounter.

As you learned in the previous chapter, most clinicians use a Problem List at some point during the examination. The ability to quickly view and cite from a flow sheet specific to the problem not only can speed up the documentation process but also can ensure that the clinician recalls significant findings from previous visits.

Step 6

Locate and click the Details button on the Toolbar to restore the Details Entry section.

Locate the following finding in the flow sheet and click on the red button in the column dated **05/24/2012**.

● (red button) recent weight change

Locate the Value field in the Entry Details section and type **-2 lbs**. Press the enter key on your keyboard.

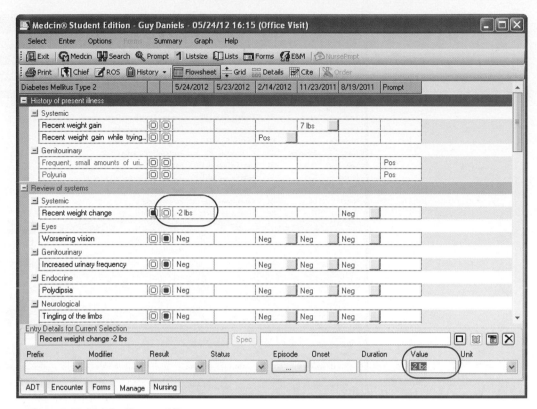

► Figure 9-26 Weight Change -2 lbs.

Compare your screen to Figure 9-26.

Step 7

Ask your instructor if you should print another copy of Guy Daniels's encounter note. If so instructed, follow the directions in step 25 of the previous exercise. Note that if you did not continue from the previous exercise, your print out will contain less data. This is acceptable for the purposes of this exercise.

Guided Exercise 59: Creating a Flow Sheet from a Nursing Care Plan

Flow sheets can also be created based on the nursing care plan. In this view the nurse can not only see what actions have been performed on previous shifts, but also easily cite those that he or she performs during the current encounter. In this exercise you will learn to generate a flow sheet based on the nursing care plan and record nursing actions using the Flow Sheet view.

Case Study

Judy Dean is a 29-year-old female who was recently injured when her motorcycle fell on her, fracturing her right hip. She was admitted for surgical repair of the fracture right femoral head with posterior dislocation. She has no significant prior medical or surgical history and this is her first hospitalization. She has no known allergies and was not taking any medications at home. She is in her third day of postoperative care. She has been placed on postoperative advancing activity protocol with physical therapy using appropriate assistive devices and advancing from walker to crutches today. You will document her care in this encounter using a flow sheet created from an interactive nursing plan of care.

Step 1

If you have not already done so, start the Student Edition software.

Click on the ADT tab at the bottom of your screen.

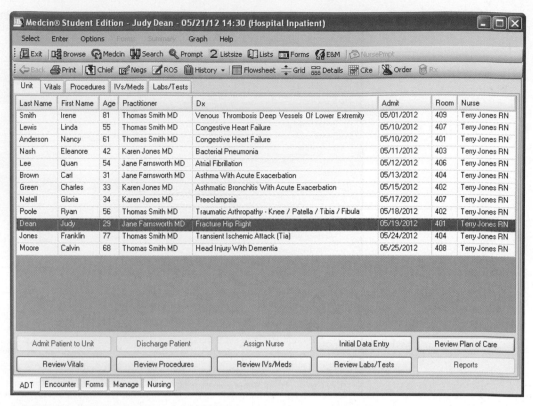

▶ **Figure 9-27 Select Judy Dean on the ADT tab.**

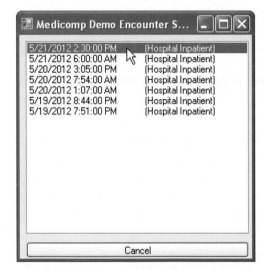

▶ **Figure 9-28 Select Existing encounter May 21, 2012, 2:30 PM.**

In the ADT window, locate and click on **Judy Dean** as shown in Figure 9-27.

Locate and click on the button labeled "Review Plan of Care."

Step 2

Click Select on the Menu bar at the top of your screen and then click Existing Encounter.

Locate and click on the encounter dated **May 21, 2012**, the time **2:30 PM**, as shown in Figure 9-28.

Step 3

Scroll the left pane downward to locate the heading "**Current and Active Nursing Diagnosis**," and then click the **right-click** button on the mouse.

Locate and select "**Flow Sheet Active**" from the drop-down menu as shown in Figure 9-29. A flow sheet similar to Figure 9-30 should be displayed.

Step 4

If the Entry Details fields are currently displayed at the bottom of the flow sheet, you can locate and click on the button labeled "Details" in the Toolbar at the top of your screen. This will hide the Entry Details section and allow you to see more rows of the flow sheet.

Take a moment to study the flow sheet. The left column lists the nurse actions related to the nursing diagnosis and nursing interventions in the plan of care as well as symptoms and physical findings related to the nursing intervention CCC code. The column next to it, dated 5/21/2012, is your current encounter, into which you will record data. The remaining columns to the right of it contain the findings

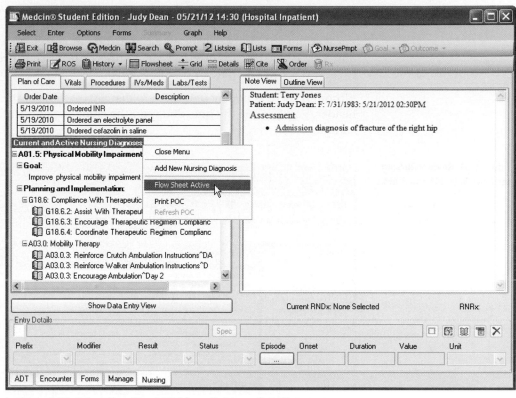

► Figure 9-29 Select Flow Sheet POC from the drop-down list.

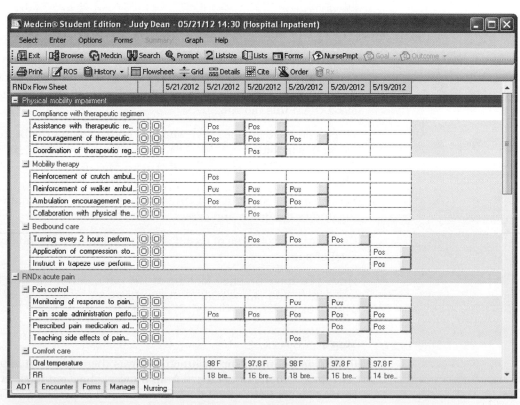

► Figure 9-30 Flow sheet created from Active Nursing Diagnosis.

recorded by nurses on previous shifts. In this type of flow sheet, not all encounters are displayed only those containing nursing assessments, interventions, or actions. For example, there is a prior encounter note in the client's chart from the surgeon dated 5/19/2012 containing clinical orders. Because it precedes the nursing plan of care, it does not display in this flow sheet view.

Although there is not enough room to display the time of the encounter in the column header, you can see the time and read the complete encounter note by clicking on the column date.

▶ **Figure 9-31 Review nursing notes from 5/21/2012 6:00 AM.**

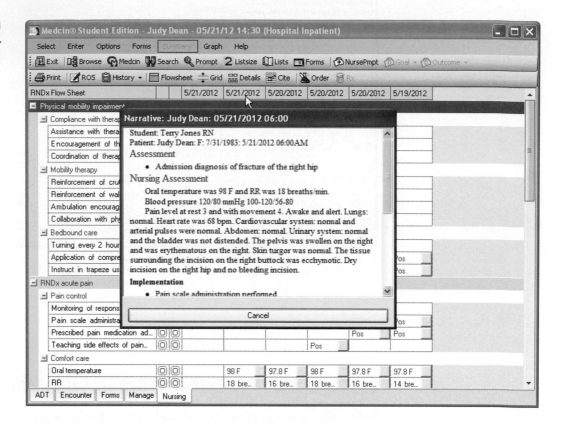

Locate and click on the date 5/21/2012 in the third column from the left. A small window will open as shown in Figure 9-31. This is the nursing notes from the nurse on shift at 6:00 AM this morning.

When you have finished reviewing the note, click on the button labeled "Cancel" to close the note window.

Step 5

Scroll the flow sheet downward so you can compare the data from each shift, concerning Judy's condition and care.

Compare the columns of recent shifts to evaluate the stability of her vitals and reported level of pain.

Once you have finished looking at the data, scroll the flow sheet upward or downward until you can see all of the findings for vital signs on your screen as shown in Figure 9-32.

Step 6

Judy was up in a chair for lunch and was then transported to the physical therapy department. When she returned from therapy she went back to bed, where she has been resting since. She reports fatigue from the therapy and a current pain rating of 5. You will now record her vital signs using the flow sheet.

► **Figure 9-32 Vital signs data entered into the nursing flow sheet.**

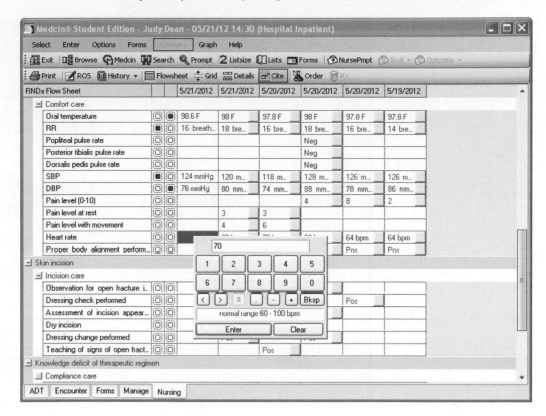

Locate and click on the Cite button in the Toolbar at the top of your screen. It will turn orange, as shown in Figure 9-32.

Locate the blank column dated 5/21/2012, immediately to the right of the finding descriptions. Although there is a second column of the same date, it already contains data; that is the data from the morning shift.

When you double-click your mouse in the empty cell of a vital sign, a pop-up window will appear, such as the one shown for heart rate in Figure 9-32. For each of the vital signs listed below, double-click your left mouse button in the empty cell, type the value indicated into the pop-up window, and then click the button labeled "Enter" or press the Enter key on your keyboard.

Temperature:	**98.6**
Respiration:	**16**
Blood Pressure	
SBP:	**124**
DBP:	**76**
Heart Rate:	**70**

Compare you screen to the flow sheet shown in Figure 9-32.

Step 7

Only the vital signs findings will automatically invoke the pop-up entry window. If you need to record a value, free text, or other field, you can do so by using the Details button to redisplay the Entry Details fields.

In this case, Judy reports that she is in pain. After administering the pain scale, record the value.

Locate and click on the Details button in the Toolbar at the top of your screen.

Locate and click the empty cell in the 5/21/2012 column for the finding "Pain Level at rest." Locate the Entry Details field labeled "Value," type the numeral "**5**" in the field, and then press the Enter key.

▶ Figure 9-33 Enter pain level 5 in the Entry Details value field.

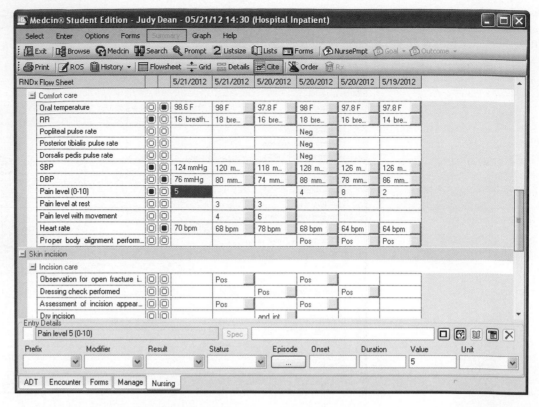

Compare your screen to Figure 9-33.

Step 8

Any field in the Entry Details section can be used to add data to a finding in the flow sheet view.

You have checked Judy's surgical dressing, which is dry and intact, and observed her incision is healing well.

▶ Figure 9-34 Adding Status "improving" to a finding in the flow sheet.

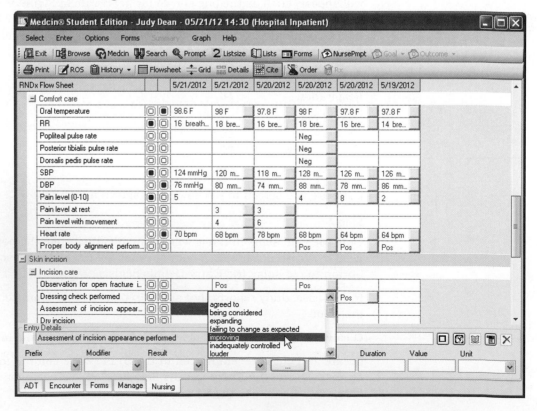

Locate and click your mouse in the empty cell for the finding "Assessment of incision appearance" (under Incision Care).

Locate and click on the down arrow in the Entry Details field "Status." Click on "Improving" in the drop-down list as shown in Figure 9-34.

The finding will be recorded in the encounter with the status. In the Flow Sheet view you will not see the text of the status in the cell, but you should verify that the red button for the finding has been selected. You will see the status text in the encounter note, in step 14.

▶ **Figure 9-35 Cited findings "Dressing check performed" and "Dry incision."**

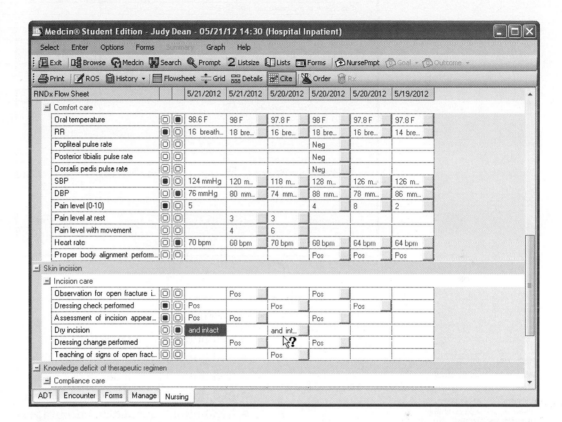

Step 9

As you have experienced with other types of flow sheets, the Cite function can also be used to cite findings from previous encounters into the current encounter. If the findings have Entry Details associated with them, that data is cited as well.

Because we will not need the Entry Details section for this step, hide it so that you can see more rows of the flow sheet. Locate and click the Details button on the Toolbar at the top of your screen.

Locate the finding "Dressing check performed" and click on the cell in the column dated 5/20/2012 on the text "POS."

Locate the finding "Dry incision" and click on the cell in the column dated 5/20/2012 on the text "and intact" as shown in Figure 9-35.

Compare your screen to Figure 9-35.

In one step, not only has the finding been recorded, but the free text as well.

Step 10

Cite is not the only method to record data in a flow sheet. Findings can also be recorded by simply clicking the red or blue buttons as you would in the encounter view.

Locate and click the Cite button in the Toolbar at the top of your screen. Verify that the button is no longer orange; Cite is off.

▶ **Figure 9-36 Charting additional nursing action findings into the flow sheet.**

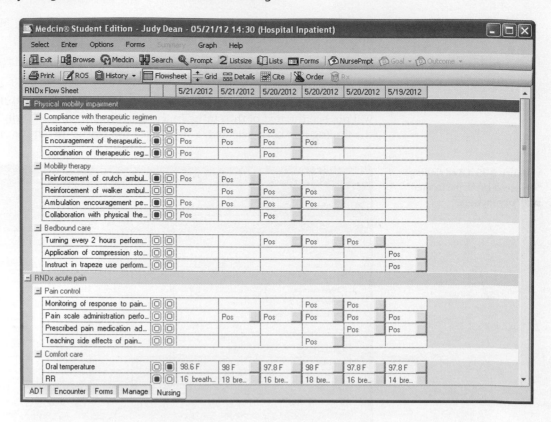

Scroll to the top of the flow sheet to locate and click the red buttons next to the descriptions of the following findings:

- (red button) Assistance with therapeutic regimen
- (red button) Encouragement of therapeutic regimen
- (red button) Coordination of therapeutic regimen
- (red button) Reinforce crutch ambulation instructions
- (red button) Ambulation encouragement performed
- (red button) Collaboration with physical therapist

Compare your screen to the flow sheet shown in Figure 9-36.

Step 11

Thus far we have been using the flow sheet for the full plan of care; however, it is also possible to flow sheet an individual nursing diagnosis or even a nursing intervention.

Return to the Plan of Care view by locating and clicking the button labeled "Flowsheet" in the Toolbar at the top of your screen. It is highlighted orange in Figure 9-36. The plan of care should still be displayed in your left pane.

You will recall that Judy's pain level increased following her therapy session.

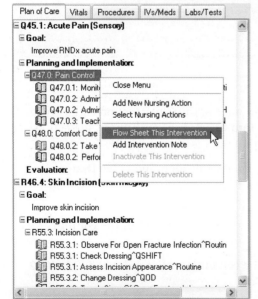

▶ **Figure 9-37 Select Flow Sheet This Intervention for Pain Control.**

Scroll the left pane to locate the nursing intervention "Pain Control." Right click on the intervention and then click on "**Flow sheet this intervention**" in the drop-down menu as shown in Figure 9-37.

The flow sheet shown in Figure 9-38 will be displayed. Notice that it has only the findings for this intervention.

Step 12

Locate and click on the Cite button on the Toolbar at the top of your screen. Verify it has turned orange, as shown in Figure 9-38.

▶ **Figure 9-38 Citing nurse actions using the flow sheet based on an intervention.**

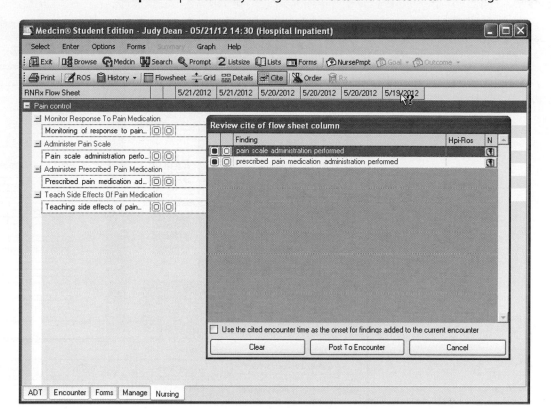

With the Cite button on, the mouse pointer will change to resemble a large question mark. Position the mouse pointer on the header of the rightmost column, dated **05/19/2012**, as shown in Figure 9-38, and click the mouse. (Remember, you must click on the date itself, not on the row or spaces adjoining it.)

A window of pain control interventions recorded in the May 19, 2012 encounter will be invoked. Compare your window to the "Review cite of flow sheet column" window shown in Figure 9-38.

If your window matches the figure, click the button labeled "Post to Encounter." If your window does not match the figure, click the Cancel button and then re-click on the correct column.

Locate and click the Cite button on the Toolbar at the top of your screen to turn Cite mode **off**.

Step 13

In the previous step you learned to flow sheet an intervention and to Cite a column of data. In the next step you will learn how to print a flow sheet. However, we will want to print the full Plan of Care flow sheet. Therefore we will need to redisplay the full sheet. To do this, locate and click the button labeled "Flowsheet" in the Toolbar at the top of your screen. The Plan of Care should display in your left pane.

Scroll the Plan of Care upward to locate the heading "Current and Active Nursing Diagnoses," as you did in step 3.

Locate and select "**Flow Sheet Active**" from the drop-down menu. If you need assistance, refer to Figure 9-29.

Step 14

When the full Plan of Care flow sheet is redisplayed, click on the Print button on the Toolbar at the top of your screen to invoke the Print Data window.

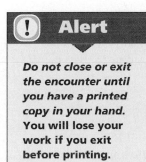

(!) Alert

Do not close or exit the encounter until you have a printed copy in your hand. You will lose your work if you exit before printing.

▶ **Figure 9-39 Print Data window with Current Encounter and RNDx Flow Sheet selected.**

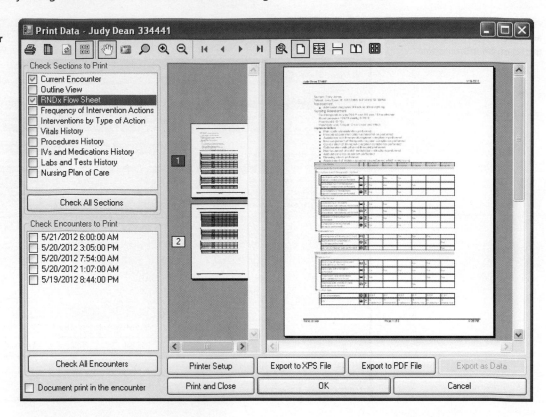

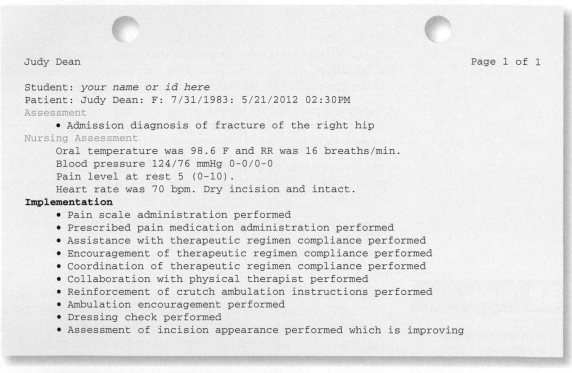

▶ **Figure 9-40a Printed encounter note for Judy Dean.**

Be certain there are check marks in the boxes next to both "Current Encounter" *and* "RNDx Flow Sheet," as shown in Figure 9-39, and then click on the appropriate button to either print or export a file, as directed by your instructor.

Compare your printout or file output to Figure 9-40a and Figure 9-40b. The paging will be different from the textbook figures. If there are any differences, other than pagination, review the previous steps in the exercise and find your error. When it is correct, hand it in to your instructor.

Compliance with therapeutic regimen

Assistance with therapeutic regimen compliance performed	■ ☐	Pos	Pos	Pos			
Encouragement of therapeutic regimen compliance performed	■ ☐	Pos	Pos	Pos	Pos		
Coordination of therapeutic regimen compliance performed	■ ☐	Pos		Pos			

Mobility therapy

Reinforcement of crutch ambulation instructions performed	■ ☐	Pos	Pos				
Reinforcement of walker ambulation instructions performed	☐ ☐		Pos	Pos	Pos		
Abulation encouragement performed	■ ☐	Pos	Pos	Pos	Pos		
Collaboration with physical therapist performed	■ ☐	Pos		Pos			

Bedbound care

Turning every 2 hours performed	☐ ☐			Pos	Pos	Pos	
Application of compression stockings performed	☐ ☐						Pos
Instruct in trapeze use performed	☐ ☐						Pos

RNDx acute pain

Pain control

Monitoring of response to pain medication performed	☐ ☐				Pos	Pos	
Pain scale administration performed	■ ☐	Pos	Pos	Pos	Pos	Pos	Pos
Prescribed pain medication administration performed	■ ☐	Pos				Pos	Pos
Teaching side effects of pain medication performed	☐ ☐				Pos		

Comfort care

Oral temperature	☐ ■	98.6 F	98 F	97.8 F	98 F	97.8 F	97.8 F
RR	■ ☐	16 breaths/min	18 breaths/min	16 breaths/min	18 breaths/min	16 breaths/min	14 breaths/min
Popliteal pulse rate	☐ ☐				Neg		
Posterior tibialis pulse rate	☐ ☐				Neg		
Dorsalis pedis pulse rate	☐ ☐				Neg		
SBP	■ ☐	124 mmHg	120 mmHg	118 mmHg	128 mmHg	126 mmHg	126 mmHg
DBP	☐ ■	76 mmHg	80 mmHg	74 mmHg	88 mmHg	78 mmHg	86 mmHg
Pain level 0-10	☐ ☐				4	8	2
Pain level at rest	■ ☐	5	3	3			
Pain level with movement	☐ ☐		4	6			
Heart rate	☐ ■	70 bpm	68 bpm	78 bpm	68 bpm	64 bpm	64 bpm
Proper body alignment performed	☐ ☐				Pos	Pos	Pos

Skin incision

Incision care

Observation for open fracture infection performed	☐ ☐		Pos		Pos		
Dressing check performed	■ ☐	Pos		Pos		Pos	
Assessment of incision appearance performed	■ ☐	Pos	Pos		Pos		

▶ **Figure 9-40b Printed flow sheet based on plan of care for Judy Dean (page 1 of 2).**

RNDx Flow Sheet			5/21/2012 02:30PM	5/21/2012 06:00AM	5/20/2012 03:05PM	5/20/2012 07:54AM	5/20/2012 01:07AM	5/19/2012 08:44PM
Dry incision	▣	☐	and intact		and intact			
Dressing change performed	☐	☐		Pos		Pos		
Teaching of signs of open fracture wound infection performed	☐	☐			Pos			
Knowledge deficit of therapeutic regimen								
Compliance care								
Assessment of compliance with therapeutic regimen performed	☐	☐		Pos	Pos			
Teaching of compliance care techniques performed	☐	☐			Pos	Pos		
Teaching of methods to compensate for limitations performed	☐	☐			Pos	Pos		
Compliance with safety precaution								
Fall risk assessment performed	☐	☐			Pos	Pos		Pos
Education about safety precautions performed	☐	☐				Pos		Pos

▶ **Figure 9-40b Printed flow sheet based on plan of care for Judy Dean (page 2 of 2).**

Real-Life Story

Nurse Who Uses Flow Sheets and Trending

By Kourtnie Sitarz, RN

Kourtnie Sitarz is a registered nurse working in a community health system in the Midwest. Kourtnie worked as a staff nurse on a pulmonary medical unit before joining the informatics department.

I began my career in healthcare when I was only 18 as a pharmacy technician in a small retail pharmacy. I had just started taking general education classes at the nearby community college, but was still undecided on my major. Because I was working in a pharmacy, it was natural for me to start taking classes with a major in mind. A pharmacy technician position opened up at a local hospital, so I decided to take it, figuring it would help open my eyes to the other world of pharmacy—the clinical pharmacist.

It wasn't long before I realized I was more interested in what the nurses were doing on the units, and began dreading having to go back to my little area so far away from the nurses and clients. Luckily, the classes I had taken in preparation for a career as a pharmacist were above and beyond what I needed for the nursing program. I was accepted into the associate's degree nursing program on my first try, and never looked back. I have since gone on to pursue my bachelor's degree in nursing, and I am one class away from completion.

I have been exposed predominately to electronic documentation and medical records throughout my nursing career. I have charted on paper, but only during clinical rotations while in nursing school and the occasional downtime at my current hospital. On those rare occasions of downtime, I would hold out as long as I could to document, hoping the electronic system would become available so I wouldn't have to document on paper. It was also difficult for me to find the multiple tests and labs on paper, let alone trend them. Electronic medical records put all the information I needed to see the full picture of my client, not only from this visit but from past visits, at my fingertips in a centralized location.

My background as a pharmacy technician, coupled with my nursing degree, as well as my love of electronic medical records, opened a door for me I never realized existed. I was asked to join the Clinical Information Systems Department of my hospital as a clinical systems analyst. When I was asked to consider bidding on the job, I honestly had no idea what the position involved. As a nurse, I never thought about how the screens I documented on or the orders I entered into the system were developed. They were just there, and that was all I needed to know.

As a clinical systems analyst, my responsibility is to be the "voice of nursing in IT". It doesn't make sense for a person who has never taken care of a client to decide how a nurse should document client care. That is where I come in. As one of my fellow co-workers says, we are "techno nurses." We understand how nurses practice and what will work best for them, but we also understand how the technology works.

Although I spend a great deal of my time at a desk, my position still allows me to be involved in clinical work. I participate in my hospitals' Professional Practice Model, interact with the staff nurses during a monthly orders and documentation workgroup, attend a monthly meeting to minimize medication errors, teach classes to help familiarize staff with our IT solutions, and act as the voice of the registered nurse while evaluating new IT solutions. Knowing I am able to be the voice of my fellow registered nurses, as well as shape how nurses care for clients using IT solutions, is the most rewarding part of my job.

Use of Anatomical Drawings in the EHR

Another method of entering data about the client into the EHR involves the use of anatomical drawings of the body and body systems. These drawings are used in two different ways, as an alternative method of navigating the nomenclature or by actually annotating a drawing and including it in the client record. In this chapter we will discuss both. Anatomical drawings are particularly easy to navigate or annotate on a Tablet PC, but the same or similar result can be achieved on a laptop or workstation computer using a mouse.

Navigation by Body System

Some EHR systems have navigation pages that allow the nurse to quickly locate findings by pointing to a particular body part in a drawing that opens a list of findings relevant to that

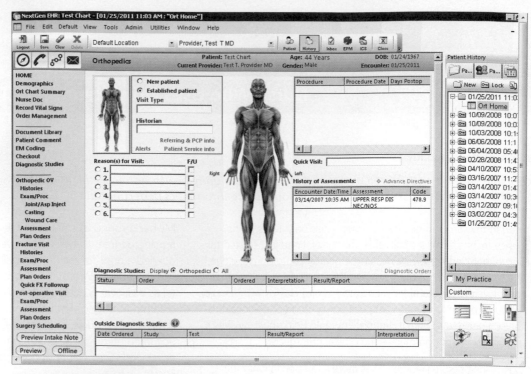

Courtesy of NextGen Healthcare www.nextgen.com

▶ **Figure 9-41 Entering findings using an image on a Tablet PC.**

body system. The nurse then selects the findings appropriate to the visit. In this case, the pictures do not become part of the client note; they are just a visual tool for navigation (see Figure 9-41 for an example). Think of this as searching with pictures rather than words.

Annotated Drawings as EHR Data

Another type of EHR data is the visual representation of the finding. Certain specialties routinely record information about the physical exam in the form of drawings or sketches. Two examples are dermatologists, who sometimes note the location of nevi (moles) on an outline of the body, and ophthalmologists, who frequently document observations on a drawing of the eye. Similarly, a nurse working in a nursing home might document the location of pressure ulcers on a bed-bound resident's skin. These types of annotated drawings have long been a part of the client's paper chart and most EHR systems today support a tool to annotate drawings in the computer. The images created using the tools in the EHR become part of the electronic encounter. Annotated drawings are also useful for client education, as we shall see in a later exercise.

Some EHR systems actually embed the annotated image in the encounter note while other EHR systems attach or associate the image with the note. Although annotated images might contain descriptive text, the text within the image is not codified data. This means that for the purpose of subsequent analysis of the EHR records, the computer will be able to locate encounter records that have an attached or embedded image, but it will not be able to know what data the image contains unless the nurse enters findings for the data as well. You will see this in the next exercise.

Guided Exercise 60: Annotated Dermatology Exam

This exercise will give you an opportunity to practice the annotation of a drawing using a simplified tool in the Student Edition software. As with previous exercises, the purpose here is to let you experience a function often available in commercial EHR systems. The drawing tools you will use here will be similar in principle but not identical to those you might use in your workplace. The method of invoking the annotation tooland the manner in which a drawing is subsequently merged into the encounter note will vary by EHR vendor as well.

Case Study

Arnie Greensher is a 66-year-old male who has a large number of moles on his back, the result of years of working in the sun without a shirt. The clinic has been monitoring them through regular follow-up visits. In addition to the encounter notes created at those visits, the clinic finds it useful to save annotated drawings, which show the placement of the moles. In subsequent visits, the nurse will compare the drawings from past encounters to the current state of the Mr. Greensher's skin to quickly identify new moles or changes from a previous visit.

Step 1

If you have not already done so, start the Student Edition software.

Click Select on the Menu bar, and then click Patient.

In the Patient Selection window, locate and click on **Arnie Greensher**, as shown in Figure 9-42.

Step 2

Click Select on the Menu bar, and then click Existing Encounter.

A small window of previous encounters will be displayed. Compare your screen to the window shown in Figure 9-43.

Select the encounter dated **5/24/2012 5:00 PM** (Follow-Up).

The encounter note from that date will be displayed as shown in Figure 9-44.

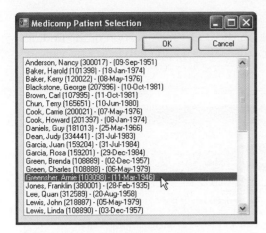

► **Figure 9-42 Select Arnie Greensher.**

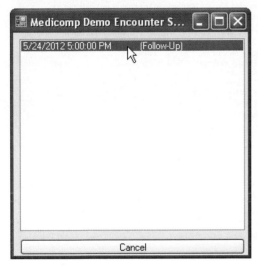

► **Figure 9-43 Select existing encounter for May 24, 2012.**

► **Figure 9-44 Arnie Greensher's encounter note for May 24, 2012 encounter.**

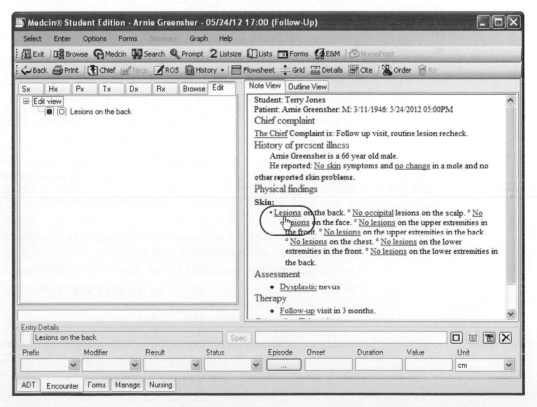

Step 3

In the right pane of your screen, locate and click on the underlined portion of the finding labeled "Lesions on the back" (circled in red). The left pane should change to Edit view, as shown in Figure 9-44.

▶ **Figure 9-45 Click the Context button (circled in red) and select "Add Object to Finding."**

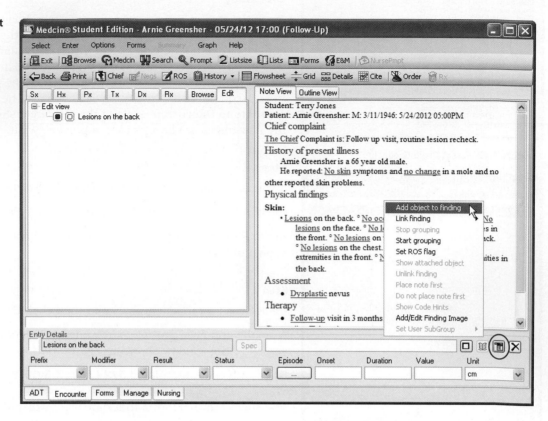

Step 4

Locate the four buttons in the lower right corner of the window. The Context button is the second button from the right (circled in red in Figure 9-45).

Click on the Context button to display a list of advanced actions that can be used with a finding.

Click the first option in the list labeled "Add object to finding." This will invoke the annotation tools in the right pane of the window (shown in Figure 9-46).

The software contains various anatomical illustrations, which may be selected for annotation. The right pane displays one of the images.

Above the image is a navigational bar consisting of three fields with drop-down lists. These are used to select images of other body systems and views.

▶ The first field can be used to select the body system to be presented (skin, circulatory, skeletal, and so on).

▶ The center field is used to select the image region within that system (full body, head and neck, lower extremities, and so on).

▶ The third field is used to select the view of the image (front, back, left, and so on).

▶ The gender of the image as well as the age range of the image is automatically determined by the demographics of the current client. The default body system for the image is automatically determined by the selected finding.

Compare your screen to Figure 9-46; if the image is not of the back of a man's trunk, click the down arrow of the center or right field to change the view. Select Trunk and Back from the respective drop-down lists.

► **Figure 9-46 Template image of trunk and back.**

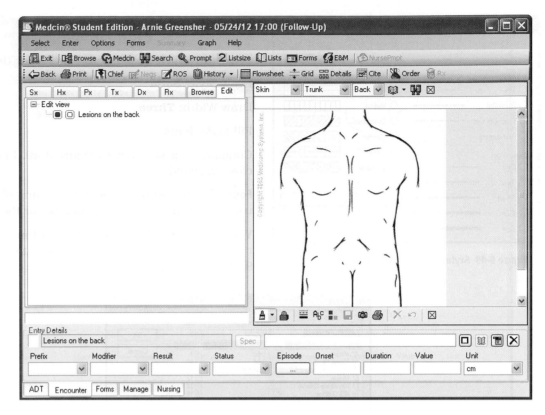

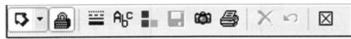

► **Figure 9-47 Draw toolbar (enlarged to show detail).**

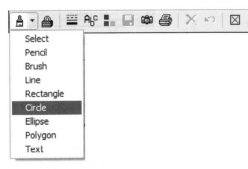

► **Figure 9-48 Select the shape "Circle" from the drop-down list.**

At the bottom of the image is the drawing toolbar, which is shown enlarged in Figure 9-47. We will discuss each of the buttons on the drawing toolbar, from left to right.

Select Tool The first icon on the Toolbar shows the currently selected drawing shape or tool. The icon of the button will change according to the current selection. The down arrow next to the button displays a drop-down list of tools.

Step 5

Click the down arrow next to the Select button to display the list of tools.

Figure 9-48 shows the drop-down list of shapes of the drawing tool. Most are self-explanatory, except the first one, Select. The Select option is used to select items that have been added to the drawing so they can be deleted or modified.

Locate and click on the word "Circle." The drawing tool button will display a circle in place of the pointer.

Step 6

Lock Button The icon resembles a padlock. This is used to "lock" the selected shape. When it is "locked," the button background will be white and the selections you have made for shape or the other drawing tool buttons (discussed later) stay set. When it is not "locked" the drawing toolbar buttons return to their default state after each use.

Locate and click on the "lock" button in the drawing toolbar.

Step 7

Style This button icon consists of different horizontal lines. This button invokes the Style Selection window, which sets the pattern and thickness of the tools you will use to annotate the drawings. The style sets not only the line but also the solidity and thickness of other shapes.

▶ **Figure 9-54 Draw 15 small moles on the back.**

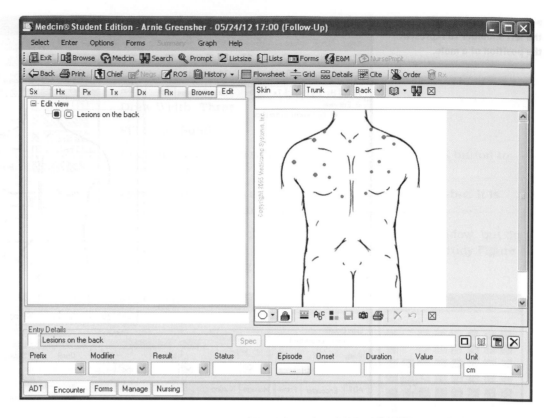

Click on the down arrow in the toolbar and reselect the circle from the drop-down list as you did in step 5. Locate and click on the padlock to lock the circle shape.

Draw **15** small moles on the back, as shown in Figure 9-54. You do not have to place them exactly as they are in the figure; just get reasonably close.

> **Note**
>
> **If at any time during this step your Shape tool reverts to the mouse pointer, just unlock the padlock, reselect the Circle shape, and click on the padlock to relock the shape.**

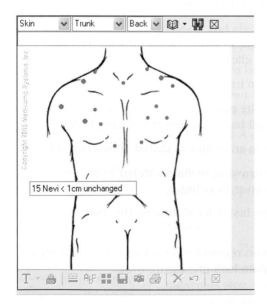

▶ **Figure 9-55 Type "15 Nevi < 1 cm. Unchanged" in text box.**

Step 12

Nurses also can annotate the images by adding text directly on the drawing canvas with the Text tool. The nurse also can select a different color for the text. It is wise to do so, as it will help the text stand out from the color and the background of the drawing.

Locate and click on the down arrow next to the Select button. Choose Text from the drop-down list.

Locate and click on the Color button in the drawing toolbar. When the Color pallet window is displayed, select blue, and then click OK.

Now click over an empty portion of the drawing and a text box will appear, as shown in Figure 9-55.

If the text box is not positioned where you would like it, click elsewhere. It will move to wherever you click your mouse.

Type the following text in the box: **15 Nevi < 1 cm. unchanged.**

Step 13

When you have finished typing, merge the text into the drawing by clicking the right mouse button anywhere on the drawing except in the text box. A drop-down menu will appear, as shown in Figure 9-56.

Locate and click on the option "Complete Text Entry," as shown in Figure 9-56.

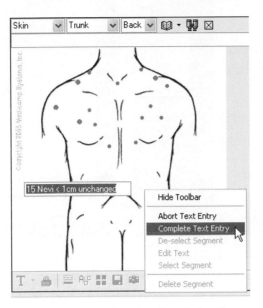

▶ **Figure 9-56 Right click elsewhere in drawing and select "Complete Text Entry."**

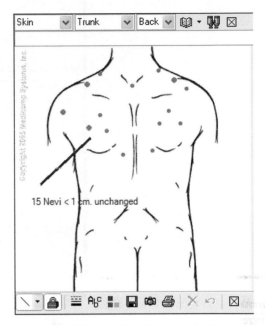

▶ **Figure 9-57 Draw a blue line from text to region of the moles.**

Step 14

Another useful drawing tool is the Line, which can be used to connect text to the drawing points.

Click on the down arrow in the toolbar and select Line from the drop-down list.

Position your mouse on the drawing just above the text. Hold down the left mouse button as you drag the mouse upward toward the moles on the back. When you release it, the line will end.

Compare your drawing to Figure 9-57.

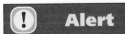

Alert

Do not close or exit the drawing tool or change tabs until you have a printed copy in your hand. **You could lose your work if you exit the drawing before printing has completed.**

Step 15

In commercial EHR systems, you can merge your finished drawing into the narrative encounter notes for the visit. In the Student Edition you will only print your drawing, not merge it, because students from other classes share the data.

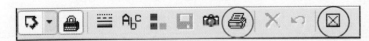

▶ **Figure 9-58 Print button circled in blue and Exit button circled in red on the drawing toolbar.**

Click the Print button on the *drawing toolbar*, **not** the Print button on the main Toolbar. The print button for images is circled in blue in Figure 9-58.

The familiar Print Data window shown in Figure 9-59 will be invoked.

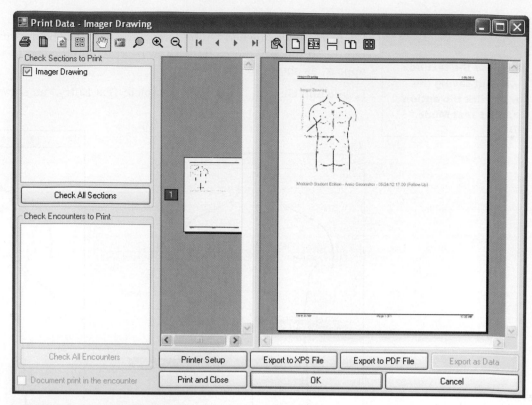

▶ **Figure 9-59 Print Data window is invoked from drawing toolbar.**

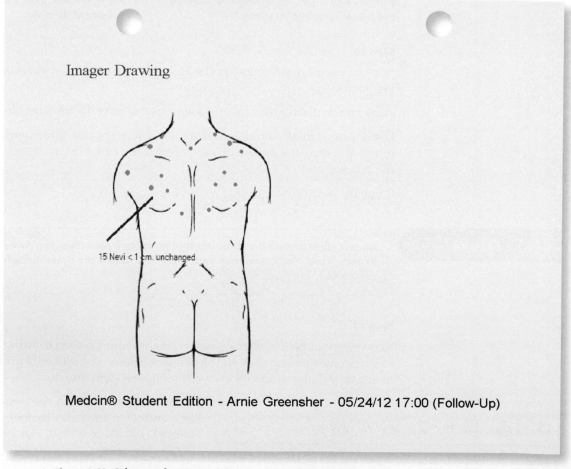

▶ **Figure 9-60 Printout of annotated drawing for Arnie Greensher.**

Be certain there is a check mark in the box next to "Imager Drawing" and then click on the appropriate button to either print or export a file, as directed by your instructor.

Compare your printout or file output to Figure 9-60.

When you have a printout of your annotated drawing in hand, close the Print Data window. Save the printed copy to give to your instructor along with the encounter note you will print in step 18.

Step 16

Return to the encounter note view by exiting the drawing tool.

Locate and click on the Exit button in the drawing toolbar (circled in red in Figure 9-58). Use only this button in this step, not any other Exit button in the window.

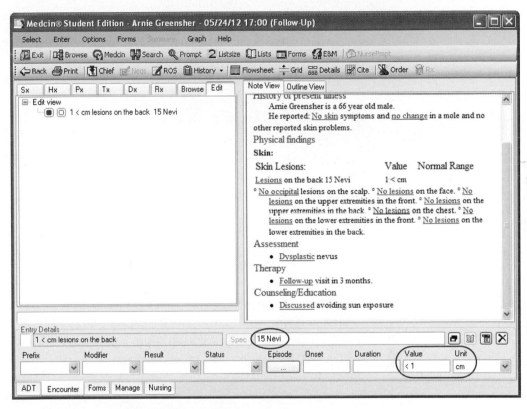

▶ **Figure 9-61 Recording free text and value in the encounter.**

Step 17

Annotated drawings provide an excellent means of recording the location and size of certain observed findings in a physical exam. However, as we have discussed several times the contents of the image are not codified, searchable records. In this example, the text added to the drawing became part of the image and as such can only be read by a person, not the computer.

Therefore, the nurse also will record the text of the findings in the encounter note. This will result in the best of both worlds; codified data for the computer and a visual record of the location of moles for use in future exams.

With the finding "Lesions on the back" still selected for edit, you will add data to the finding.

Locate the Entry Details free-text field just below the right pane and type **15 Nevi**.

Locate the Value field in the Entry Details section at the bottom of the screen and type: **<1**.

Press the enter key. Compare your screen to Figure 9-61.

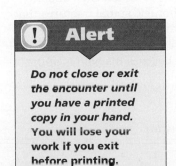

```
Arnie Greensher                                          Page 1 of 1

Student: your name or id here
Patient: Arnie Greensher: M: 3/11/1946: 5/24/2012 05:00PM
Chief complaint
The Chief Complaint is: Follow up visit, routine lesion recheck.
History of present illness
    Arnie Greensher is a 66 year old male.
He reported: No skin symptoms and no change in a mole and no other reported skin
problems.
Physical findings
Skin:
Skin Lesions:                  Value Normal Range
Lesions on the back 15 Nevi < 1 cm
° No occipital lesions on the scalp. ° No lesions on the face. ° No lesions on
the upper extremities in the front. ° No lesions on the upper extremities
in the back. ° No lesions on the chest. ° No lesions on the lower extremities
in the front.
° No lesions on the lower extremities in the back.
Assessment
    • Dysplastic nevus
Therapy
    • Follow-up visit in 3 months.
Counseling/Education
    • Discussed avoiding sun exposure
```

▶ **Figure 9-62 Printed encounter note for Arnie Greensher.**

Step 18

Click on the Print button on the Toolbar at the top of your screen to invoke the Print Data window.

Be certain there is a check mark in the box next to "Current Encounter" and then click on the appropriate button to either print or export a file, as directed by your instructor.

Compare your printout or file output to Figure 9-62. If it is correct, hand it in to your instructor. If there are any differences, review the previous steps in the exercise and find your error.

Critical Thinking Exercise 61: Examination of a Client with Pressure Sores

In this exercise, you will use the skills you have acquired in the previous exercise to document a client with pressure sores.

Case Study

Raj Patel is an 80-year-old male, who presents complaining of sores on his back and buttocks. Two months ago he had surgery to repair cervical and thoracic spinal fractures that were the result of a motor vehicle crash. He was initially discharged to rehab, but has become sedentary post-therapy and is developing pressure sores on his shoulder blades and buttocks. Because he cannot see his sores, he mistakenly believes his pain is at the sites of his spinal and iliac incisions.

 Alert

Make certain you set the date and time correctly for this exercise.

Step 1

If you have not already done so, start the Student Edition software.

Click Select on the Menu bar, and then click Patient.

In the Patient Selection window, locate and click on **Raj Patel**.

Step 2

Click Select on the Menu bar, and then click New Encounter.

Select the date **May 24, 2012**, the time **5:15 PM**, and the reason **Office Visit**.

Compare your screen to the date, time, and reason printed in bold type before clicking on the OK button.

Step 3

Enter the Chief complaint: "**Post-surgical sores on back and buttocks**."

When you have finished typing, click on the button labeled "Close the Note Dialog."

Step 4

Begin the visit by taking Mr. Patel's vital signs and history.

Locate the Forms button on the Toolbar and select the form labeled "**Vitals**." Enter Mr. Patel's vital signs in the corresponding fields on the form as follows:

Temperature:	**98.6**
Respiration:	**28**
Pulse:	**78**
BP:	**150/90**
Height:	**67**
Weight:	**210**

When you have finished, check your work; if it is correct, click on the Encounter tab at the bottom of your screen.

Step 5

Click on the Hx tab.

Expand the past medical history tree by clicking the small plus signs next to "past medical history," and "surgical/procedural."

Locate and click on following finding

● (red button) prior surgery

Locate and click in the Entry Details field "Onset" and type **60 days**

Press the Enter key and the software will automatically calculate the date 3/25/2012 and add it to the finding in the encounter note.

Step 6

Scroll the left pane downward to locate "social history" expand the tree by clicking the small plus signs next to "social history," "habits," and "exercise habits."

Locate and click on following finding

● (red button) sedentary

Step 7

Click on the Dx tab.

Locate and click on the small plus signs next to "Orthopedic Disorders" and "Fracture."

Click on the description "Vertebral Column" to highlight it. Locate and click the History button on the Toolbar at the top of your screen.

In the free text below the right pane type "**C7, T1, T2, T3**" and press the Enter key.

Click on the description "Ribs" to highlight it. Locate and click the History button on the Toolbar at the top of your screen.

Step 8

Locate and click on the Search button on the Toolbar at the top of your screen. The Search String window will be invoked.

Type the search string "**pressure sores**" and click on the Search button in the window.

Step 9

Click on the Sx tab.

Locate and click on following finding:

- (red button) red sore blanches with pressure

Step 10

Click on the Hx tab.

Locate and click on following findings:

- (red button) difficulty inspecting body for pressure sores

Step 11

Click on the Px tab.

Locate and click on following finding:

- (red button) Lesions tender to direct pressure

Locate and click on the button labeled "Medcin" on the Toolbar at the top of your screen to restore the full nomenclature.

Scroll the left pane downward to locate and click on the small plus signs next to "Skin" and "Ulcer _cm."

Locate and click on following findings:

- (red button) On Shoulders
- (red button) Buttocks

Step 12

Click on the Dx tab.

Click again on the Search button on the Toolbar at the top of your screen. The Search String window will be invoked and should still display the search string "**pressure sores**." Click on the Search button in the window.

Locate and click on the small plus signs next to "Chronic Cutaneous Ulcer Decubitus," and "Lower Back."

Locate and click on following findings:

- (red button) Upper Back
- (red button) Coccyx

Step 13

Click on the Rx tab.

Locate and click on following finding:

- (red button) ADL Inspect body for pressure sores Short-Term

Locate and click on the button labeled "Medcin" on the Toolbar at the top of your screen to restore the full nomenclature.

Locate and click on the small plus sign next to "Basic Management Procedures and services."

Scroll the left pane downward and click on the small plus sign next to "Orthopedic services."

Locate and click on following finding:

- (red button) Regular exercise

Scroll the left pane further downward to locate and click on the small plus signs next to "Home care," "Visit," and "For Clinical Assessment."

Locate and click on the finding description "Skin" to highlight it.

Locate and click on the Order button in the Toolbar at the top of your screen.

      🔺 (order button) Skin

Step 14

Create an annotated drawing to illustrate the position of his incision scars and pressure sores for the client.

Scroll the encounter note in the right pane to locate and click on the underlined finding "Lesions." The left pane should change to the Edit tab.

Locate the Context button (the second button from the right in the lower right corner of your window) and click on it. From the drop-down list displayed, choose "Add Object to Finding."

The drawing window will be invoked in the right pane.

If the drawing of the trunk is not displayed, use the fields at the top of the drawing to select the Skin, Trunk, Back view from the drop-down lists.

Step 15

Once the correct illustration template is displayed, use the toolbar in the drawing tool to set up the tool.

Locate and click on the down arrow next to the first button; then select "Ellipse" from the drop-down list.

Locate and click on the Lock button (with the padlock). It should have a white background.

Locate and click on the Style button in the drawing toolbar. A window similar to Figure 9-49 will be invoked.

Locate and click on the following:

    Draw Style: **Solid**

    Draw Width: **Three**

    Fill Style: **Solid**

Click on the OK button to close the Style window.

Locate and click on the Color pallet button in the drawing toolbar. When the color pallet window is displayed, select red. Click OK to close the Color pallet window.

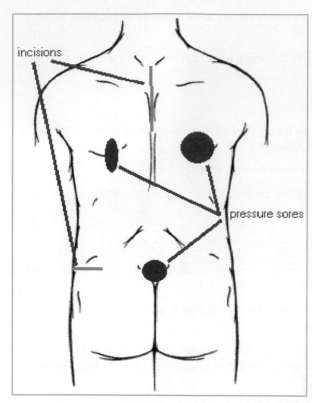

Anatomical Figure © MediComp Systems, Inc.

▶ **Figure 9-63 Drawing of incisions and pressure sores.**

Step 16

As closely as possible, replicate the drawing in Figure 9-63.

Draw a large red circle over the right shoulder blade, a red circle over the coccyx, and a vertical oval over the left shoulder blade (as shown in Figure 9-63).

Change the drawing tool.

Locate and click on the down arrow next to the first button, then select "Line" from the drop-down list.

Locate and click on the Color pallet button. When the window is displayed, select orange. Click OK to close the Color pallet window.

Draw a short horizontal line from the edge of the left hip toward the coccyx as shown in Figure 9-63.

Draw a long vertical line from the base of the neck to the center of the shoulder blades as shown in Figure 9-63.

Change the drawing tool to annotate the drawing.

Locate and click on the down arrow next to the first button in the drawing toolbar, then select "Text" from the drop-down list. Next, change the color to blue by selecting the Color pallet button.

Click in the upper left of the drawing and type "incisions" in the text box.

Right-click anywhere on the drawing except in the text box to display a list of options; click on "Complete Text" from the list displayed.

Click on the right side of the drawing and type "**pressure sores**" in the text box.

Right-click anywhere on the drawing except in the text box to display a list of options;

Change the drawing tool.

Locate and click on the down arrow next to the first button, then select "line" from the drop-down list.

Draw two blue lines from the word "incisions" to the orange lines you drew earlier.

Draw three blue lines from the phrase "pressure sores" to the red circles.

Compare your drawing to Figure 9-63. If you need to correct the line or circle, change the tool button to "Select" and click on the object. Use the Delete button in the Toolbar and then redraw the correct element.

 Alert

Do not exit the drawing or change tabs until you have a printed copy in your hand. **You will lose your work if you exit the drawing tool before printing is complete.**

Step 17

Click the Print button on the *drawing toolbar*, **not** the Print button on the main toolbar. The familiar Print Data window will be invoked.

Be certain there is a check mark in the box next to "Imager Drawing" and then click on the appropriate button to either print or export a file, as directed by your instructor.

Compare your printout or file output to Figure 9-63.

When you have a printout of your annotated drawing in hand, close the Print Data window. Save the printed copy to give to your instructor along with the encounter note you will print in step 18.

Raj Patel   Page 1 of 1

Student: *your name or id here*
Patient: Raj Patel: M: 3/05/1932: 5/24/2012 05:15PM
Chief complaint
The Chief Complaint is: Post-surgical sores on back and buttocks.
History of present illness
    Raj Patel is an 80 year old male.
    He reported: A red sore which blanches with pressure.
Past medical/surgical history
Reported History:
    Surgical / Procedural: Prior surgery 3/25/2012.
Diagnosis History:
    Fracture of the vertebral column C7, T1, T2, T3
    Rib fracture
Personal history
Habits: Sedentary.
Functional: Inspecting body for pressure sores with difficulty.
Physical findings
Vital Signs:

Vital Signs/Measurements	Value	Normal Range
Oral temperature	96.8 F	97.6 - 99.6
RR	28 breaths/min	18 - 26
PR	78 bpm	50 - 100
Blood pressure	150/90 mmHg	100 - 120/60 - 80
Weight	210 lbs	121 - 205
Height	67 in	64.57 - 73.23

Skin:
- Lesion was tender to direct pressure.
- An ulcer was seen on the shoulders.
- An ulcer was seen on the buttocks.

Assessment
- Decubitus ulcer of the upper back
- Decubitus ulcer of the coccyx

Therapy
- Regular exercise.
- Short-term goals for inspecting the body for pressure sores.

Plan
- Home care visit for skin assessment

▶ **Figure 9-64 Printed encounter note for Raj Patel.**

Step 18

Locate and click on the Exit button in the *drawing toolbar* to close the drawing tool and redisplay the encounter note.

Click on the Print button on the Toolbar at the top of your screen to invoke the Print Data window.

Be certain there is a check mark in the box next to "Current Encounter" and then click on the appropriate button to either print or export a file, as directed by your instructor.

Compare your printout to Figure 9-64. If anything is missing, review steps 1 to 13 and correct your mistake.

Hand in the printed encounter note or file output of Raj Patel's encounter and the annotated drawing of his pressure sores to your instructor.

Chapter Nine Summary

This chapter showed how codified data in the EHR could be displayed in a format called a flow sheet.

Flow sheets present data from multiple encounters in column form. This format allows for a side-by-side comparison of findings over a period of time.

The flow sheet view resembles a spreadsheet made up of rows and columns of "cells." The first column displays descriptions as well as red and blue buttons to record findings in the current encounter. The date of the current encounter is at the top of the column. The remaining columns to the right display encounter data from previous visits.

The flow sheet rows are grouped vertically into logical sections that match the sections you are accustomed to seeing in the encounter note. The title of each section is printed in blue on a teal background.

The Student Edition software allows you to create flow sheets four different ways based on:

▶ List

▶ Problem

▶ Form

▶ Nursing Plan of Care

You also used multiple forms during a single exam to document a client with multiple chronic conditions. From this you have learned that you can change forms as often as you like during an examination without losing any of the data.

In this chapter you learned that some EHR systems have navigation pages that allow the nurse to quickly locate findings by pointing to a particular body part in a drawing, which opens a list of findings relevant to that body system. This was described as searching with pictures rather than words.

You also learned another method of entering data about the client into the EHR with the use of anatomical drawings of the body and body systems. Annotated drawings often are included in the EHR at ophthalmology, dermatology practices, nursing homes, and by home care nurses. Annotated images created in the EHR become part of the electronic encounter, and are useful for client education as well as documentation.

The Student Edition software includes a set of simple drawing tools for creating annotated drawings and associating them with findings in the encounter notes. The tools are invoked by clicking on a finding in the right pane, then clicking on the Context button and then selecting Add Object to Finding from the drop-down list.

The software contains various anatomical illustrations, which may be selected for annotation. A special toolbar allows you to select the shape, line, thickness, and color of the drawing tool. You can also add text annotations to the drawing. A Print button on the drawing toolbar (not the Print button on the main Toolbar) is used to print your finished drawing.

Task	Exercise		Page No.
How to use a flow sheet	57		338
How to cite findings in a flow sheet	57		339
How to create a flow sheet from a problem list	58		351
How to create a flow sheet from a nursing plan of care	59		355
How to print a flow sheet	59	Step 14	363
How to create annotated drawings	60		368
How to print annotated drawings	60	Step 15	375

Test Your Knowledge

1. What were the two chronic diseases for which Mr. Daniels was being monitored?

2. Why did the hypertension and diabetes forms create different flow sheets?

3. Why were some items already filled in when you loaded the second form?

4. What form did you use to record dietary orders?

5. What is a flow sheet?

6. What does it mean to cite a finding?

7. Describe how to create a flow sheet from a form.

8. Describe how to create a problem-oriented flow sheet.

9. Describe how to create a flow sheet for a nursing plan of care.

10. Describe how to cite a finding from a flow sheet.

11. Name two medical specialties that typically incorporate annotated drawings in an encounter note.

12. If you click the date of a flow sheet column when the Cite button is *off*, what data is displayed?

13. If you click the date of a flow sheet column when the Cite button is *on*, what data is displayed?

14. How do you print an annotated drawing?

15. You should have produced narrative documents for four clients and two annotated drawings. If you have not already done so, hand these in to your instructor with this test. These will count as a portion of your grade.

Ask your instructor for answers to Test Your Knowledge

nursing.pearsonhighered.com

Prepare for success with animated examples, practice questions, challenge tests, and interactive assignments.

10 Subacute Care, Nursing Homes, and Home Care

Learning Outcomes

After completing this chapter, you should be able to:

1. Identify at least seven long-term care options
2. Describe aspects of care unique to nursing homes
3. Understand and use a Resident Assessment Instrument
4. Discuss the provision of home care
5. Understand and use OASIS-C
6. Compare an OASIS plan of care synopsis and a nursing plan of care

Postdischarge Nursing Care

Thus far you have explored how nurses document their work in acute care hospitals, outpatient clinics, and medical offices. This chapter will discuss healthcare delivered after the client is discharged from an acute care facility. Clients are typically discharged to either their home or to a long-term care facility (LTC).

Long-term care facilities include skilled nursing facilities (SNF), long-term acute care facilities (LTAC), nursing homes, residential care facilities, and rehabilitation hospitals. One difference between acute care and long-term care facilities is the average length of stay (ALOS). In an acute care hospital, the ALOS is less than 30 days. In a long-term care facility, the ALOS is greater than 30 days.

Another difference is that the level of care required by LTC clients or residents is generally less. For this reason, long-term care facilities are sometimes referred to as "subacute care." Subacute care facilities and home care services are appropriate for clients whose nursing care needs are less frequent and less intensive than the care offered in an acute care facility.

As the baby-boomer generation ages, our nation's demographic population will shift to a higher percentage of elderly clients. Traditionally, the elderly are the highest consumers of subacute care, skilled nursing facilities, nursing homes, and home health care. It is anticipated that there will be a greater need for nurses in these areas. This chapter will focus on nursing homes and home care, but first let us briefly review various venues of subacute care delivery.

Long-Term Care Facilities

Long-term care facilities, also called extended care facilities, offer nursing care to clients who need inpatient services, but at a less intense level than that provided at an acute care facility. Long-term care clients generally have a length of stay greater than 30 days. Examples of long-term care facilities include LTAC, rehabilitation hospitals, SNF, residential care facilities, and nursing homes. In most of these facilities, the term *resident* is used instead of *patient* or *client*.

Long-Term Acute Care Facilities

A LTAC provides a subacute level of care to inpatients who have postintensive care needs for an extended period of time before they are well enough to qualify for moving to a rehabilitation facility or skilled care facility. These clients may need a variety of nursing care support similar to that given in a hospital intensive care but are no longer in their acute risk phase of recovery. Their nursing care needs are generally too extensive to qualify for other levels of long-term care. The goal of care is for the client to improve sufficiently to qualify for either rehabilitation or a skilled care facility.

Rehabilitation Facilities

Rehabilitation facilities strive to help clients return to their maximum possible functionality. Different facilities help clients with different conditions. Some specialize in physical medicine, physical therapy, and occupational therapy, helping clients recover from the effects of accidents, severe injuries or illnesses, strokes, or serious surgery. To qualify for care in these facilities, the client must meet a specific activity tolerance sufficient to benefit from rehabilitation therapy. Clients may be discharged from acute care to another type of long-term care facility until they have sufficiently recovered to be able to tolerate and participate in the offered rehabilitation. Rehabilitation facilities often offer both inpatient and outpatient therapy levels of care to meet the changing care requirements of their clients, as their level of independence progresses.

A different type of rehabilitation facility is one that helps clients detoxify and recover from dependence on alcohol or drugs. Treatment includes counseling and therapy by psychiatrists, psychologists, and other mental health workers.

Rehabilitation facilities can be privately owned, not-for-profit, or affiliated with a hospital or university.

Skilled Nursing Facilities

A SNF is an institution, or a distinct part of an institution (skilled care unit), that has a transfer agreement in effect with one or more participating hospitals. A SNF is appropriate for residents whose acuity levels require a higher level of nursing care such as tube feeding, intravenous therapy, chronic wound therapy, or mechanical ventilators.

A SNF located within a hospital must consist of a physically identifiable separate unit. Although a SNF in a hospital may span several floors or buildings, the residents of the SNF must be located in units that are physically separate from those units housing all other clients of the institution. This separation of units does not apply to swing bed hospitals.

Swing bed hospitals are rural hospitals with fewer than 100 beds that receive a special classification by Medicare. This is done to address the shortage of rural SNF beds. Such a hospital can "swing" its beds between hospital and SNF levels of care, on an as needed basis. Swing bed hospitals must meet other requirements that apply to SNF. Nursing services provided to a resident in a skilled nursing facility or a resident in a swing bed are the same.

Residential Care Facilities

Residential care facilities provide residents with a living environment that is more apartment-like than a nursing home. Residents are independent, yet have access to the level of assistance they need. Group meals, activities, and transportation are often provided by the facility. Residents have the ability to notify management of a medical or other emergency at the touch of a button. Most residential care facilities have nurses on staff and a "nurse's office" where residents can consult with a nurse. However, nurses do not have "rounds" and typically nursing care is provided only when requested by the resident.

Hospice

Hospice provides end-of-life care for terminally ill clients. Hospice care may be delivered in a residential hospice facility or in the client's home. Nurses are the principal hospice care provider. If the client is at home, their family is designated as the primary caregiver. The goal of care is focused on client comfort, quality of life, and support of the client and family holistically throughout the dying process. Hospice support to the family extends beyond the demise of the client.

Home Care

Although not a subacute facility, home care is a form of postdischarge care. As the name implies, home care allows clients to remain in their homes, yet receive the services of nurses, physical therapists, occupational therapists, or other healthcare providers. The home care provider visits the client's home on a regularly scheduled basis and provides services based on a physician's orders. Nurses providing home care are employed by home care agencies that may be independently owned or affiliated with a hospital.

Home care provides an important component of healthcare delivery, but tracking the records of the visits provides a challenge with regard to integration of home care visit notes into a comprehensive health record. Often the visiting nurse or therapist carries only a small portion of the client's record. These home care providers record notes concerning the home care visit, the client's progress, and any measurements taken such as vital signs, range of motion, and so forth; they then transfer their notes to the client record at the Home Health Agency. This is changing. Wireless connectivity is making it possible to access and update client records remotely.

Home care nursing will be covered in-depth later in this chapter.

Assessment Instruments

One thing all LTC venues have in common is that each of them has a special form that the nurse must use to document an assessment of the client or resident and that person's anticipated care needs. Each type of long-term care uses a different assessment instrument (form) to gather a standardized set of data, but regardless of which form is used, the law requires the assessments to be completed at specific milestones or intervals, such as at start of care, discharge, or transfer. Funding, duration of care and services that will be authorized for the client are based on data gathered by these assessment instruments. Although there is an assessment form for each type of long-term care, in the interest of time the chapter will examine only two: the Residential Assessment Instrument (RAI) and Outcome and Assessment Information Set (OASIS).

Study of these two forms is useful because the charting requirements for a client in a skilled nursing facility or other type of LTC hospital are more similar to acute care hospitals, although the frequency and type of documentation varies with each level of care. The difference for nursing home and home care documentation is that there are additional requirements that must be met. The government-mandated forms are different from those you have worked with so far and their LTC care plans concern both long-term and short-term goals.

Like acute care settings, the nurse's ability to document accurately and *completely* the assessment, goals, and risks in the required forms is important, but in the long-term setting these forms will determine how much will be reimbursed for that care, the length of stay, how much assistance from a certified nursing aide is needed, and the amount of time a licensed professional is needed. Because this is the first time we have discussed these concepts, here are a few examples:

▶ Nurses are required to assess both nursing home residents and home care clients in a timely manner and to complete required forms documenting the assessment. The forms are different but have a similar purpose. Billing cannot begin until the forms are complete in all aspects. Additionally, the forms must be completed within a specified time frame. Nurses must reevaluate the residents and update the records at mandated intervals.

▶ Both forms contain a section to assess activities of daily living (ADL). The answers are important because they not only document how much oversight the nurse will have to do, but how much time and how many certified nursing aides are needed to care for the client—for example, if it takes two people to help the resident.

▶ Funding for the resident's stay may be dependent on charting that indicates the degree of dependency and rate of improvement.

▶ If a client comes into a nursing home with a history of falling and then falls while a resident there, is it documented in the assessment that the resident has fallen before? The nurse's documentation will directly affect the nursing home's liability.

Nursing Homes

Nursing homes provide a level of care beyond assisted living or residential care facilities. Many residents of nursing homes are there because they can no longer live independently either due to physical debilitation or neurological conditions such as Alzheimer's disease, or other types of dementia. Federal law regulates care in nursing homes and many elements of that regulation are concerned with documentation. Here are some examples:

▶ "Patients in nursing homes shall be called residents."

▶ "Each resident must have his or her rights and responsibilities explained at the time of admission."

▶ "There must be written documentation of the investigation into any possible violation of residents' rights or standard of care" (Centers for Medicare & Medicaid Services, n.d., *Conditions of Participation*).

▶ "Minimum Data Set 3.0 (MDS) must be used to assess the resident's needs and desires, accomplished by direct interview of the individual resident and or family member."

▶ "Comprehensive care plans must include outcomes and target dates for needs identified in the MDS."

▸ "A quality assurance committee must monitor the maintenance of residents' medical records."

▸ "Any transfers, discharges, accidents, or changes in medical condition must be thoroughly documented."

▸ "Residents must have an updated assessment upon admission, a brief one each quarterly, with any significant change in the resident's condition and a more comprehensive annual assessment. Assessments are done even more frequently for residents covered by Medicare" (Centers for Medicare & Medicaid Services, n.d., *Nursing Home Quality*).

Resident Assessment Instrument

Providing care to residents with posthospital and long-term care needs is complex and challenging work. Clinical competence, observational, interviewing and critical thinking skills, and assessment expertise from all disciplines are required to develop individualized care plans. The Resident Assessment Instrument (RAI) correctly and effectively helps provide appropriate care. The RAI helps the nursing home staff to gather definitive information on a resident's strengths and needs, which must be addressed in an individualized care plan. It also assists staff with evaluating goal achievement and revising care plans accordingly by enabling the nursing home to track changes in the resident's status. As the process of problem identification is integrated with sound clinical interventions, the care plan becomes each resident's unique path toward achieving or maintaining his or her highest practical level of well-being.

The RAI helps nursing home staff look at residents holistically—as individuals for whom quality of life and quality of care are mutually significant and necessary. Interdisciplinary use of the RAI promotes this emphasis on quality of care and quality of life. Nursing homes have found that involving disciplines such as dietary, social work, physical therapy, occupational therapy, speech language pathology, pharmacy, and activities in the RAI process has fostered a more holistic approach to resident care and strengthened team communication. This interdisciplinary process also helps to support the spheres of influence on the resident's experience of care, including: workplace practices, the nursing home's cultural and physical environment, staff satisfaction, clinical and care practice delivery, shared leadership, family and community relationships, and Federal/State/local government regulations.

Persons generally enter a nursing home because of problems with functional status caused by physical deterioration, cognitive decline, the onset or exacerbation of an acute illness or condition, or other related factors. Sometimes, the individual's ability to manage independently has been limited to the extent that skilled nursing, medical treatment, and/or rehabilitation is needed for the resident to maintain and/or restore function or to live safely from day-to-day. Although there are often unavoidable declines, particularly in the last stages of life, all necessary resources and disciplines must be used to ensure that residents achieve the highest level of functioning possible (quality of care) and maintain their sense of individuality (quality of life). This is true for both long-term residents and residents in a rehabilitative program anticipating return to their previous environment or another environment of their choice. (Adapted from Centers for Medicare & Medicaid Services, 2010b.)

Content of the RAI for Nursing Homes

The RAI consists of three basic components: The Minimum Data Set (MDS) Version 3.0, the Care Area Assessment (CAA) process, and the RAI utilization guidelines. The utilization of the three components of the RAI yields information about a resident's functional status, strengths, weaknesses, and preferences, as well as offering guidance on further assessment once problems have been identified. Each component flows naturally into the next as follows.

Minimum Data Set: A core set of screening, clinical, and functional status elements, including common definitions and coding categories, forms the foundation of a comprehensive assessment for all residents of nursing homes certified to participate in Medicare or Medicaid. The items in the MDS standardize communication about resident problems and conditions within nursing homes, between nursing homes, and between nursing homes and outside agencies. The required subsets include data items for each MDS assessment and tracking document (e.g., admission, quarterly, annual, significant change, discharge, entry).

Care Area Assessment Process: This process is designed to assist the nurse in systematically interpreting the information recorded on the MDS. Once a care area has been triggered, nursing home providers use current, evidence-based clinical resources to conduct an assessment of the potential problem and determine whether or not to care plan for it. The CAA process helps the clinician to focus on key issues identified during the assessment process so that decisions as to whether and how to intervene can be explored with the resident. Specific components of the CAA process include:

▶ Care Area Triggers are specific resident responses for one or a combination of MDS elements. The triggers identify residents who have or are at risk for developing specific functional problems and require further assessment.

▶ CAA Resources are a list of resources that may be helpful in performing the assessment of a triggered care area.

▶ CAA Summary (Section V of the MDS 3.0) is used for documentation of the care area(s) that have been triggered from the MDS and the decisions made during the CAA process regarding whether or not to proceed to care planning.

Utilization Guidelines provide instructions for when and how to use the RAI. These include instructions for completion of the RAI as well as structured frameworks for synthesizing MDS and other clinical information (Adapted from Centers for Medicare & Medicaid Services, 2010b). The nurse should consult these guidelines when unsure how to answer a question as examples are provided in the guidelines.

Nursing home care is multidisciplinary by its nature, employing the services of physical therapists, speech therapists, respiratory therapist, and registered dietitians, in addition to registered nurses and certified nursing assistants. Although various members of the resident's care team may be asked to contribute parts of the assessment related to their discipline, in the end it is the registered nurse's responsibility to ensure the RAI is completed on time.

Guided Exercise 62: Studying the MDS 3.0 RAI

This exercise will examine the MDS 3.0 Resident Assessment Instrument form. Although nearly all nursing homes submit the MDS 3.0 electronically, many gather the data using this form and then enter it into a computer. We have elected to use the PDF form instead of a computer form for this exercise because the descriptive instructions within sections of the PDF form will help you understand the concepts and rules of the MDS.

You will need Adobe Reader installed on your computer and access to the Internet. If you normally submit your work as an output file, you will also need Microsoft XPS Document writer installed.

Case Study

After experiencing TIAs earlier in the month, Franklin Jones subsequently suffered a stroke and was admitted to an acute care hospital. He has been discharged from the hospital to the nursing home to meet his extended care needs, related to the residual effect of his recent stroke. Franklin has residual left-sided weakness, has difficulty swallowing, and is unable to grasp objects easily with his left hand. He still becomes short of breath with activity, but has no skin lesions. Franklin and his wife ran a family business before their retirement and he is accustomed to be independent and in control. Before his hospitalization he was the primary caregiver for his wife of 50 years who has been diagnosed with Alzheimer's disease.

Step 1

Start your web browser, go to the Online Student Resources web site, and log in.

Locate and click the link for Exercise 62.

You will need Adobe Reader. If your computer does not already have it, a link is provided on the browser tune-up web page to download and install it.

If you normally submit your work as an output file, you will also need Microsoft XPS Document Writer installed. If your computer does not already have it, a link is provided on the Exercise 62 web page to download and install it.

Step 2

When you are ready to proceed, locate and click the link for "MDS 3.0 RAI form."

The nursing home assessment form will be displayed in Adobe Reader.

If you wish to complete the steps below while you remain online, proceed to step 4.

If you wish to work offline, you can save a blank copy of the form by following the directions in step 3.

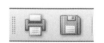

► **Figure 10-1 Print and Save icon button on the Adobe toolbar.**

Step 3

To save a blank copy of the form on your computer so that you can work offline, locate the Adobe toolbar and click on the "Save" button (shown on the right in Figure 10-1). The button icon resembles a computer disk. You can also save by clicking on word "File" on the menu bar. When a drop-down menu is displayed, click on "Save as . . ."

A warning dialog (shown in Figure 10-2) may appear to remind you that the copy does not save any data that you typed into your form.

Locate and click on the button within the dialog labeled "Save a Blank Copy."

A window will be displayed showing the folder where the file is being saved. Write down the folder name as you will need it in a moment.

When the file has been saved, you can close your browser.

Open the folder where the file was saved; locate the file named "MDS3.pdf" and double-click on it.

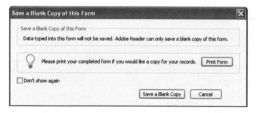

► **Figure 10-2 Save a Blank Copy warning that it does not save data.**

The form will open in Adobe Reader if that program has been installed on your computer.

Step 4

As discussed earlier, the complete assessment of a resident is a lengthy and detailed multiple disciplinary process. This form is 38 pages long; because you cannot save your work except by printing it, we are only going to complete the first 11 pages. You will then print your work or output it to an XPS file. Once you have your printout in hand, you will review the remaining pages of the form without entering data.

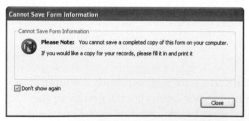

► **Figure 10-3 Cannot Save Form Information reminder.**

The first section of the form contains fields for identifying the facility. Normally, these fields would contain the nursing home ID numbers. We are going to usurp them for your student ID.

You can type directly into the boxes on the form. Locate and click your mouse on the first empty square in section A0100, field C, State Provider Number. The warning reminder shown in Figure 10-3 will be displayed.

The first time you type in the form you will receive a reminder that you cannot save the data you type into it. Locate and click on the check box labeled "Don't show again," to prevent this warning from being displayed again, and then click on the Close button.

Type your name or student ID in section A0100, field C. As you type, letters will appear in the next empty box. If your name or student ID is too long for field C, use additional fields A and B as directed by your instructor.

Step 5

The remaining items on this page are completed by typing a code into boxes in the left column. Where there are two adjacent boxes, you must enter a two-digit code—for example, 01 not 1.

Enter codes into the white boxes for the sections of the form indicated below by clicking on the box and typing the number listed in the left column:

1	A0200 A Type of Provider 1. Nursing home (SNF/NF)
01	A0310.A Federal OBRA Reason for Assessment 01. Admission Assessment (required by day 14)
01	A0310.B PPS Assessment 01. 5-day scheduled assessment
0	A0310.C PPS Other Medicare Required Assessment - OMRA 0. No
1	A0310.E Is this assessment the first assessment since the most recent admission? 1. Yes
01	A0310.F Entry Discharge reporting 01. Entry Record

When you have verified that your entries are correct, scroll the form downward to page 2 of the form.

Step 6

The second page contains demographic information about the resident.

As you have done on the previous page, enter codes into the white boxes in the left column; where a name or ID is required, type text into the appropriate boxes on the form using the information printed in bold below:

3	A0410.A Submission Requirement 3. Federal required submission
	Legal Name of Resident A0500.A First Name **Franklin** A0500.C Last Name **Jones**
	A0600.A Social Security number **999-99-9999** A0600.B Medicare number **999-99-9999B**
1	A0800. Gender 1. Male
	A0900 Birth Date **02 28 1935**
☒	A1000. Race/Ethnicity C. Black or African American
0	A1100.A Does the resident need or want an interpreter to communicate with a doctor or healthcare staff? 0. No

When you have verified that your entries are correct, scroll the form downward to page 3 of the form.

Step 7

The third page continues demographic and admission information about the resident.

As you have done on the previous pages, enter codes into the white boxes in the left column; where a name or ID is required, type text into the appropriate boxes on the form using the information printed in bold below:

2	A1200 Marital Status 2. Married
	Optional Resident Items A1300.A Medical record number **380001** A1300.D Lifetime occupation(s) **Businessman**
0	A1500. Preadmission Screening and Resident Review (PASRR) Has the resident been evaluated by Level II PASRR and determined to have a serious mental illness and/or mental retardation or a related condition? 0. No
	A1600 Entry Date **05 25 2012**
1	A1700. Type of Entry 1. Admission

When you have verified that your entries are correct, scroll the form downward to page 4 of the form.

Step 8

The fourth page requires only one item. Mr. Jones was admitted following his discharge from an acute care hospital.

03	A1800 Entered From 3. Acute hospital

Verify that your entry is correct and scroll the form downward to page 5 of the form.

Step 9

The fifth page begins the nursing assessment about the resident.

Case Study

Franklin is awake and responsive, although he tires easily. Upon his arrival, he was wearing glasses and hearing aids, which are effective in correcting any sensory deficits. Following his stroke, his speech continues to be somewhat slurred and he sometimes struggles to find words to finish his thoughts. He usually comprehends conversations with a minimal assistance.

As you have done on the previous pages, enter codes into the white boxes in the left column of the form using the information below:

0	B0100 Comatose 0. No
1	B0200 Hearing 1. Minimal difficulty
1	B0300. Hearing Aid 1. Yes
1	B0600 Speech Clarity 1. Unclear speech (slurred or mumbled words)
1	B0700. Makes Self Understood 1. Usually understood - difficulty communicating some words or finishing thoughts but is able if prompted or given time
1	B0800 Ability to Understand Others 1. Usually understands - misses some part/intent of message but comprehends most conversation
0	B1000 Vision 0. Adequate
1	B1200 Corrective Lenses 1. Yes

When you have verified that your entries are correct, scroll the form downward to page 6 of the form.

Step 10

The nurse performs a mental status exam and documents it on the sixth page.

As you have done on the previous pages, enter codes into the white boxes in the left column of the form using the information below:

1	C0100. Should Brief Interview for Mental Status be Conducted? 1. Yes
2	C0200. Repetition of Three Words. 2. Two
3	C0300.A. Able to report correct year. 3. Correct
2	C0300.B. Able to report correct month 2. Accurate within 5 days
1	C0300.C. Able to report correct day of the week 1. Correct
1	C0400.A. Able to recall "sock". 1. Yes, after cueing ("something to wear")
1	C0400.B. Able to recall "blue". 1. Yes, after cueing ("a color")
2	C0400.C. Able to recall "bed". 2. Yes, no cue required
	C0500. Summary Score. Add and fill in total score (00-15).

When you have verified that your entries are correct, sum the resident's scores for questions C0200 to C0400 (do not include C0100). Type your answer into the two boxes in the left column at the bottom of page 6. Scroll the form downward to page 7 of the form.

Step 11

Because Mr. Jones was able to complete the interview for mental status, enter a 0 in the first field.

0	C0600. Should the Staff Assessment for Mental Status be Conducted? 0. No (resident was able to complete interview)

Verify that your entry is correct and then scroll downward to section C1300, Signs and Symptoms of Delirium.

Case Study

Over the course of the last 5 days in the facility Franklin Jones has remained alert and oriented, but demonstrated trouble concentrating on the task at hand. He was easily distracted but responded well to cueing. Although he is able to participate in conversation, he often exhibits an inability to find the word to finish his thoughts and requires some prompting to create coherent sentences.

In this portion of the form, the selection of codes the nurse is to use is in the left column and the white boxes are in the center column of the form. The same three codes: 0, 1 or 2 are used for each of the questions C1300.A to C1300.D. To complete this section, the staff member must review the resident's status over the previous 5 days. To better understand the answers, read the full text of the questions in the PDF form as you enter the data. Enter the nurse's assessment using the information below:

1	C1300.A Inattention 1. Behavior continuously present, does not fluctuate.
2	C1300.B Disorganized thinking 2. Behavior present, fluctuates
0	C1300.C Altered level of consciousness 0. Behavior not present.
0	C1300.D Psychomotor retardation 0. Behavior not present.
0	C1600. Acute Onset Mental Status Change. 0. No

When you have verified that your entries are correct, scroll the form downward to page 8 of the form.

Step 12

The eighth page is used to record the resident's mood interview.

Case Study

Within the last 2 weeks Mr. Jones has seemed sad and frustrated. He has eaten well and slept through the night, but consistently demonstrated a reluctance to participate in any activities with the other residents or show any interest in TV or current events. He becomes easily discouraged with his limitations and exhibits anger at himself when he can't express his ideas or complete independent tasks. He has repeatedly verbalized to the nurse aide that he felt useless and didn't want to live any longer. Despite his reactions to his disabilities, he has been cooperative with staff and shown no signs of aggressive behavior.

1	D0100. Should Resident Mood Interview be Conducted? 1. Yes

The format for questions in section D0200 is different in several ways. The interview questions are on the left and the code for the answer is entered to the right of it. Additionally, for each question the resident answers in the affirmative, the nurse asks, "About how often have you been bothered by this?" The resident's response is entered in a box in the Symptom Frequency column of the form. If a resident is non-responsive to a question, a 9 is entered in the Symptom Presence column and the Symptom Frequency column is left blank.

As you read the questions on the form, enter the resident's answers given below. If the resident's response is "0 No," then enter a 0 in both columns. If the resident's response is "1 Yes," then type the value provided in the table below in the Symptom Frequency column.

D0200. Resident Mood Interview	Symptom Presence	Symptom Frequency
A. Little interest or pleasure in doing things. 1. Yes, Frequency: 3.	1	3
B. Feeling down, depressed, or hopeless. 1. Yes, Frequency: 2.	1	2
C. Trouble falling or staying asleep, or sleeping too much. 0. No, Frequency: 0.	0	0
D. Feeling tired or having little energy. 1. Yes, Frequency: 1.	1	3
E. Poor appetite or overeating. 0. No, Frequency: 0.	0	0
F. Feeling bad about yourself - or that you are a failure or have let yourself or your family down. 1. Yes, Frequency: 3.	1	3
G. Trouble concentrating on things, such as reading the newspaper or watching television. 1. Yes, Frequency: 1.	1	1
H. Moving or speaking so slowly that other people could have noticed. Or the opposite - being so fidgety or restless that you have been moving around a lot more than usual. 0. No, Frequency: 0.	0	0
I. Thoughts that you would be better off dead, or of hurting yourself in some way. 1. Yes, Frequency: 1.	1	1

When you have completed questions D0200.A to D0200.I, sum the numbers in the "Symptom Frequency" column to calculate his Total Severity score. Enter your answer in the boxes for field D0300. Complete box D0350 as shown below.

	D0300. Total Severity Score. Add scores for all frequency responses in Column 2.
1	D0350. Was responsible staff or provider informed that there is a potential for resident self harm? 1. Yes

When you have verified that your entries are correct, scroll the form downward to page 10 of the form. (The ninth page is being skipped because it is only used in cases where a resident's mood interview cannot be conducted.)

Step 13

The tenth and eleventh pages are used to assess behavior. Using what you have learned so far and the information provided below, complete the tenth and eleventh pages.

Z	E0100. Psychosis (Check all that apply) Z. None of the above.
0	E0200.A. Physical behavioral symptoms directed toward others 0. Behavior not exhibited
0	E0200.B. Verbal behavioral symptoms directed toward others 0. Behavior not exhibited
0	E0200.C. Other behavioral symptoms not directed toward others 0. Behavior not exhibited
0	E0300. Were any behavioral symptoms in questions E0200 coded 1, 2, or 3? 0. No (skip to section E0800)
0	E0800. Did the resident reject evaluation or care (that is necessary to achieve the resident's goals for health and well-being? 0. Behavior not exhibited
0	E0900. Has the resident wandered? 0. Behavior not exhibited (skip to section E1100)
3	E1100. How does resident's current behavior status, care rejection, or wandering compare to prior assessment (OBRA or PPS)? 3. N/A because no prior MDS assessment.

Verify that your entries are correct.

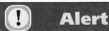
Alert

Do not close your browser or exit Adobe Reader until you have your printed RAI document in your hand. **You will lose your work if you exit before printing.**

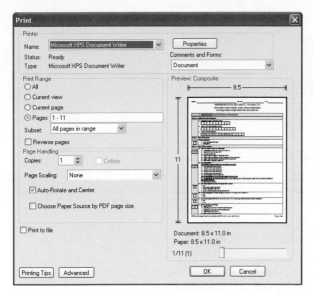

▶ **Figure 10-4 Printer dialog, showing XPS printer selected and a range of pages 1 to 11.**

Step 14

Print out or export an XPS file, as directed by your instructor.

Locate and click the button with a printer icon in the Adobe toolbar shown earlier in Figure 10-1. A printer dialog window similar to Figure 10-4 will be displayed.

Locate the section of the window labeled "Print Range." Locate and click on the circle next to the word "Pages." In the field next to it, type **1 - 11**, as shown in Figure 10-4. This will limit the printing to only the first 11 pages.

If you are printing to a printer, locate and click on the button labeled OK and then proceed to step 16.

If you are printing to a file proceed to step 15.

Step 15

Print to an XPS file:

If your instructor has directed you to print to a file, locate and click on the down arrow button in the field at the top of the window labeled "Name." A list of printers on your computer will be displayed.

Locate and click on "Microsoft XPS Document Writer" in the list. (You installed this in step 1.)

Locate and click on the button labeled OK.

A "Save File" window will be displayed. When this window appears, locate the field labeled "File Name" and type your name or student ID in it; then click on the button labeled "Save."

Step 16

When your RAI document has printed or your XPS file has been saved, give your work to your instructor. A sample of the first page of the printout is shown in Figure 10-5.

Step 17

Review the remaining pages of the MDS 3.0 RAI form, studying the type of information being gathered in the resident assessment.

If there is not sufficient class time remaining to complete your review of the form, your instructor may assign it as homework. You can access the form again anytime by following the instructions in steps 1 and 2 of this exercise.

Step 18

Scroll the PDF through the remaining pages of the MDS 3.0 RAI form and study each section. Information about the purpose of each section is contained within the form.

▶ Section F. Preferences for Customary Routine and Activities.

▶ Section G. Functional Status.

▶ Section H. Bladder and Bowel.

▶ Section I. Active Diagnoses.

▶ Section J. Health Conditions.

▶ Section K. Swallowing/Nutritional Status.

▶ Section L. Oral/Dental Status.

▶ Section M. Skin Conditions.

▶ Section N. Medications.

▶ Section O. Special Treatments, Procedures, and Programs.

▶ Section P. Restraints.

▶ Section Q. Participation in Assessment and Goal Setting.

▶ Section V. Care Area Assessment (CAA) Summary.

▶ Section X. Correction Request.

▶ Section Z. Assessment Administration.

When you have completed your review, you may close the form without printing, unless otherwise directed by your instructor.

▶ **Figure 10-5 Sample page of printed MDS 3.0 RAI form.**

Resident _____ Identifier _____ Date _____

MINIMUM DATA SET (MDS) - Version 3.0
RESIDENT ASSESSMENT AND CARE SCREENING
Nursing Home Comprehensive (NC) Item Set

Section A	Identification Information

A0100. Facility Provider Numbers

A. National Provider Identifier (NPI):

☐☐☐☐☐☐☐☐☐☐

B. CMS Certification Number (CCN):

☐☐☐☐☐☐☐☐☐☐☐☐

C. State Provider Number:

| T | e | r | r | y | | J | o | n | e | s | | | |

A0200. Type of Provider

Enter Code [1]

Type of provider
1. **Nursing home (SNF/NF)**
2. **Swing Bed**

A0310. Type of Assessment

Enter Code [0][1]

A. Federal OBRA Reason for Assessment
01. **Admission** assessment (required by day 14)
02. **Quarterly** review assessment
03. **Annual** assessment
04. **Significant change in status** assessment
05. **Significant correction** to **prior comprehensive** assessment
06. **Significant correction** to **prior quarterly** assessment
99. **Not OBRA required** assessment

Enter Code [0][1]

B. PPS Assessment
PPS Scheduled Assessments for a Medicare Part A Stay
01. **5-day** scheduled assessment
02. **14-day** scheduled assessment
03. **30-day** scheduled assessment
04. **60-day** scheduled assessment
05. **90-day** scheduled assessment
06. **Readmission/return** assessment
PPS Unscheduled Assessments for a Medicare Part A Stay
07. **Unscheduled assessment used for PPS** (OMRA, significant or clinical change, or significant correction assessment)
Not PPS Assessment
99. **Not PPS** assessment

Enter Code [0]

C. PPS Other Medicare Required Assessment - OMRA
0. **No**
1. **Start of therapy** assessment
2. **End of therapy** assessment
3. **Both Start and End of therapy** assessment

Enter Code [ ]

D. Is this a Swing Bed clinical change assessment? Complete only if A0200 = 2
0. **No**
1. **Yes**

Enter Code [1]

E. Is this assessment the first assessment (OBRA, PPS, or Discharge) **since the most recent admission?**
0. **No**
1. **Yes**

Enter Code [0][1]

F. Entry/discharge reporting
01. **Entry** record
10. **Discharge** assessment-**return not anticipated**
11. **Discharge** assessment-**return anticipated**
12. **Death in facility** record
99. **Not entry/discharge** record

Guided Exercise 63: Assessing Functional Status

In this exercise you will complete three additional sections of the MDS 3.0 RAI data set using the Student Edition software instead of the PDF form. These are Section G. Functional Status, which includes activities of daily living, bathing, balance during transitions and walking, functional limitation in range of motion, mobility devices, and functional limitation potential; Section H. Bladder and Bowel; and Section I. Active Diagnoses.

Case Study

Franklin was ambulatory with the use of a walker in the halls and his room, requiring limited assistance to manage turning corners or maneuvering around doorways and furniture. Because of his weakened left side, he has some difficulty rising from a sitting position to a standing position and has required supervision or minor assistance to manage these transitions safely. Because he is right-handed, he has managed his personal hygiene, fed and dressed himself, requiring only assistance with cutting his food and managing some clothing items such as tying his shoes. He has been continent for both bladder and bowel and has no evidence of constipation. His appetite has remained good.

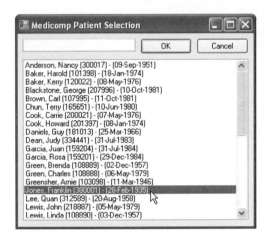

▶ **Figure 10-6 Select Patient Franklin Jones.**

Step 1

If you have not already done so, start the Student Edition software.

Click Select on the Menu bar, and then click Patient.

In the Patient Selection window, locate and click on **Franklin Jones** as shown in Figure 10-6.

Step 2

Click Select on the Menu bar, and then click New Encounter.

Select the reason **Initial Chart Entry-Existing Patient** from the drop-down list. You may use the current date.

Step 3

Locate and click on the Forms button in the Toolbar at the top of your screen, as you have done in previous exercises.

Select the form labeled "Partial MDS 3.0" as shown in Figure 10-7.

The form (shown later in Figure 10-8) will be displayed. You will notice that it has three tabs labeled "Functional Status," "Bladder and Bowel," and "Active Diagnoses." These tabs allow you to record findings that correspond to sections G, H, and I of the PDF form you reviewed in Exercise 62. The Partial MDS 3.0 form was created just for this exercise. The Student Edition software does not contain the entire MDS 3.0 form.

The first tab contains the different portions of Section G. Functional Status. The left column is used to report the resident's performance of ADL. Numerical codes are entered into two value fields: the first field codes the

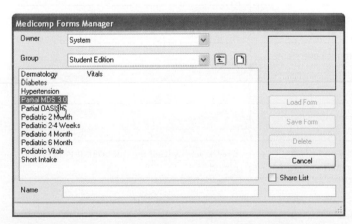

▶ **Figure 10-7 Select Partial MDS 3.0 in the Form Manager.**

▶ **Figure 10-8 Functional Status tab of the Partial MDS 3.0 form.**

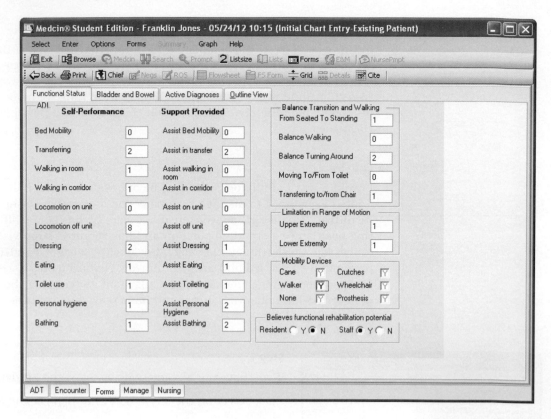

resident's ability to perform the activity, and the second field codes the level of support provided by the staff. The codes are defined as follows:

ADL Self-Performance Codes	ADL Support Provided Codes
When Activity Occurred 3 or More Times:	*Code for Most Support Provided Over All Shifts:*
0. Independent no help or staff oversight at any time.	0. No setup or physical help from staff.
1. Supervision—oversight, encouragement or cueing.	1. Setup help only.
2. Limited assistance—resident highly involved in activity; staff provides guided maneuvering of limbs or other nonweight-bearing assistance.	2. One person physical assist.
3. Extensive assistance—resident involved in activity, staff provide weight-bearing support.	3. Two or more persons physically assist.
4. Total dependence—full staff performance every time during entire 7-day period.	
Activity Occurred 2 or Fewer Times:	
7. Activity occurred only once or twice—activity did occur but only once or twice.	
8. Activity did not occur—activity (or any part of the ADL) was not performed by resident or staff.	8. ADL activity itself did not occur during entire period.

When coding ADL, the nurse follows the "rule of 3" to code the most dependent level. For example, if while dressing the resident required extensive assistance three times and limited assistance three times, the nurse would code extensive assistance (3).

> ### Rule of 3

▶ When an activity occurs three times at any one given level, code that level.

▶ When an activity occurs three times at multiple levels, code the most dependent level. Exceptions are:

 ▶ Total dependence (4)—activity must require full assist every time.

 ▶ Activity did not occur (8)—activity must not have occurred at all.

▶ When an activity occurs at various levels, but not three times at any given level, apply the following:

 ▶ When there is a combination of full staff performance and extensive assistance, code extensive assistance.

 ▶ When there is a combination of full staff performance, weight-bearing assistance, and/or nonweight-bearing assistance code limited assistance (2).

If none of the above are met, code supervision (1).

Step 4

Following the "rule of 3," the nurse records the following information about the resident's self-performance and the support provided:

Activity of Daily Living	Self-Performance Code	Support Code
Bed mobility—how resident moves to and from lying position, turns side to side, and positions body while in bed or alternate sleep furniture.	0	0
Transfer—how resident moves between surfaces including to or from: bed, chair, wheelchair, standing position (excludes to/from bath/toilet).	2	2
Walk in room—how resident walks between locations in his/her room.	1	0
Walk in corridor—how resident walks in corridor on unit.	1	0
Locomotion on unit—how resident moves between locations in his/her room and adjacent corridor on same floor. If in wheelchair, self-sufficiency once in chair.	0	0
Locomotion off unit—how resident moves to and returns from off-unit locations (e.g., areas set aside for dining, activities, or treatments). If facility has only one floor, how resident moves to and from distant areas on the floor. If in wheelchair, self-sufficiency once in chair.	8	8
Dressing—how resident puts on, fastens, and takes off all items of clothing, including donning/removing a prosthesis or TED hose. Dressing includes putting on and changing pajamas and housedresses.	2	1
Eating—how resident eats and drinks, regardless of skill. Do not include eating/drinking during medication pass. Includes intake of nourishment by other means (e.g., tube feeding, total parenteral nutrition, IV fluids administered for nutrition or hydration).	1	1
Toilet use—how resident uses the toilet room, commode, bedpan, or urinal; transfers on/off toilet; cleanses self after elimination; changes pad; manages ostomy or catheter; and adjusts clothes. Do not include emptying of bedpan, urinal, bedside commode, catheter bag, or ostomy bag.	1	1

Personal hygiene—how resident maintains personal hygiene, including combing hair, brushing teeth, shaving, applying makeup, washing/drying face and hands (excluding baths and showers).	1	2
Bathing—how resident takes full-body bath/shower, sponge bath, and transfers in/out of tub/shower (excludes washing of back and hair). Note: does not follow rule of 3; code 0–4 for most dependent in self-performance and support or 8, did not occur.	1	2

Step 5

After observing the resident's balance during walking and transition, the nurse enters codes for the highest level of support that the resident required.

In this step, you will determine what value to enter using the following codes:

Codes for Balance
0. Steady at all times.
1. Not steady, but able to stabilize without human assistance.
2. Not steady, only able to stabilize with human assistance.
8. Activity did not occur.

Select the appropriate code from the list and enter it in the section of the form labeled "Balance Transition and Walking" for each of the following items:

☐ Moving from sitting to standing position Mr. Jones was unsteady, but able to stabilize himself.

☐ Walking (with assistive device) Mr. Jones was steady.

☐ Turning around and facing the opposite direction while walking, required someone to assist him.

☐ Moving on and off toilet he was steady every time.

☐ Surface-to-surface transfer (transfer between bed and chair or wheelchair) he was unsteady, but able to do it himself.

Step 6

The next section records any Functional Limitation in Range of Motion that interfered with daily functions or placed resident at risk of injury using the following codes:

Codes for Limitation
0. No impairment.
1. Impairment on one side.
2. Impairment on both sides.

Mr. Jones's stroke has left him with a partial paralysis on his left side. Select the correct code for Mr. Jones and enter it in the Limitation In Range of Motion fields:

☐ Upper Extremity

☐ Lower Extremity

Step 7

Mr. Jones is currently using a mobility device to get around. Click on the check box next to "Walker."

Step 8

For the last section on this tab, Functional Rehabilitation Potential, two questions are used to record the opinion of the resident and the staff as to whether the resident will be able to increase independence in at least some activities of daily living. You will recall from the case study that Mr. Jones is experiencing despair over his condition; therefore he does not believe he is going to improve. However, his direct care staff believes he is capable of improvement.

In the PDF form, codes are used for Yes and No; on the computer form, Y and N radio buttons are used. The full questions are:

Resident believes he or she is capable of increased independence in at least some ADLs. Yes, No, or Unable to determine.

- Click on the circle next to the **N**

Direct care staff believe resident is capable of increased independence in at least some ADLs. Yes or No.

- Click on the circle next to the **Y**

Compare your screen to Figure 10-8.

► Figure 10-9 Bladder and
Bowel tab of the Partial MDS
3.0 form.

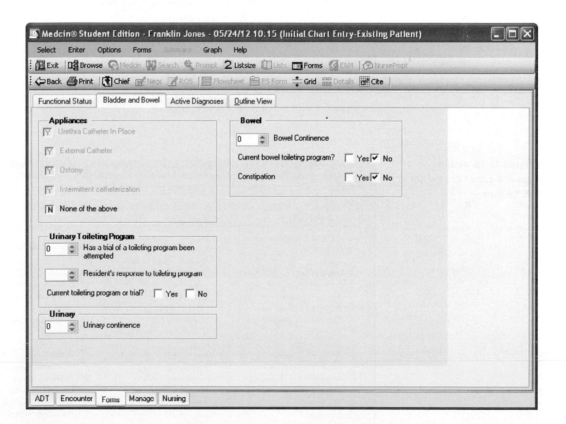

Step 9

Click on the tab at the top of the form labeled "Bladder and Bowel." The items on this tab are found in Section H of the PDF form; they are used to record data about the resident's urinary and bowel continence and whether that resident has a catheter or ostomy appliance. The onscreen findings are slightly abbreviated to fit the screen. The full text of a question is provided below where necessary. Complete the form using the information below. Where a code is used, enter the number printed in bold.

Appliances

✓   **N** None of the Above

Urinary Toileting Program

Has a trial of a toileting program (e.g., scheduled toileting, prompted voiding, or bladder training) been attempted on admission/reentry or since urinary incontinence was noted in this facility?

0 No Skip to H0300, Urinary Continence

Urinary Continence

0 Always continent.

Bowel Continence

0 Always continent.

Bowel Toileting Program

Is a toileting program currently being used to manage the resident's bowel continence?

✓   No

Bowel Patterns

Constipation present?

✓   No

Compare your screen to Figure 10-9.

▶ **Figure 10-10 Active Diagnoses tab of the Partial MDS 3.0 form.**

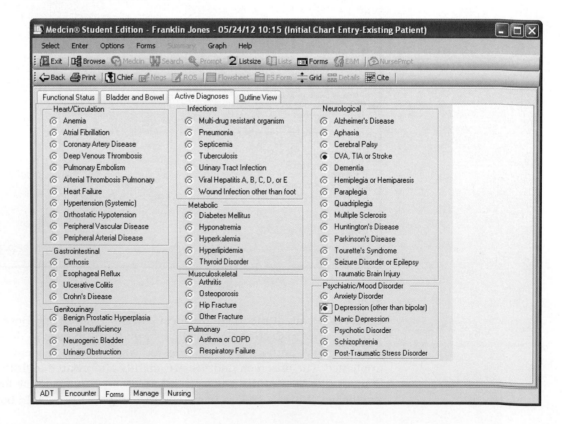

Step 10

Click on the tab at the top of the form labeled "Active Diagnoses." This tab is used to record all diagnoses that the resident had in the last seven days. In many cases a single item on the MDS 3.0 form represents multiple diagnoses and does not represent a particular ICD-9-CM diagnosis. For example, the form has one entry representing three different diagnoses: cerebrovascular accident (CVA), transient ischemic attack (TIA), and stroke.

Mr. Jones was transferred from the hospital after a TIA and resulting stroke.

Clicking on the circle next to a diagnosis will turn the button red and record the finding. Locate and click on the following diagnoses for Mr. Jones:

- CVA, TIA, or Stroke
- Depression (other than bipolar disorder)

Compare your screen to Figure 10-10.

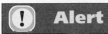

Alert

Remain on the Form tab, during printing. Do not change tabs or exit the program until you have a printed copy in your hand. You will lose your work if you exit before printing.

▶ **Figure 10-11 Print Data window with three forms selected for printing.**

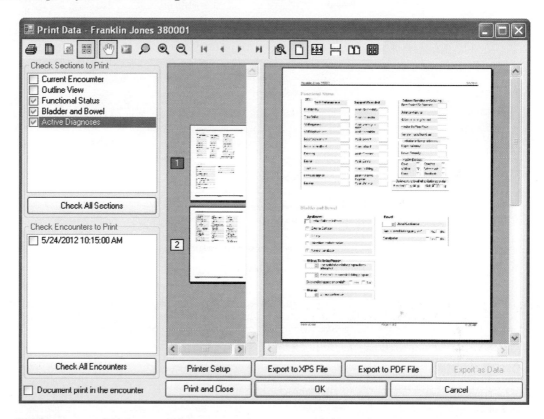

Step 11

In this step you are going to print the form pages. To do this, remain on the form tab and click on the Print button on the Toolbar at the top of your screen to invoke the Print Data window.

When the Print Data window is displayed, do not check the "Current Encounter" box. Instead, check the boxes next to:

✓ Functional Status

✓ Bladder and Bowel

✓ Active Diagnoses

Compare your screen to Figure 10-11, and then click on the appropriate button to either print or export a file, as directed by your instructor.

Compare your printout or file output to Figure 10-12. If there are any differences, review the previous steps in the exercise and find your error. When it is correct, hand it in to your instructor.

▶ **Figure 10-12a Printed RAI Form for Franklin Jones (page 1 of 2).**

Functional Status

ADL

	Self-Performance		Support Provided	
Bed Mobility	0	Assist Bed Mobility	0
Transferring	2	Assist in transfer	2
Walking in room	1	Assist walking in room	0
Walking in corridor	1	Assist in corridor	0
Locomotion on unit	0	Assist on unit	0
Locomotion off unit	8	Assist off unit	8
Dressing	2	Assist Dressing	1
Eating	1	Assist Eating	1
Toilet use	1	Assist Toileting	1
Personal hygiene	1	Assist Personal Hygiene	2
Bathing	1	Assist Bathing	2

Balance Transition and Walking

From Seated To Standing	1
Balance Walking	0
Balance Turning Around	2
Moving To/From Toilet	0
Transferring to/from Chair	1

Limitation in Range of Motion

Upper Extremity	1
Lower Extremity	1

Mobility Devices

Cane	Y	Crutches	Y
Walker	Y	Wheelchair	Y
None	Y	Prosthesis	Y

Believes functional rehabilitation potential
Resident ○ Y ● N   Staff ● Y ○ N

Bladder and Bowel

Appliances

- Y Urethra Catheter In Place
- Y External Catheter
- Y Ostomy
- Y Intermittent catheterization
- N None of the above

Urinary Toileting Program

0 Has a trial of a toileting program been attempted

[ ] Resident's response to toileting program

Current toileting program or trial? ☐ Yes ☐ No

Urinary

0 Urinary continence

Bowel

0 Bowel Continence

Current bowel toileting program? ☐ Yes ☑ No

Constipation ☐ Yes ☑ No

▶ **Figure 10-12b Printed RAI Form for Franklin Jones (page 2 of 2).**

Active Diagnoses

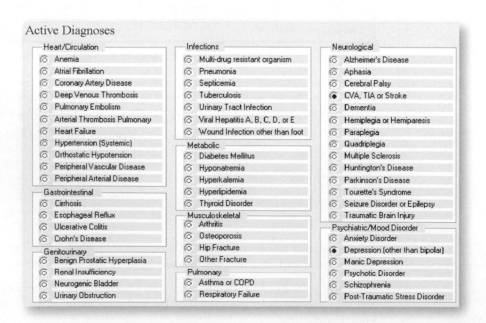

Heart/Circulation
- ⊙ Anemia
- ⊙ Atrial Fibrillation
- ⊙ Coronary Artery Disease
- ⊙ Deep Venous Thrombosis
- ⊙ Pulmonary Embolism
- ⊙ Arterial Thrombosis Pulmonary
- ⊙ Heart Failure
- ⊙ Hypertension (Systemic)
- ⊙ Orthostatic Hypotension
- ⊙ Peripheral Vascular Disease
- ⊙ Peripheral Arterial Disease

Gastrointestinal
- ⊙ Cirrhosis
- ⊙ Esophageal Reflux
- ⊙ Ulcerative Colitis
- ⊙ Crohn's Disease

Genitourinary
- ⊙ Benign Prostatic Hyperplasia
- ⊙ Renal Insufficiency
- ⊙ Neurogenic Bladder
- ⊙ Urinary Obstruction

Infections
- ⊙ Multi-drug resistant organism
- ⊙ Pneumonia
- ⊙ Septicemia
- ⊙ Tuberculosis
- ⊙ Urinary Tract Infection
- ⊙ Viral Hepatitis A, B, C, D, or E
- ⊙ Wound Infection other than foot

Metabolic
- ⊙ Diabetes Mellitus
- ⊙ Hyponatremia
- ⊙ Hyperkalemia
- ⊙ Hyperlipidemia
- ⊙ Thyroid Disorder

Musculoskeletal
- ⊙ Arthritis
- ⊙ Osteoporosis
- ⊙ Hip Fracture
- ⊙ Other Fracture

Pulmonary
- ⊙ Asthma or COPD
- ⊙ Respiratory Failure

Neurological
- ⊙ Alzheimer's Disease
- ⊙ Aphasia
- ⊙ Cerebral Palsy
- ● CVA, TIA or Stroke
- ⊙ Dementia
- ⊙ Hemiplegia or Hemiparesis
- ⊙ Paraplegia
- ⊙ Quadriplegia
- ⊙ Multiple Sclerosis
- ⊙ Huntington's Disease
- ⊙ Parkinson's Disease
- ⊙ Tourette's Syndrome
- ⊙ Seizure Disorder or Epilepsy
- ⊙ Traumatic Brain Injury

Psychiatric/Mood Disorder
- ⊙ Anxiety Disorder
- ● Depression (other than bipolar)
- ⊙ Manic Depression
- ⊙ Psychotic Disorder
- ⊙ Schizophrenia
- ⊙ Post-Traumatic Stress Disorder

Real-Life Story

A Nurse's Experiences with MDS in Nursing Homes

By Xiaoqiu Hu RN, MSN

Xiaoqiu Hu is a registered nurse with a master's degree in nursing informatics. She has over 15 years experience in long-term care nursing and has in recent years set up a number of nursing homes on electronic records.

I think the move to electronic health records is coming to nursing homes. Larger corporations that operate many nursing facilities might implement more of the electronic chart, but smaller nursing homes (especially stand alone "mom and pop" shops) will at least have some computerization, even if they don't have a complete electronic chart.

I was recently involved in implementing an electronic charting system in three nursing homes. In those facilities we had mobile computers and encouraged all the MDS nurses and social workers to take one of the mobile computers to a resident's room and chart while talking with the resident. Some of the employees were comfortable using the computer while conducting interview, but some still preferred to jot down notes on paper and enter the data in the computer later. Others felt like inputting data into the computer was more work. They wanted to just pull out a paper chart and use a pen. In the end, however, there are real advantages to electronic records. For one, the chart is more legible in electronic charts. In addition, the electronic chart is more accessible and easily shared.

In long-term care, everybody needs the chart: doctors, nurses, and managers. With electronic charts, you can access the data more efficiently, more quickly; this is especially true for the management team. It is very easy to query the report for diagnosis, medications, and incontinent status. When paper records were in use, you had to carry the residents' charts to the morning staff meeting. With electronic charts, all you need is a computer at the meeting. In our facility we have a projector in our conference room, so that everybody can see the chart as it is being discussed. It is very convenient.

One reason even small nursing homes will have computer systems is for MDS reporting. MDS, which has been around for about 20 years, must be electronically submitted to the state. This is a requirement of CMS. Even a small nursing home that can't afford a complete electronic chart, purchases a computer system for MDS and the financial parts of the business.

Even if a nursing home does use electronic charts, it frequently won't have a computer at the bedside of the resident. In that case the nurses and social workers use a notebook to interview and assess the resident on paper. On the floor, there is an ADL flow sheet, medication administration records, and treatment administration records. The charge nurse documents the resident's condition, and signs the treatment administration and the medication administration records. The nurses will sign the record for medications as these are administered. The nurses at my current facility record this information in our electronic system. At facilities without electronic charts, they collect this information on paper on the floor and then enter it into the computer later.

In the past, members of the care team also filled out the MDS forms on paper and gave them to the MDS coordinator to enter the data into a computer, so it could be submitted electronically. Now it is standard for each discipline's team members to enter their own data into the system because they also have to write a summary of the care area triggers and decisions made during the process to proceed to care planning.

Direct care to the residents provided by Geriatric Nursing Assistants (GNA) is documented on a flow sheet. The GNA documents the percentage of assistance with meals, ADL care, and so on, but the GNA does not enter data in the MDS system.

The ADL information is entered into the system by an MDS coordinator. The level of assistance that the resident requires may be coded as total, extensive assistance, limited assistance, with supervision, or independent. The challenge is to train the GNA to document the ADL in a manner consistent with the MDS.

To understand this problem better, take dressing for example. The definition of this ADL category includes a lot of activities: putting on shoes, putting on socks, putting on pants, putting on upper body dress. These activities are combined together and assigned one code. Perhaps the resident can put everything on personally, but that person can't tie his or her shoes. The GNA thinks "tying shoes is nothing." If I ask the GNA "How does the resident dress himself?" the GNA will respond "very independently, the resident can do everything but tie his shoes." But according to the MDS rule of three, if you have to tie the resident's shoes three or more times, the level should be coded as extensive, not independent.

Home Health Care

Home care involves a wide range of healthcare providers, including professionals such as registered nurses and therapists, paraprofessionals such as home health aides, and businesses known as durable medical equipment (DME) providers who supply oxygen, infusion pumps, beds, wheelchairs, and such to homebound clients. Here we are going to focus on the nurse's role in home care and will therefore not be covering DME or other providers except to discuss the nurse's role supervising or collaborating with other home care providers.

What these diverse types of home care providers have in common is that they are delivering care in a home setting instead of a medical facility, and that means they have little control over the healing environment. Contrast this with a nurse who works in an acute care hospital where:

▶ Safety and hygiene standards are the norm.

▶ Hospital rules govern visitors and pets.

▶ Response to a client in distress is only seconds away.

▶ A variety of medical, nursing, and ancillary support staff are available around the clock.

Although a registered nurse in both environments is responsible for developing the plan of care, in a home care setting the client's family members and supporting care givers are the ones who implement it. This puts the plan's outcomes beyond the nurse's control.

Home care clients may be recovering from an acute illness or injury; others maybe disabled or have a chronic condition. Although home health clients include children and adults, the elderly make up a larger portion of the client census. Traditionally, home care has followed discharge from an acute care hospital; however, there is an increase in use of home care to avoid hospitalization. Home care may be an effective way to avoid admission or readmission to the hospital.

Clients may be referred to home health providers by a physician, nurse, social worker, therapist, discharge planner, or even a family member. Families often initiate the process by directly approaching one of these referral sources or by directly contacting the home health agency. Home care cannot begin, however, without a physician's order and a physician-approved treatment plan. This is a legal and reimbursement requirement (Berman, Snyder, Krosier, & Erb, 2012).

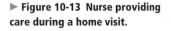

▶ **Figure 10-13 Nurse providing care during a home visit.**

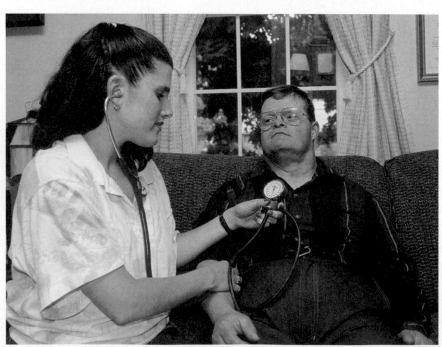

Home care is typically paid for by a third-party payer (Medicare, Medicaid, Blue Cross, or other health insurance plans). CMS has strict guidelines governing reimbursement. These include what data must be collected about the client's medical condition, health status, functional status and home environment, as well as a written treatment or care plan. Other payers tend to follow the CMS guidelines, or have similar requirements. In respect to documentation, like the registered nurse in a nursing home, a registered nurse at a home health agency has a similar obligation. Accurate and complete documentation is critical to the nurse's employer being paid for services; moreover, the nurse's documentation affects whether the client will be authorized for the level of care required.

Home Health Care Nursing

Home health care nurses are sometimes called "visiting nurses" for the obvious reason that they make "house calls." Most home health nurses work for a home health agency (HHA). Some agencies are owned by a hospital or large healthcare organization; others are companies that specialize in home health.

Home health agencies offer coordinated professional, skilled, and paraprofessional services. Because clients often require the services of several professionals, case coordination (case management) is essential. This responsibility generally rests with the registered nurse (Berman, et al., 2012).

Home health nurses work more independently than nurses in other settings, but in a sense they have greater responsibility as well. The registered nurse is not only responsible for reporting, coordinating home health aides, other care professionals, and all the required paperwork, but teaching is a critical part of their job. Because the delivery of care is going to be provided by a family member, neighbor, friend, or support person after the nurse leaves, education of the client and supporting caregivers takes on more importance than in other nursing settings.

Although home health nurses follow the same six steps of the nursing process discussed in Chapter 6, their assessment is not limited to their client, but includes identifying risks, dangers, hygiene, environmental concerns, or other issues that negatively affect care in the home. The home visit allows the nurse to become aware of client needs such as laundry, transportation, child or pet care and help the client find solutions.

The time the nurse has for a home care visit is limited, usually no longer than one hour. The interval between visits can be lengthy; this means the nursing process does not occur as quickly as it would in a healthcare facility. Still, many believe that clients' respond to care better in the familiar setting of their own home.

Home care nurses get to know the client's family as they are often the caregivers and support team that the nurse is training. In cases of particularly difficult or prolonged medical conditions, the nurse must also assess and provide support to family members who become stressed in the caregiver role.

As mentioned earlier, the larger portion of home care clients are elderly. This means that their caregiver may be a spouse of similar age. This can present challenges for the nurse educator as the spouse may have difficulties seeing or hearing, or may not be physically able to lift or assist the client.

The older age of home care clients also means that the majority of home care clients are covered by Medicare and therefore the home health agency must follow CMS rules called "condition of participation" which includes collecting and submitting required data within strict timelines. The home care data set required for that is called OASIS.

OASIS

Medicare-certified home health agencies are required to use a standard set of data items, known as OASIS (Outcome and Assessment Information Set), as part of a comprehensive assessment for all clients who are receiving skilled care that is reimbursed by Medicare or Medicaid. OASIS data are submitted by home health agencies to the States, and subsequently transmitted to the Centers for Medicare & Medicaid Services.

OASIS is a group of data elements that:

► Represent core items of a comprehensive assessment for an adult home care client

► Form the basis for measuring outcomes for purposes of outcome-based quality improvement (OBQI)

"The Outcome Assessment Information Set (OASIS) was developed by the Centers for Medicare & Medicaid Services (CMS) to set a standardized protocol for assessing the clinical characteristics of Home Health Agency (HHA) patients" (Centers for Medicare & Medicaid Services, 2010a, p.4).

Originating in 1999, OASIS has evolved over the last decade based on recommendations of the Institute of Medicine (IOM), National Quality Forum (NQF) and Medicare Payment Advisory Commission (MedPAC). The current version, OASIS-C, became required January 2010. The new version eliminated items not used for payment, quality measures, case mix, or risk adjustment, and added items to increase clarity in measurement and measure the processes of care. Several evidence-based screening tools and interventions that can be considered best practices in home health care were added to focus on high-risk, high-volume, problem-prone conditions in home health care. Data items were created to measure processes of care in the following domains:

► Date of referral and physician-ordered start of care (timeliness)

► Patient-specific parameters for physician notification (care coordination)

► Influenza and pneumococcal vaccines (population health and prevention)

► Formal pain assessment, pain interventions, and pain management steps (effectiveness of care)

► Pressure ulcer risk assessment, prevention measures, and use of moist healing principles (effective care and prevention)

► Diabetic foot care plan, education and monitoring (disease specific: high risk, high volume, problem prone)

► Heart failure symptoms of volume overload and follow-up (disease specific: high risk, high volume, problem prone)

► Depressive symptom screening and intervention/referral (influences self-management abilities)

► Falls risk assessment, planning, and interventions (safety)

► Medication adverse events/reaction, reconciliation and follow-up; drug education (high priority for safety—care coordination) (Centers for Medicare & Medicaid Services, 2010c)

There are particular time points at which this data must be gathered. These include:

► Start of care

► Resumption of care

► Resumption of care (after inpatient stay)

► Follow-up

► Recertification (follow-up) assessment

► Other follow-up assessment

► Transfer to an inpatient facility

► Transferred to an inpatient facility—patient not discharged from an agency

► Transferred to an inpatient facility—patient discharged from agency

► Discharge from agency—not to an inpatient facility (patient died or discharged from agency)

"Because most OASIS items describe patient health and functional status, they are useful in assessing the care needs of adult patients. HHAs will find it necessary to supplement the OASIS items in order to comprehensively assess the health status and care needs of their patients (for example, the OASIS does not include vital signs which are typically included in patient assessments)" (Centers for Medicare & Medicaid Services, n.d., *Using OASIS Items*).

The sections of OASIS are:

▶ Patient Tracking

▶ Clinical Record Items

▶ Patient History & Diagnoses

▶ Living Arrangements

▶ Sensory Status

▶ Integumentary Status

▶ Respiratory Status

▶ Cardiac Status

▶ Elimination Status

▶ Neuro/Emotional/Behavioral Status

▶ ADLs/IADLs

▶ Medications

▶ Care Management

▶ Therapy Need and Plan of Care

▶ Emergent Care

▶ Discharge/Transfer data

"These data form the basis for case-mix profile reports and outcome reports that are used by home health agencies for quality improvement and quality monitoring purposes and by state survey staff in the certification process. Home health agency quality measures that appear on the CMS Home Health Compare web site are also based on OASIS data, and the data are used for case-mix adjustment of per-episode payment (Centers for Medicare & Medicaid Services, n.d., *Oasis-Based Home Health Agency*).

Critical Thinking Exercise 64: OASIS-C Form for Head Injury with Residual Dementia

CMS makes available the HAVEN software program to home health agencies to enable the agencies to gather and report OASIS-C data electronically. Rather than have students learn a different software program at this point in the course, we have replicated several pages of HAVEN screens as a form in the Student Edition software. In this exercise you will review the client's case as a home care nurse and complete sections of the home visit assessment and determine the plan of care.

Case Study

Calvin Moore is a widowed 68 year old male who was recently discharged from the hospital, where he was treated for a head injury with residual dementia. Before his injury he was retired but living independently and competently managing his own affairs. Although his long-term prognosis for recovery is good, his discharge plan included Calvin staying with his granddaughter Denya Moore, as she is the only family living in the area. Denya is single and works during the day. At the time of discharge, Calvin's discharge plan included a referral to home care nursing to support his daily care, safety needs, and evaluate ongoing occupational therapy interventions. Because of his current dementia symptoms, Denya is concerned for his safety while she is at work. Denya participates in the interview with the home care nurse.

Step 1

If you have not already done so, start the Student Edition software.

Click Select on the Menu bar, and then click Patient.

In the Patient Selection window, locate and click on **Calvin Moore**.

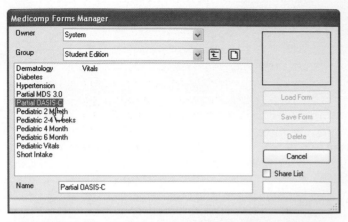

Step 2

Click Select on the Menu bar, and then click New Encounter.

Select the reason **Initial Chart Entry-Existing Patient** from the drop-down list. You may use the current date.

Step 3

Locate and click on the Forms button in the Toolbar at the top of your screen, as you have done in previous exercises.

Select the form labeled "Partial OASIS-C," as shown in Figure 10-14.

▶ **Figure 10-14 Select Partial OASIS-C in Form Manager.**

▶ **Figure 10-15 ADL/IADL tab of the Partial OASIS-C form (shown without data).**

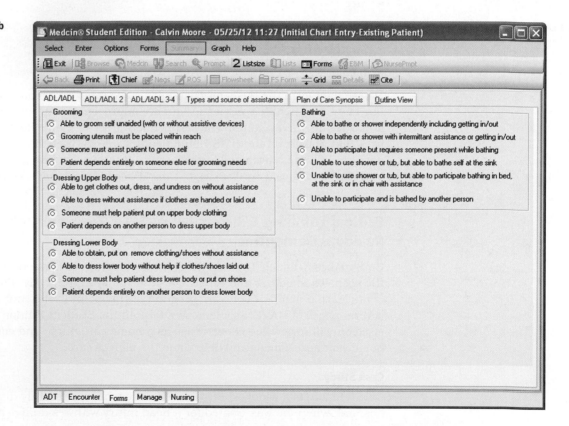

The form (shown in Figure 10-15) will be displayed. You will notice that it has three tabs labeled ADL/IADL, which are used to record activities of daily living. Two more tabs record the types and source of assistance available, and a plan of care synopsis. The Partial OASIS-C form was created just for this exercise and does not replicate all of the HAVEN screens.

Step 4

Read the following case information and determine how you would assess the client. Record your responses by clicking on a red button in each of the four sections. Note that this tab allows only one assessment in each section; to change an entry, simply click on a different red button in the same section.

Case Study

Mr. Moore is independent in his toileting needs, is ambulatory and transfers from bed to standing with no assistance needs. He is dressing himself, but Denya noticed he kept putting on the same clothes he wore on the previous day. She has started laying out clean clothes and removing the soiled clothes—this has helped. Denya tells the nurse that her grandfather had always been very fastidious in his appearance, but now doesn't shave unless she reminds him. Once reminded he completes the task using his electric razor. Denya also believes that he isn't bathing. He has body odor that is noticeable and she is certain he didn't bathe because she ran the water, but he never used the towel. Denya states that she would feel uncomfortable helping him with his bath beyond a reminder that it is bath time. He is continuing to exhibit mild confusion as to date and time and has poor short-term memory. He is easily distracted and forgetful. Denya doesn't feel he can safely participate in meal preparation and has been preparing his breakfast and supper. For lunch she leaves his a "packed" lunch that requires no cooking.

► **Figure 10-16 ADL 2 tab of the Partial OASIS-C form (shown without data).**

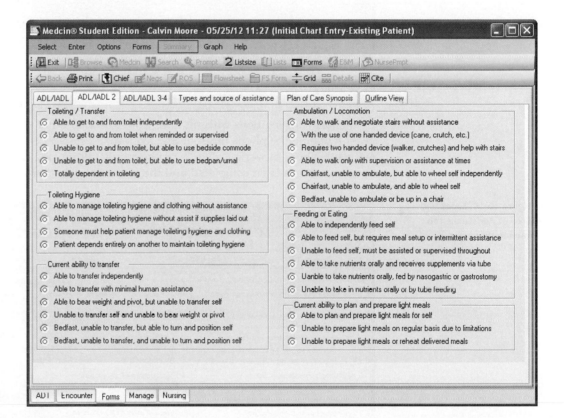

Step 5

Locate and click on the second tab, labeled "ADL/IADL 2." The form shown in Figure 10-16 will be displayed. Record your responses by clicking on a red button in each of the six sections, using the information from the case study in step 4.

Step 6

Locate and click on the third tab, labeled "ADL/IADL 3-4." The form shown in Figure 10-17 will be displayed.

Read the following case information and determine how you would assess the client. Record your responses by clicking on a red button in each of the six sections.

► **Figure 10-17 ADL 3-4 tab of the Partial OASIS-C form (shown without data).**

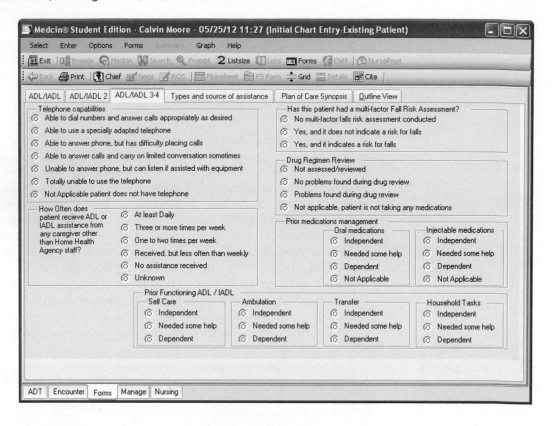

Case Study

Calvin's granddaughter worries because he will answer the telephone when it rings and hold short conversations with his son, who lives in another state, but he hasn't been successful dialing the phone himself. She fears that if he needed help, he wouldn't be able to call while she is at work. Calvin is not currently taking medications or injections. The fall assessment has been completed and the nurse believes there is a risk he could fall.

► **Figure 10-18 Types and Source of Assistance tab (shown without data).**

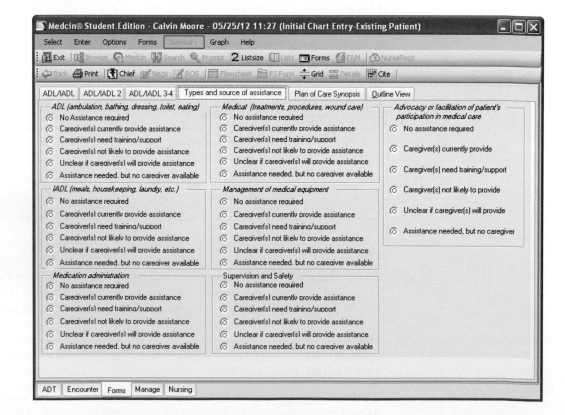

Step 7

Locate and click on the fourth tab, labeled "Types and Source of Assistance." The form shown in Figure 10-18 will be displayed.

Read the following case information and determine what data you would record and then click on the appropriate red button in each of the seven sections.

Case Study

Denya is not likely to give her grandfather a bath. She currently prepares his meals, and he does not use prescribed medications, treatments, or medical equipment and therefore does not require assistance in those areas. The nurse recommends further training for Denya concerning safety and fall prevention. Denya strongly encourages her grandfather's participation in his care.

▶ **Figure 10-19 Plan of Care Synopsis tab of the Partial OASIS-C form (shown with data).**

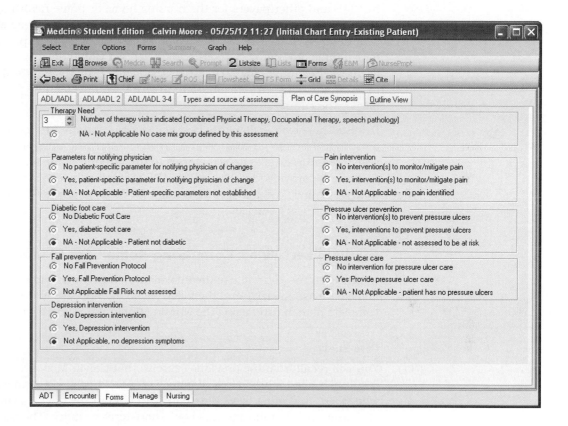

Step 8

Locate and click on the fifth tab, labeled "Plan of Care Synopsis." The form shown in Figure 10-19 will be displayed.

Read the following case information and determine what data you would record and then click on the appropriate red or blue button in each of the seven sections.

Case Study

Calvin needs his occupational therapy continued. He is authorized for three visits related to phone use, hygiene, and memory skills. He also needs an aide to assist with his bath. He is not diabetic nor on any pain medication. He does not have any pressure ulcers. His physician has not established parameters for notification.

When you have finished, compare your screen to Figure 10-19.

Alert

Remain on the Form tab during printing. *Do not change tabs or exit the program until you have a printed copy in your hand.* You will lose your work if you exit before printing.

Step 9

Print your completed encounter note, but remain on the Form tab. Click on the Print button on the Toolbar at the top of your screen to invoke the Print Data window.

Be certain there is a check mark in the box next to "Current Encounter" and then click on the appropriate button to either print or export a file, as directed by your instructor.

When your printing has completed and you have your printout or output file in hand, turn it into the instructor and exit the software.

Data the Nurse Needs

Thus far we have studied two standard instruments for collecting data about the resident or client, MDS 3.0 and OASIS-C. Each of these respective data sets are required by CMS and other payers for the nursing home or home health agency to get paid. However, these instruments represent the minimum data; they obviously do not represent detailed nurses' notes that would be useful for a nurse providing care. Vital signs, for example, are not part of either data set, yet would always be recorded by the nurse. In another example, the MDS 3.0 assessment of the resident's ability to dress does not differentiate between someone with arthritis who needs help tying his shoes and a paraplegic who cannot dress.

Despite this obvious disparity between what is gathered to meet regulatory requirements and what needs to be charted at every encounter, the nurse must do both. In particular, registered nurses are the signatories to the nursing home and home care documentation of care provided by CNA, LPN, LVN, and home health aides. In these settings more than any other, registered nurses must do their "paperwork" well or their clients may be denied necessary services.

Guided Exercise 65: Comparing Home Care Planning Data

In this exercise, you will use the information from the previous exercise case studies, your home care assessment, and the following additional case information to create a more complete plan of care, using the Nursing tab in the Student Edition.

Case Study

You will recall from the previous exercise that Calvin Moore, 68, has dementia as the result of a head injury. He is staying with his 23-year-old granddaughter Denya Moore, who works and must leave him alone throughout the day. Calvin exhibits mild confusion from time to time and has poor short-term memory. The nurse must provide clearly spoken directions and give the client ample time to communicate.

The nurse evaluates his memory, administers a mental status exam, and evaluates his ability to manage the home environment during the home care visit. The nurse plans to help the client set realistic goals and teach him to compensate for limitations, but believes he is at risk for a fall because of his confusion and lack of attention to his surroundings and plans to teach his granddaughter safety precautions. Calvin needs his occupational therapy continued. He is authorized for three visits related to phone use, hygiene, and memory skills. The nurse will coordinate his ongoing care and encourages Calvin to continue improving his activities of daily living as a means to restore his cognitive thought processes.

Denya is a willing participant in his care and the nurse encourages her. However, she tells the nurse she would be uncomfortable bathing her grandfather and so the nurse orders a weekly visit by a home health aide to bathe him. The nurse assesses his social network and invites Denya to call for advice or assistance in solving any additional problems.

▶ **Figure 10-20 Select Calvin Moore on the ADT tab.**

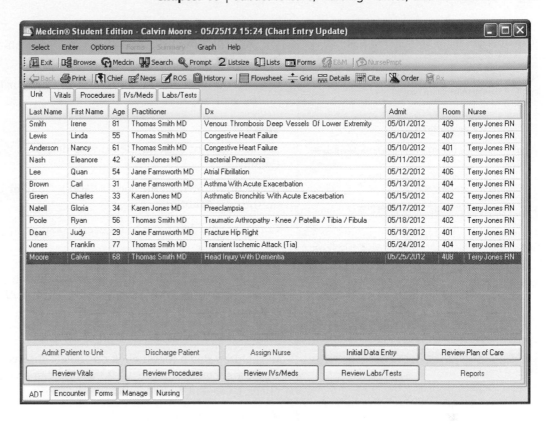

Step 1

If you have not already done so, start the Student Edition software.

Click Select on the ADT tab at the bottom of your screen.

Locate and click on **Calvin Moore** in the ADT tab, as shown in Figure 10-20.

Locate and click on the button labeled "Initial Data Entry."

Step 2

The nursing tab will automatically be displayed. (Ignore the fact that "Hospital Inpatient" is at the top of your screen; the type of encounter is not relevant to this exercise.)

Locate and click on the following nursing diagnoses in the left pane:

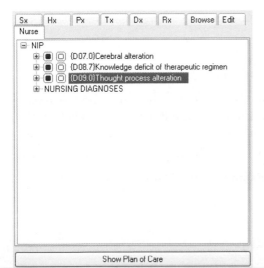

- ● (red button) RNDx Cerebral Alteration
- ● (red button) RNDx Knowledge deficit of therapeutic regimen
- ● (red button) RNDx Thought Process Alteration

▶ **Figure 10-21 Select Nursing Diagnoses.**

Compare your left pane to Figure 10-21.

Locate and click on the long button below the left pane labeled "Show Plan of Care."

Step 3

Now that the nursing diagnoses have been identified, the next phase in the nursing process is to identify an expected outcome for each of the nursing diagnoses.

Locate and right-click on the nursing diagnosis "Cerebral Alteration" in the left pane.

In the drop-down menu, locate "Add a Goal for this Diagnosis," and click on the goal **Stabilize**.

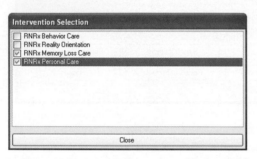

▶ **Figure 10-22 Expected outcome goals for Calvin Moore.**

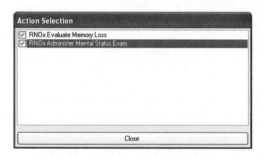

▶ **Figure 10-23 Interventions selected for cerebral alteration.**

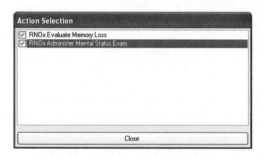

▶ **Figure 10-24 Actions selected for memory loss care.**

Step 4

Locate and right click on the nursing diagnosis "Knowledge Deficit of Therapeutic Regimen."

In the drop-down menu, locate "Add a Goal for this Diagnosis," and click on the goal **Improve**.

Step 5

Locate and right click on the nursing diagnosis "Thought Process Alteration Cognitive."

In the drop-down menu, locate "Add a Goal for this Diagnosis," and click on the goal **Stabilize**.

Compare your left pane to Figure 10-22.

Step 6

The next step is to identify the interventions and actions for each diagnosis. Starting with the diagnosis of Cerebra Alteration, identify desired interventions.

Right-click on "Cerebral Alteration" again.

In the drop-down menu click on "Select Interventions" and the small window shown in Figure 10-23 will be displayed. Locate and click on the check boxes for the following interventions:

✓ Memory Loss Care

✓ Personal Care

Compare your window with Figure 10-23; when it is correct, click on the Close button.

Step 7

Now, add the actions for the first intervention.

Right-click on the intervention "Memory Loss Care."

In the drop-down menu click on "Select Nursing Actions" and the small window shown in Figure 10-24 will be displayed. Locate and click on the check boxes for the following nursing actions:

✓ Evaluate memory loss

✓ Administer Mental Status Exam

Click on the Close button.

Step 8

Add the actions for the Personal Care intervention.

Right-click on the intervention "Personal Care," and then click "Select Nursing Actions" in the drop-down menu.

Locate and click on the check boxes for the following nursing actions:

✓ Provide Ample Time to Communicate

✓ Provide Clearly Spoken Directions

✓ Encourage Participation By Family

✓ Assess Ability to Bathe Independently

✓ Assess Ability to Manage Home Environment

✓ Collaborate with Occupational Therapist

Click on the Close button.

Step 9

Complete the plan by adding interventions and actions for two remaining diagnoses.

Right-click on the nursing diagnosis "Knowledge Deficit of Therapeutic Regimen" and then click "Select Interventions" on the drop-down menu.

Locate and click on the check box for the following nursing intervention:

✓ Compliance Care

Click on the Close button.

Right-click on the intervention "Compliance Care," and then click "Select Nursing Actions" in the drop-down menu.

Locate and click on the check boxes for the following nursing actions:

✓ Assess Perceptions

✓ Assist Family with Problem Solving

✓ Assist With Setting Realistic Individual Goals

✓ Assess Healthcare Beliefs

✓ Teach Methods to Compensate For Limitations

✓ Assess Social Network

✓ Coordinate Ongoing Care

Click on the Close button.

Step 10

Right-click on the nursing diagnosis "Thought Process Alteration" and then click "Select Interventions" on the drop-down menu.

Locate and click on the check box for the following nursing intervention:

✓ Reality Orientation

Click on the Close button.

Right-click on the intervention "Reality Orientation" and then click "Select Nursing Actions" in the drop-down menu.

Locate and click on the check boxes for the following nursing action:

✓ Encourage ADLs

Click on the Close button.

Step 11

Calvin's granddaughter is uncomfortable bathing him. Add an action to the plan.

Scroll the left pane to the top to locate and right-click on the intervention "Personal Care."

Select "Add New Nursing Action" from the drop-down menu. The full RNOx list will be displayed.

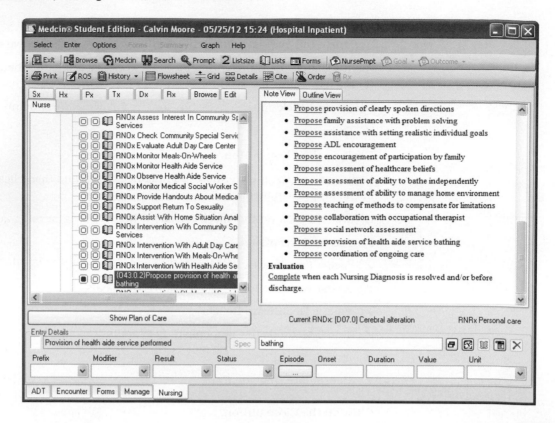

Locate and click the small plus sign next to "RNOx Home Care."

Scroll the expanded tree downward to locate and click the red button for the following finding:

- (red button) Provide Health Aide Service

In the free-text field located below the right pane, type **bathing** and press the enter key.

Compare your screen to Figure 10-25.

▶ **Figure 10-26 SIG: home health aide service window.**

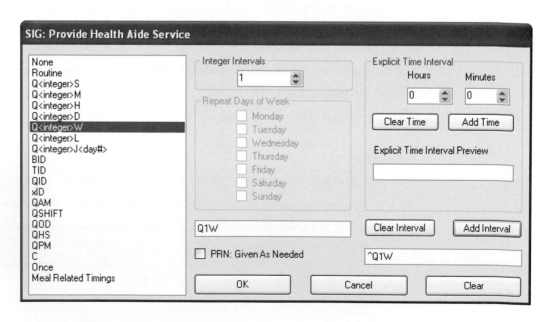

Step 12

Click on the long button below the left pane labeled "Show Plan of Care."

Locate the new nursing action you have just added, "Provide Health Aide Service."

Right-click on it and select "Change Sig" from the drop-down menu. The Sig window show in Figure 10-26 will be displayed.

Locate and click the button labeled "Clear Interval."

Locate and click on the timing "Q<integer>W" in the left column. The integer field at the top of the screen should default to 1. If it does not, enter a 1 in the field.

Locate and click on the OK button at the bottom of the Sig window.

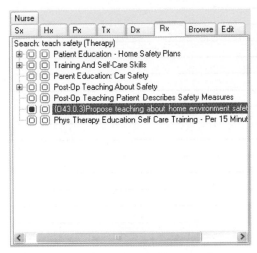

▶ **Figure 10-27 Teach About Home Environment Safety selected from the search results.**

Step 13

Because Calvin is at risk for a fall, the nurse will teach about home environment safety.

Locate and click on the Search button on the Toolbar at the top of your screen.

When the search window is displayed, type "teach safety" and then click the button labeled "Search" the search dialog window.

Locate and click on the red button for the following finding:

● (red button) RNOx Teach About Home Environment Safety

Compare your left pane with Figure 10-27.

Click on the long button below the left pane labeled "Show Plan of Care."

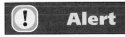

Alert ▶ *Do not close or exit the Encounter or change tabs.* **You will lose your work if you do.**

Step 14

Remain on the Nursing tab while you print the plan of care.

Click on the Print button on the Toolbar at the top of your screen to invoke the Print Data window.

Click on the check box next to Nursing Plan of Care, and then click on the appropriate button to either print or export a file, as directed by your instructor.

Compare your printout or file output to Figure 10-28. If it is correct, hand it in to your instructor. If there are any differences, review the previous steps in the exercise to find and correct your error.

Step 15

Compare and contrast the output of Exercises 64 and 65 to answer the following questions:

1. What role did the Oasis-C play in determining the home care services plan of care in Exercise 64?

2. How was the home care services plan in Exercise 64 different from the nursing plan of care developed in Exercise 65?

Give your answers to your instructor.

Nursing Plan of Care

Plan of Care	
Clinical Diagnoses	
Admission diagnosis of head injury with dementia	
Clinical Orders	
Current and Active Nursing Diagnoses	
D07.0: Cerebral Alteration (Cognitive)	
Goal:	Stabilize cerebral alteration
D64.0: Memory Loss Care	
D64.0.1: Evaluate Memory Loss^Routine	
D64.0.2: Administer Mental Status Exam^Routine	
O43.0: Personal Care	
O43.0.1: Assess Ability To Bathe Independently^Routine	
O43.0.1: Assess Ability To Manage Home Environment^Routine	
O43.0.2: Provide Ample Time To Communicate^Routine	
O43.0.2: Provide Clearly Spoken Directions^Routine	
O43.0.2: Provide Health Aide Service^Q1W	
O43.0.3: Encourage Participation By Family^Routine	
O43.0.4: Collaborate With Occupational Therapist^Routine	
O43.0.3: Teach About Home Environment Safety^Routine	
Evaluation:	
D08.7: Knowledge Deficit Of Therapeutic Regimen (Cognitive)	
Goal:	Improve knowledge deficit of therapeutic regimen
G18.0: Compliance Care	
G18.0.1: Assess Perceptions^Routine	
G18.0.2: Assist Family With Problem Solving^Routine	
G18.0.2: Assist With Setting Realistic Individual Goals^Routine	
G18.0.1: Assess Healthcare Beliefs^Routine	
G18.0.3: Teach Methods To Compensate For Limitations^Routine	
G18.0.1: Assess Social Network^Routine	
G18.0.4: Coordinate Ongoing Care^Routine	
Evaluation:	
D09.0: Thought Process Alteration (Cognitive)	
Goal:	Stabilize thought process alteration
D11.0: Reality Orientation	
D11.0.3: Encourage ADLs^Routine	
Evaluation:	
Inactive Nursing Diagnoses with Interventions	

▶ **Figure 10-28 Plan of care printed for Calvin Moore.**

Chapter Ten Summary

This chapter discussed examples of the care provisions options available to clients who require care on a long-term basis in a subacute setting. Clients with complex health issues may require prolonged care following discharge from an acute care hospital; these care needs are termed long-term care (LTC). LTC may be delivered in a residential or inpatient facility or as home health care. The average length of stay (ALOS) in an acute care facility is normally under 30 days. In long-term care facilities the ALOS is greater than 30 days.

Normally the level of professional care needs and the expected recovery outcomes of the client help determine which level of long-term care is implemented upon discharge from an acute care hospital. Other factors that help determine the client's long-term care includes the restrictions of their health care insurance coverage, the wishes of the family and client, and the outcome of the LTC nursing assessment. Various types of LTC were discussed in this chapter including:

► Long-term acute care facilities that provide acute care on a long-term basis for clients who no longer require this care at the level of intensity and frequency necessary in the acute care hospital.

► Rehabilitation facilities offer therapeutic interventions to support the long-term needs of their clients and these facilities specialize in specific types of rehabilitation such as neuromuscular rehabilitation or substance abuse recovery.

► Skilled nursing facilities (SNF) provides a variety of skilled and nonskilled support to their residents.

► Nursing homes and residential care facilities support the more maintenance-type care needs of their residents.

► Hospice specializes in care of clients in the end stage of life. Hospice care is delivered in an inpatient facility or as home care service.

► Home care provides for care needs of clients discharged from either acute care or long-term care where the care is provided in the client's home situation.

To qualify for payment for care, the nurse and other care staff observations contribute to the completion of various assessment criteria the nurse uses to determine if and how much care the client's needs require. In nursing homes the assessment instrument that must be completed is the MDS 3.0, which is documented by the nurse and reassessed at prescribed intervals. This chapter used portions of the Residential Assessment Instrument to illustrate the process of documentation required for long-term facility care.

The home care agencies nurses use a similar instrument, the Outcome and Assessment Information Set (OASIS), which documents the nursing assessment and determines the type and frequency of home care visits that required by the client. OASIS summarizes an agency's plan of care, but does not include the nursing plan of care to accomplish the identified nursing goals. That must be created separately.

References

Berman, A. J., Snyder, S., Krosier, B. J., & Erb, G. (2012). *Fundamentals of nursing*. Upper Saddle River, NJ: Pearson Education.

Centers for Medicare & Medicaid Services. (2010a, October 1). *Home assessment validation and entry system reference manual*. Washington, DC: Author.

Centers for Medicaid and Medicare Services. (2010b, December). *Long-term care facility resident assessment instrument user's manual*. Washington, DC: Author.

Centers for Medicare & Medicaid Services. (2010c, December). *OASIS-C guidance manual*. Washington, DC: Author.

Centers for Medicare & Medicaid Services. (n.d.). *Conditions of participation and requirements for long-term care facilities*. Washington, DC: Author. Retrieved from http://www.cms.gov

Centers for Medicare & Medicaid Services. (n.d.). *Nursing home quality initiatives*. Washington, DC: Author. Retrieved from http://www.cms.gov/NursingHomeQualityInits/

Centers for Medicare & Medicaid Services. (n.d.). *OASIS based home health agency patient outcome and case mix reports (41 measures)*. Retrieved from http://www.cms.gov/OASIS.

Centers for Medicare & Medicaid Services. (n.d). *Using OASIS items in assessment and care planning*. Washington, DC: Author. Retrieved from http://www.cms.gov/OASIS

Test Your Knowledge

1. What is the difference in length of stay between an acute care and a long-term care facility?

2. What is a subacute facility?

3. What is the MDS?

4. What is an LTAC?

5. List three types of LTC facilities.

   True or False Questions

6. A person receiving care in a nursing home is referred to as a resident.

   True or False

7. Both certified long-term care facilities and home care agencies are required to meet the CMS regulations.

   True or False

8. Any hospital may swing beds from acute care to long-term care use when their inpatient acute care census declines.

   True or False

9. The frequency and timing of completion and reassessment for the RAI is determined by the CMS requirements.

   True or False

10. The MDS 3.0 RAI requires precise codified completion by the health care team be completed at the time of admission before a resident's care can begin.

    True or False

11. How is the "rule of 3" used to help the nurse determine the ADL needs of the resident in the RAI?

12. Why is there a growing need for nurses to enter the field of long-term care?

13. In what circumstances must a nurse complete an OASIS?

14. Why is teaching such a major role of nursing care in the home care setting?

15. You should have produced an eleven-page form, and two additional pages from the student edition for Franklin Jones, one narrative document, and one plan of care for Calvin Moore. If you have not already done so, hand these in to your instructor with this test. These will count as a portion of your grade.

Ask your instructor for answers to Test Your Knowledge

nursing.pearsonhighered.com

Prepare for success with animated examples, practice questions, challenge tests, and interactive assignments.

11

Using the Internet to Expedite Care

Learning Outcomes

After completing this chapter, you should be able to:

1. Discuss the effect of the impact of Internet technology on healthcare

2. Explain how EHR systems use the Internet

3. Describe decision support available on the web

4. Understand how the Internet works

5. Discuss methods of remote access and secure Internet communications

6. Compare different types of telemedicine

7. Describe the advantages and workflow of client-entered data

8. Contrast differences between provider-to-client e-mail and secure messaging

9. Understand the workflow of an E-visit

The Impact of Technology

Not only is healthcare delivery is being changed by the EHR, but by the Internet as well. Perhaps the last time the introduction of new technology caused such a powerful unforeseen change to our society was the emergence of the automobile. Comparing the two transition periods can provide some useful lessons.

A hundred years ago, the most common means of transportation was the horse and carriage. As the first automobiles began to appear, people referred to them as "horseless carriages." The people of that era conceptualized this new invention in terms of the existing technology. Even the inventors of the technology were not immune to this viewpoint. Isn't the engine in the front of a car today because that's where the horse was yesteryear?

As the automobile began to appear across the country, many people did not rush to adopt it or understand the full potential of the change that society was about to undergo. The new vehicles seemed to some to be fancy toys, inferior to the horse and carriage in many ways.

▶ The supply chain of the period was built to feed and water the horse, not fuel the car.

▶ The condition of the roads, which were passable by horse, often caused cars to become stuck.

Viewed within the existing infrastructure of their time, the critics were right; driving an automobile instead of a horse seemed like a lot of work for very little gain.

People of our era use the term *electronic medical records* because they are thinking in terms of paper medical records. However, the opinion in a report by the IOM is that "Merely automating the form, content, and procedures of current patient records will perpetuate their deficiencies and will be insufficient to meet emerging user needs" (Dick & Steen, 2000, pp. 178–179).

Reexamining the workflow of paper versus electric charts in Chapter 1, we can see that the healthcare workflow has been designed around the infrastructure of a paper chart. Adapting the electronic chart to fit the old technology provides a level of comfort during the transition to the new system, but it also prevents us from seeing the full potential of the EHR. In Chapter 1, Drs. Bachman and Wenner stated that adopting an EHR changes the way clinicians' work.

Using the horseless carriage analogy of driving early automobiles on inadequate roads, we see that implementing an EHR without considering the landscape can make it seem like a lot of work for very little gain. Implementation of an EHR enables the client records to be used in ways that paper medical records cannot. To achieve these benefits, nurses must make it part of their workflow that is as natural as driving their car.

Chapter 1 named the Internet as one of the social forces driving EHR adoption. If you are a nursing student today, the Internet as we know it did not exist when you were born. It is our newest technology. While we continue to evolve what we can do with it, the Internet changes the way we work.

The flexibility of the Internet and its ability to get information to and from almost any point in a worldwide network obviously has a lot of potential for healthcare. Providers can access their clients' charts, communicate with clients, transmit medical images, consult with a specialist at a distant location, and work from anywhere. In this chapter we are going to discuss how Internet-related technologies are changing client's expectations and changing the way healthcare is delivered. To conclude our analogy of the automobile, the Internet has been called the Information Highway and it is changing the 21st-century practice of medicine as surely as the interstate system changed the habits of 20th-century drivers and spawned the suburbs (*Note.* Automobile analogy paraphrased from T. Stein, 2005, *The Electronic Physician*, p. 41. © 2005 Allscripts Healthcare Solution.)

The Internet and the EHR

The Internet is one of the key technologies impacting our society in general. It has changed the way that people communicate, research, shop, and conduct business. It also is influencing changes in healthcare.

People shop for doctors online, insurance companies provide online participating provider lists, physician specialty associations, and state and local medical societies all offer web sites that help clients locate a provider near them.

Clients also use the Internet for research. Many nurses are finding their clients are coming to visits armed with printouts about their conditions gathered from web sites. Some of these web sites provide reliable information, some do not. One of the most trusted sources of consumer information on the web is webMD Health® (www.webmd.com). On the webMD Health consumer portal, clients can access health and wellness news, support communities, interactive health management tools, and more. Online communities and special events allow individuals to participate in real-time discussions with experts and with other people who share similar health conditions or concerns. The clients' insurance provider also may offer a wealth of wellness information and interactive tools

Courtesy of MedFusion, Inc
Figure 11-1 Web site of Karen Smith, MD, FAAFP

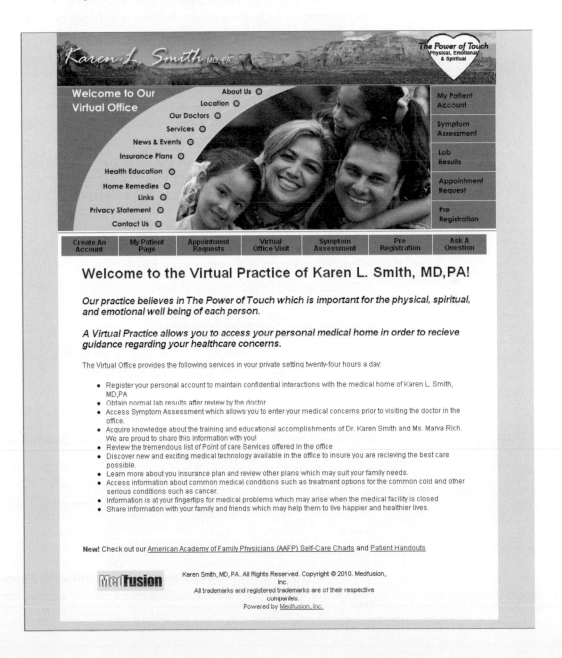

to help them evaluate and manage their controllable health risks. By using sites such as these, clients can play an active role in managing their own healthcare.

It is important for nurses to teach clients how to evaluate the information they find on the internet. Here are some suggested criteria:

▶ The article or information includes the author and credentials.

▶ The article or web site lists the date the information was last updated.

▶ The article or web site does not have a bias toward selling a treatment, therapy, drug or book.

▶ The web site is known to be reliable or from a trusted medical institution (a university, hospital, or the client's regular doctor).

A reliable source of health information on the Internet is a web site set up by a hospital or medical practice. Many medical practices today have their own web sites. An example is shown in Figure 11-1. Although some of these sites are limited to information about the medical practice, clinicians, and office hours, the site shown in Figure 11-1 includes online information about preventative health measures, diseases, and conditions that the practice treats as well as other features we will discuss later. Client educational information on a clinic's web site has the advantage of being consistent with the medical philosophy of the practice.

Additionally, the ONC strategies discussed in Chapter 1 call for the use of technology to make health information available to the client. "Consumer-centric information helps individuals manage their own wellness and assists with their personal health care decisions" (Brailer, 2004, p. c). The HITECH Act, also discussed in Chapter 1, establishes criteria for providers that includes "engaging patients and families" through the use of web portals for their clients.

The ONC committee helping to define meaningful use objectives stated: "The ultimate vision is one in which all clients are fully engaged in their health care, providers have real-time access to all medical information and tools to help ensure the quality and safety of the care provided while also affording improved access and elimination of health care disparities" (Meaningful Use Workgroup, 2009, p. 1). The committee recommendation included the following criteria:

▶ Patient access to self-management tools

▶ Patient access to personal health records, populated with patient health information in real time

▶ Secure patient–provider messaging

▶ Access to comprehensive patient data from all available sources

▶ Participation in a health information exchange (HIE)

Critical Thinking Exercise 66: Internet Search for Client Education Materials

In this exercise you will need access to the Internet. You will visit two web sites to obtain information for client education.

Case Study

Arnie Greensher is a 66-year-old male who is beginning cancer treatment.

Step 1

Start your web browser.

Enter the following URL address: **www.careindividualized.com**.

Step 2

Locate and click on the link for **Patient**.

Step 3

Choose from any of the patient information documents, and click on it. When the document is displayed, review it and print only the first page. Give the printout to your instructor.

Case Study

Brenda Green is a 54-year-old established client with a history of hypertension and possible peripheral arterial disease of the legs. She has been prescribed Coumadin, a drug that has specific risks. Follow the steps below to locate the answers to the questions in step 6.

Step 4

Start your web browser, if it is not already running.

Enter the following URL address: www.webmd.com.

Step 5

When the web page is displayed, type **Coumadin** in the search field and click on the button labeled "Search."

A page of search results will be displayed. Locate and click on the link "Drug Information."

Locate and click on the link "Coumadin Oral."

Step 6

From the information displayed on the page, answer the following questions:

What is the generic drug name for Coumadin?

What is a very serious (possibly fatal) effect of this drug?

What lab test is used to monitor the effect of this drug?

Decision Support Via the Web

The rapidly expanding body of medical and nursing information challenges the nurse to continuously keep current with all the changes in healthcare practices. Regardless of the clinical setting where a nurse works, the need for up-to-date clinical support information is needed. Sometimes a nurse may be caring for a client who offers a health problem with which the nurse has little or no care experience or who requires new and unfamiliar medications. In other situations, nurses may be called upon to share their expertise with committees in their work setting to develop new care programs or policies to support developing best practice guidelines. Nurses may also be involved in new program development to meet needs in their community or be involved in research to improve client outcomes.

The quantity of information available to nurses regarding conditions, disease management, protocols, case studies, and treatments far exceeds their available time to read it. Although the Internet offers easy access to a myriad of web sites that can quickly provide information to help support any knowledge deficit, it is important to obtain information from sites that can be depended on for accurate and quality information to guide their care. It may be quick and easy to use a general search engine to look up information about a drugs or diseases, but it is important to use professional quality sites to obtain best practice, up-to-date, and quality research-based information.

Nursing professional organizations have many web sites offering information on professional practice and best practice guidelines. Nursing professional web sites also provide information on continuing education credits for nurses, upcoming conferences, and online opportunities for nurses to network. Two examples are www.nursingworld.org and www.ana.org; both offer information on professional practice and include areas specifically designed to for student nurses.

An increasing number of nursing journals publish research articles online. Here are three examples:

The Internet *Journal of Advanced Nursing Practice*:

www.ispub.com/journal/the_internet_journal_of_advanced_nursing_practice.html

Online *Journal of Issues in Nursing*: www.ana.org/ojin

Online *Journal of Rural Nursing and Healthcare*: www.rno.org/journal

If the nurse is working within a particular clinical specialty, the professional nursing organization associated with the specialty will contain information clinically relevant and supportive of best practice standards. The following exercise lists web sites that help nurses locate quality information. This is not intended to be a comprehensive list, but a few examples of specialty nursing sites to explore.

Critical Thinking Exercise 67: Internet Nursing Research

In this exercise you will need access to the Internet.

Step 1

Read the following case studies and select three that are of most interest to you.

Case Study

As a registered nurse working in the perioperative area of a hospital, you have agreed to work on a task force to prevent postoperative infections. Research the topic of infection on the Association of periOperative Registered Nurses, www.aorn.org, to obtain information on infection control practices.

Case Study

As a home care nurse, you have a client who is newly diagnosed with a cancerous lesion on his neck. Research the Oncology Nursing Society web site, www.ons.org, to obtain information designed specifically for the nurse to increase understanding of how to meet the care or education needs of the client.

Case Study

A nurse working in a critical care unit visits the American Association of Critical Care Nurses web site, www.aacn.org, to identify the most recent practice alerts. Using the web site, locate and read one practice alert that may help you in your clinical practice.

Case Study

As a nurse working in a medical/surgical unit, research the Academy Medical-Surgical Nurses web site, www.amsn.org, to locate an article within its electronic library that addresses one care issue of your patient experiencing pain.

Case Study

As a nurse working in an OB clinic, research the Association of Women's Health, Obstetric and Neonatal Nurses site, www.awhonn.org, and locate one the latest information of health policy and legislation that may impact your nursing practice and the care of obstetric clients.

Case Study

As a nurse interested in the national trends for nursing data to demonstrate consistency in meeting and improving client outcome standards, visit the National Database of Nursing Quality Indicators web site, www.nursingquality.org, and read the FAQ on quality indicator measurements.

Step 2

For each of the three chosen scenarios, use the designated web site to locate the information described in the case; print out and bring to class something relevant to the case study that you found there to share with your fellow students.

Integrated Decision Support

Although continuing education classes, nursing journals, and web sites are useful, they are not always at hand in the exam room or at the bedside.

Decision support in an EHR refers to the ability of systems to store or quickly locate materials relevant to the findings of the current case. Clinics can imbed links in their forms that, when selected, display any type of helpful material. These might include defined protocols, results of case studies, or standard care guidelines prepared by departments within the hospital, medical or nursing organizations, or government-sponsored research.

In current EHR systems, the decision support documents are selected and linked to the system by each individual healthcare organization. (The authors are not aware of any system that automatically installs standard decision support documents or links into the EHR.) The selection of decision support items is generally one of the responsibilities of the hospital or clinic when setting up the EHR. Therefore, the support content of EHR systems will differ from facility to facility.

However, the health organization where a nurse is working may have paid subscriptions to web sites that provide decision support information about drugs consistent with their pharmacy standards, web sites that offer research-based order entry standards for physicians and nurses, or web sites to obtain approved education materials to assist the nurse with client education. These sites usually offer education materials consistent with the ethnically diverse population of their normal client base as well as client-friendly reading levels to promote better client understanding.

Many healthcare organizations also have departments for clinical quality, infection control, or clinical nurse specialists—all of whom can assist the staff nurses and students to locate quality, clinically relevant web sites; of course, your nursing college faculty can help you find sound research-based sites that can offer valid nursing decision support.

Students can explore the research sites subscribed by their collegiate libraries and nursing education programs. Another way to locate quality web sites is to read the resource list of nursing research articles. Often the bibliography lists will cite online resources worth exploring. For example, the CCC System used in this course can be explored further on the web site www.sabacare.com.

Understanding the Internet

Most people know the Internet because of the services they use on it such as e-mail, research, games, and web pages. However, before proceeding further it may be helpful to understand how it works.

Multiple computers can be connected together to exchange data in private networks that can be accessed only by the users in that network. These are called local-area networks (LAN) or wide-area networks (WAN). In a LAN, data flows to and from specific computers using cables in a wired building.

The Internet is a worldwide public network that can be accessed by any computer anywhere. The Internet was created by interconnecting millions of smaller business-, academic-, and government-run networks. It is really a very large network of networks. In a network schematic it is sometimes referred to as a "cloud" because data does not necessarily follow a consistent path.

To understand the difference between a private network and the Internet, let us compare the post office and the phone company. When you make a phone call (on a land line), the wires and circuits must establish an electrical connection with the phone of the person you are calling before that person's phone rings and the call can go through. When you write a letter, you address the envelope and deposit it in the mailbox. You do not know how the post office will transport it or what roads the trucks will take, but in the end it is delivered to the address on the envelope.

The Internet Protocol encloses data in packets that have an address on them. The packets are sent through the various networks making up the Internet until they arrive at their address. The sending computer does not have to establish a wired connection with the receiving computer for this to occur and does not know how the packets will be routed.

Secure Internet Data

The problem is that the Internet is not secure. The packets of data pass through many computers and networks on their way to their destination. They can be copied, opened, and read by anyone with enough technical savvy.

How do we secure the information so we can use the accessibility of the Internet, but protect the information? When Congress enacted the Health Insurance Portability and Accountability Act (HIPAA), a subsection of that law established rules and regulations to protect the privacy and security of medical records (Health Insurance Portability and Accountability Act, 1996). Under the HIPAA security rule, protected health information that is transmitted over an open network such as the Internet must be encrypted (Centers for Medicare & Medicaid Services, 2005). Encryption uses a mathematical algorithm to convert readable data into encoded or scrambled data. The authorized recipient decrypts the message back to its original form using a mathematical key.

Secure transmission of data over the Internet usually relies on either of two methods. These are secured socket layer (SSL) or a virtual private network (VPN). Both of these rely on encrypting the transmission. There are additional secure transmission schemes not covered here.

SSL adds security by encrypting the content of web pages and automatically decrypting it when it is received to display the web page. This prevents anyone intercepting the transmitted packets from making sense of them. SSL, however, is limited to the type of things you can do on a web page. Some providers and organizations want to run software or view records that are on their office network computers from elsewhere. To do this, a VPN may be used.

The VPN uses the Internet to transport packets of data, but it has its own software that encrypts and decrypts the packets between the sending and receiving systems. The VPN also verifies the identity of the person signing on, ensuring access only to those who are permitted to use the system. A VPN is not limited to web pages and may be used to secure the data being transmitted for other application software, such as an electronic health record system.

Remote Access to the EHR

As we discussed earlier, providers increasingly want access to their EHR when they are away from the hospital or office. Many medical facility networks are configured to allow authorized providers to access their clients' medical records. This is often is referred to as "remote access."

The benefits to the provider and the client are tremendous. If the clinician receives an emergency call from or about a client, the client's records can be accessed from home, helping the clinician to make better decisions. In home health, enabling nurses to connect wirelessly to the home health agency computers allows a nurse to view and update a client's records from the point of care. Figure 11-2 shows a nurse using a laptop computer and wireless connection to record the OASIS-C assessment in real time.

Remote access must be secure. In the past this was facilitated by having the provider direct dial the modem at the medical facility or home health agency. In the age of the Internet, remote access is more likely to accomplished using the SSL or VPN encryption methods just discussed. Using a VPN, the provider connects to the network and logs in

Photo courtesy of Kourtnie Sitarz

▶ Figure 11-2 A nurse remotely accesses the home health agency system from the client's home.

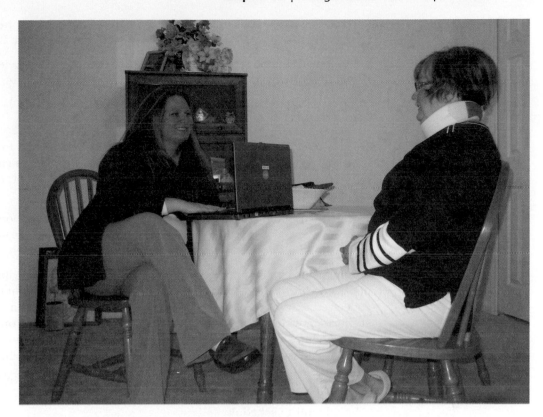

just as if he or she were in the facility. This method allows the provider to run the actual EHR system remotely.

Where SSL is used, the remote access is usually through a web portal. The portal is not the actual EHR application that the provider would see at work, but a rendition of EHR data presented in an interactive web page. Using a portal, authorized medical personnel can view (and sometimes update) selected records in chart. A portal can allow providers to retrieve medical records, and review and sign lab results and charts. Some portals also allow the provider to place electronic care orders or input electronic prescriptions. This approach is popular with hospitals and large healthcare organizations that wish to avoid the technically more complicated VPN setup or want to provide remote access to only selected aspects of the chart.

Practicing Medicine Online

Although the banking, brokerage/investing, and travel industries have made Internet-based transactions readily available to consumers, healthcare as a whole has not. That seems to be changing. An annual Survey of Health Care Consumers, conducted by the Deloitte Center for Health Solutions, found that "65 percent of consumers are interested in home monitoring devices that enable them to check their condition and send the results to their doctor" and "42 percent want access to an online personal health record connected to their doctor's office. E-visits with physicians, personal health records, self-monitoring devices, personalized physician referrals and customized insurance products are innovations that consumers support. They are willing to try new services, change providers and hospitals and use their money in different ways to obtain better value from the healthcare system. And they are highly receptive to technology-enabled care that eliminates redundant paperwork, replaces unnecessary tests and saves time and money" (Deloitte Center for Health Solutions, 2009, p. 11).

The leading organization in healthcare informatics, the Health Information Management Systems Society (HIMSS) has formed a Special Interest Group to study *e-health*, which the Society defines as "The application of Internet and other related technologies in the healthcare industry to improve the access, efficiency, effectiveness, and quality of clinical and business processes utilized by healthcare organizations, practitioners, patients, and consumers to improve the health status of patients" (Grehalva, 2010, p. 12).

Let us now examine several of the ways that the Internet is being used not only as a research tool, but as a tool for the actual process of client care.

Telemedicine

Telemedicine uses communication technology to deliver care to a client in another location. A consulting health professional studies the client's case and offers an opinion to the referring physician or instructions directly to the client, neither of whom are at the consultant's location.

Telemedicine can take many forms, ranging from a simple phone call between two doctors to a videoconference between a nurse and a client, as shown in Figure 11-3. Even examinations or surgical procedures have been conducted remotely.

Telemedicine can be practiced in real time or asynchronously (independent sessions not occurring at the same time). Before the Internet, early pioneers of telemedicine conceived of it terms of the technology of their time, television. They imagined a scenario in which the doctor and client could see each other on television sets at each end. Satellites that carry television signals would securely transmit the bidirectional video sessions. There were several drawbacks to this approach.

▶ Real-time telemedicine requires the presence of all parties at the same time. When participants are located in different time zones, real-time telemedicine sessions can be difficult to schedule.

▶ Television cannot transmit or display at a sufficient resolution for diagnostic images, such as x-rays or CAT scans.

▶ State laws can prohibit treatment of clients by providers licensed in another state.

Telemedicine in Nursing

One area where real-time telemedicine seems to work well is home health nursing. Home health agencies and their clients are typically in the same time zone and always licensed in the same state as their clients. Although home care nurses have been monitoring clients using the telephone for a long time, the availability of faster Internet speeds has made video conferencing via computer possible. It has been reported that the older generation is among the fastest growing segment of computer users. Because this group is the larger portion of home health clients, the field is ready for telemedicine nursing.

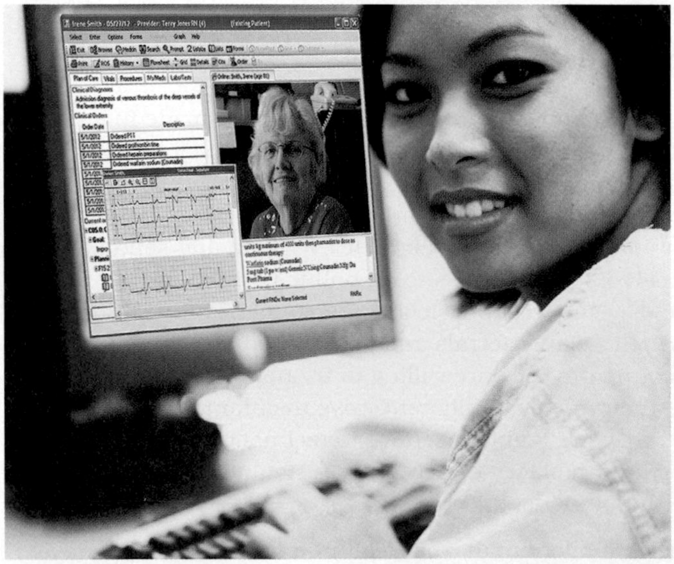

There are many advantages for the client. As we discussed in Chapter 10, home nurses do not see clients as frequently as they would in other healthcare settings. Using Internet video conferencing, the client can not only talk to but can also see the nurse between visits. Questions can be answered and issues addressed sooner. Nurses can download data from home medical devices that monitor the client's heart rate, blood pressure, glucose, and other measures.

Using the downloaded data and the nurse's impressions from face-to-face video communication, the nurse can determine the client's progress. In addition to the elderly, telemedicine works well for home care nursing for clients with AIDS and for monitoring women at risk for preterm labor. Telemedicine does not replace, but supplements, home visits and thereby home care is improved.

▶ **Figure 11-3 Home health nurse video conferences with client, while monitoring her heart rate.**

Asynchronous Telemedicine at Mayo Clinic

Known worldwide for their medical expertise, specialists at Mayo Clinic in Rochester, Minnesota, are in great demand. However, doctors and clients seeking consultations are frequently in other time zones or even other countries. In those cases, real-time telemedicine is impractical.

Rather than trying to get participants on each end into real-time video conferences, they decided to conduct telemedicine asynchronously. Marvin Mitchell, division chair of Media Support Services at Mayo Clinic, calls this *store-and-forward telemedicine*. It allows a doctor requesting a consult to send case information that is then reviewed and responded to later by a specialist at Mayo.

If a video conference is an example of real-time telemedicine, voice mail would be a simple analogy of store-and-forward telemedicine. One doctor leaves a message stating the facts of the case; the other doctor listens to the message and then calls back, leaving a detailed response for the original doctor. In practice, however, telemedicine is not that simple.

In the Mayo Clinic's practice, the client's physician in a remote location does the necessary examinations and diagnostic tests he or she would normally do. Then the doctor creates an electronic package including high-resolution images, scanned paper documents, motion image capture, angiography, and anything else that the specialist at Mayo might need to review. The information is then transmitted with a consultation request to the Mayo telemedicine office via a secure Internet connection.

The Mayo telemedicine system follows the same workflow as if the client were at the clinic. When the Mayo Clinic telemedicine office receives the electronic package, the client is registered and given a Mayo Clinic patient number, and then an electronic medical record is created. The diagnostic images from the package are stored in the Mayo PAC system and orders to the radiologist are created. Other records are imported into the EHR.

One of the principal advantages of this workflow is that it is as transparent to the Mayo physicians as possible. Specialists at Mayo see the remote client's records in the same system they use every day. A Mayo radiologist views the diagnostic images, interprets them, and dictates a report. Similarly, other specialties look at the imported EHR data and dictate their second opinion into Mayo's clinical notes system.

When all the subspecialists' reports have been completed, a comprehensive second-opinion document is compiled and sent back to the remote physician. That physician can use the second opinion to work up the diagnosis and treatment plan for the client. In the Mayo Clinic's case, real-time interactions between remote physicians are not necessary.

Although store-and-forward telemedicine works well for consults, it can involve delays when additional information or tests are needed and one must wait for the response to arrive. Also, it is not suitable to remote, robotic, or even guided surgery, all of which must be conducted in real time.

The benefit of telemedicine is that it makes high-level medical expertise available to remote and rural areas. Many communities do not have medical specialists. Even fewer places in the world have subspecialists, or sub-subspecialists who can recognize and treat rare or complex medical problems. Using telemedicine, it is possible for a local physician to get advice from a distant expert and guidance in treating the client.

Teleradiology

One form of telemedicine that is specifically concerned with the transmission of diagnostic images from one location to another is teleradiology. Usually this is for the purpose of having the images "read" by a radiologist at the receiving end. This may be to obtain a second opinion or consult, or because the sending facility does not have sufficient radiologists on staff and has contracted to have radiology interpretations done by another facility. In the latter case, state laws may require the radiologist to be licensed by the state from which the images are sent.

Currently, most states require a physician to be licensed by that state to treat clients in that state. The Mayo Clinic's method of telemedicine solves the problem of licensure that has hindered telemedicine in the United States. At Mayo, the telemedicine consultation is physician to physician as a resource for the client's doctor. Because they are not giving advice directly to a client in another state, no laws are broken. This method also has the additional advantage of keeping the client's local physician in control of the care at all times.

Entry of Symptoms and History by the Client

Contributed by Allen R. Wenner, MD (*Note.* Courtesy of Primetime Medical Software and Instant Medical History. Used by permission.)

A day in a medical clinic is a busy stream of clients ranging in age from newborn to geriatric. Their presenting complaints are as varied as their age range. Because clients may have a minor illness or a life-threatening condition, it is very hard to predict exactly how long each client will take. As a result, the schedule falls behind. Clients from the morning often spill over into lunch, which often becomes abbreviated.

In contrast to the hectic pace of the clinic staff, time seems to drag for the clients who are waiting. A major challenge for the staff is keeping the clients from waiting too long in the waiting room or exam rooms.

In a traditional office, by the time the clinician (physician or nurse practitioner) enters the examination room and greets the client, there is still little or no information about the client except for vital signs and a few notes from the medical assistant who brought the client to the room. The clinician has to begin by asking why the client has sought care. The bulk of the visit is spent querying the client about symptoms and the history of present illness, by a review of systems, and then finally performing the physical exam. Because of time pressures or fatigue as the day wears on, the clinician may forget to ask about vital pieces of data including essential symptoms, family or social history, or habits such as alcohol or drug use.

EHR systems facilitate documentation at the point of care, but only the client has the information about what symptoms were present at the outset of the illness and what the outcome of medical treatment of those symptoms was. The client is also typically the source of past medical, family, and social history. The clinician's time with the client is spent entering the client's symptom into the visit documentation, leaving too little time to provide client education about the diagnosis or answer questions about the treatment and care plan.

In the late 1980s, Allen Wenner, MD, a physician in Columbia, South Carolina, wondered if history couldn't be taken by a computer. The medical literature was replete with academic efforts at patient computer dialog, beginning with Warner Slack at Harvard (Slack, Hicks, Reed, & Van Cura, 1966) and John Mayne at Mayo Clinic (Mayne, Weksel, & Sholtz, 1968). If the patients entered their own data, it would free up clinical staff and allow more of the clinician's time to be focused directly on the important issues identified by the patient. Dr. Wenner confirmed the theories of the academics that given the opportunity to add information to their medical chart while waiting was readily accepted by most clients. Working with his colleagues at Primetime Medical Software, he developed Instant Medical History™, an automated component for recording client-entered data that is available in many commercial EHR systems today.

Dr. Wenner decided that the computer could ask all the necessary questions intelligently if it was given a limited set of initial information. A nurse would start the interview by entering the client's age and sex, and selecting the symptoms and organ systems for review. At that point, the computer could pose questions that simulated a live client interview. The knowledge-based approach of the computer's artificial intelligence changed the questions based on the client's answers, simulating a live clinical interview. The software sought to collect the necessary prerequisite data for the clinical interview.

Another important element of history taking is the depth to which a client is asked questions. Dr. Wenner found the use of computer interviews improves the quality of the information presented by the client because it is more complete. For example, an ideal interview about the upper respiratory tract and sinuses should include questions about unusual causes such as psittacosis, an infection acquired from raising birds, query about prevention such as use of tobacco, and consideration of the risk for pregnancy in determining treatment options. The clinician may forget or just not have enough time to ask these questions; the computer will not forget. Because the computer never forgets details, it allows the clinician to converse casually with a client while clarifying the objective information needed to make a confident diagnosis.

In the earliest days of computers, a study at Cornell University had clients answer questions on a punch card that was processed by a computer. The study found that "it collects for appraisal a large and comprehensive body of information about the patient's medical history at no expenditure of the physician's time; it facilitates interview by making available to the physician a preliminary survey of the patient's total medical problems; its data, being systematically arranged, are easier to review than those on conventional medical histories; and, by calling attention to the patient's symptoms and significant items of past history, it assures that their investigation will not be overlooked because the physician lacked time to elicit them" (Brodman et al., 1949, pp. 530–534).

Because clients want their providers to arrive at the best diagnosis, Dr. Wenner found they are willing to answer questions. Also, because the clinician can review the information entered by the client, more time is available for explaining the diagnosis and educating the client; the client's time and effort to enter the data are rewarded.

Workflow Using Client-Entered Data

Instant Medical History can be administered on a kiosk or Tablet PC in the waiting room, in a subwaiting area, in the exam room, or at home via the web. Figure 11-4 illustrates one workflow of an office using Instant Medical History. As you will see in Exercise 68, it is also easily administered over the Internet.

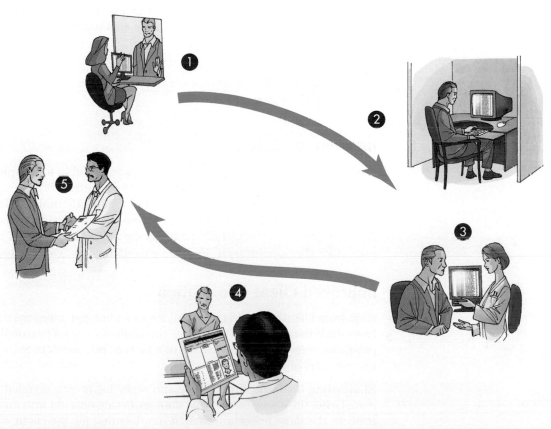

▶ Figure 11-4 Workflow of client entering his own data.

❶ When the client arrives, a receptionist, medical assistant, or nurse asks the client to complete a medical history and reason for today's visit using a computer in a private area of the waiting room.

❷ The client is given access to a kiosk or other computer to enter his or her own history and symptom information using a computer-guided questionnaire. The questions are asked one at a time and can dynamically branch to other question sets based on the answers provided by the client.

The client completes the questions at his or her own pace and has an opportunity to change answers. Clients can review their histories and are better prepared to interact with the physician.

❸ When the client has completed the questionnaire, the system alerts a nurse that the client is ready to move to an exam room. The nurse and client review the client-entered symptoms and history together. Where necessary, the nurse edits the record if there is additional information.

The computer organizes the client-entered information in a succinct and easy-to-read format that becomes the starting point for the encounter. After review of the data, the nurse merges it into the EHR encounter note.

❹ The clinician examines the client and can and discusses the reason for the visit and reviews with the client the HPI information now in the chart. Having a complete history in the EHR in advance of the exam provides the clinician with a great deal of useful information to begin making the proper diagnosis and considering appropriate treatment. It also allows the physician to spend less time documenting and more time with client discussing the effects of the illness on the client. It also allows the clinician time to discuss the treatment plan with the client.

Because interview software records subjective information from the client, the data represents a more complete and accurate reflection of a client's complaints.

After asking a few confirmatory questions, clinician completes the physical exam, assessment, and plan portions of the encounter note in the examination room while the client is still present.

❺ The encounter note has been completed at the point of care. As the client leaves, the client is given a copy of the encounter note along with any client education materials or prescriptions.

Internet Workflow

Providers and clients soon realized that it was possible to complete the symptom and history interview before the visit by using the Internet. Today many clinics enable the client to complete the Instant Medical History questionnaire online before the visit. This saves time during the office visit and allows the client to give more thought to his or her answers when completing the interview from the comfort of home. When the client arrives for the appointment, the data will already be available to the clinician.

Improved Client Information

Data from client screening is useful for providing pertinent information that allows an immediate diagnosis. Not only does the clinician have a reasonable idea of the client's problems even before the examination begins, but the data are also instantly ready to become part of the medical record.

Eliminating the bulk of data entry and replacing it with detailed, client-entered data transforms the encounter from a data-gathering session into an opportunity to concentrate on the most important task at hand: caring for the client.

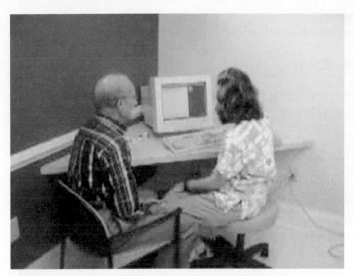

Courtesy of Primetime Medical Software & Instant Medical History.

▶ **Figure 11-5 Exam room computer positioned so client (on left) and nurse (on right) share information.**

The increased efficiency that computer screening can make office visits more enjoyable because the clinician has more time to explain the diagnosis and educate the client.

Dr. Wenner and his peers have found most clients willing and eager to answer a computer interview about their reason for the visit. The client benefits because the time the clinician has saved from having to input the symptoms and history can be focused fully on the client and used for counseling and education.

When the exam room is configured as shown in Figure 11-5, so that the client and provider can both see the screen, the client is able to engage in the mutual process of documenting the visit. The client benefits from this arrangement because when the client and provider share information, the client feels a part of the decisions and has a vested interest in following the plan of care.

John Mayne at the Mayo Clinic observed, "If the time physicians spend collecting, organizing, recording, and retrieving data could be reduced, at least in part, by information technology, more time would be available for actual delivery of medical care (and, thus, in effect increase the number of physicians) and at the same time the physician's capabilities for collecting information from patients would be extended" (Mayne et al., 1968, pp. 1–25). Likewise, this is the same observation commonly voiced by nurses.

Guided Exercise 68: Experiencing Client-Entered HPI

In this exercise you will have an opportunity to experience what we have been discussing, by taking on the role of a client who is completing his "paperwork" for an upcoming appointment online. You will need access to the Internet for this exercise.

Case Study

Tomas Martiniz is a 24-year-old male who injured his knee when he jumped off a loading dock at work. He has an upcoming appointment at the Family Care medical clinic and is going online to complete his medical questionnaire in advance.

Step 1

Start your web browser program and follow the steps listed inside the cover of this textbook to access Online Student Resources.

When the welcome page is displayed, click on the link "**Exercises and Activities**" or select "Exercises and Activities" from the drop-down list and click on the button labeled "Go."

Step 2

A menu on the left of the screen will list various activities and exercises. Locate and click on the link **Exercise 68**.

Information about the exercise will be displayed.

Locate and click the link "Click here to start the web portal program."

▶ **Figure 11-6 Simulated provider web page used for exercises in Chapter 11.**

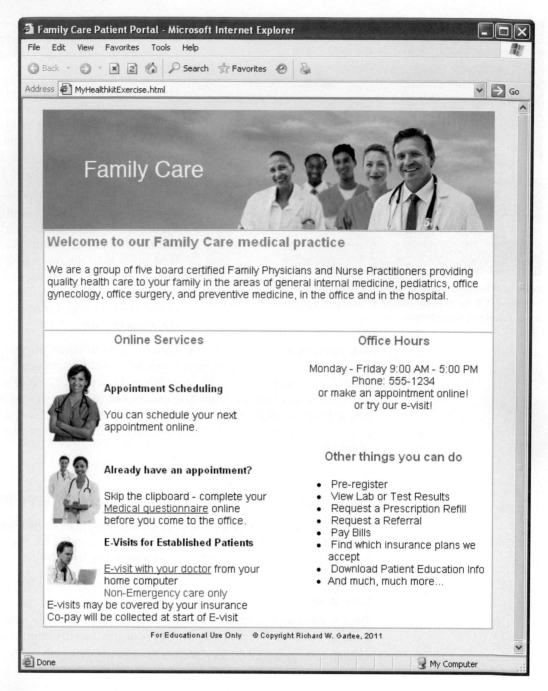

Step 3

The sample provider web portal shown in Figure 11-6 will be displayed.

Locate the section of the web page labeled "Already have an appointment?" and click on the link "Medical Questionnaire."

The interview web page, "Get started preparing for your next doctor's visit," will be displayed.

Step 4

Locate and click on the button labeled "Start Interview."

Step 5

The center portion of the web page will display the Interview dialog as shown in Figure 11-7.

▶ **Figure 11-7 Student ID and patient information portion of the interview.**

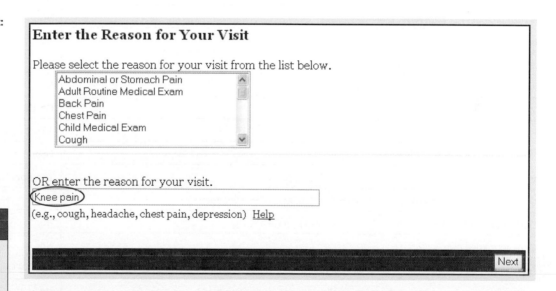

Please enter your information and click Next.

Student Name or ID	Terry Jones

Patient Information

First name	Tomas
Last name	Martiniz
Gender	⦿ Male ◯ Female
Date of birth	October ▾ 7 ▾ 1987 ▾

Next

Enter the following:

Student Name or ID: Enter either your name or student ID as directed by your instructor.

Patient Information:

First Name: **Tomas**

Last Name: **Martiniz**

Click on the circle next to **Male**.

Click on the down arrow buttons in each of the Date of Birth fields and select from the drop-down lists: **October**, **7**, and **1987**.

Compare your screen to Figure 11-7. When everything has been entered correctly, locate and click on the button labeled "Next."

▶ **Figure 11-8 Reason for visit: Knee pain.**

Enter the Reason for Your Visit

Please select the reason for your visit from the list below.

> Abdominal or Stomach Pain
> Adult Routine Medical Exam
> Back Pain
> Chest Pain
> Child Medical Exam
> Cough

OR enter the reason for your visit.

Knee pain

(e.g., cough, headache, chest pain, depression) Help

Next

Step 6

The reason for visit screen will be displayed.

The interview on the web page is functionally identical to online questionnaires on the web sites of doctors such as Karen Smith, MD (shown in Figure 11-1), and many other forward-thinking doctors.

Locate the free text field (circled in red in Figure 11-8) and type: **Knee pain**.

Compare your screen to Figure 11-8. When you have finished typing, locate and click on the button labeled "Next."

Step 7

The software at the web site will conduct the interview by asking Mr. Martiniz the questions listed below, one question at a time. For each question there will be buttons labeled with various answers to the question. Additional buttons allow you to skip a question or go back to the previous question.

For each question in the table below, locate and click on the indicated button. If you make an error, click on the button labeled "Previous Question" and correct your error.

Interview Question	Click on the button labeled
What kind of problem are you having with your knee (or knees)?	**Pain**
What were you doing when the problem or pain began?	**Fell**
How long ago did your knee symptoms begin?	**3 to 4 days**
How did your knee symptoms begin?	**Suddenly or quickly**
Please select the best answer which most closely describes the pace of your knee problem.	**My symptoms seem to be getting better but improvement is slow**
Has your knee symptoms caused you to stop or reduce work, exercise, or other activities?	**Yes**
On a scale of 0 (no pain) to 10 (severe), how severe is your knee problems?	**5 to 6 moderate**
What time of day does your knee problem occur?	**No specific time of day**
Do your knee problems improve with activity?	**No**
Are your knee problems made worse by walking, running or other movement?	**Yes**
Are your knee problems worse when at rest or not moved?	**No**
Does your knee swell?	**Yes**
Is your painful knee joint red?	**No**
Is the painful knee joint warm?	**No**
Is the painful knee joint tender when you touch it?	**Yes**
Is the skin of the knee draining or open?	**No**
Which best describes where your knee is tender?	**On the outside of the knee**
How long have you had knee pain?	**1 to 3 days**
Which knee is painful?	**Left knee**
Which part of your knee hurts?	**The part towards the outside**
Does your painful knee joint creak or make a grating noise when you move it?	**No**
Does your painful knee joint lock when it is moved in certain ways?	**No**
Does your knee give way?	**No**
Are you able to completely bend and extend your knee?	**Yes**
Is the skin around your knee red, warm, swollen, tender, or draining fluid?	**No**
Have you noticed any lumps under the skin around your knee along with the pain?	**No**
Does your knee(s) seem to be enlarged or larger on one or both sides?	**Yes**
When do you have knee pain?	**Only during activity**
Does your knee pain become worse when climbing up stairs?	**Yes**
Does your knee pain become worse when going down stairs?	**No**
Is your knee pain worse when you are bearing weight on your legs?	**Yes**
Is your knee pain worse when you are kneeling?	**Yes**

Interview Question	Click on the button labeled
Is your knee pain worse when you turn or twist on your leg with your foot planted?	**Yes**
What happens to your painful knee joint when you are active?	**Joint pain become worse during use**
Does your knee pain become worse if you actively move the knee joint (that is if you make the knee joint move as you would during activity but without any stress or pressure on the knee joint)?	**No**
Does your knee pain become worse if you move the knee joint passively (that is if you make the knee joint move by having someone else move it for you)?	**No**
Have you ever injured the knee joint that is now painful?	**Yes**
Have you ever had the knee joint that is now painful immobilized (motionless) for 3 days or more?	**No**
Did this episode of knee pain start at the same time as an injury to the knee?	**Yes**
Which best describes the way that you injured your knee?	**I jumped or fell from a high place**
Which best describes how quickly your knee pain has come on?	**Suddenly and worsened quickly over hours**
What time of day does your knee pain occur?	**No specific time of day**
How would you describe the pain you usually have in your knee?	**Moderate**
On a scale of 0 (no pain) to 10 (severe), how is your knee pain with walking on flat surfaces?	**5 to 6 (moderate)**
On a scale of 0 (no pain) to 10 (severe), how is your knee pain with walking up stairs?	**7 to 8 (severe)**
On a scale of 0 (no pain) to 10 (severe), how is your knee pain with walking up hills?	**Skip this question**
On a scale of 0 (no pain) to 10 (severe), how is your knee pain with walking down stairs?	**5 to 6 (moderate)**
On a scale of 0 (no pain) to 10 (severe), how is your knee pain with walking down hills?	**Skip this question**
On a scale of 0 (no pain) to 10 (severe), how is your knee pain while running?	**Skip this question**
On a scale of 0 (no pain) to 10 (severe), how is your knee pain while kneeling?	**9 to 10 (unbearable)**
On a scale of 0 (no pain) to 10 (severe), how is your knee pain sitting with knee straight?	**3 to 4 (mild)**
On a scale of 0 (no pain) to 10 (severe), how is your knee pain at night?	**3 to 4 (mild)**
Do you have a skin rash?	**No**
Have you had any fever in the past 4 weeks?	**No**
Do you have discolored blood vessels or varicose veins in your skin?	**No**
Do you have tenderness, swelling, redness, or pain anywhere on your leg in addition to around your knee?	**No**
Do you have a new hard lump or mass anywhere on your leg?	**No**
Do you have pain from your back shooting down your leg?	**No**
Have you tried any treatments for your knee problem?	**No**
Do you have rheumatoid arthritis?	**No**
Do you have osteoarthritis also known as degenerative arthritis?	**No**
Has a doctor ever diagnose you as having bursitis?	**No**
Has a doctor or other health professional ever told you that you had back problems?	**No**
Have you ever broken a bone of your lower extremity (thigh, knee, calf, ankle etc.)?	**No**
Have you ever dislocated a joint of your lower extremity (hip, knee, ankle, foot, etc.)?	**No**
Have you ever had a problem with phlebitis?	**No**
Have you had knee surgery?	**No**
Have you ever had an injury to your knee ligaments, knee tendons, or knee cartilage problem?	**No**
Have you ever had an infection in your knee?	**No**

Chief Complaint
Tomas Martiniz is a 24 year old male. His reason for visit is "Knee Pain".

History of Present Illness

#1. "Knee Pain"

Location
He reported: Left knee joint pain. Tenderness on the outside of the knee. Pain towards the outside of the knee.

Quality
He reported: Knee larger than normal.
He denied: Knee unstable when stressed. Painful knee joint locks in certain positions. Back pain moves down the leg. Knee joint movement associated with grating noise. Lumps under the skin. Leg redness, swelling, or tenderness. New lump on leg. He reported: No limitation of range of motion of the knee.

Severity
He reported: Knee pain moderate. Knee pain moderate (5-6/10) walking on flat surfaces and walking down stairs. Knee pain mild (3-4/10) sitting with knee straight and at night. Knee problem slowly improving and moderate (5-6/10). Knee pain severe (7-8/10) walking up stairs. Knee pain unbearable (9-10/10) while kneeling.

Duration
He reported: Knee pain 1 to 3 days. Knee problem 3 to 4 days.

Timing
He reported: Knee pain occurs at no specific time of day. Knee problem started with a fall, started suddenly or quickly, and at no specific time of day. Knee pain began with injury. Knee pain starting suddenly and quickly worsening over hours.

Context
He reported: Knee pain only with movement.
He denied: Previous immobilization of painful knee joint.

Modifying Factors
He reported: Knee pain becomes worse during use. Knee pain worse when climbing stairs, bearing weight, kneeling, and twisting.
He denied: Knee pain worse when descending stairs. Knee problem improved with activity. Knee problem worsened by activity. Knee pain worsened by active motion. Knee pain worsened by passive motion.

Associated Signs and Symptoms
He reported: Knee swells and tender.
He denied: Knee red and warm.

Past, Family, and Social History

Past Medical History
He denied: Bursitis. Rheumatoid arthritis. Back pain. Inflamed blood vessel. Internal derangement of knee. Knee infection.

Surgical History
He denied: Knee surgery.

Accidents and Injuries
History of: Previous injury to painful knee joint. Knee injured by jumping from a high place.
He denied: Broken hip or leg. Lower extremity dislocation.

Social History
History of: Treatment for knee problem.

Activities for Daily Living
History of: Knee problem reduced activity.

Review of Systems

Constitutional
He denied: Fever in the last month.

Cardiovascular
He denied: Varicose veins.

Skin
He denied: Knee draining. Rash.

Additional Comments
I jumped off a loading dock at work

[Save] [Print] [Next]

▶ **Figure 11-9 Completed interview for Tomas Martiniz.**

Step 8

When you have reached the end of the interview, a free-text note box is displayed to allow the client to enter additional comments in his or her own words.

Type: "**I jumped off a loading dock at work**."

Locate and click on the button labeled "Next."

Step 9

The final screen of the interview allows you to review your work.

Compare your screen to Figure 11-9 by scrolling the window as necessary. If there are any differences (other than the client's age), repeat the exercise, making certain you answer each of the questions in steps 6 and 7 correctly.

Step 10

At the bottom of the interview report screen are two buttons labeled "Save" and "Print." The Save button will save the report to a file, similar to the Export button you have used in other exercises.

When everything in your report is correct, locate and click on the appropriate button to either print or save to a file, as directed by your instructor. Once you have your printout or file output in hand, close your browser and proceed to Exercise 69.

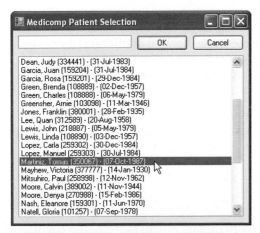

▶ **Figure 11-10 Select patient Tomas Martiniz.**

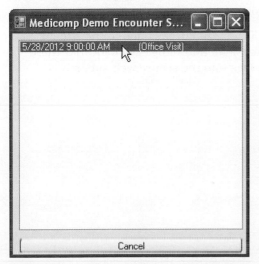

▶ **Figure 11-11 Select existing encounter for May 28, 2012.**

Critical Thinking Exercise 69: Reviewing Client-Entered Data

It is important to note that a client entering medical history either in the medical clinic or via the Internet is not accessing the actual EHR, but rather a separate application. This protects the security and integrity of the EHR.

Once the data is reviewed by the nurse, the data can be imported or merged directly into the EHR to become part of the encounter note. In this exercise you will take on the role of the nurse, to review the data Mr. Martiniz has entered.

Case Study

Tomas Martiniz is a 24-year-old male who has an appointment May 28, 2012, at 9:00 AM. He has used the Internet to complete his medical questionnaire in advance. The data has been merged into the EHR to initiate the encounter note for his visit.

Step 1

If you have not already done so, start the Student Edition software.

Click Select on the Menu bar, and then click Patient.

In the Patient Selection window, locate and click on Tomas Martiniz as shown in Figure 11-10.

Step 2

Click Select on the Menu bar again, and then click **Existing Encounter**.

Select **5/28/2012 9:00 AM Office Visit** as shown in Figure 11-11.

The encounter note from that date will be displayed.

Step 3

Click on the Print button on the Toolbar at the top of your screen to invoke the Print Data window.

Be certain there is a check mark in the box next to "Current Encounter" and then click on the button labeled "Print and Close," even if you normally exported a file in previous exercises. You will need a printed copy for the next step.

Step 4

Compare the answers from the interview report you printed in the previous exercise with the encounter note you have just printed. On your printed encounter note identify and draw a circle around any instances where the terminology is different.

If there were any differences, why would the client's terminology and the medical nomenclature be different?

When you are finished, give your interview report or output file to your instructor.

Provider-to-Client E-Mail Communication

The HIPAA Security Rule does not expressly prohibit the use of e-mail for sending electronic protected health information (EPHI). The Security Rule allows for EPHI to be sent over an open network as long as it is adequately protected. However, the security rule standard for transmission security includes specifications for integrity controls and encryption.

The catch is that the HIPAA Privacy Rule permits the client to disclose information to anyone whom the client likes, but the covered entity cannot. This means a client can e-mail a doctor, nurse, or medical facility any information he or she wants about his or her medical condition, even if the e-mail is not encrypted. However, the provider has to be very guarded in replying through unencrypted e-mail—that is, neither a copy of the client's message should be included nor any specific information revealed. Most importantly, the client should consider whether he or she should send private health information using unencrypted e-mail.

Although e-mail can be secured by encryption, managing separate encryption keys for thousands of clients and using the appropriate key each client would be untenable. The preferred alternative is to use a secure web site for communication between the client and provider.

Secure Messaging

Instead of sending an e-mail message from his or her usual e-mail system, the client logs on to the clinic's web site and types the information in an e-mail screen on the web page. The web site handles all the security, protecting the EPHI as required by HIPAA.

Responses to the client are handled similarly. The client checks back to the site for messages, or receives a benign message via regular e-mail informing the client that there is a reply to the query waiting. The client then logs into the secure web site, reads the message and, if necessary, writes a reply.

Real-Life Story

Using the Internet to Build a Client-Centered Practice

By Karen Smith, MD, FAAFP

I practice medicine in Raeford, North Carolina, which is located in the second-most impoverished county in our state. We are close to a military base, so we have a culturally diverse mix of patients, those native to this area as well as people from all over who are stationed here.

After graduating from family medicine residency, my family relocated to Raeford. There were only three doctors in town caring for the whole population. The first two practices that I worked at used paper medical records. When I set up my own practice, I knew EHR was a necessary tool. That is when I met Dr. Alan Wenner. I went to his lecture symposium titled the "High-Performing Physician."

We simultaneously implemented both an EHR and a practice management system in place from day one. In 2008, the NCQA introduced the recognition process for the "medical home." We reviewed the criteria and the requirements for Patient-Centered Medical Home (PCMH) status (covered in Chapter 12). We already had most of it. The last component we needed was the virtual health office.

Our practice web site (shown in Figure 11-1) allows patients to register online, request an appointment, complete their Instant Medical History (IMH) symptom assessment before their appointment, review health insurance information, obtain their lab results, access medical information for common medical conditions, and have a virtual office visit with their doctor online.

IMH is readily accepted by our patients, especially military families. Because of a base realignment of the military, we have 30,000 new military personnel coming into our community and a lot of them already registered online and completed their IMH before they come into the office.

Workflow of Our Office

Our patients' have several ways of contacting us; some call on the telephone and some just walk in. Our preferred first point of contact, however, is our web site. We automate a lot of our previsit activity. I have already mentioned they can complete the IMH symptom assessment over the Internet. We also have an automated system that telephones patients to remind them of their appointments. Once the Televox system has confirmed their appointment, one of my staff reviews their chart to see if their immunizations are up to date, if they have a balance due, or need anything else before their visit. In addition, we have now introduced a live operator system via the practice portal and Athena communicator, which is a very important combination of the web with a person who is familiar with the office systems.

When a patient shows up, existing demographic information is verified as that person is checked in on the computer. Once the patient is checked into the system, the nurse is automatically notified on her computer that the patient is checked in. She then goes to the lobby and gets the patient. She takes the patient's vital signs and then brings the patient into the exam room. There she starts her nursing intake. She will start the IMH and then leave the patient in the room to do his or her own entry, unless the person did the entry from home via our web site before coming. About 15 percent of our patients do it in advance.

If the patient did it at home, the nurse would extract it and bring it into the HPI section of the note. If the patient does it in the office, the nurse will return when that person is finished and then paste it into the note. In either case, when that is done I will see a color change on my computer and know that the patient is ready for me.

I go into the exam room and log on to the EHR. I have computers in every exam room, so I do not have to carry anything around. I have the patient elaborate a little more on the purpose of the visit. I perform the exam and go over any issues the patient may have. Then I sit down with that person so that we are both on the same level and can both see the computer screen. The computer is positioned where we can both see it at the same time and yet I can maintain eye-to-eye contact. My exam room computers are set up the way Dr. Wenner recommends (as shown in Figure 11-5) and it works well.

Many of my patients have hypertension or hyperlipidemia. By sharing the screen, the patient can actually see the objective information: "Here is your cholesterol and what you have been doing is working well." To get the patient to be compliant with the treatment plan, we put it in together. I am literally entering the orders in front of the patient as a way of emphasizing "I am putting this in the way we mutually agreed." When I have everything ordered, I look at the patient and ask, "Did we cover everything today, or is there anything else we need to take care of?" When the person answers no, then I close the encounter note. I stand up and we walk out the room together.

All of our office systems are interfaced. For example, if I had ordered labs when I wrote the order, the lab system automatically printed the labels and if an ABN (advanced beneficiary notices) is necessary, it printed out as well. Many times I will walk the patient to the lab and the phlebotomist already has the tubes ready. Because I use a bidirectional interface, the lab orders have already gone to the lab company.

When the patient is finished, he or she is taken to the front desk where my instructions to the patient, follow-up visit information, and a summary of today's visit is already prepared—all of this from the click of a button on the exam room computer. By the time the patient gets to the front desk to check out, his or her already has an appointment card ready for the next appointment, the billing information for the claim has gone into the billing system, the charges have been posted, the patient due has been calculated and ready for the front desk to collect balance due, including any deductible that has not been met.

Even after the patient goes home, if he or she has a question about treatment, medication, or just forgot to ask something, the patient can go online to our web site and send me a secure message.

Virtual Office Visits

We also offer patients the ability to use our web portal to have their office visit online instead of coming into the office. What we had to do was make it clear to the patient that "using the virtual office means the doctor is going to see and take care of your problems online; you do not need to be physically present to the office." Our virtual office visit uses an interview question format similar to the IMH symptom assessment.

▶ The patient logs in and chooses Virtual Office Visit. The normal E-visit workflow is to collect the payment on the web site at the time of service; however, we initially had an issue with the electronic payment process to be resolved.

▶ The patient confirms personal information and answers the health questions specific to the topic of the consultation, which normally takes about five minutes.

▶ Upon completion of their Virtual Office Visit, the system sends me a message.

▶ I log on and review the visit. I can see everything that the patient put in. I then create the response. I can reply with any further questions, but in most cases the online interview has gathered sufficient data. I also have access to my patient's medical history in the EHR. If I put in a prescription, it is sent to the pharmacy and adds information to the patient message that this is the patient's medication and the name of the drug store where it has been sent. Alternatively, I can say that the patient needs to come into the office in person.

▶ The patient then receives an e-mail notification from us. The confidential e-mail message does not disclose any information about the nature of the visit to our site. It simply asks the patient to return to our site for more information.

▶ Upon revisiting our site, the patient logs in and views the message from the physician. This message contains the treatment plan or a request for additional information. If the treatment plan involves prescription medications, the patient is given the pharmacy information.

In most cases, that completes the E-visit because very specific conditions and treatments can be done this way. Also, because these are my patients, I know what their health conditions are. I usually do not have to ask patients for further information and can close out the E-visit.

The utility of the E-visit occurring is very useful for our group. We promote the use of our web site everywhere, including our practice policies and patient care information sheets, but using the web portal and virtual office visits has been a learning curve in our community. I think in part this is because of the impoverishment in our county; only 30 percent of the households have Internet access within the home. I have noticed our military patients and their families use E-visits more than my other patients, but the Army has given the families computers and Internet access, so that may be a factor.

E-Visits

Even when using secure messages, clinics have concerns about the potential for medical liability, the lack of structure in the messages, and the difficulty of keeping the e-mail exchange as part of the client's medical record. Also, the clinic does not receive payment for the e-mail exchange.

One solution that enhances the efficiency of providers and improves the accessibility of healthcare for the clients is the E-visit. An E-visit allows the client to be treated by a clinician for nonurgent health problems without the client having to come into the office.

An E-visit has all the advantages that e-mail lacks: not only are E-visits secure but the E-visit also gathers symptom and HPI information, creating a documented medical encounter. When the E-visit data is imported into the EHR, it becomes a part of the client's chart, just like any other visit.

Equally as important to the clinician, E-visits are reimbursed as a legitimate visit. At the time that this book was published, E-visits were being paid by Blue Cross/Blue Shield™ plans and other private insurance carriers in numerous states. A study by Price-Waterhouse-Coopers predicted that more than 20 percent of all office visits could be replaced by an online equivalent (PricewaterhouseCooper, 1999).

Workflow of an E-Visit

The basic workflow of an E-visit begins with client-entered symptom, history, and history of present illness information. Some E-visit web sites use IMH to gather HPI data from the client. Other E-visit web sites use a combination of check boxes and free-text messages, similar to secure messaging discussed earlier. Some E-visit web sites such as the one at the Mayo Clinic allow the client to upload digital photos.

The workflow begins when a client accesses the clinic web site and signs on. The client must already be an established client with the practice and have medical records on file. E-visits are not generally permitted for a new client who has never been seen at the practice.

The client answers a few simple questions and selects the reason for the visit from a list. This allows the software to determine which question sets would be appropriate to ask. The client also could just enter a free-text complaint.

The client answers online interview questions related to his or her reported complaint, as shown later in Exercise 69. Answers to certain medically significant questions could cause the software to ask different sets of medically related questions automatically. The client can add free-text clarification at various points in the interview.

E-visits are only used for nonurgent visits. If the software detects that the condition seems urgent, the client is advised to seek immediate medical care and the provider is notified. If the software determines that although the condition is not urgent, it is one for which the client should be seen in person, the client is given a message to that effect and automatically offered a choice of available appointments.

When the interview is complete, the data entered by the client is recorded in the EHR and the clinician is notified that an E-visit is ready to review. Even in the event that the client must come in for the visit, the provider is better prepared because the symptom and history information is already at hand.

Unlike e-mail, which is directed at a particular individual and therefore not likely to be accessible by another provider, E-visits can be directed to the "provider on call," allowing practicing partners to share "E-visit" duty, just like they share other on-call services. Providers usually respond promptly after being notified. A study of E-visits that was done in California (Relay Health Corporation, 2003, *Relay Health webVisit Study: Final Report.* © 2002–2003, Relay Health Corporation) found a majority of clients were happy if the provider responded by the next morning. Remember, E-visits are for nonurgent matters.

The clinician reviews the client-entered data and any relevant client medical records, then replies to the client. The system allows the provider and client to continue to exchange messages, much as a question-and-answer session in the exam room, except for the factor of time, which is sometimes delayed by one or both parties' responses.

The clinician also can prescribe electronically during the E-visit, just as he or she would during an office visit. When the client receives the clinician's reply to the E-visit, that client is prompted to select a preferred pharmacy from a list (if it is not already known to the EHR) and the prescription is electronically transmitted to the pharmacy by the EHR system.

The provider's response also can include client education material and comments or care instructions, all of which are recorded in the care plan. The clinic's practice management system can verify the client eligibility for the E-visit, and submit the claim electronically.

Mayo Clinic Study of E-Visits

The largest study of Internet use for online care (E-visits) using a structured history was conducted in the Department of Family Medicine at Mayo Clinic in Rochester, Minnesota. Here are excerpts from the study (Adamson & Bachman, 2010).

"Patients in the department preregistered for the service and then were able to use the online portal for consultations with their primary care providers."

"After completing (data entry for) the e-visit, the patients received an e-mail stating that their clinician would review their consultation within 24 hours. Another e-mail was forwarded to the clinician informing him or her of an e-visit waiting in the secure portal. The portal allowed the clinician to use templated encounter forms for many common illnesses so that information such as diagnostic codes, links to patient education, and treatment plans could be stored and reused. This standardization of treatment greatly speeded the process of reviewing an online visit. Medications were often prescribed during the process and faxed to the pharmacy. At the conclusion of the online visit, patients received an e-mail stating that the results of their encounter could be found on the portal. Patients would then log in and view the materials."

"Generally, online consultations were completed by clinicians within 24 hours of the e-visit submission; only 11 were not completed. E-visits were completed by the patient's primary provider 89% of the time; 11% of the consultations were provided by an on-call clinician for absent providers or if the patient selected 'first available doctor.'"

"Because patients could enter any symptom or concern, ask questions, and add additional comments, the e-visits eliminated the need for clinicians to ask for further information in most instances. . . . This was because the patient's history was organized and pertinent information including all medications, allergies, and vital signs such as weight were always obtained. The volume of exchanges could be decreased further by emphasizing the need to send pictures of rashes. . . ."

"Some consultations for patients with chronic disease seemed to show promise. Patients with diabetes mellitus first had laboratory tests and then were asked to complete an online visit regarding their diabetes. If all was well according to the interview and laboratory results, the patients did not need to visit the office. Hypertension was also managed online; patients sent in their blood pressure responses and clinicians managed their medications and laboratory studies online."

"During the 2-year study, 4,282 patients were registered for the service. Patients made 2,531 online visits, and billings were made for 1,159 patients."

"E-visits were made primarily by working-aged women who completed e-visits for themselves, their dependents, and their older parents during office hours and involved 294 different conditions. Two percent of the visits included uploaded photographs, and 16% of the e-visits replaced nonbillable telephone protocols with billable encounters. The e-visits made office visits unnecessary in 40% of cases; in 12.8% of cases, the patient was asked to schedule an appointment for a face-to-face encounter."

"[T]he . . . study . . . showed the feasibility of online visits to educate, treat, and bill patients. The extent of conditions possible for treatment by online care was far ranging and was managed with a minimum of message exchanges by using structured histories" (pp.1–14).

California Study

In an independent study sponsored by Blue Shield of California, most clients and doctors in the study preferred a web visit to an office visit for nonurgent medical needs. Providers found that the E-visit gathered the important details and eliminated multiple messages back and forth that occur when trying to provide client care via e-mail. The clients found that the time spent scheduling, driving, parking, and waiting was saved with an E-visit (Relay Health Corporation, 2003, *Relay Health webVisit Study: Final Report.* © 2002–2003, Relay Health Corporation).

Guided Exercise 70: Client Requests an E-Visit

Case Study

Jacob Silverstein is a 46-year-old male with a history of hypertension and diabetes. He is on medication and has regular checkups at his family practice. He has an issue with his medication and is going to try an online E-visit instead of coming to the office.

Step 1

Start your web browser program and log in to Online Student Resources for this book.

When the welcome page is displayed, click on the link "**Exercises and Activities**" or select "Exercises and Activities" from the drop-down list and click on the button labeled "Go."

Step 2

A menu on the left of the screen will list various activities and exercises. Locate and click on the link Exercise 70.

Information about the exercise will be displayed.

Locate and click the link "Click here to start the web portal program."

Step 3

The sample provider web page shown in Figure 11-6 will be displayed.

Locate the section labeled "E-visits for Established Patients" and click on the link "E-visit."

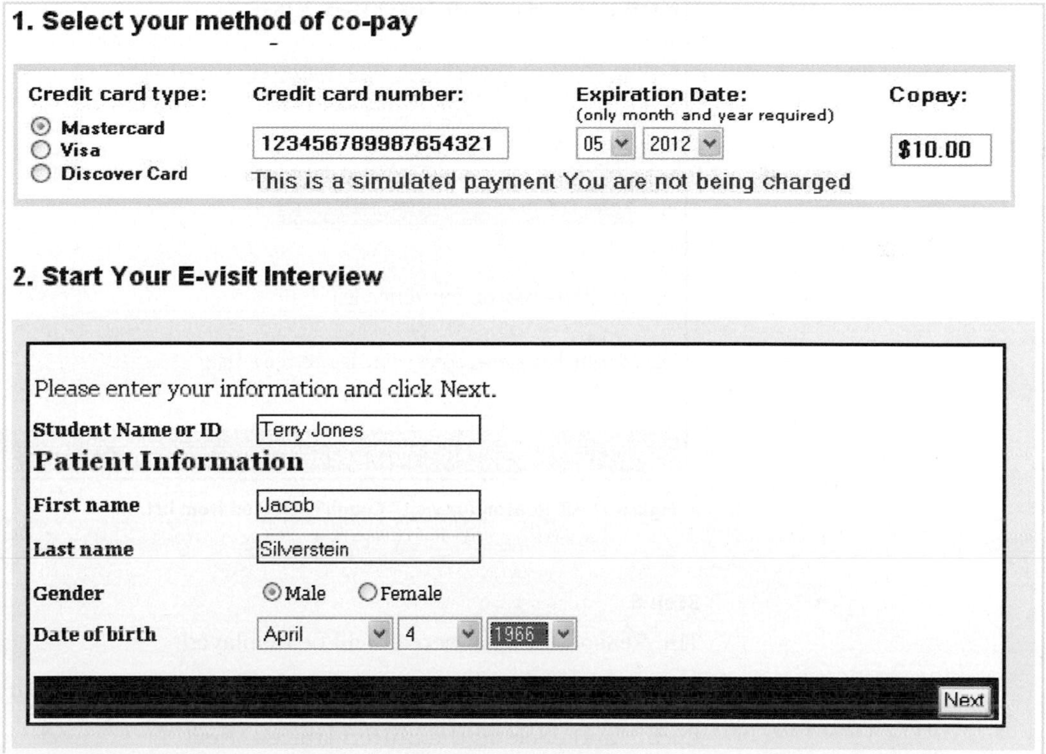

▶ Figure 11-12 Client interview screen for an E-visit.

Step 4

The "Welcome to Family Care E-visit" web page is displayed. It includes simulated payment information as shown at the top of Figure 11-12. A key difference between an

E-visit and a pre-visit questionnaire is that providers collect a copay at the time of the E-visit. It is not necessary to collect the copay on the previsit questionnaire page as the client will be coming into the office, where the payment will be collected.

This is a student exercise; you will not be charged. Do not enter any personal credit card data; simply complete the student ID and patient information fields shown below.

Locate and click on the button labeled "Start Interview." The center portion of your web page will look similar to Figure 11-12.

Step 5

Enter the following:

Enter your name or student ID as you have in the previous exercise.

Enter the follow information about the client:

First Name: **Jacob**

Last Name: **Silverstein**

Click the circle next to **Male**

Click on the down arrow buttons in each of the Date of Birth fields and select from the drop-down lists: **April**, **4**, and **1966**

Compare your screen to Figure 11-12. When everything has been entered correctly, locate and click on the button labeled "Next."

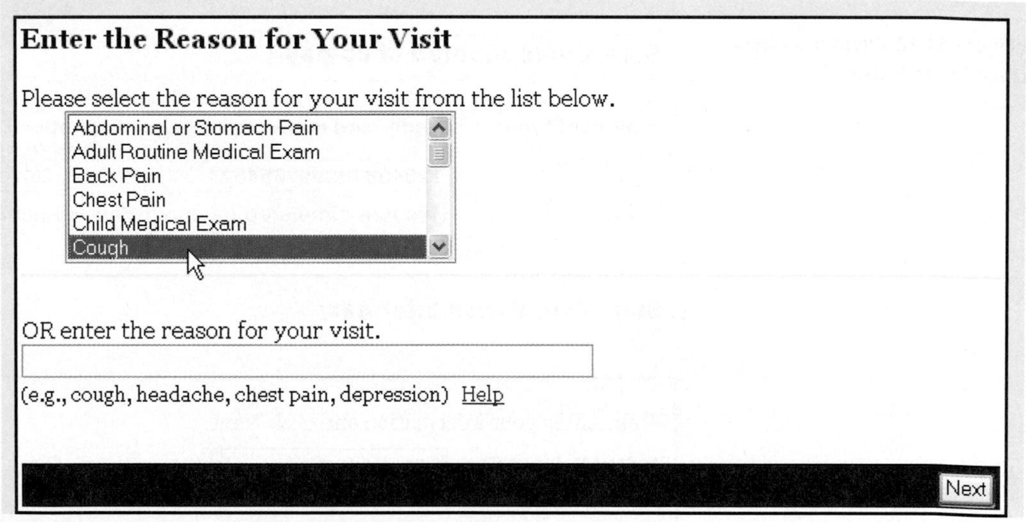

► Figure 11-13 Reason for visit "Cough" selected from list.

Step 6

The Reason for Visit screen will be displayed.

Locate and click on "Cough" in the list of reasons as shown in Figure 11-13.

Locate and click on the button labeled "Next."

Step 7

The interview process will start. For each question in the table below, locate and click on the indicated button. If you make an error, click on the button labeled "Previous Question," and correct your error.

Interview Question	Click on the following buttons
Do you have a cough?	**Yes**
How long have you had a cough?	**16 - 20 days**
Have you had a cold, flu, or cough within the last month that seemed to improve and then worsen?	**No**
Do you cough all day long?	**Yes**
Does your cough sometimes wake you up at night?	**No**
Does your cough seem to occur in spasms or episodes of multiple coughs?	**No**
When you cough, are you bringing up any sputum or phlegm from deep in your chest other than a small amount early in the morning?	**No**
Is your cough worse after exercise?	**No**
Is your cough worse when you lie down?	**No**
Are you having a major problem with shortness of breath right now?	**No**
Do you have chest discomfort when you breathe?	**No**
Do you have any wheezing when you breathe?	**No**
Do you sound hoarse?	**No**
Do you have post-nasal drip or are you always clearing the back of your throat?	**No**
Have you had a fever in the past week?	**No**
Do you sometimes wake up with soaking sweats at night?	**No**
Did your cough begin after any change in your medications?	**Yes**
Do you have a cough at certain seasons of the year?	**No**
Have you ever had pneumonia?	**No**
Have you ever kept or raised birds?	**No**
Describe your use of tobacco	**Never used**

Step 8

When you have reached the end of the interview, a free-text note box is displayed to allow the client to enter messages in their own words. Leave the box empty.

Locate and click on the button labeled "Next."

Step 9

The final screen of the interview allows you to review your work.

Compare your screen to Figure 11-14 by scrolling the window as necessary. If there are any differences (other than the client's age), repeat the exercise, making certain you answer each of the questions in steps 6 through 8 correctly.

Step 10

At the bottom of the Interview Report screen are two buttons labeled "Save" and "Print."

When everything in your report is correct, locate and click on the appropriate button to either print or save to a file, as directed by your instructor. Once you have your printout or file output in hand, close your browser and proceed to Exercise 71.

Chief Complaint

Jacob Silverstein is a 44 year old male. His reason for visit is "Cough".

History of Present Illness

#1. "Cough"

Severity

He reported: Cough continuously throughout the day.

Duration

He reported: Cough 16 to 20 days.

Timing

He denied: Nocturnal cough. Seasonal cough.

Context

He reported: Cough nonproductive. Cough started after any medication change.

He denied: Cough seems to occur in spasms or episodes, stopping in between. Deep breathing causes chest pain.

Modifying Factors

He denied: Cough after exercise. Cough worse lying down.

Associated Signs and Symptoms

He denied: Wheezing. Shortness of breath. Recent cold improved then worsened.

Past, Family, and Social History

Past Medical History

He denied: Pneumonia.

Social History

He denied: Cough associated with history of exposure to birds.

Tobacco Use

He reported: Never used tobacco.

Review of Systems

Constitutional

He denied: Cough associated with fever. Night sweats.

Ear, Nose, and Throat

He denied: Nasal drainage. Hoarseness.

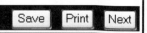

▶ **Figure 11-14 Completed interview for E-visit.**

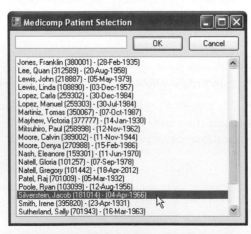

▶ **Figure 11-15 Select patient Jacob Silverstein.**

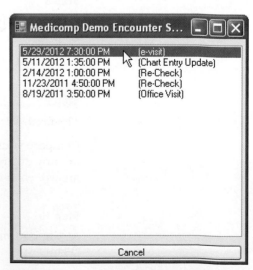

▶ **Figure 11-16 Select the E-visit encounter for 5/29/2012.**

Guided Exercise 71: Clinician Completes the E-Visit

Step 1

If you have not already done so, start the Student Edition software.

Click Select on the Menu bar, and then click Patient.

In the Patient Selection window, locate and click on **Jacob Silverstein** as shown in Figure 11-15.

Step 2

Click Select on the Menu bar again, and then click **Existing Encounter**.

Select **5/29/2012 7:30 PM e-Visit** as shown in Figure 11-16.

The encounter note containing the client-entered data from the E-visit will be displayed.

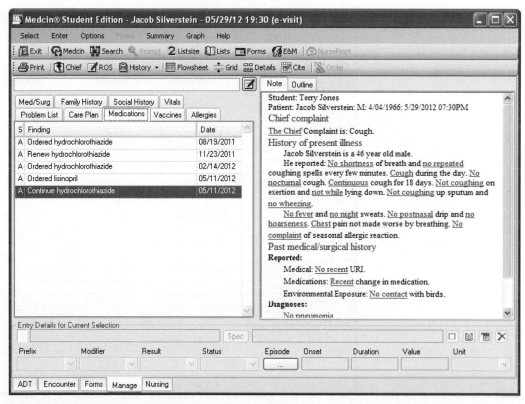

▶ Figure 11-17 Medications tab showing prescription history.

Step 3

When the encounter is displayed, locate and click on the Manage tab at the bottom of your screen. Review the HPI data supplied by the client displayed in the right pane and then locate and click on the tab labeled "Medications" in the left pane. Compare your screen to Figure 11-17. Review Mr. Silverstein's prescription history. Note that a new drug was prescribed on 5/11/2012.

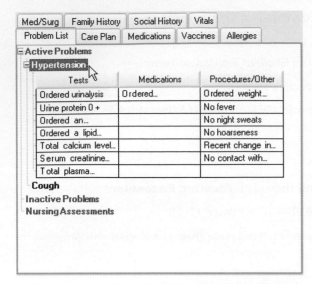

► **Figure 11-18 Problem tab with Hypertension highlighted.**

Step 4

Locate and click on the tab labeled "Problem List" and then click on "Hypertension" to highlight it, as shown in Figure 11-18.

Locate and click on the Flowsheet button on the Toolbar at the top of your screen (highlighted orange in Figure 11-19).

Step 5

Scroll the Flowsheet downward until your screen looks like Figure 11-19. Locate and click on the red button for the Assessment:

● (red button) Hypertension

Locate the heading Medications, Vaccines in the Plan section near the bottom of the Flowsheet. Click on the description "Ordered Lisinopril" (circled in Figure 11-19). The entire row will become highlighted. Do not click the red or blue buttons.

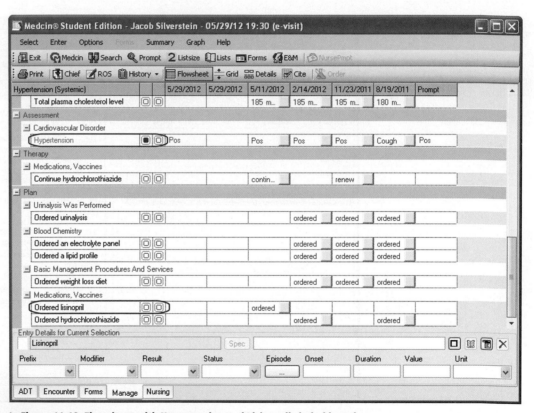

► **Figure 11-19 Flowsheet with Hypertension and Lisinopril circled in red.**

Step 6

Locate and click on the down arrow in the Entry Details "Prefix" field. Select "discontinue" from the drop-down list.

Locate and click on the Flowsheet button on the Toolbar to close the Flowsheet.

Locate and click on the Encounter tab at the bottom of your screen.

Step 7

Click on the Dx tab in the left pane.

▶ **Figure 11-20 Select "discontinue" from the Prefix drop-down list.**

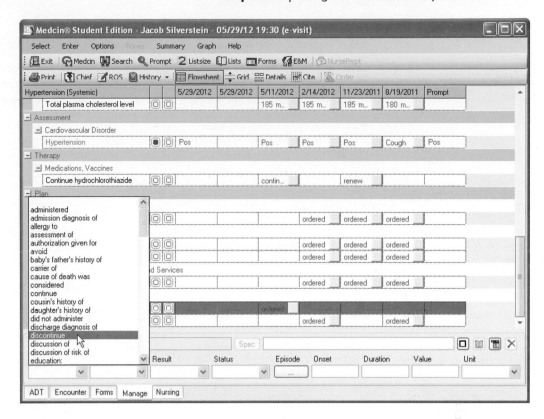

▶ **Figure 11-21 Dx: Adverse effect of drug therapy.**

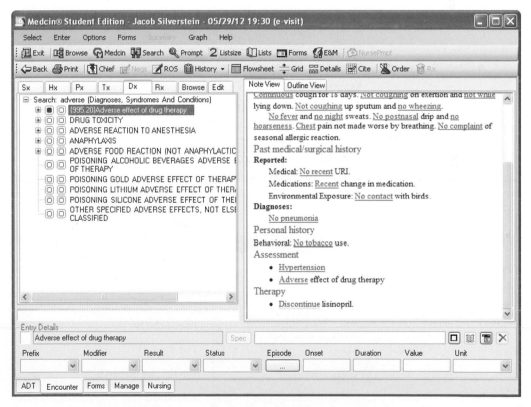

Locate and click on the Search button on the Toolbar at the top of your screen. When the Search dialog window is displayed, type "**adverse**," and then click on the button in the dialog window labeled "Search." Compare your results to the left pane of Figure 11-21.

Locate and click on the red button for the following finding:

● (red button) Adverse effect of drug therapy

Step 8

Click on the Rx tab in the left pane.

Locate and click on the Search button on the Toolbar at the top of your screen. When the Search dialog window is displayed, type "**Amlodipine**," and then click on the button in the dialog window labeled "Search." Compare your results in the left pane of your screen to Figure 11-22.

Highlight the finding "Calcium Channel Blockers Amlodipine Maleate," and then click the Rx button on the Toolbar at the top of your screen. This will invoke the Rx Writer.

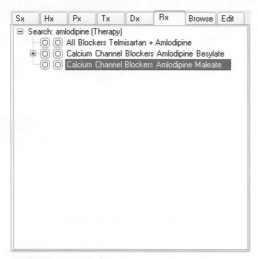

▶ **Figure 11-22 Highlight Calcium Channel Blockers Amlodipine Maleate.**

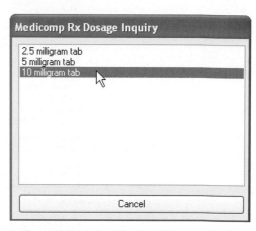

▶ **Figure 11-23 Select the 10 milligram tablet in the Rx Dosage Inquiry window.**

Step 9

Select the dosage "10 milligram tab," as shown in Figure 11-23, and then double-click on it.

Step 10

The Rx Brand window will be displayed (not shown). There is only one brand, "Amvaz"; double-click on it.

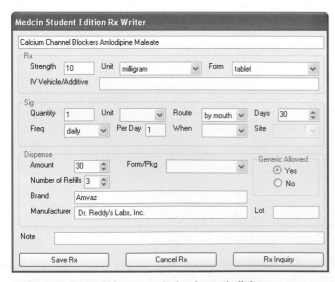

▶ **Figure 11-24 Rx Writer prescription for Amlodipine.**

Step 11

The Rx Writer will display the selected dosage and manufacturer. Complete the prescription by entering the remaining information in the following fields:

Quantity: **1**

Freq: **daily**

Per Day: **1**

Route: **by mouth**

Days: **30**

Amount: **30**

Refills: **3**

Generic: **Y**

Compare your screen to Figure 11-24. When everything is correct, locate and click the button labeled "Save Rx."

```
Jacob Silverstein                                          Page 1 of 1

Student: your name or ID here
Patient: Jacob Silverstein: M: 4/04/1966: 5/29/2012 07:30PM
Chief complaint
The Chief Complaint is: Cough.
History of present illness
     Jacob Silverstein is a 46 year old male.
     He reported: No shortness of breath and no repeated coughing spells every
     few minutes. Cough during the day. No nocturnal cough. Continuous cough for
     18 days. Not coughing on exertion and not while lying down. Not coughing up
     sputum and no wheezing.
     No fever and no night sweats. No postnasal drip and no hoarseness. Chest pain
     not made worse by breathing. No complaint of seasonal allergic reaction.
Past medical/surgical history
Reported History:
Medical: No recent URI.
Medications: Recent change in medication
Environmental Exposure: No contact with birds.
Diagnosis History:
No pneumonia
Personal history
Behavioral: No tobacco use.
Assessment
     • Hypertension
     • Adverse effect of drug therapy
Therapy
     • Discontinue lisinopril.
Plan
     • Amlodipine maleate
10 mg tab (1 po qd 30) DISP:30 Refill:3 Generic:Y Using:Amvaz Mfg: Dr. Reddy's
Labs, Inc.
```

▶ **Figure 11-25 Printout of E-visit encounter for Jacob Silverstein.**

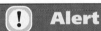

Alert

Do not close or exit the Encounter until you have a printed copy in your hand. You will lose your work if you exit before printing.

Step 12

Click on the Print button on the Toolbar at the top of your screen to invoke the Print Data window.

Be certain there is a check mark in the box next to "Current Encounter" and then click on the appropriate button to either print or export a file, as directed by your instructor.

Compare your printout or file output to Figure 11-25. If it is correct, hand it in to your instructor. If there are any differences, review the previous steps in the exercise and find your error.

Chapter Eleven Summary

The Internet is one of the key technologies impacting healthcare. It not only facilitates remote access, but gives the nurse instant access to medical research and best practice nursing guidelines for decision support.

Clients research their conditions using the Internet and bring the information with them to their clinic visits. Clients are also sending e-mail to their providers asking medical questions about their conditions. However, the Internet is really a large network of public computers, which is sometimes referred to as a "cloud." EPHI, which is sent over the Internet, needs to be secured.

Remote provider access to the EHR via the Internet usually involves setting up a VPN or using a web portal that has SSL encryption. Telemedicine provides home nursing and specialist consultation to clients in remote locations. Similarly, teleradiology allows a radiologist to interpret diagnostic images from another location.

Providers are setting up secure web sites, where clients can see their medical information and consult with their doctors and nurses using secure messaging. One feature of these web sites is the ability for clients to use the Internet to enter information about their history and symptoms before arriving at a scheduled appointment.

Numerous studies have shown that client-entered data can become a significant contributor to the EHR, for some of the following reasons:

▶ Only the client has the information about what symptoms were present at the outset of the illness.

▶ Only the client knows the outcome of medical treatment of those symptoms.

▶ The client is also the source of past medical, family, and social history.

▶ Client-entered data is a more accurate reflection of a client's complaints.

▶ Clients who can review their histories are better prepared for the visit.

▶ Up to 67% of the nurse or clinician's time with the client is spent entering the client's symptom into the visit documentation.

▶ A computer can be used by the client over the Internet or in the waiting room to enter the same symptom and history information that the nurse or clinician would have entered.

▶ Client-entered data is organized by the computer for the provider in a succinct and easy-to-read format that becomes the starting point for the encounter.

▶ Having a complete history in advance of the visit allows the clinician to ask fewer questions about the diagnosis and concentrate more on the effects of the illness on the client. It also allows the clinician more time to discuss the treatment plan with the client.

Other features found on clinic web sites allow clients to request an appointment time or a prescription renewal, provide secure access to information from their medical record, and securely communicate with the provider. However, even using secure messaging, merging the e-mail threads into clients' EHR, or filing an insurance claim for e-mail consults would be a challenge. A preferred alternative is the E-visit, which allows clients to be treated for nonurgent health problems without having to come into the clinic.

The E-visit gathers symptom and HPI information and creates a documented encounter. It can be integrated into the EHR to become part of clients' chart, and equally important to the clinician, E-visits are reimbursed in some states.

References

Adamson, M. D., Steven, C., Bachman, M. D., & John, W. (2010). *Pilot study of providing online care in a primary care setting.* Rochester, MN: Department of Family Medicine, Mayo Clinic.

Brailer, D. J. (2004, July 21). *The decade of health information technology: Delivering consumer-centric and information-rich healthcare.* Washington, DC: U.S. Department of Health and Human Services.

Brodman, K., Erdmann, A. J., Jr., Lorge, I. et al. (1949). The Cornell Medical Index: An adjunct to medical interview. *Journal of the American Medical Association, 140,* 530–534.

Centers for Medicare & Medicaid Services. (2005, May). *HIPAA Security Series No. 4: Security standards: Technical safeguards.* Baltimore, MD: Author. (Revised March 2007

Deloitte Center for Health Solutions. (2009). *2009 Survey of Health Care Consumers.* Washington, DC: Deloitte, LLP.

Dick, R. S., & Steen, E. B. (2000). *The computer-based patient record: An essential technology for health care.* Washington, DC: Institute of Medicine, National Academy Press. (Originally published 1991, revised 1997)

Grehalva, R. (2010). *eHealth patterns in the 21st century.* Birmingham, AL: MEDSEEK.

Health Insurance Portability and Accountability Act, Title 2, Pub. L. 104-191, subsection f (1996).

Mayne, J. G., Weksel, W., & Sholtz, P. N. (1968). Toward automating the medical history. *Mayo Clinic Proceedings, 43,* 1–25.

Meaningful Use Workgroup to the HIT Policy Committee, U.S. Department of Health and Human Services Office of National Coordinator. (2009, June 16). *Meaningful use: A definition.* Washington, DC: Author.

PricewaterhouseCoopers. (1999, November). *HealthCast 2010: Smaller world, bigger expectations.* Retrieved April 28, 2011, from http://www.pwc.com/us/en/healthcast/past-reports.jhtml

RelayHealth Corporation. (2003, January). *The Relay Health webVisit Study: Final Report.* Retrieved from www.relayhealth.com .

Slack, W. V., Hicks, G. P., Reed, C. E., & Van Cura, L. J. (1966). A computer-based medical-history system. *New England Journal of Medicine, 274,* 194–198.

Stein, T., Ed. (2005). *The electronic physician.* Chicago: Allscripts Healthcare Solution.

Test Your Knowledge

1. Name the two methods of securing information sent over the Internet described in this chapter.

2. List three examples of changes in healthcare related to the Internet.

3. What percentage of the nurse's time is spent entering client symptoms and history into the chart?

4. What is an E-visit?

5. Name three things the home health nurse did for the client using telemedicine.

6. Where was the largest study of using the Internet for E-visits conducted?

7. Describe the differences between provider-to-client e-mail and E-visits.

8. What were the two types of telemedicine described in this chapter?

9. What does HIPAA require when sending EPHI by e-mail?

10. Why did the Mayo Clinic need to develop a different method of telemedicine?

11. What is the risk to a client who e-mails information about his or her condition to the provider?

12. Name two criteria for assessing the reliability of information found on a web site.

13. Give three examples of decision support information available via the web.

14. Does the Internet function more like the telephone or the post office? Explain your answer.

15. You should have produced two Internet research documents, a report of three nursing web sites, one printed encounter note, and one printed interview report. If you have not already done so, give these to your instructor.

Ask your instructor for answers to Test Your Knowledge

nursing.pearsonhighered.com

Prepare for success with animated examples, practice questions, challenge tests, and interactive assignments.

12 Using the EHR for Prevention and Health Maintenance

Learning Outcomes

After completing this chapter, you should be able to:

1. Document a well-baby checkup using a wellness form
2. Explain the relationship between vital signs and growth charts
3. Create a pediatric growth chart
4. Understand Body Mass Index
5. Calculate Body Mass Index
6. Understand immunization schedules
7. Order immunizations for a child
8. Describe how clients can be involved in their own health
9. Discuss preventive care guidelines
10. Understand how EHR preventive care systems work
11. Discuss client access to electronic health records
12. Explain the criteria for Patient-Centered Medical Home
13. Understand and compare Personal Health Records

Prevention and Early Detection

The value of the EHR as a longitudinal record increases with use. As more of the client's health record is stored in a codified EHR, more can be done with it. The previous chapters have shown that data from past encounters can be used to improve care through disease management, trending, and creating graphs for client education and counseling. Trending allows early recognition and intervention of the client's health changes. Still, it is always better to prevent a disease than to treat it.

An important aspect of nursing practice is health promotion; educating clients to maintain a state of wellness. Health promotion is not necessarily disease related. Although prevention focuses on protection against specific health problems, health promotion is collaboration between the nurse and client to educate and encourage increased responsibility for personal health and self-care. Prevention is focused on avoiding potential threats to health. The nurse's role in prevention includes educating clients to decrease the risk of injury or disease, immunization to prevent contagious diseases, early detection of disease, and helping clients identify behaviors that can affect their health.

In this chapter, we will discuss various ways in which preventive care, immunization, preventive screening, client education, and clients' participation in their healthcare can help people live longer, healthier lives. One setting in which a nurse experiences all of that is pediatrics; therefore we shall begin with several exercises in a pediatric clinic.

Pediatric Wellness Visits

Those of us who are adults may someday have an electronic health record, but we may never have a completely codified personal health record, because too much of our medical history is isolated in paper records at medical offices that we no longer visit. Those who are just being born, however, have an excellent chance that their medical records are being created and stored electronically even today.

The care we receive in the early years is fundamental to lifelong health. Early screening, detection, education, and immunizations have all contributed to increased life spans of the population as a whole. Nowhere does this have more support than in the pediatric practice, where regular examinations are recommended for wellness visits, not just when the child is ill.

In the next exercises, you will use the Student Edition software to record a pediatric visit, create a different kind of graph called a *growth chart*, and learn about childhood immunizations. This is a lot of material to cover, and for that reason the pediatric visit will span several exercises.

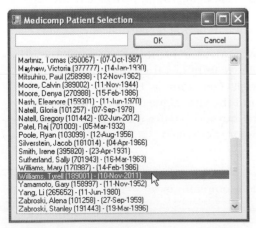

▶ **Figure 12-1 Selecting Tyrell Williams from the Patient Selection window.**

Guided Exercise 72: A Well-Baby Checkup

Case Study

Tyrell Williams is a 6-month-old male who is brought by his mother to the pediatric clinic where he has always been seen. As a result, the clinic has a lifelong history of his care and growth.

Step 1

If you have not already done so, start the Student Edition software.

Click Select on the Menu bar, and then click Patient.

In the Patient Selection window, locate and click on **Tyrell Williams** as shown in Figure 12-1.

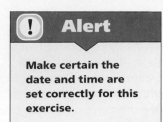

Alert

Make certain the date and time are set correctly for this exercise.

Step 2

Click Select on the Menu bar, and then click New Encounter.

Use the date **May 25, 2012**, the time **11:00 AM**, and the reason **Well-Baby Check**.

(You will need to scroll the drop-down list of reasons to find Well-Baby Check.)

Compare your screen to Figure 12-2; when it is correct, click on the OK button.

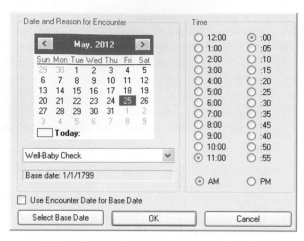

▶ Figure 12-2 New encounter for a well-baby check, May 25, 2012 11:00 AM.

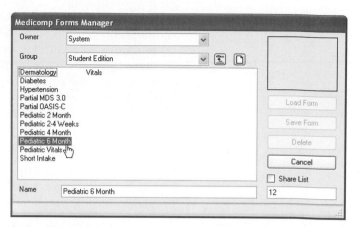

▶ Figure 12-3 Selecting the pediatric 6-month from the Form Manager window.

Step 3

Locate and click on the Forms button on the Toolbar.

Notice that there are several pediatric forms. Because there are different developmental milestones and therefore different questions appropriate to different ages, pediatric clinics typically have a form for each age-appropriate visit. In an actual pediatric practice, there would be more forms than are shown in the Student Edition.

Locate and click on the form labeled "**Pediatric 6 Month**."

Step 4

The pediatric form will be displayed. Take a moment to orient yourself. You will notice that there are quite a few tabs on the form.

Well-baby checkups are usually quite extensive, and involve the social history of the parents as well as of the baby. This form contains the items that a pediatric clinic might cover during a checkup for a 6-month-old baby. In the interest of time, you will not enter data for every question, although you would during an actual pediatric wellness visit.

Whereas nurses interviewing clients with chronic illnesses might use several different forms for a single visit, the designer of this pediatric form has tried to combine in one form all the elements required for a well-baby visit. For example, the form has a button for the chief complaint imbedded in the form, and the vital signs also are imbedded in the form. This type of design allows the pediatric nurses to move through the encounter quickly, while ensuring that nothing is forgotten or overlooked.

Step 5

Locate the finding in the form labeled "The Chief Complaint is:"

Click on the note button to the right of the finding (circled in red in Figure 12-4). The Chief complaint dialog window will be invoked.

In the dialog window, type "**6 month check up**."

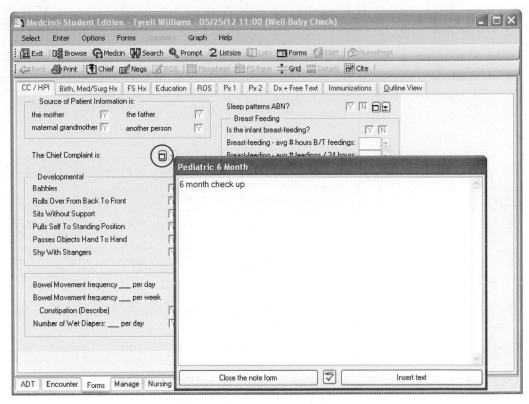

▶ Figure 12-4 Pediatric form—CC/HPI tab with Chief complaint dialog invoked.

Compare your screen to Figure 12-4, then click on the button labeled "Close the note form."

Step 6

This form uses check boxes to record the findings. Notice that the letters "Y" and "N" are gray. When you click on a "Y" check box the letter will turn red; clicking on an "N" check box will turn the letter blue.

The first thing the form asks is the source of information. Tyrell is accompanied by his mother. Click your mouse in the check box:

✓ **Y** "the mother"

Locate sleep patterns on the top right of the form and click on the check box:

✓ **N** Sleep patterns ABN

Locate and click the button labeled "Negs" (Auto Negative) in the Toolbar at the top of your screen.

Step 7

Complete the HPI by locating and clicking the check boxes indicated for the following findings about the infant's feeding:

✓ **Y** Is the infant breast-feeding

✓ **N** Any difficulties w/breast-feeding

✓ **Y** Is rice cereal introduced

✓ **Y** Fruits oz/day

✓ **Y** Vegetables oz/days

▶ **Figure 12-5 Pediatric form—HPI findings recorded with Auto Negative.**

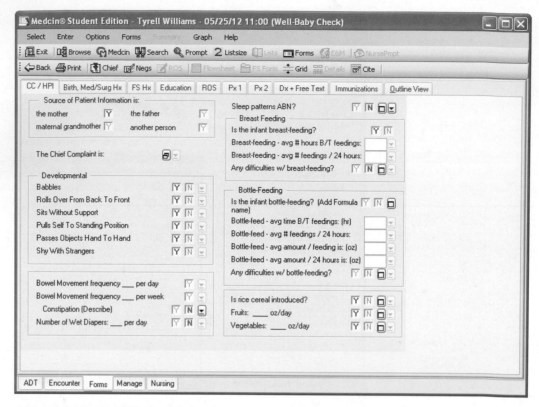

Compare your screen to Figure 12-5.

▶ **Figure 12-6 Pediatric form—Birth, Med/Surg Hx.**

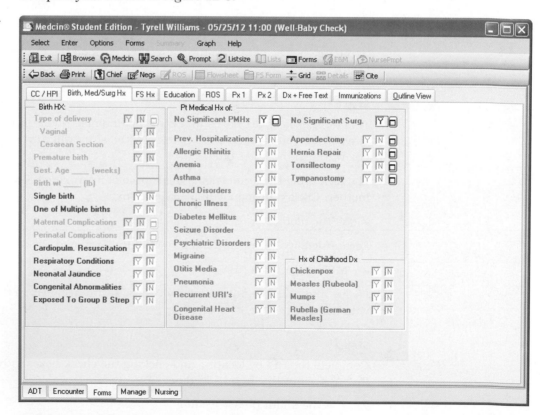

Step 8

Locate and click on the tab labeled "Birth, Med/Surg Hx" at the top of the form.

Tyrell has no previous medical or surgical history. This is indicated by findings at the top of the middle and right columns, as shown in Figure 12-6. Locate and click on the following check boxes:

✓ **Y** No Significant PM Hx

✓ **Y** No Significant Surg Hx

Compare your screen to Figure 12-6.

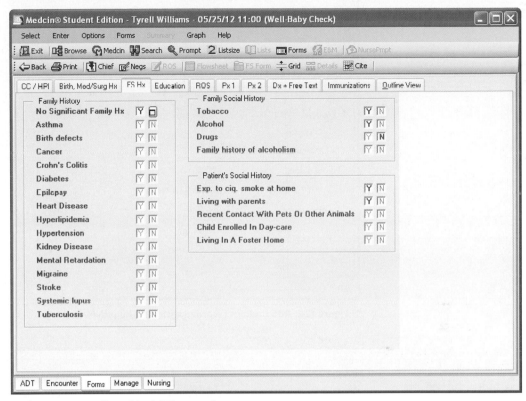

▶ **Figure 12-7 Family and Social History tab.**

Step 9

Locate and click on the tab labeled "FS Hx" at the top of the form.

FS Hx stands for Family and Social History. In pediatric visits, the parent's social habits and environment are seen as health factors that can affect the child. This page of the form is used to record findings about the family history, the child's environment, and the parents' behavioral habits. The Family Social History section is not asking if the baby uses tobacco, alcohol, or drugs, but if the parents do.

Locate and click on the check boxes indicated for the following findings:

Family History:

✓ **Y** No Significant Family Hx

Parent's Social History:

✓ **Y** Tobacco

✓ **Y** Alcohol

✓ **N** Drugs

Child's Social History:

✓ **Y** Exposure to cig. smoke at home

✓ **Y** Living with parents

Compare your screen to Figure 12-7.

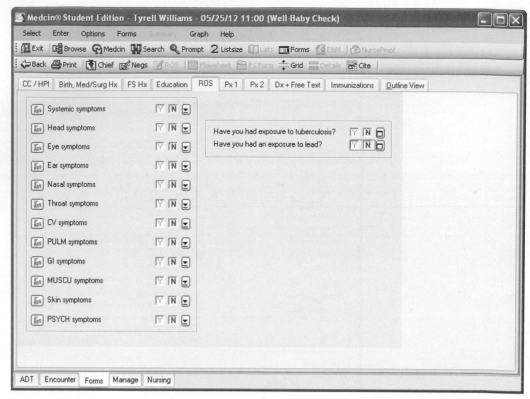

▶ Figure 12-8 ROS findings recorded with Auto Negative.

Step 10

Locate and click on the tab labeled "ROS" at the top of the form.

Locate and click the button labeled "Negs" (Auto Negative) in the Toolbar at the top of your screen.

Complete the ROS by clicking the check boxes for the following findings:

✓ **N** GI Symptoms

✓ **N** Have you had exposure to tuberculosis?

✓ **N** Have you had exposure to lead?

Compare your screen to Figure 12-8.

Step 11

This form uses two tabs to record the physical exam.

Locate and click on the tab labeled "Px 1" at the top of the form. The first page of the Physical Exam form will be displayed.

The Px 1 tab allows the vital signs to be entered without leaving the form. Notice that there are several differences between pediatric and adult vital signs:

▶ Infant growth is measured in length not height.

▶ The temperature is measured in the ear (tympanic).

▶ The circumference of the head is also recorded.

▶ Blood pressure readings are not typically taken in healthy children under the age of 3.

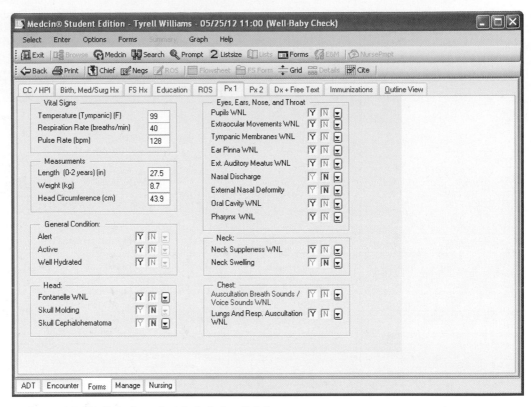

▶ **Figure 12-9 The first of two Px tabs includes vital signs.**

Enter the following measurements for Tyrell in the corresponding Vital Signs fields:

Temperature: **99**

Respiration Rate: **40**

Pulse: **128**

Length (in):   **27.5**

Weight (kg):   **8.7**

Head Circumference (cm):   **43.9**

Click the button labeled "Negs" (Auto Negative) in the Toolbar at the top of your screen to record the rest of the physical exam findings for this page.

Compare your screen with Figure 12-9.

Step 12

Record the remainder of the physical exam.

Locate and click on the tab labeled "Px 2" at the top of the form. The second page of the Physical Exam form will be displayed.

Locate and click the button labeled "Negs" (Auto Negative) in the Toolbar at the top of your screen.

Locate and click the check box for the physical exam finding:

✓ **Y** Growth and Development WNL

▶ **Figure 12-10 The second Px tab completes the physical exam.**

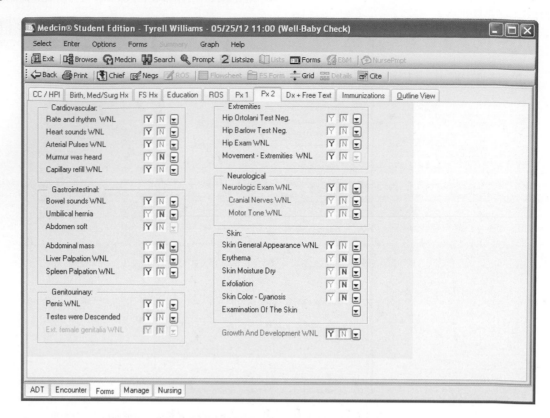

Compare your screen with Figure 12-10.

▶ **Figure 12-11 The Dx tab with free-text findings.**

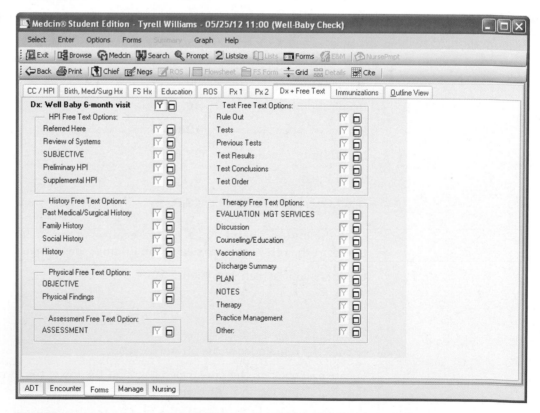

Step 13

Locate and click on the tab labeled "Dx + Free Text" at the top of the form.

Unless the child is ill, the diagnosis for a well-baby checkup is the same for each child; therefore, the form designer has included an option to record it via the form, saving the clinician the time it would take to search the nomenclature.

Additionally, there are many possible areas of the exam in which the pediatric nurse may wish to record additional free text. In this form, the nurse can add notes to any section of the encounter from this one tab. The type of finding and the section of the note in which it will appear have been clearly labeled.

Locate and click on the check box for the diagnosis:

✓ **Y** Dx: Well Baby 6-month visit

Compare your screen to Figure 12-11.

▶ **Figure 12-12 Parent Education tab.**

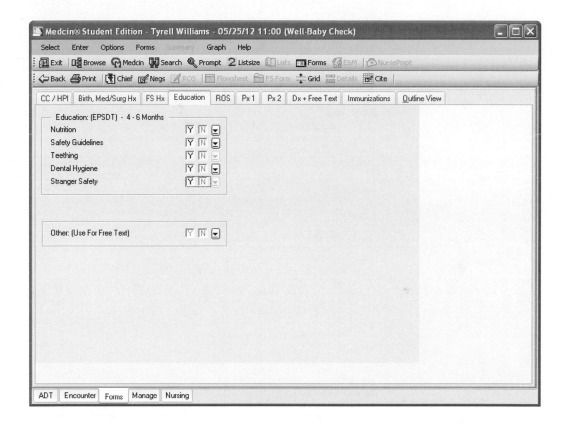

Step 14

During well-baby visits, the pediatric nurse provides educational information to the mother about the child's development, nutrition, immunizations, and safety.

Locate and click on the tab labeled "Education" at the top of the form.

Locate and click on the "Y" check box for each of the following to indicate that these points were covered during the visit:

✓ **Y** Nutrition

✓ **Y** Safety Guidelines

✓ **Y** Teething

✓ **Y** Dental Hygiene

✓ **Y** Stranger Safety

Compare your screen to Figure 12-12.

Step 15

Click on the Encounter tab at the bottom of your screen.

Click on the Print button on the Toolbar at the top of your screen to invoke the Print Data window.

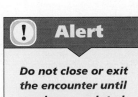

Alert

Do not close or exit the encounter until you have a printed copy in your hand. You will lose your work if you exit before printing.

Be certain there is a check mark in the box next to "Current Encounter" and then click on the appropriate button to either print or export a file, as directed by your instructor.

Compare your printout or file output to Figure 12-13. If there are any differences, other than page breaks, review the previous steps in the exercise and find your error.

If sufficient class time remains, you may continue with the next exercise.

Tyrell Williams   Page 1 of 2

Student: *your name or id here*
Patient: Tyrell Williams: M: 11/10/2011: 5/25/2012 11:00AM
Chief complaint
The Chief Complaint is: 6 month check up.
History of present illness
     Tyrell Williams is a 6 month old male. Source of patient information
     was mother.
     No constipation. A normal number of wet diapers per day.
Past medical/surgical history
Reported:
     Past medical history - No significant past medical history.
     Surgical / Procedural: Prior surgery - No significant surgical history.
     Exposure: No exposure to tuberculosis.
     Environmental Exposure: No exposure to lead.
     Dietary: Infant is breast-feeding.
     Pediatric: No difficulty breast-feeding, rice cereal introduced, with pureed
     fruit introduced, and with pureed vegetables introduced.
Personal history
Habits: A normal sleep pattern.
Home Environment: Lives with parents and the living environment has secondhand
tobacco smoke.
Family history
     Family medical history - No significant family history
     Tobacco use
     Alcohol
     Not using drugs.
Review of systems
Systemic: No systemic symptoms.
Head: No head symptoms.
Eyes: No eye symptoms.
Otolaryngeal: No ear symptoms, no nasal symptoms, and no throat symptoms.
Cardiovascular: No cardiovascular symptoms.
Pulmonary: No pulmonary symptoms.
Gastrointestinal: No gastrointestinal symptoms.
Musculoskeletal: No musculoskeletal symptoms.
Psychological: No psychological symptoms.
Skin: No skin symptoms.
Physical findings
Vital Signs:

Vital Signs/Measurements	Value	Normal Range
Tympanic membrane temperature	99 F	99 - 101
RR	40 breaths/min	36 - 44
PR	128 bpm	110 - 175
Weight	8.7 kg	6.136 - 10
Body length	27.5 in	25.59 - 29.13
Head circumference	43.9 cm	42 - 47

General Appearance:
     ° Alert. ° Well hydrated. ° Active.
Head:
     Injuries: ° No cephalohematoma.
     Appearance: ° No skull molding was seen. ° Fontanelle was normal.
Neck:
     Appearance: ° Neck was not swollen.
     Suppleness: ° Neck demonstrated no decrease in suppleness.
Eyes:
     General/bilateral:
     Extraocular Movements: ° Normal.
     Pupils: ° Normal.

▶ **Figure 12-13a Printed encounter note for Tyrell Williams 6-month checkup (page 1 of 2).**

Tyrell Williams   Page 2 of 2

Ears:
    General/bilateral:
    Outer Ear: ° Auricle normal.
    External Auditory Canal: ° External auditory meatus normal.
    Tympanic Membrane: ° Normal.
Nose:
    General/bilateral:
    Discharge: ° No nasal discharge seen.
    External Deformities: ° No external nose deformities.
Oral Cavity:
    ° Normal.
Pharynx:
    ° Normal.
Lungs:
    ° Clear to auscultation.
Cardiovascular:
    Heart Rate And Rhythm: ° Normal.
    Heart Sounds: ° Normal.
    Murmurs: ° No murmurs were heard.
    Arterial Pulses: ° Equal bilaterally and normal.
    Venous Filling Time: ° Normal.
Abdomen:
    Auscultation: ° Bowel sounds were normal.
    Palpation: ° Abdomen was soft. ° No mass was palpated in the abdomen.
    Liver: ° Normal to palpation.
    Spleen: ° Normal to palpation.
    Hernia: ° No umbilical hernia was discovered.
Genitalia:
    Penis: ° Normal.
    Testes: ° No cryptorchism was observed.
Musculoskeletal System:
    General/bilateral: ° Normal movement of all extremities.
    Hips:
    General/bilateral: ° Hips showed no abnormalities.
Neurological:
    ° System: normal.
Skin:
    ° General appearance was normal. ° Showed no erythema. ° No cyanosis. ° Not
    dry. ° No exfoliation was seen.
Growth And Development:
    ° Normal. ° Babbles. ° Rolls over from back to front. ° Passes objects from
    hand to hand. ° Sits independently. ° Pulls self to a standing position.
    ° Shy with strangers.
Counseling/Education
    • Discussed safety practices
    • Discussed stranger safety
    • Discussed nutritional needs
    • Discussed concerns about teething
    • Discussed concerns about dental hygiene
Reason for Visit
    Visit for: 6-month visit.

▶ Figure 12-13b Printed encounter note for Tyrell Williams 6-month checkup (page 2 of 2).

Understanding Growth Charts

Childhood growth depends on nutritional, health, and environmental conditions. Changes in any of these influences how well a child grows and develops. A child's vital signs can be compared against statistical information of the general population. The National Center for Health Statistics (NCHS) has created a set of graphs used to track the growth of the child and compare him or her to statistical information that has been gathered about the growth rate of babies in the general population. These are called *growth charts.*

Pediatric growth charts have been used by pediatricians, nurses, and parents to track the growth of infants, children, and adolescents in the United States since 1977. The 1977 growth charts were developed by the NCHS as a clinical tool for health professionals to determine if the growth of a child is adequate. The 1977 charts also were adopted by the World Health Organization (WHO) for international use.

Today, 16 pediatric growth charts are maintained and distributed by the Centers for Disease Control and Prevention (CDC), 8 for boys and 8 for girls. The charts were revised in 2000, when 2 new charts were added. The new charts are body mass index-for-age for boys and girls ages 2 to 20 years. Body Mass Index (BMI) is explained later.

The CDC provides the following clinical growth charts:

Infants, birth to 36 months:

▶ Length-for-age and Weight-for-age

▶ Head circumference-for-age and Weight-for-length

Children and adolescents, 2 to 20 years:

▶ Stature-for-age and Weight-for-age

▶ BMI-for-age

Preschoolers, 2 to 5 years:

▶ Weight-for-stature

You may recall from Chapter 1 that the HITECH Act requires hospitals and physician offices to use electronic systems to not only create electronic records for their clients but also to demonstrate meaningful use of those records. One of the definitions of meaningful use is the creation and use of growth charts for clients who are under age 20.

What Is a Percentile?

Figure 12-14 shows a blank paper form of one of the CDC growth charts. This form would be used by a clinic to manually record two graphs on one page. The age of the child is indicated horizontally across the top of the graph and the height and weight measurements are listed vertically down the sides of the graph. The curved blue lines printed across the face of the graph are called *percentiles*. The curved lines represent what percent of the reference population that the individual would equal or exceed. This graph includes the 5th through 95th percentiles; the CDC also has a version available that widens the spectrum by showing a 3rd and 97th percentile.

The child's weight and height (or length) measurements can be marked on the chart under each age for which readings are available. By finding the percentile line closest to the child's vitals, the pediatric nurse can assess the size and growth patterns of the individual as compared with other children in the United States.

For example, a 2-year-old boy whose weight is at the 25th percentile weighs the same or more than 25 percent of the reference population of 2-year-old boys, but weighs less than 75 percent of the 2-year-old boys.

Guided Exercise 73: Creating a Growth Chart

As you have learned in previous chapters, when vital signs are routinely entered in an EHR, those measurements can be used to create graphs. Most popular EHR systems have the ability to graph children's' measurements over an image of the CDC percentiles, similar to the paper form in Figure 12-14. Using the age of the client, the EHR software determines if the graph should include the CDC growth chart. Because the growth charts are gender specific, the software also uses the child's age and sex to determine which of the 16 growth charts to display.

Pediatric growth charts often are used for parent education during well-baby checkups. Graphing the height and weight measurements recorded in the EHR to create growth

▶ **Figure 12-14 Boys birth to 36 months Length-for-age/ Weight-for-age growth chart.**

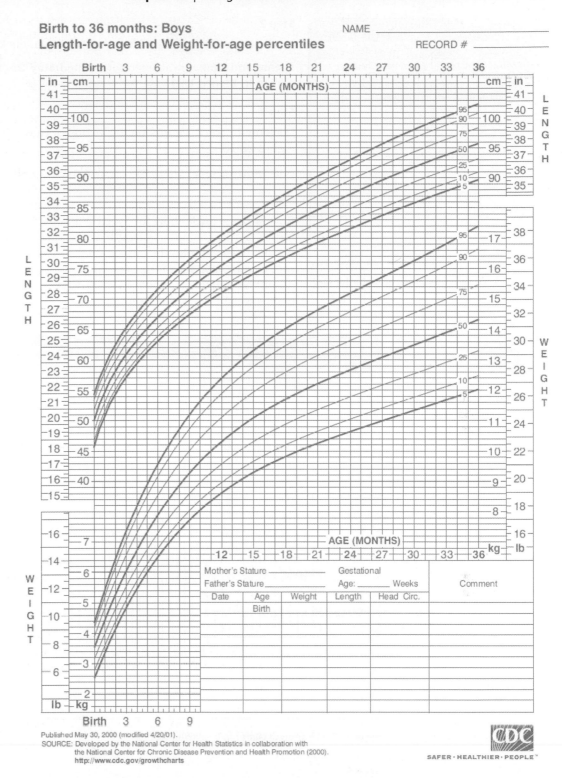

Published May 30, 2000 (modified 4/20/01).
SOURCE: Developed by the National Center for Health Statistics in collaboration with the National Center for Chronic Disease Prevention and Health Promotion (2000).
http://www.cdc.gov/growthcharts

charts is useful in two areas: measuring the growth rate of children and fighting obesity in our society by determining if a person's weight is appropriate for his or her height.

In this exercise, you will create a growth chart for Tyrell Williams.

Step 1

If you are continuing from the previous exercise, proceed to step 3; otherwise, click Select on the Menu bar, and then click Patient.

In the Patient Selection window, locate and click on **Tyrell Williams**, as shown in Figure 12-1.

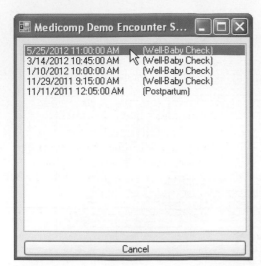

▶ **Figure 12-15 Select existing encounter for May 25, 2012 11:00 AM.**

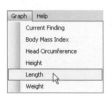

▶ **Figure 12-16 Select length from graph menu to generate a growth chart.**

Step 2

Again, click Select on the Menu bar and then click Existing Encounter.

Locate and click on the encounter dated **May 25, 2012**, at **11:00 AM**, as shown in Figure 12-15.

Step 3

Click on the word "Graph" on the Menu bar, then click "Length" as shown in Figure 12-16.

A pediatric growth chart will be displayed, as shown in Figure 12-17.

Step 4

Review the growth chart for Tyrell Williams displayed on your screen. The blue X marks the infant's length at the various months, listed across the bottom of the graph. The curved lines represent the comparable growth rate as a percentage of the general population. This is the percentile described previously. Similar growth charts also can be generated for a child's weight and head circumference.

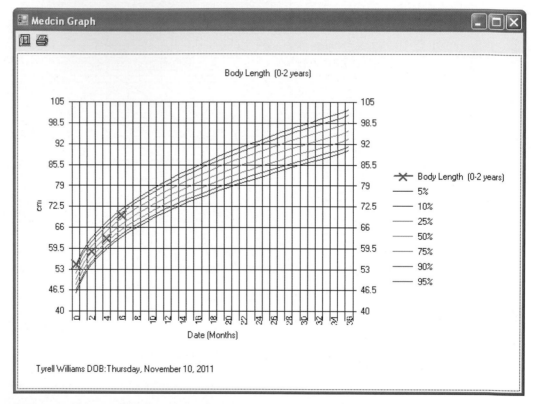

▶ **Figure 12-17 Growth chart for Tyrell Williams.**

Step 5

Print out Tyrell's growth chart. Locate and click on the Print button in the upper left corner of the graph window to invoke the Print Data window.

In the left column of the Print Data window make sure there is a check mark in the box next to "Body length (0-2 years)" and then click on the appropriate button to either print or export a file, as directed by your instructor.

When your graph has printed successfully, click on the Exit button in upper right corner of the window displaying the growth chart.

This completes Exercise 73.

Body Mass Index

BMI stands for Body Mass Index. It is a number that shows body weight adjusted for height. BMI can be calculated with a simple math formula wt/ht^2 using metric measurements (wt = kilograms and ht = meters) or $wt/ht^2 \times 703$ using English measurements (wt = pounds and ht = inches).

The CDC encourages pediatric clinics to replace use of the older weight-for-stature charts with the new BMI-for-age charts (U.S. Department of Health and Human Services, Centers for Disease Control, n.d.). There are several advantages to using BMI-for-age as a screening tool for overweight and underweight children. BMI-for-age provides a reference for adolescents, which was not available previously. Another advantage is that the BMI-for-age measure is consistent with the adult index, so BMI can be used continuously from two years of age to adulthood. This is important, as BMI in childhood is a determinant of adult BMI.

Because BMI changes substantially as children get older, BMI is gender specific and age specific for children ages 2 to 20 years. Adults of both genders age 20 years or older share the same BMI chart. Adult BMI falls into one of four categories: underweight, normal, overweight, or obese.

Guided Exercise 74: Graphing BMI

BMI can be easily calculated for adults using the EHR. In this exercise you are going to graph an adult client's BMI. The EHR software calculates the BMI for you and creates the graph in one operation.

Case Study

Sally Sutherland is a 48-year-old female with hypertension and borderline diabetes. She has been struggling with her weight and in Chapter 9 you created a graph of her weight gain. In this exercise, you are going to create a graph of Sally's BMI.

Step 1

If you have not already done so, start the Student Edition software.

Click Select on the Menu bar, and then click Patient.

In the Patient Selection window, locate and click on **Sally Sutherland** as shown in Figure 12-18.

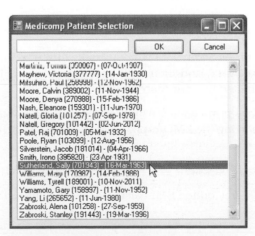

▶ **Figure 12-18 Selecting Sally Sutherland from the Patient Selection window.**

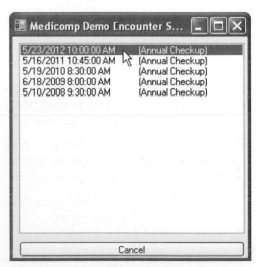

▶ **Figure 12-19 Select existing encounter for May 23, 2012 10:00 AM.**

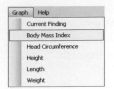

▶ **Figure 12-20 Select Body Mass Index from the Graph menu.**

Step 2

Again, click Select on the Menu bar and then click Existing Encounter.

Locate and click on the encounter dated **5/23/2012**, at **10:00 AM**, as shown in Figure 12-19.

Step 3

Click on the word "Graph" on the Menu bar, then click "Body Mass Index" as shown in Figure 12-20.

A graph of her BMI will be displayed, as shown in Figure 12-21.

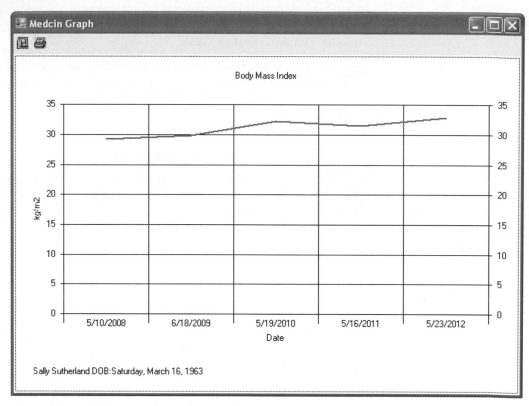

▶ **Figure 12-21 Graph of Sally Sutherland's Body Mass Index.**

Step 4

Compare your screen to Figure 12-21 and then print out Ms. Sutherland's BMI graph.

Locate and click on the Print button in the upper left corner of the graph window to invoke the Print Data window.

In the left column of the Print Data window make sure there is a check mark in the box next to "Body Mass Index" and then click on the appropriate button to either print or export a file, as directed by your instructor.

When your graph has printed successfully, click on the Exit button in upper right corner of the window displaying the BMI graph.

Critical Thinking Exercise 75: Adult BMI Categories

The CDC provides a free online BMI calculator. You will need access to the Internet for this exercise.

Step 1

Start your web browser, and type the following URL in the address:
www.cdc.gov/healthyweight/assessing/bmi/index.html

Step 2

Locate and click on "Adult BMI Calculator."

Step 3

As mentioned previously, there are four categories of adult BMI. At her most recent visit, Sally Sutherland's measurements were:

Height: **5** feet **0** inches

Weight: **168** lbs.

Enter Sally's data, following the on-screen instructions.

When Sally's category is displayed, write the category on your printout of her BMI graph and give it to your instructor. If your BMI graph has been printed to a file, report Ms. Sutherland's category to your instructor separately.

Step 4

Because BMI is a useful measurement for adults as well, you may have an interest in seeing how you measure up.

Repeat step 1.

Step 5

Locate and click on "Adult BMI Calculator" if you are at least 20 years old.

If you are not yet 20, locate and click on the "Children and Teen BMI Calculator."

Follow the on-screen instructions.

The Importance of Childhood Immunizations

Immunization slows down or stops disease outbreaks. Vaccines prevent disease in the people who receive them and protect those who come into contact with unvaccinated individuals.

Although it is true that newborn babies are immune to many diseases because they have antibodies they obtained from their mothers, the duration of this immunity may last only a month to about a year. If a child is not vaccinated and is exposed to a disease germ, the child's body may not be strong enough to fight the disease. Before vaccines, many children died from diseases that vaccines now prevent.

Through childhood immunization, we are now able to control many infectious diseases that were once common in this country, including polio, measles, diphtheria, pertussis (whooping cough), rubella (German measles), mumps, tetanus, and Haemophilus influenzae type b (Hib) (Centers for Disease Control and Prevention, n.d.).

One of the standard components of well baby checkups is to compare the child's immunization history against a recommended schedule of immunizations. At regular intervals, the well baby will receive one or more vaccines. Ideally by the age of 2 years, the child is then protected against a vast array of diseases that once caused the death of many children.

When the pediatric clinic uses an EHR system, the information from all previous immunizations is readily at hand. The clinician can then easily order the next scheduled vaccines appropriate to the client's age and vaccine history.

Health maintenance systems, such as the one shown in Chapter 2, Figure 2-24, automatically calculate and display the next recommended immunizations. The Student Edition software does not have that feature, but EHR systems used in a pediatric clinic quite likely will.

Guided Exercise 76: Reviewing and Ordering Vaccines

In this exercise, you will use the Manage tab to verify what immunizations the child has had, and in a subsequent step you will order vaccines that are required.

Case Study

Before concluding Tyrell Williams's six-month checkup, the clinic will compare his immunization records with the immunization schedule recommended by the CDC and administer any vaccines for which he is due.

Step 1

If you have not already started the Student Edition software, do so at this time.

Locate and click Select on the Menu bar, and then click Patient.

In the Patient Selection window, locate and click on **Tyrell Williams** as you have previously (see Figure 12-1).

Step 2

Click Select on the Menu bar, and then click Existing Encounter.

Position your mouse pointer on the first encounter in the list, dated **5/25/2012 11:00 AM** and click on it (as shown in Figure 12-15).

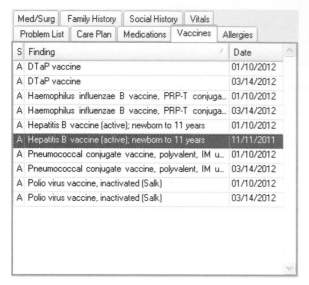

▶ **Figure 12-22 Patient Management Vaccines tab history for Tyrell Williams.**

Step 3

Locate and click on the tab labeled "Manage" at the bottom of your screen. Click on the tab in the left pane labeled "Vaccines."

The vaccine list can be sorted in two ways. If you click the mouse on the column header labeled "Finding," the vaccines are sorted into groups, allowing you to see easily how many doses have been given of each vaccine. If you click the mouse on the column header for date, the list will be reordered so that you can see exactly which vaccines were administered during each well-baby checkup.

Click the mouse on the column header labeled "Finding" so that the vaccines are sorted by type. Compare your screen to Figure 12-22.

Immunization Schedules from the CDC

Immunizations must be acquired over time. Vaccines cannot be given all at once. Several require repeated applications over a period of time, and some, such as the measles vaccine, cannot be given to children under the age of 1 year. Therefore, the

Recommended Immunization Schedule for Persons Aged 0 Through 6 Years—United States • 2010

For those who fall behind or start late, see the catch-up schedule

Vaccine ▼ Age ▶	Birth	1 month	2 months	4 months	6 months	12 months	15 months	18 months	19–23 months	2–3 years	4–6 years
Hepatitis B[1]	HepB	HepB			HepB						
Rotavirus[2]			RV	RV	RV[2]						
Diphtheria, Tetanus, Pertussis[3]			DTaP	DTaP	DTaP	see footnote[3]	DTaP				DTaP
Haemophilus influenzae type b[4]			Hib	Hib	Hib[4]	Hib					
Pneumococcal[5]			PCV	PCV	PCV	PCV				PPSV	
Inactivated Poliovirus[6]			IPV	IPV		IPV					IPV
Influenza[7]						Influenza (Yearly)					
Measles, Mumps, Rubella[8]						MMR		see footnote[8]			MMR
Varicella[9]						Varicella		see footnote[9]			Varicella
Hepatitis A[10]						HepA (2 doses)				HepA Series	
Meningococcal[11]										MCV	

Range of recommended ages for all children except certain high-risk groups

Range of recommended ages for certain high-risk groups

▶ **Figure 12-23 Immunization schedule from the CDC.**

CDC and state health departments have designed a schedule to immunize children and adolescents from birth through 18 years. The Recommended Immunization Schedules for Persons Aged 0 through 18 Years are approved by the (CDC) Advisory Committee on Immunization Practices, the American Academy of Pediatrics, and the American Academy of Family Physicians.

Figure 12-23 shows the immunization schedule recommended by the CDC for children age 0 to 6 years old. Age categories are shown across the top of the schedule. The full names of recommended vaccine combinations are shown down the left column. An abbreviation for the vaccine name is shown within the grid under the ages at which it should be administered.

Yellow bars within the grid indicate the ideal interval at which a particular series should be completed. Blue bars indicate the ages that should be given special attention if the series has not been completed. The fact that colored bars extend over multiple age categories indicates the flexibility that is built into the recommended schedule.

For example, the chart shows that the CDC recommends that infants should receive the first dose of Hepatitis B vaccine (HepB) soon after birth and ideally before hospital discharge. The second dose would be administered at least 4 weeks after the first dose. The third dose should be given at least 16 weeks after the first dose and at least 8 weeks after the second dose. The last dose in the vaccination series (third or fourth dose) should not be administered before the age of 24 weeks.

Step 4

Compare the vaccine list on your screen to the CDC schedule, as shown in Figure 12-23. Notice the following:

Tyrell was born November 10, 2011.

> He had his first dose of Hepatitis B (HepB) before leaving the hospital on 11/11/2011.

> He had his second dose during his 2-month checkup on 01/10/2012.

> He could receive his third dose during this visit or at his 12-month visit.

Compare his DTaP (Diphtheria, Tetanus, Pertussis) vaccines with the CDC schedule.

> He had his first dose of DTaP during his 2-month checkup on 01/10/2012.

> He had his second dose during his 4-month checkup on 03/14/2012.

> He is due for his third dose during this visit.

Compare his Haemophilus influenzae type B (Hib) doses to the CDC schedule.

> He had his first dose of Hib during his 2-month checkup on 01/10/2012.

> He had his second dose during his 4-month checkup on 03/14/2012.

> He is due for his third dose during this visit.

Compare his IPV (Inactivated Polio Virus) doses to the CDC schedule.

> He had his first dose of IPV during his 2-month checkup on 01/10/2012.

> He had his second dose during his 4-month checkup on 03/14/2012.

> He is due for his third dose during this visit.

Compare his Pneumococcal Conjugate (PCV) doses to the CDC schedule.

> He had his first dose of PCV during his 2-month checkup on 01/10/2012.

> He had his second dose during his 4-month checkup on 03/14/2012.

> He is due for his third dose during this visit.

Of the vaccines remaining on the CDC schedule, he is too young for the Varicella vaccine as well as the Measles, Mumps, Rubella (MMR) vaccine, which is not administered before 12 months.

He is old enough for a flu shot, but the well checkup occurs in May and annual flu shots are not available until fall.

Step 5

Now that you have a clear picture of the client's immunization needs, they can be ordered and administered.

Locate and click on the Forms button on the Toolbar.

Locate and click on the form labeled "**Pediatric 6 Month**." as you did in Exercise 72. If you need assistance, refer to Figure 12-3.

► Figure 12-24 Pediatric 6-month form—Immunization tab.

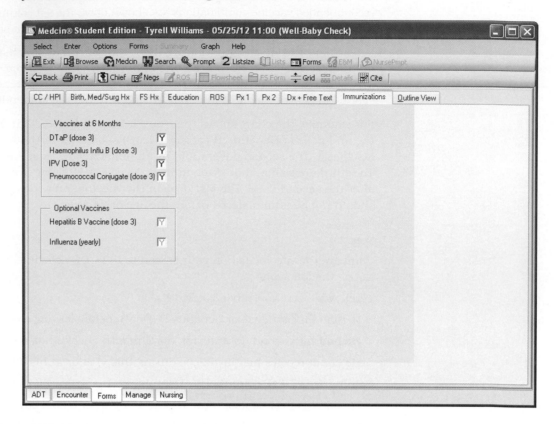

Step 6

Locate and click on the tab labeled "Immunizations" at the top of the form.

Locate the section labeled "Vaccines at 6 Months" and click the check box for each of the following:

✓ **Y** DTaP (dose 3)

✓ **Y** Haemophilus influ B (dose 3)

✓ **Y** IPV (dose 3)

✓ **Y** Pneumococcal Conjugate (dose 3)

Compare your screen to Figure 12-24.

Locate and click on the tab labeled "Encounter" at the bottom of your screen.

Step 7

Click on the Print button on the Toolbar at the top of your screen to invoke the Print Data window.

Be certain there is a check mark in the box next to "Current Encounter" and then click on the appropriate button to either print or export a file, as directed by your instructor.

Compare your printout or file output to Figure 12-25. If it is correct, hand it in to your instructor. If there are any differences other than pagination, review the previous steps in the exercise and find your error.

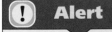 **Alert**

Do not close or exit the encounter until you have a printed copy in your hand. You will lose your work if you exit before printing.

Student: *your name or id here*
Patient: Tyrell Williams: M: 11/10/2011: 5/25/2012 11:00AM
Chief complaint
The Chief Complaint is: 6 month check up.
History of present illness
    Tyrell Williams is a 6 month old male. Source of patient information was mother.
No constipation. A normal number of wet diapers per day.
Past medical/surgical history
Reported History:
    Past medical history - No significant past medical history.
    Surgical / Procedural: Prior surgery - No significant surgical history.
    Exposure: No exposure to tuberculosis.
    Environmental Exposure: No exposure to lead.
    Dietary: Infant is breast-feeding.
    Pediatric: No difficulty breast-feeding, rice cereal introduced, with pureed
    fruit introduced, and with pureed vegetables introduced.
Personal history
Habits: An abnormal sleep pattern.
Home Environment: Lives with parents and the living environment has secondhand
tobacco smoke.
Family history
    Family medical history - No significant family history
    Tobacco use
    Alcohol
    Not using drugs.
Review of systems
Systemic: No systemic symptoms.
Head: No head symptoms.
Eyes: No eye symptoms.
Otolaryngeal: No ear symptoms, no nasal symptoms, and no throat symptoms.
Cardiovascular: No cardiovascular symptoms.
Pulmonary: No pulmonary symptoms.
Musculoskeletal: No musculoskeletal symptoms.
Psychological: No psychological symptoms.
Skin: No skin symptoms.
Physical findings
Vital Signs:

Vital Signs/Measurements	Value	Normal Range
Tympanic membrane temperature	99 F	99 - 101
RR	40 breaths/min	36 - 44
PR	128 bpm	110 - 175
Weight	8.7 kg	6.1 - 10
Body length	27.5 in	25.6 - 29.1
Head circumference	43.9 cm	42 - 47

General Appearance:
    ° Alert. ° Well hydrated. ° Active.
Head:
    Injuries: ° No cephalohematoma.
    Appearance: ° No skull molding was seen. ° Fontanelle was normal.
Neck:
    Appearance: ° Neck was not swollen.
    Suppleness: ° Neck demonstrated no decrease in suppleness.
Eyes:
    General/bilateral:
    Extraocular Movements: ° Normal.
    Pupils: ° Normal.

▶ **Figure 12-25a Printed encounter note for Tyrell Williams with immunizations (page 1 of 2).**

Ears:
> General/bilateral:
> Outer Ear: ° Auricle normal.
> External Auditory Canal: ° External auditory meatus normal.
> Tympanic Membrane: ° Normal.

Nose:
> General/bilateral:
> Discharge: ° No nasal discharge seen.
> External Deformities: ° No external nose deformities.

Oral Cavity:
> ° Normal.

Pharynx:
> ° Normal.

Lungs:
> ° Clear to auscultation.

Cardiovascular:
> Heart Rate And Rhythm: ° Normal.
> Heart Sounds: ° Normal.
> Murmurs: ° No murmurs were heard.
> Arterial Pulses: ° Equal bilaterally and normal.
> Venous Filling Time: ° Normal.

Abdomen:
> Auscultation: ° Bowel sounds were normal.
> Palpation: ° Abdomen was soft. ° No mass was palpated in the abdomen.
> Liver: ° Normal to palpation.
> Spleen: ° Normal to palpation.
> Hernia: ° No umbilical hernia was discovered.

Genitalia:
> Penis: ° Normal.
> Testes: ° No cryptorchism was observed.

Musculoskeletal System:
> General/bilateral: ° Normal movement of all extremities.
> Hips:
> General/bilateral: ° Hips showed no abnormalities.

Neurological:
> ° System: normal.

Skin:
> ° General appearance was normal. ° Showed no erythema. ° No cyanosis. ° Not
> dry. ° No exfoliation was seen.

Growth And Development:
> ° Normal. ° Babbles. ° Rolls over from back to front. ° Passes objects from
> hand to hand. ° Sits independently. ° Pulls self to a standing position.
> ° Shy with strangers.

Assessment
- Normal routine history and physical well-baby (birth - 2 yr)

Vaccinations
- Received dose of polio virus vaccine, inactivated (Salk)
- Received dose of DTaP vaccine
- Received dose of haemophilus influenzae B vaccine, PRP-T conjugate (4 dose schedule), for intramuscular use
- Received dose of pneumococcal conjugate vaccine, polyvalent, IM use

Counseling/Education
- Discussed safety practices
- Discussed stranger safety
- Discussed nutritional needs
- Discussed concerns about teething
- Discussed concerns about dental hygiene.

▶ **Figure 12-25b Printed encounter note for Tyrell Williams with immunizations (page 2 of 2).**

Critical Thinking Exercise 77: Determine Your Adult Immunizations

The CDC also publishes a recommended immunization schedule for adults. Because adult immunizations are different from those you had as a child, you may have an interest in seeing what you need as an adult. You will need access to the Internet for this exercise.

Step 1

The CDC provides a free online service to determine your adult immunization needs.

Start your web browser, and type the following URL in the address:
www.cdc.gov/vaccines/recs/schedules/adult-schedule.htm

Step 2

Locate and click on the link "Adolescent & Adult Vaccine Quiz," and then on the link "Take the Quiz."

Step 3

Follow the on-screen instructions.

Step 4

Optionally, you may print out your immunization schedule. You do not have to turn it into your instructor.

Client Involvement in Their Own Healthcare

Clients must become involved in their own healthcare to effectively manage and prevent diseases. One such example was the immunization quiz you completed in Exercise 77. Other examples are the use of client-specific graphs, growth charts, and BMI that are useful in client education and counseling. Doctors Wenner and Bachman discussed in Chapter 1 the concept of giving the client a copy of the encounter note at the conclusion of the visit. One effect of that is to stimulate compliance by giving the client written documentation of the diagnosis, therapy, and plan of care discussed during the visit. The other effect is that it improves the client's recollection of the clinician's advice.

Client-Entered Data Graphs

Clients can also be engaged in their own healthcare by measuring their own blood pressure at home and keeping a log that they bring to the doctor's office when they have a checkup. Although vital signs such as blood pressure readings from quarterly office visits can be graphed by the EHR software, as you have done in Chapter 9, it is also possible for clients with home computers who keep their daily blood pressure log on a computer to create a graph themselves or to bring the log as a computer file when they have their checkup and let the clinician graph it.

During a client's office visit, the clinician and the client can discuss the graph of the daily blood pressure readings compared with the regimen of blood pressure medicine, and the parameters of control, for example, 140/90 for most hypertensive clients and 130/80 for diabetics. The client also can view the graph at home as he or she enters data. Following the graph on his or her home computer, the client knows whether the therapy is working.

Figure 12-26 shows an example of a graph created in Excel by the client using a template supplied by the clinic. Notice during the Hyzaar treatment that the client's blood pressure is tending higher than 140 over 90. The graph indicates the medication needs to be changed. Once the client is educated by the clinic nurse on how to read the graph within the context of the normal and abnormal range, the client will know when to call the clinic for advice rather than wait until the next appointment. This shared information results in shared decision making. The interaction is transformed from one of

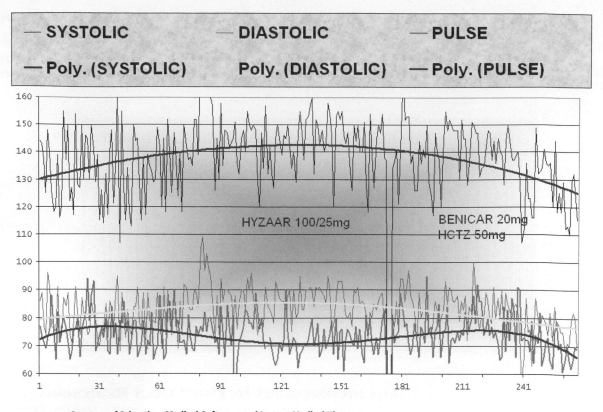

Courtesy of Primetime Medical Software and Instant Medical History.

▶ Figure 12-26 Graph of blood pressure readings from February to May.

gathering information to one of managing the client's problem. Clients can now look actively at issues of the illness, the treatment regime, and the desired outcome.

This is an example of clients' involvement in their own health care by using technology to improve blood pressure management. Research has shown that controlling blood pressure will reduce stroke, heart attack, and vascular disease. Nearly 200 medications are approved for use. There is a combination of drugs that will work for most clients without side effects. Currently in the United States, only about one-third of hypertensive clients have their illness under good control. A number of reasons contribute to this, but an increased clients' involvement can improve their health.

Preventative Care Screening

The U.S. Preventive Services Task Force is an independent panel of experts in primary care and prevention that systematically reviews the evidence of effectiveness and develops recommendations for clinical preventive services. The task force recommendations about preventive services are based on age, sex, and risk factors for disease (see U.S. Prevention Services Task Force, 2005).

Research has shown that the best way to ensure preventive services are delivered appropriately is to make evidence-based information readily available at the point of care. As far back as 1990, EHR systems were developed to compare client information in a medical office computer with age, sex, and risk factors. The system generated a list of preventive care measures individualized to the client based on the U.S. Preventive Services Task Force guidelines at the point of care. The task force recommendations have now been incorporated in EHR systems from several vendors.

Evidence-based guidelines are created by analyzing scientific evidence from current research and studies to determine the effectiveness of preventive services. The

Real-Life Story

First Patient Whose Life Was Saved by Expert System Software He Operated Himself

Jack Gould of Columbia, South Carolina, became the first person in medical history to save his own life with software he operated himself using a preventive medicine screening configuration of Instant Medical History, similar to the exercise in the previous chapter. (Note. Courtesy of Primetime Medical Software and Instant Medical History. Used by permission).

One day Mr. Gould came to his physician's office to pick up a prescription renewal for his wife, who was also a patient there. In the waiting room was a computer kiosk running a patient-operated medical expert system. A sign posted near the system read, "Stay Healthy: Take our Prevention Questionnaire." While waiting for the prescription refill to be authorized, he decided to try it out.

In addition to eating and exercise recommendations, the software suggested that he needed the standard procedure to check for colon cancer because he could not recall having been checked within the time frame suggested by standard guidelines. Normally, after the patient completes the questionnaire, the physician reviews the information with the patient. Because in this case he was not there to see the physician, he spoke with the triage nurse, who confirmed it was a wise preventive action to take and scheduled an appointment.

A few weeks later, the patient returned for his appointment. The doctor was surprised that the patient was there for such a specific preventative procedure months before his annual physical examination. The doctor asked who scheduled the procedure. In a tone reflecting his expectation that it was common for patients to schedule proctosigmoidoscopies on their own volition, he replied, "Well, your computer did."

No physician can be expected to remember the thousands of recommended interventions for each patient. The preventive health screening software queried the patient for the appropriate items based on his sex, age, and risk factors and compared them to the preventive guidelines of the U.S. Preventive Services Task Force. In the case of Mr. Gould, a flexible sigmoidoscopy was scheduled and a resectable severely dysplasic polyp was removed easily from his colon.

The large precancerous polyp that was discovered might have gone completely undetected without the intelligent prompting of the Instant Medical History program. Mr. Gould knew the importance of his decision to take the interview after his physician explained that he would not have thought to do this test until his routine annual complete medical examination. The polyps were removed without complication, before they could develop into colon cancer.

He was totally unaware of his risk for other conditions until he took the preventive interview. Now he strongly believes that Instant Medical History saved his life.

guidelines recommend both for and against certain measures, including screening, counseling, and preventive medications. However, the guidelines are not set in stone. They vary not only by age and sex but change at recommended intervals based on the individual client. For example, a blood test measuring total cholesterol and high-density lipoprotein (HDL-C) is recommended every five years for a male over 35, but the interval shortens to every two years if the client has additional risk factors such as high blood pressure, abnormal lipid levels on previous tests, or a family history of cardiovascular disease before age 50.

Using data in the EHR, the computer is able to find the appropriate guideline based on the client's age and sex, add to it based on the client's problem list and history findings, and then reduce the intervals based on abnormal values of previous test results. The system then generates a guideline unique to the client and delivers it to the clinician's computer screen. Using this information, the clinician can order tests, discuss important health care options, and recommend lifestyle changes to the client at the point of care.

Preventive care screening programs, such as the health maintenance program shown in Chapter 2, Figure 2-24, makes effective use of the EHR to present the provider with recommended tests for early detection and immunizations for prevention.

Client Access to Electronic Health Records

Although HIPAA guarantees clients right to obtain copies of their health record, the HITECH Act went further. As we discussed in Chapter 1, CMS "meaningful use" criteria for EHR incentives included:

▶ Providing clients with timely electronic access to their health information (including lab results, problem list, medication lists, allergies, and so on) within 96 hours of the information being available to the provider.

▶ Providing clients with an electronic copy of their health information upon request.

▶ Providing inpatients with an electronic copy of their discharge instructions and procedures at time of discharge, upon request.

▶ Sending reminders to clients for preventive/follow-up care.

The Agency for Healthcare Research and Quality (AHRQ) created the Hospital Consumer Assessment Healthcare Providers and Systems (HCAHPS) as a standardized survey instrument and data collection methodology for measuring clients' perspectives on care. In 2008, AHRQ reported that clients in the HCAHPS survey indicated that they preferred to go online to access records, results, and scheduling (Grehalva, 2010).

The number of medical offices with interactive web sites is growing. Practice web sites provide a secure means of communication. As discussed in Chapter 11, practice web sites allow the client to request an appointment time or a prescription renewal, and provide secure access to results of recent lab tests and other information in the client record.

Among primary care clinicians, much of this change is being fueled by the implementation of the Patient-Centered Medical Home.

The Patient-Centered Medical Home

"The Patient-Centered Medical Home (PCMH) is an approach to providing comprehensive primary care for children, youth and adults. The PCMH is a healthcare setting that facilitates partnerships between individual patients, and their personal physicians, and when appropriate, the patient's family" (American Academy of Pediatrics, American Academy of Family Physicians, American College of Physicians, & American Osteopathic Association, 2007).

Practices qualify for PCMH status by meeting the Physicians Practice Connections Patient-Centered Medical Home criteria, developed and owned by the National Committee for Quality Assurance (NCQA). There are three levels of recognition, with the higher levels achieved by increased use of electronic communication and web portals. The nine PCMH standards (adapted from National Committee for Quality Assurance, 2010) are:

1. Access and Communication—processes for scheduling appointments, communicating with patients, and data showing that the practice meets this standard.

2. Patient Tracking and Registry Functions—organizes patient-population data using an electronic system that includes searchable patient clinical information used to manage patient care. The practice applies electronic or paper-based charting tools to organize and document clinical information consistently using standard data fields and uses the system to identify the following:

   ▶ Most frequently seen diagnoses

   ▶ Most important risk factors

   ▶ Three clinically important conditions

   The practice uses electronic information to generate patient lists and remind patients or clinicians about necessary services, such as specific medications or tests, preventive services, previsit planning, and follow-up visits.

3. Care Management—implement evidence-based guidelines for the three identified clinically important conditions, and use guideline-based reminders to prompt

physicians about a patient's preventive care needs at the time of the patient's visit. Maintain a team approach to managing patient care, use various components of care management for patients with one or more of the clinically important conditions, and coordinate care with external organizations and other physicians.

4. Patient Self-Management Support—establish a system to identify patients with unique communication needs and facilitate self-management of care for patients with one of the three clinically important conditions.

5. Electronic Prescribing—eliminate handwritten prescriptions, use drug safety alerts when prescribing, and improve efficiency by using cost (drug formulary) information when prescribing.

6. Test Tracking—order and view lab test and imaging results electronically, with electronic alerts; manage the timely receipt of information on all tests and results.

7. Referral Tracking—coordination of care and following through critical consultations with other practitioners.

8. Performance Reporting and Improvement— measures or receives performance data by physician or across the practice and reports on:

   ▶ Clinical process

   ▶ Clinical outcomes

   ▶ Service data

   ▶ Patient safety

   Collects data on patient experience with and reports on:

   ▶ Access to care

   ▶ Quality of physician communication

   ▶ Patient/family confidence in self-care

   ▶ Patient/family satisfaction with care

   Uses performance data to set goals based on measurement results and, where necessary, act to improve performance. Produces reports using nationally approved clinical measures and electronically transmits them to external entities.

9. Advanced Electronic Communication—maximizes electronic communication with patients via the web to support patient access and self-management. Sends patients e-mail about specific needs and clinical alerts. Uses electronic communication among the care management team for patients with one of the three identified clinically important conditions.

The Personal Health Record

As we discussed in Chapter 1, even with growing adoption of EHR in many medical facilities, connectivity between the EHR systems of those entities is often lacking. Although the ONC strategies may eventually address this deficiency, there is one entity central to the record who can bring records from multiple sources together—that is the client. The client is also the person most likely to recognize discrepancies or differences in records from different providers.

Online services independent of any one medical group have sprung up to offer clients the ability to maintain their own medical records online. This is called a Personal Health Record (PHR). The ONC strategies discussed in Chapter 1 encourage the use of PHR.

A PHR is an online service that allows clients to log on to a secure web site and to create and update their records. Clients control who has rights to access the information and can add or remove permission for clinicians they might visit to view the online record.

The clinics, of course, retain their own records, but the clinic's EHR typically contains only the information gathered at that facility or practice. The record maintained online by a client can contain data from visits at multiple practices. Another advantage of the online PHR is that it is available everywhere. Whether clients are traveling and need medical care, or are just being treated at a different medical practice, clients can retrieve their own records using the Internet and share them with the provider.

Early attempts to develop secure PHR solutions sometimes included stand-alone computer programs or flash drives that contained copies of the client's records. The problem with these solutions is that if clients need urgent care and do not have their computer or flash drive with them, then they do not have access to their PHR. The trend for most PHR systems today is to provide the PHR as an Internet service, making it almost universally available.

Kaiser-Permanente, one of the largest healthcare providers in the United States, has implemented what is perhaps the largest PHR to date. Their comprehensive web site securely connects more than 8.6 million members to a personal health record that includes timely access to lab results, medication information, summaries of their health conditions, and other important health information. Using the web site, Kaiser-Permanente clients can securely communicate with their physicians, nurses, and pharmacists, perhaps avoiding the need to make a trip to the clinic in person. The web site also provides access to the up-to-date medical knowledge and client education information.

As Kaiser-Permanente has shown, the PHR can be more than just a repository of client records. Sophisticated PHR services can present the client with preventive health alerts, reminders to renew prescriptions, and links to evidence-based articles related to PHR data that can help clients better manage their own health.

There are numerous organizations developing and sponsoring web-based PHR. Although there may be differences between their offerings, there are some fundamental basics that clients should look for in every PHR:

▶ Data is secure and private

▶ Data is managed by the client

▶ Client controls who can have access

▶ Universally accessible via the Internet

▶ PHR contains information for one's lifetime

▶ Client can see who entered each data record and when

▶ (And ideally) the PHR should be able to exchange data with provider systems

Critical Thinking Exercise 78: Researching the PHR

You will need access to the Internet to complete this exercise.

Step 1

Start your web browser.

Listed below are five URL for PHR web sites. Additionally, your local hospital, health insurance plan, or certain government programs may also offer PHR that you may use for this exercise. Select at least two sites to use for your will research.

www.healthvault.com   www.mymediconnect.net

www.ihealthrecord.org   www.webmd.com/phr

www.myphr.com

Step 2

Type the URL of your first choice in the address field of your web browser.

When the web site is displayed, read the information provided about that organization's PHR. Many of the sites offer a demonstration version; if one is available, click on it.

Take notes or print pages of the web site. You will use these in step 4.

Step 3

Type the second URL your have chosen in the address field of your web browser. Study the information presented on the second site, taking notes or printing pages as you did in step 2.

Step 4

Write a comparative analysis of the web sites you have visited. Include the following information in your report:

What entity owns or operates the PHR web site?

Is the owner a nonprofit or for-profit corporation?

Compare the features offered by the two PHR.

Were there any significant advantages of one over the other?

Compare the two PHR for ease of use.

When you have finished, give your completed report to your instructor.

Chapter Twelve Summary

In this chapter you learned to create a pediatric growth chart. You also learned about pediatric forms and to document a well-baby checkup using a wellness form.

The baby's length, weight, and head circumference are measured on each visit. These measurements can be plotted on a graph called a growth chart that compares the individual's growth to statistical information from the general population. Lines on the chart called percentiles represent the percentage of the reference population that was the same size at the same age. A child who is at the 50th percentile weighs the same or more than 50 percent of the reference population at that age.

For older children, the CDC now recommends using Body Mass Index (BMI). BMI is a number (wt/ht^2) that represents body weight adjusted for height. BMI can be calculated with inches and pounds or meters and kilograms. BMI is gender specific and age specific for children, but a single BMI chart is used for adults of both genders. The CDC has replaced the older weight-for-stature charts with the new BMI charts.

Immunizations must be acquired over time. Vaccines cannot all be given at once. CDC recommended immunizations are aligned with the well-baby visit intervals. You learned how to compare a child's immunization history to the schedule recommended by the CDC (or state health department) to determine what is required each visit.

Disease prevention through periodic screening and early detection also can save lives. Preventive guidelines, also known as health maintenance guidelines, can be generated by an EHR system. Tailored by the computer, these guidelines recommend tests and preventative measures based on the client's age and sex, and also dynamically modify the recommendations based on past history and problems unique to the individual. Using this information, the clinician can order tests, discuss important healthcare options, and recommend lifestyle changes to the client at the point of care.

A Patient-Centered Medical Home is a model for providing primary care. PCMH standards encourage electronic orders, results, and communication with clients.

PHR, or Personal Health Records, enable clients to better manage their health by maintaining their own electronic copies of their health records. The PHR is secure, private, owned, and managed by clients; clients control who can access their records. The most popular type of PHR is universally accessible by the Internet and many are able to exchange data with a provider's EHR system.

Task	Exercise	Page No.
How to document a well-baby visit	72	465
How to create growth charts	73	476
How to calculate Body Mass Index	74	479

References

American Academy of Pediatrics, American Academy of Family Physicians, American College of Physicians, & American Osteopathic Association. (2007, February 21). *Joint principles of the patient centered medical home*. Retrieved from http://www.pcpcc.net/content/joint-principles-patient-centered-medical-home.

Centers for Disease Control and Prevention. (n.d.). Retrieved from http//www.cdc.gov/vaccines

Grehalva, R. (2010). *eHealth patterns in the 21st century*. Birmingham, AL: MEDSEEK.

National Committee for Quality Assurance. (2010). *PPC-PCMH companion guide*. Washington, DC: Author. Retrieved from http://www.ncqa.org/ppcpcmh.aspx

U.S. Preventive Services Task Force. (2005). *The guide to clinical preventive services 2005*. Rockville, MD: Agency for Healthcare Research and Quality.

Test Your Knowledge

1. List at least three factors the EHR can use to create client-specific preventive screening or health maintenance guidelines.

2. Describe how to create a child's growth chart in the EHR.

3. Why are childhood immunizations important?

4. Describe how to change the order in which vaccines are displayed on the Manage tab.

5. Name two of the CMS criteria for EHR incentives related to clients' access of their health records.

6. What is a PHR?

7. Who controls access to the PHR?

8. What are "evidence-based" guidelines?

9. Name the organization that developed pediatric growth charts.

10. What is a growth chart percentile?

11. Adult BMI falls into one of four categories—name them.

12. Name three criteria required to qualify for Patient-Centered Medical Home status.

13. At what age is the first dose of HepB recommended?

14. Name the task force that develops preventive screening guidelines.

15. You should have produced two narrative documents of encounters, one growth chart, one BMI graph, and a report on PHR. If you have not already done so, hand these in to your instructor with this test. The printed encounter notes and graphs will count as a portion of your grade.

Ask your instructor for answers to Test Your Knowledge

nursing.pearsonhighered.com

Prepare for success with animated examples, practice questions, challenge tests, and interactive assignments.

Comprehensive Evaluation of Chapters 7–12

This comprehensive evaluation will enable you and your instructor to determine your understanding of the material covered in the second half of this book. Complete both the written test and the hands-on exercises provided below. Depending on the time provided, it may be necessary to do this in two separate sessions. Your instructor will advise you. Do not begin Part II if there will not be enough class time to complete it. You will need access to the Internet for Part III.

Part I—Written Exam

1. Where does the data that appears in the "Manage" tab come from?

2. Why would nurses use trending of lab results and what type of results can be graphed?

3. Describe the benefits of having clients entering their own symptoms and history.

4. Why are childhood immunizations important?

5. List at least three ways that codified data in the EHR can be used to manage and prevent disease.

6. Describe a problem list and provide at least two reasons why problem lists are used.

7. Describe how to record a test that was performed.

8. What does it mean to cite a finding and how would you do it from a flow sheet?

9. How does an E-visit differ from provider-to-client e-mails?

10. What are "evidence-based" guidelines?

11. What type of nurse completes an OASIS form?

12. What is a growth chart percentile?

13. Describe the closed loop of medication administration.

14. Name at least three things that are checked by a DUR alert system.

15. Give an example of a specialty that might use annotated drawings in an encounter note.

16. What month and year is the United States scheduled to begin using ICD-10?

17. Name some advantages of a PHR.

18. Describe how to create a flow sheet from a form.

19. How is the Internet changing healthcare? Give examples of changes.

20. What is the difference between synchronous and asynchronous telemedicine?

21. Describe the concept of the Patient-Centered Medical Home.

22. At what type of facility do nurses complete the MDS data entry?

For questions 23–30, select the acronym from the list below that best matches the description, and write it next to the number.

BMI	EPHI	PHR
CPOE	HPI	PKI
DUR	MMR	VPN

23. _____ Information protected by the HIPAA Security Rule

24. _____ Client-owned medical records

25. _____ Calculation for height/weight ratio

26. _____ Checks for medication contraindications

27. _____ Combination of three vaccines

28. _____ Electronic order system

29. _____ Element of an encounter note

30. _____ Method of Internet Security

Part II—Hands-On Exercise

The following exercise will require use of the Student Edition software and it may require a full class period to complete the exercise. Do not start the exercise unless there is sufficient time remaining to complete it.

Critical Thinking Exercise 79: Examination of a Client with Arterial Disease

In this exercise, you will use all of the skills you have acquired to document this client encounter. Complete each step in sequential order using the instructions and other information provided.

Case Study

Brenda Green is a 54-year-old female with a history of hypertension and peripheral arterial disease of the legs. During her last visit, she complained of pain in the legs and cold feet following exercise. After performing an ankle-brachial index test in the office, the clinician ordered an angiogram and a home visit. The nurse is visiting Brenda today to discuss the results of her test and her care plan. The nurse has a laptop computer with wireless connectivity to the EHR.

Step 1

Start the Student Edition software and log in.

Click Select on the Menu bar, and then click Patient.

In the Patient Selection window, locate and click on **Brenda Green**.

Alert

Make certain you set the date and time correctly for this exercise.

Step 2

Click Select on the Menu bar, and then click New Encounter.
Select the date **May 31, 2012**, the time **10:15 AM**, and the reason **Follow-Up**.
Compare your screen to the date, time, and reason printed in bold type before clicking on the OK button.

Step 3

Enter the Chief complaint: "**Client reports leg pain after exercise**."

When you have finished typing, click on the button labeled "Close the Note Dialog."

Step 4

After assessing Brenda's home management needs, it is apparent to the nurse that the client does not require assistance with any ADL. Begin the visit by recording that data.

Locate the Forms button on the Toolbar and select the form labeled "**Partial OASIS-C**."

Click on the tab at the top of the form labeled "Type and Source of Assistance."

Locate and click on the first item, "No Assistance Required," in each of the seven boxes.

Click the tab at the top of the form labeled "Plan of Care Synopsis."

Locate and click the blue button for "N/A Not Applicable No case mix group defined by this assessment."

Step 5

Remain on the Forms tab.

The nurse takes Brenda's vital signs and enters them.

Locate the Forms button on the Toolbar and select the form labeled "**Hypertension**." Enter Brenda's vital signs in the corresponding fields on the form as follows:

Temperature:	**98.6**
Respiration:	**16**
Pulse:	**78**
BP:	**140/90**
Weight:	**210**

Step 6

Locate and click on the "Y" check box next to hypertension. The small circle will turn red.

● Hypertension   ✓ Y

Step 7

Locate and click on the button labeled "FS Form" in the Toolbar at the top of your screen to invoke the Flowsheet view.

Locate and click on the button labeled "Cite" in the Toolbar at the top of your screen.

Move your mouse pointer over the column date "**5/17/2012**." The pointer should change to include a large question mark. Click on the column date. A window of findings from that encounter will be displayed.

Scroll the "Review cite of flow sheet column" window downward.

Locate and click on the red buttons for seven the ordered tests listed. This will deselect the orders, so that they will not be ordered again.

- ○ (red button) ordered urinalysis
- ○ (red button) ordered CBC
- ○ (red button) ordered hematocrit level

    ○ (red button) ordered hemoglobin level

    ○ (red button) ordered an electrolyte panel

    ○ (red button) ordered a lipid profile

    ○ (red button) ordered a random blood glucose level

When you have deselected all seven tests, click on the button labeled "Post To Encounter."

Locate and click on the button labeled "Cite" in the Toolbar at the top of your screen to turn off the Cite feature. Then locate and click on the button labeled "FS Form" in the Toolbar at the top of your screen to return to the Hypertension form.

Step 8

The nurse heard listened to Brenda's heart, but did not examine her eyes. Two finding were cited from the flow sheet that you should remove.

Locate the section of the Hypertension form labeled "Quick Screening Exam."

Click on the checked boxes to remove the check mark from the following findings:

✓ Optic Disk

✓ Retina

Confirm each deletion by clicking on the OK button in the confirmation dialog box that will appear.

Step 9

Locate and click on the Manage tab at the bottom of the screen.

Review the client's problem list. Locate and click on the problem "Atherosclerosis of the femoral artery" to highlight it.

Locate and click on the button labeled "Flowsheet" in the Toolbar at the top of your screen. The Flowsheet view will be invoked for the specific problem.

Locate and click on the button labeled "Cite" in the Toolbar at the top of your screen.

Locate the section of the Flowsheet with the label "Tests" (in a teal divider) by scrolling the window.

Cite an individual test result by moving your mouse pointer over the column "5/18/2012." The pointer should change to include a large question mark.

Locate the finding of Bilateral Angiography and click on the column with the abbreviation "72% blockage" (in red). The finding will be recorded in the current encounter.

Step 10

Cite the findings from the previous exam by moving your mouse pointer over the date "5/17/2012" at the top of the column, and click on the date.

A window of findings from that encounter will be displayed.

Locate and click on the red buttons for the two ordered tests to deselect them, so that they will not be ordered again:

    ○ (red button) ordered a lipid profile

    ○ (red button) ordered bilateral angiography of the extremity

When you have deselected both tests, click on the button labeled "Post To Encounter."

> **Note**
>
> **If you have difficulty locating the test finding of "Bilateral Angiography" in the problem-oriented flow sheet because it does not appear on the problem flow sheet, the most likely cause is a misstep with the Flowsheet and Cite buttons earlier in the exercise. Do the following to remedy the situation:**
>
>   **Before citing anything in step 9, locate and click on the button labeled "Cite" in the Toolbar at the top of the screen to turn off the Cite feature.**
>
>   **Then locate and click on the button labeled "Flowsheet" in the Toolbar at the top of the screen to close the flow sheet and return to the Patient Management Problem tab.**
>
>   **Locate and click on the Encounter tab to return to the encounter note view.**
>
>   **Start step 9 over again from the beginning. The "Bilateral Angiography" should then appear in the flow sheet as indicated in the directions.**

Step 11

Locate and click on the button labeled "Cite" in the Toolbar at the top of your screen to turn off the Cite feature. Then locate and click on the button labeled "Flowsheet" in the Toolbar at the top of your screen to return to Patient Management.

The nurse reviews Brenda's current medications. Locate and click on the Manage tab labeled "Medications."

When you have reviewed her medications, locate and click on the tab labeled "Encounter" at the bottom of the window to return to the encounter note view.

Step 12

The nurse learns that Brenda has not started her Coumadin because the prescription was written on paper and she lost it. The nurse contacts her physician and obtains approval to reorder the prescription. Using CPOE, she will send an electronic prescription to Brenda's pharmacy, which delivers.

Locate and click the assessment "Atherosclerosis of the femoral artery" in the encounter note (right pane). The finding will then be displayed in the left pane on the Edit tab.

Highlight the diagnosis description, then locate and click on the button labeled "Prompt" in the Toolbar at the top of your screen.

Locate and click on the Rx tab in the left pane. Locate and highlight "**Anticoagulants Warfarin sodium (Coumadin)**," and then click the Rx button on the Toolbar.

This will invoke the prescription writer.

Step 13

Enter the following prescription by selecting the following options as they are presented:

Rx Dosage:	**2 mg**
Rx Brand:	**Coumadin**

Enter the following data in the prescription fields:

Sig

Quantity:	**1**
Frequency:	**daily**
Per Day:	**1**
Days:	**30**

Dispense

Amount:	**30**
Refill:	**3**
Generic:	**Y**

Verify that you have entered the information correctly, and then click the button labeled "Save Rx." You may assume that the prescription transmitted electronically.

Step 14

Brenda needs counseling on her diet and new medication.

Locate and click the button labeled "Search" in the Toolbar at the top of your screen. The Search window will be invoked. Type "**Low fat diet**" and click the Search button.

Locate and select the following findings from the list displayed in the Rx tab:

- (red button) Low Fat Diet
- (red button) Patient Education Dietary Low Fat Cooking
- (red button) Patient Education Dietary Changing Eating Habits

Step 15

The nurse explains to Brenda that she will need to have regular blood tests, starting in about two weeks.

Click on the button labeled "Search" on the Toolbar at the top of your screen. The Search String window will be invoked.

Type the search string "**INR**" and click on the Search button in the window.

If the left pane is not on the Rx tab, click on the Rx tab.

Locate and highlight the finding "**Anticoagulants management**."

Locate and click on the down arrow in the Entry Details Prefix field. Select "**Follow-up with**" from the drop-down list.

In the Entry Details Duration field, type "**2 weeks**" and press the Enter key on your keyboard.

Step 16

Click on the Tx tab.

Highlight **Coagulation Studies: INR**

Click on the button labeled "Order" on the Toolbar at the top of your screen.

Step 17

Create an annotated drawing to explain the angiography results to the client.

Scroll the encounter note in the right pane to locate the imaging study finding "Bilateral Angiography." Click on the word "Bilateral." The left pane should change to the Edit tab.

Locate the context button (the second button from the right in the lower right corner of your window) and click on it. From the drop-down list displayed, choose "Add Object to Finding."

The drawing window will be invoked in the right pane.

If the cardiovascular drawing is not displayed, use the fields at the top of the drawing to select the Cardiovascular, Full Body, Front view from the drop-down lists.

Step 18

Once the correct illustration template is displayed, use the Toolbar in the drawing tool to set up the tool.

Locate and click on the down arrow next to the first button; then select "Circle" from the drop-down list.

Locate and click on the Lock button (with the padlock). It should have a white background.

Locate and click on the Color pallet button. When the window is displayed, select Blue.

Click OK to close the Color pallet window.

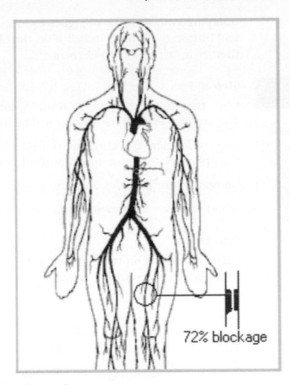

Anatomical Figure © MediComp Systems, Inc.
▶ **Figure C-1 Drawing of annotations to be performed in Exercise 79.**

Step 19

As closely as possible, replicate the drawing in Figure C-1.

Draw a blue circle over the femoral artery midway between the groin and the knee (as shown in Figure C-1).

Change the drawing tool.

Locate and click on the down arrow next to the first button, then select "Line" from the drop-down list.

Draw a horizontal line from the circle to the blank area of the drawing on the right.

Next, change the color to red by selecting the Color pallet button.

In the blank area of the drawing, draw two vertical, parallel lines to represent an enlarged view of the artery.

Change the drawing tool.

Locate and click on the down arrow next to the first button, then select "Brush" from the drop-down list.

Using the Brush, make a thick line on the interior of each of the parallel lines to represent the blockage in the artery (similar to Figure C-1).

Annotate the drawing.

Locate and click on the down arrow next to the first button, then select "Text" from the drop-down list.

Click your mouse in the image to the right of the knee and a text field will open. Type **"72% blockage."**

Right click anywhere on the drawing except in the text box to display a list of options; click on "Complete Text" from the list displayed.

Compare your drawing to Figure C-1. If you need to correct the line or circle, change the tool button to "Select" and click on the object. Use the Delete button in the Toolbar and then redraw the correct element.

Alert

Do not exit the drawing or change tabs until you have a printed copy in your hand. You will lose your drawing if you exit before printing.

Step 20

Click the Print button on the *drawing toolbar*, **not** the Print button on the main Toolbar. The familiar Print Data window will be invoked.

Be certain there is a check mark in the box next to "Imager Drawing" and then click on the appropriate button to either print or export a file, as directed by your instructor.

Compare your printout or file output to Figure C-1.

When you have a printout of your annotated drawing in hand, close the Print Data window.

Step 21

Locate and click on the Exit button in the *drawing toolbar* to close the drawing tool and redisplay the encounter note.

Step 22

Locate and click on the button labeled "Search" in the Toolbar at the top of your screen. The Search String window will be invoked.

Type the search string "Total cholesterol" and click on the Search button in the window.

Click on the Tx tab.

The left pane should display several findings with the words "Total Cholesterol" in them.

Locate and highlight the finding "Total plasma cholesterol" (the finding with the red button selected).

Click Graph on the Menu bar, and then click "Current Finding" from the drop-down list. The Graph window will be invoked with a graph of Brenda's recent cholesterol results.

Locate and click on the Print button in the upper left corner of the graph window to invoke the Print Data window.

Locate the check box for Total Cholesterol in the left column and click on it.

Locate and click on the appropriate button to either print or export a file, as directed by your instructor. When your graph has printed successfully, click on the Exit button in the window displaying the Total Cholesterol graph.

Step 23

Print a chart of Brenda's weight.

Click Graph on the Menu bar, and then click "Weight" from the drop-down list. The Graph window will be invoked with a graph of Brenda's weight measurements.

Locate and click on the Print button in the upper left corner of the graph window to invoke the Print Data window.

Locate the check box for Weight in the left column and click on it.

Locate and click on the appropriate button to either print or export a file, as directed by your instructor. When your graph has printed successfully, click on the Exit button in the window displaying the weight graph.

Step 24

Click on the Nursing tab at the bottom of your screen.

Locate and click the assessment "Atherosclerosis of the femoral artery" in the encounter note (right pane). The finding will then be displayed in the left pane on the Edit tab.

Locate and click on the button labeled "NursePmpt" in the Toolbar at the top of your screen. A list of nursing diagnoses and interventions will be displayed in the Nurse tab.

Locate and click on the red buttons for the following findings:

- (red button) RNDx Knowledge Deficit of Medication Regimen
- (red button) RNRx Compliance with Medication Regimen

Click the small plus sign next to "Compliance with Medication Regimen" to expand the list of RNOx actions.

Scroll the expanded list to locate and click the red buttons for the following nursing actions:

- (red button) RNOx Assess prescribed medications
- (red button) RNOx Provide written medication plan
- (red button) RNOx Instruct in Medication Regimen
- (red button) RNOx Teach side effects of medication

Step 25

Click on the Rx tab.

Click on the button labeled "Search" on the Toolbar at the top of your screen. The Search String window will be invoked.

Type the search string "**Counseling**" and click on the Search button in the window.

Locate and click on the following finding:

- (red button) Preventive Medicine/Risk Factor Counseling

Locate and click on the Finding Note button (in the lower right corner of your screen).

Type the following text into the Finding Note window: "**30 minutes of visit spent on dietary and Coumadin counseling.**"

When you have finished, click your mouse on the button labeled "Close the note form."

! Alert

Do not close or exit the encounter until you have a printed copy in your hand. You will lose your work if you exit before printing.

Step 26

Click on the Print button on the Toolbar at the top of your screen to invoke the Print Data window.

Be certain there is a check mark in the box next to "Current Encounter" and then click on the appropriate button to either print or export a file, as directed by your instructor.

Part III—Internet Exercise

You will need access to the Internet for this portion of your evaluation.

Critical Thinking Exercise 80: Nurse Teaches Client How to Research Medication

Case Study

Brenda Green has been prescribed a new drug. The nurse shows her how to use the Internet to look up information about it.

Step 1

Start your web browser. In the address bar type the URL: **www.webmd.com**.

Step 2

When the web site is displayed, locate the search field and type: **warfarin PAD**.

Click on the Search button.

Step 3

A list of search results will be displayed.

Locate and click on the link for "**Peripheral Arterial Disease of the Legs - Medications**."

Step 4

When the article is displayed, locate and click on the link "**Print Article**."

If your instructor normally requires printouts of your work, click the Print button.

If you normally submit your work as a file, print it to the Windows XPS printer if that is what you used in Chapter 10. Otherwise, copy the URL displayed in the WebMD print window and paste it into an e-mail. Consult your instructor as to his or her preference for this step.

Give your instructor the following printouts or files along with your written exam:

1. Annotated drawing of femoral artery

2. Graph of Total Cholesterol

3. Graph of Brenda Green's Weight

4. Encounter note for May 31, 2012, for Brenda Green

5. Printed WebMD article, the XPS file or an e-mail containing URL of WebMD print window

Glossary

ABG A medical abbreviation for arterial blood gas.

ABN An acronym for Advance Beneficiary Notice—information presented to the client in advance that the test or procedure will not be covered by Medicare or insurance. The same acronym is sometimes uses as the abbreviation for Abnormal.

Acetaminophen A medicine used as an alternative to aspirin to relieve pain and fever. The active ingredient in Tylenol.

Acute Severe, but of short duration.

Acute Self-Limiting Problems that normally resolve themselves over a short period of time.

ADL An acronym for Activities of Daily Living, which include activities such as bathing, dressing, walking, ambulation, toileting, meal preparation, eating, and grooming.

Administrative Simplification (HIPAA) The Administrative Simplification Subsection of HIPAA covers providers, health plans, and clearinghouses. It has four distinct components: Transactions and Code Sets, Uniform Identifiers, Privacy, and Security.

Adverse Effects Side effects of a drug or treatment severe enough that it may warrant discontinuing use.

AHIMA An acronym for American Health Information Management Association, the leading organization of health information professionals.

AHRQ An acronym for Agency for Healthcare Research and Quality, a Public Health Service agency in the Department of Health and Human Services to support research designed to improve the quality, safety, efficiency, and effectiveness of healthcare for all Americans.

Alert A warning, message, or reminder automatically generated by EHR systems based on logical rules.

Allergy (tab) A feature on the Patient Management tab that provides a list of the client's allergies, or the fact that the client has no known allergies. This information is reviewed before writing a prescription.

Alzheimer's Disease A disease with symptoms of memory loss, inability to care for self, and progressive dementia.

AMA An acronym for American Medical Association; also an acronym for Against Medical Advice.

Ambulatory Setting Outpatient setting.

AMI An acronym for acute myocardial infarction (heart attack).

Amoxicillin An oral antibiotic; a synthetic penicillin derived from ampicillin.

ANA An acronym for the American Nurses Association.

Angina Pectoris A disease marked by brief, recurrent pain, usually in the chest and left arm, caused by a sudden decrease of the blood supply to the heart muscle.

Angiogram An x-ray (roentgenogram) of the flow of blood after injecting a contrast material.

Angiography *See* Angiogram.

Annotated Drawing Anatomical drawings of the body and body systems on which the clinician has marked observations and text notes. Medcin-based software is capable of linking an annotated drawing to a relevant finding.

ANSI An acronym for American National Standards Institute, a private, nonprofit organization that administers and creates product and communication standards in the United States. ANSI uses a voluntary consensus process to arrive at and maintain standards not only in healthcare but also in many diverse areas of industry and manufacturing.

Apical Pulse A central pulse located at the apex of the heart.

ARRA an acronym for American Recovery and Reinvestment Act, federal legislation that included the HITECH Act. *See* HITECH Act.

Assessment (chart) The diagnosis or determination arrived at by the clinician from the medical examination, subjective and objective findings, and test results.

Asthma A generally chronic disorder often caused by an allergic origin, characterized by wheezing, coughing, labored breathing, and a suffocating feeling.

Atrial Fibrillation Irregular heartbeat.

Atherosclerosis Buildup of fatty plaque in the arteries.

Auscultation Listening (in this text, listening with a stethoscope).

Auto Negative *See* Negs (button).

BID A medical abbreviation for "twice daily."

BIPAP A medical abbreviation for Bilevel Positive Airway Pressure.

Blood Glucose Level The amount of glucose (a type of sugar) in the blood at the time the specimen is taken. A random blood glucose test is done without regard to when the client last ate. A fasting blood glucose test is done after a client has not had food or drink (except water) for 12 hours.

BMI An acronym for Body Mass Index, a number that shows body weight adjusted for height.

BMP A medical abbreviation for basic metabolic panel blood test.

Bradycardia Abnormally slow heart rate (less than 60 beats per minute).

Bronchitis A disease marked by inflammation of the bronchial tubes.

Browse (button) Displays the current finding's position in the Medcin nomenclature hierarchy. Also a tab in the software.

Button (software) A raised or indented object in the software used to invoke an action or change of state when clicked on with a mouse. Found in most Windows software programs, buttons usually contain a word or icon representing their function.

Bypass Surgery *See* Cardiac Bypass.

Cardiac Bypass A surgical shunt to divert blood supply from one circulatory path to another.

Cardiac Catheterization A test to evaluate the heart and arteries. A thin flexible tube is threaded through a blood vessel into the heart, then a contrast material is injected to trace the movement of blood through the coronary arteries.

Cardiac Output The amount of blood ejected by the heart with each ventricular contraction.

Cardiovascular The heart and the system of blood vessels.

Care Plan (tab) A feature on the Patient Management tab that provides a view of the plan from each previous encounter in a problem-oriented view. It is organized by problem and encounter date for which the client was seen for that problem.

Care Pathway *See* Nursing Care Plan.

CAT Scan Computerized Axial Tomography uses multiple x-rays and a computer to generate images of cross sections of the body.

CBC An acronym for Complete Blood Count, which is a lab test that includes separate counts for both white and red blood cells.

CC *See* Chief complaint.

CCC *See* Clinical Care Classification System.

CCHIT An acronym for Certification Commission for Healthcare Information Technology, a nonprofit organization that certifies EHR systems.

CDA An acronym for Clinical Document Architecture, an HL7 standard for incorporating clinical text reports or other information in a Claim Attachment.

CDC An acronym for the Centers for Disease Control, an agency of the U.S. Department of Health and Human Services.

CDISC An acronym for Clinical Data Interchange Standards Consortium, an organization that has created standards that enable sponsors, vendors, and clinicians to acquire and exchange data used in clinical drug trials. CDISC has become part of HL7.

CDR An acronym for Clinical Data Repository, a database used to aggregate EHR data from several disparate systems.

CHCS II An acronym for Composite Health Care System II, the U.S. Department of Defense Electronic Health Record System.

CHF A medical abbreviation for Congestive Heart Failure.

Chief Complaint A concise statement describing the symptom, problem, condition, diagnosis, or other factor that is the reason for the encounter, usually stated in the client's words.

Chronic Disease or problem that lasts a long time or recurs often.

CIS Clinical Information System Department of a hospital that develops or manages EHR applications and training.

Cite (software) A feature of the software that allows follow-up visits to be quickly documented by bringing forward findings from previous exams into the current encounter. While doing so, the clinician can update or make any changes to the finding without affecting the previous encounter.

Clinical Care Classification System Developed by Virginia Saba at Georgetown University, is used to document nursing care in hospitals, home health agencies, ambulatory care clinics, and other healthcare settings.

Clinical Terminology An organized list of medical phrases and codes. *See* Nomenclature.

Clinical Vocabulary An organized list of medical phrases and codes. *See* Nomenclature.

Closed Loop Safe Medication Administration A safety initiative to reduce medication errors, by issuing the prescription using CPOE, checking the medication order by the pharmacy, rechecking it by the nurse before administering it, verifying the correct client, validating the ordered medication matches the order, and confirmation by the nurse that the medication was administered.

CME An acronym for Continuing Medical Education, courses required to maintain licenses for licensed healthcare professionals.

CMS An acronym for the Centers for Medicare and Medicaid Services, an agency of the U.S. Department of Health and Human Services (formerly HCFA).

CNA *See* Certified Nursing Assistant.

Certified Nursing Assistant A Certified Nursing Assistant (CNA), sometimes called a nursing aide or patient care technician, works under the supervision of a registered nurse to provide assistance to residents with their daily living tasks including bathing, feeding, dressing, transfer assistance, serving meals, obtaining vital signs, skin care, assisting residents after incontinent episodes, and reporting changes in the residents' condition to medical staff.

Codified Data (chart) EHR data with each finding assigned a standard code assures uniformity of the medical records, eliminates ambiguities about the clinician's meaning, and facilitates communication between multiple systems.

Comprehensive Metabolic Chem Panel A blood test to determine blood sugar level, electrolytes, fluid balance, kidney function, and liver function. The panel measures (in blood) the sodium, potassium, calcium, chloride, carbon dioxide, glucose, blood urea nitrogen (BUN), creatinine, total protein, albumin, bilirubin, alkaline phosphatase transferase (ALP), aspartate amino transferase (AST), and alamine amino transferase (ALT).

Contraindicated A drug, treatment, or procedure that is inadvisable (used in this text regarding alerts to the risk of adverse reaction to a drug).

Covered Entity (HIPAA) HIPAA refers to healthcare providers, plans, and clearinghouses as Covered Entities. In the context of this book, think of covered entity as the medical facility and all of its employees.

CPOE An acronym for Computerized Provider Order Entry; also for Computerized Physician Order Entry.

CPR A medical abbreviation for cardio-pulmonary resuscitation.

CPRI An acronym for Computer-Based Patient Record Institute, formed to promote the universal and effective use of electronic healthcare information systems to improve health and the delivery of healthcare, was merged into HIMSS in 2002.

CPT-4 An acronym for Current Procedural Terminology, fourth edition. CPT-4 is standardized codes for reporting medical services, procedures, and treatments performed for clients by the medical staff. CPT-4 is owned by the American Medical Association.

CQM An acronym for Clinical Quality Measures, data reported to CMS by a provider that indicates the quality of care provided by measuring the quantity of clients assessed or successfully treated according to evidence-based best practices.

Cross-Walk (codes) A reference table for translating a code from one set to a code with the same meaning in another code set. For example, the Medcin and SNOMED-CT nomenclatures each have tables for translating a finding code to an ICD-9-CM or ICD-10 code.

Cruciate Ligament (of the knee) Two ligaments in the knee joint that cross each other from the femur to the tibia. The anterior one limits extension and rotation.

CT (codes) An acronym for Clinical Terms. *See* Read codes.

CT Scan Computerized Tomography (*see* CAT scan).

CVA A medical abbreviation for Cerebrovas-cular Accident (stroke).

CVP A medical abbreviation for cerebral vascular pressure.

DAW The acronym for Dispensed As Written is used on a prescription as an instruction to dispense the exact brand of medication specified. Do not substitute a generic equivalent drug.

Decision Support Computer- or Internet-based systems used to improve the process and outcome of medical decisions by delivering evidence-based information to the clinician who is determining the diagnosis or treatment orders.

Decryption A method of converting an encrypted message back into regular text using a mathematical algorithm and a string of characters called a "key." *See also* Encryption.

Description (entry detail) The Description field (in entry details) presents the text of the currently selected finding exclusive of any attached free text. The user cannot enter or modify the description in this field.

Diabetes Mellitus A chronic form of diabetes, characterized by an insulin deficiency, an excess of sugar in the blood and urine, and by hunger, thirst, and gradual loss of weight.

Diagnosis A disease or condition, or the process of identifying the diseased condition. Generally codified using ICD-9-CM.

DICOM An acronym for Digital Imaging and Communication. It is a standard for communication and file structure for transfer of digital images between equipment and computer systems.

Digital Images (chart) EHR data in image format. This includes diagnostic images, digital x-rays, as well as documents scanned into the EHR. *See also* Scanned Images. Image data usually requires specific software to view the image.

Discrete Data (chart) EHR data in computer format. Discrete data is typically either Fielded or Codified. Fielded data identifies the type of information by its position in the EHR record. Codified data pairs each piece of information with a code that identifies the information in uniform way.

Dorsalis Pedis (pulse) Pulse at the artery on top of the foot.

Drop-Down List A standard feature in most Windows software, which displays a list of items the user may select when a mouse is clicked in the field or on a down-arrow button next to the field.

Drug Formulary Drug formularies are used to look up drugs by names or therapeutic class, provide an updated list of the drugs that are available in the inventory, provide information on costs, indications for use, treatment recommendations, dosage, guidelines, and prescribing information. Health insurance programs use the term *formulary* for plan-specific drug lists.

DTaP An acronym for Diphtheria, Tetanus, acellular Pertussis (whooping cough); a combination vaccine.

DUR An acronym for Drug Utilization Review, which is the process of comparing a prescription drug to a client's history and recent medications for contraindications, overdosing, underdosing, allergic reactions, drug-to-drug interactions, and drug/food interactions.

Duration (entry detail) The Duration field is used to enter a number and a unit of time related to the duration of the currently selected finding. The time unit can be "second," "minute," "hour," "day," "week," "month," "year," or their plurals. A window with key-pad for entering duration can be invoked by double-clicking the mouse in the Duration field.

DVT Deep Vein Thrombosis, a blood clot in a vein deep within a muscle, typically in the lower extremities.

Dx An abbreviation for Diagnosis (also Diagnosis tab in the software).

Dysplasic Polyp Abnormal growth, a tumor.

Dyspnea Difficulty breathing or shortness of breath.

ECG An acronym for Electrocardiogram.

EDI An acronym for Electronic Data Interchange. Information exchanged electronically as data in codified transactions.

EHR An acronym for Electronic Health Records—the portions of a client's medical records that are stored in a computer system as well as the functional benefits derived from having an electronic health record. Also known as Electronic Medical Records, Computerized Patient Records, or Electronic Chart.

Electrolyte Panel A blood test that measures the levels of the minerals sodium, potassium, and chloride in the blood. The test also measures the level of carbon dioxide, which takes the form bicarbonate when dissolved in the blood. Certain medications can create in electrolyte imbalance, which is often the reason an Electrolyte Panel is ordered for clients on those medications.

Electronic Signature A method of marking an electronic record as "signed" having the same legal authority as a written signature. The electronic signature process involves the successful identification and authentication of the signer at the time of the signature, binding of the signature to the document, and nonalterability of the document after the signature has been affixed.

Eligible Professionals Providers designated as eligible to receive incentive payments under the HITECH Act.

EMR An acronym for Electronic Medical Record.

Encounter The medical record of an interaction between a client and a healthcare provider.

Encryption A method of converting an original message of regular text into encoded text, which is unreadable in its encrypted form. The text is encrypted by means of an algorithm using a private "key." *See also* Decryption.

Endoscopy Examination of the digestive tract using a flexible tube with a light and camera.

ENT An acronym for Ears, Nose, and Throat.

Entry Details The bottom portion of the Student Edition software window contains 10 fields that can be used to enter additional information about, or modify the meaning of, the finding that is selected at that time. *See* Description, Prefix, Modifier, Results, Status, Episode, Onset, Duration, Value, Units, or Note Textbox.

EPHI (HIPAA) Protected Health Information in electronic form.

Episode (entry detail) The Episode button is used to display the episode dialog window. This window is used to enter or edit data regarding the frequency or interval of occurrence of the currently selected finding.

ER An abbreviation for Emergency Room or emergency department.

Etiology The causal relationship between a problem and its related or risk factors.

E-Visit An E-visit is a client encounter conducted over the Internet, without an office visit. The client enters symptom, history, and HPI information, which is then reviewed by a clinician, who communicates via the Internet to ask additional questions, and provides a diagnosis, treatment orders, and client education. E-visits are used only for nonurgent visits and are reimbursed by a growing number of insurance plans.

Exacerbate To cause a disease or its symptoms to become more severe; to aggravate the condition.

Family History (tab) A feature on the Patient Management tab that provides a list of the client's family history items recorded in the EHR during all previous encounters.

FDA An acronym for Food and Drug Administration, an agency of the U.S. Department of Health and Human Services. This federal agency regulates prescription and nonprescription drugs.

Finding A precorrelated combination of terms from a nomenclature or clinical terminology into a clinically relevant phrase.

Flow Sheet (software) A feature of the software that presents data from multiple encounters in column format resembling a spreadsheet. Flow sheets allow findings from any previous encounter to be cited into the current note. Flow sheets can be created based on a list, a form, plan of care, or a problem.

Forms (software) Forms are used to consistently display a desired group of findings in a presentation that allows for quick entry of not only the selected findings but of any entry details as well. Forms are selected from the Forms Manager on the Forms tab. Multiple forms may be used to document an encounter.

Forms Manager A window in the EHR software used to organize and select Forms. *See* Forms.

Formulary *See* Drug Formulary.

Free Text EHR data that is not codified; may be attached to a codified finding as supplemental notes.

Gallop An abnormal heartbeat marked by three distinct sounds, like the gallop of a horse.

Gastrointestinal The stomach and the intestines.

Generalized Pallor An unusual paleness, a lack of color especially in the face.

Genitourinary The genital and urinary organs.

GI/GU An acronym for Gastrointestinal/Genitourinary body systems.

Glucose Monitors Home device used by diabetes clients to monitor glucose levels.

GMDN An acronym for Global Medical Device Nomenclature, used to identify the medical devices for ordering, inventory, or regulatory purposes, but does not provide for the codification of data from the devices.

H&P An acronym for History and Physical.

HAC An acronym for Hospital Acquired Condition, an infection or other medical problem occurring after admission.

HCAHPS is an acronym for Hospital Consumer Assessment Healthcare Providers and Systems, a standardized survey instrument and data collection methodology developed by NCQA for measuring clients' perspectives on care.

HCFA An acronym for the Health Care Financing Administration, which has since been renamed CMS. *See* CMS.

HCPCS An acronym for Healthcare Common Procedure Coding System. HCPCS is an extended set of billing codes for reporting medical services, procedures, and treatments including codes not listed in CPT-4 codes.

HDL High Density Lipoprotein cholesterol in blood plasma, sometimes referred to as good cholesterol because of its tendency to pull LDL cholesterol out of the artery wall.

Health Maintenance EHR system component to provide preventative health recommendations.

HEENT An acronym for Head, Eyes, Ears, Nose, Mouth, Throat (body system).

Hematocrit A blood test to determine the ratio of packed red blood cells to the volume of whole blood; also the result of the test.

Hematologic Blood and blood-forming organs (discussed in the text as a component of a physical exam).

Hemoglobin A1c A test that measures the average amount of sugar in the client's blood over the past three months.

Hepatic Function Panel A blood test used to determine liver function and liver disease. The panel measures total protein, albumin, bilirubin, alkaline phosphatase transferase (ALP), aspartate amino transferase (AST), and alamine amino transferase (ALT).

HepB An acronym for Hepatitis B (vaccine).

HHS An acronym for U.S. Department of Health and Human Services.

Hib An acronym for Haemophilus Influenza Type B (vaccine).

HIMSS An acronym for Healthcare Information and Management Systems Society, which is an organization that provides leadership in healthcare for the management of technology, information, and change through member services, education and networking opportunities, and publications. Members include healthcare professionals, hospitals, corporate healthcare systems, clinical practice groups, HIT supplier organizations, healthcare consulting firms, and government agencies.

HIPAA An acronym for Health Insurance Portability and Accountability Act (of 1996). HIPAA law regulates many things; however, healthcare workers often use the term HIPAA when they actually mean only the Administrative Simplification Subsection of HIPAA. *See* Administrative Simplification (HIPAA).

HIT An acronym for Health Information Technology; also Healthcare Information Technology.

HITECH Act An acronym for the Health Information Technology for Economic and Clinical Health Act, federal legislation that promotes the widespread adoption of EHR systems by authorizing incentive payments for providers that use EHR and financial penalties for those who continue using paper charts.

HIV An acronym for Human Immunodeficiency Virus (disease).

HL7 An acronym for Health Level Seven, the leading messaging standard used to exchange clinical and administrative data between different healthcare computer systems.

Holter Monitor A device worn by the client to record the heart rhythm continuously for 24 hours. This provides a record that can be analyzed by a cardiologist to determine any irregular or abnormal activity of the heart. Named for Dr. Norman Holter, its inventor.

HPI An acronym for History of Present Illness, which is a chronological description of the development of the client's present illness from the first sign or symptom or from the previous encounter to the present.

Hx An abbreviation for History. (Also the History tab in the software.)

Hyperlipidemia High levels of fat in the blood, such as cholesterol and triglycerides.

Hypertension A disease of abnormally high blood pressure.

Hypotension Abnormally low blood pressure.

ICD-9-CM An acronym for International Classification of Diseases, Ninth Revision, Clinical Modifications, a system of standardized codes to classify mortality and morbidity. ICD-9-CM is currently published in three volumes. The first two volumes provide a listing and an index of diagnosis codes. The third volume, however, lists codes for hospital inpatient procedures.

ICD-10 An acronym for International Classification of Diseases, Tenth Revision, a revision of the ICD-9 codes; scheduled to replace ICD-9-CM as the standard diagnoses codes for the United States in October 2013.

ICD-10-PCS International Classification of Diseases, Tenth Revision, Procedure Coding System (but not derived from the ICD-10 codes). PCS stands for Procedure Coding System, and it is intended to replace inpatient procedure codes in ICD-9-CM volume 3. The ICD-10-PCS is not used for billing at this time.

ICNP An acronym for International Classification for Nursing Practice, which is intended as an organizing structure for mapping other nursing terminologies.

Icon (software) In computer software, a small image usually used on a button to represent the purpose of the button—for example, a picture of a printer on the Print button.

ICU An acronym for Intensive Care Unit, a special section of the hospital with monitoring equipment and staff for seriously ill clients.

IHS An acronym for Indian Health Service, an agency of the U.S. Department of Health and Human Services responsible for providing federal health services to American Indians and Alaska natives.

Illeostomy A colostomy that empties from the distal end of the small intestine.

Immunologic The immune system; discussed as a component of evaluation during a physical exam.

INR A medical abbreviation for international normalized ratio is a frequently used reference to a Prothrombin time (PT/INR) blood test that measures how long it takes blood to clot.

Inpatient A hospital client who stays overnight.

IOM An acronym for Institute of Medicine of the National Academies, a nonprofit organization created to provide unbiased, evidence-based, and authoritative information and advice concerning health and science policy.

IPV Inactivated Polio Virus (Salk vaccine).

JCAHO Joint Commission on Accreditation of Healthcare Organizations; renamed simply as the Joint Commission.

Kiosk An unattended computer terminal for use by the clients in the waiting area.

LAN An acronym for Local Area Network, a network of computers that share data and programs located on a central computer called a server.

Laparoscopy Examination of the abdominal cavity through a small incision using a fiber-optic instrument.

Laptop Computer A self-contained, battery-operated computer, which typically includes the screen, keyboard, mouse, and speakers, in a package about the size of a standard notebook.

LDL Low Density Lipoprotein cholesterol in blood plasma; sometimes referred to as bad cholesterol, it is often associated with clogged arteries.

Leapfrog Group A coalition of 150 of the largest employers who created a strategy that tied purchase of group health insurance benefits to quality care standards, promoted Computerized Provider Order Entry, and the use of an EHR.

Lipids Test Panel A blood test that measures the levels of lipids (fats) in the bloodstream. A lipids profile measures total cholesterol, tri-glycerides, HDL (high density lipoprotein), and LDL (low density lipoprotein).

LIS An acronym for Laboratory Information System, a computer system that connects to and collects data from lab test instruments.

List A subset of findings (typically) used for a particular condition or type of exam, making it easier to read and navigate.

List (button) A button on the Student Edition software Toolbar that invokes the List Manager. *See* List Manager.

List Manager A window from which the user may select and load a List.

List Size (button) A feature of the software that controls how many findings are displayed in the nomenclature tree. List Size 1 displays the least number of findings; List Size 3 displays the most.

Login A computer screen requiring users to enter their name or ID (and password) before gaining access to the programs; or the action of entering a program through such a screen. EHR software typically requires users to "log in." Note that some systems use the term "log on" for this function.

LOINC An acronym for Logical Observation Identifier Names and Codes. LOINC was created and is maintained by the Regenstrief Institute, affiliated with the Indiana University School of Medicine, and is an important clinical terminology for laboratory test orders and results.

Lymphatic System A network of lymph nodes and small vessels that collects lymph and returns it to the bloodstream.

Macular Degeneration A disease marked by the loss of central vision in both eyes.

Mammogram An x-ray of the breast that can be used to detect tumors before they can be seen or felt.

Mammography *See* Mammogram.

MDS Minimum Data Set. *See* Resident Assessment Instrument.

Meaningful Use Criteria providers must meet to qualify for incentive payments under the HITECH Act.

Med/Surg Med/Surg is an abbreviation for Medical/Surgical History on a tab in the Patient Management feature. It provides a list of the client's past medical or surgical history items recorded in the EHR during all previous encounters.

MEDCIN A medical nomenclature and knowledge base developed by Medicomp Systems, Inc. Recognized as a national standard, it is incorporated in many commercial EHR systems as well as the U.S. Department of Defense CHCS II system.

Medication List (tab) A feature on the Patient Management tab that provides a list of the medications that the client currently is taking. The Medication list is always reviewed before writing new prescriptions.

Menu Bar The Menu bar consists of a row of words across the top of the Student Edition software screen: File, Select, Enter, Options, Forms, Summary, Graph, and Help. Clicking the mouse on any of the words on the Menu bar will display list of related software functions. Clicking the mouse on an item in the list will invoke that function.

Metformin An oral medication used along with a diet and exercise program to control high blood sugar in diabetic clients.

Microscopy Studies or images of studies performed using a microscope.

MMR An acronym for a combination of vaccines to immunize against Measles, Mumps, Rubella (German measles).

MODEM An acronym for Modulate-Demodulate. It is a device that converts computer data into signals that can be sent over a standard telephone connection. A second modem on the receiving end converts the signals back to data for the receiving computer.

Modifier (entry detail) The Modifier field (in entry details) is used to modify a selected finding. For example, the finding "Pain" may be qualified as mild, severe, and such.

Morbidity A diseased state or symptom.

MOU An acronym for Memorandum of Understanding (between government entities). It can be used between government agencies to meet the HIPAA Security Rule requirement in lieu of Business Associate agreements.

Mouse (computer) A computer device for moving the pointer or cursor on the screen, selecting items, and invoking actions in Windows software.

Mouse Button A button on the mouse that when pressed causes a Windows software program to invoke some action. The Student Edition software requires a mouse that has at least two buttons (left and right click). The left button is most frequently used to highlight items (single-click) or select items. Some programs require a double-click of the left mouse button to invoke an action. (Double-click is to press the left button twice in quick succession.) The right button generally invokes a small drop-down list or menu of options related to a particular item or area of the Window program. In most software, the right-click option is only available for selected areas of the program.

Mouse Pointer Typically an arrow shape that moves over the Window program in relationship to the movements of the mouse by the user. It also is sometimes referred to as a "cursor." When using flow sheets or forms, the Student Edition software may change the shape of the mouse pointer to a large question mark or the shape of a hand, indicating a different mode of functionality is temporarily in effect.

MPI an acronym for Master Person Index, a central database of demographic information for persons registered in a healthcare facility or organization.

MRI An acronym for Magnetic Resonance Imaging, which uses magnetic fields and pulses of energy to create images of organs and structures inside the body that cannot be seen by x-ray or CAT scan.

Musculoskeletal Components of the physical exam involving both the musculature and the skeleton.

NANDA An acronym for the North American Nursing Diagnosis Association, which has developed the Taxonomy II Nursing Diagnosis code set. It can be used to identify and code a client's responses to health problems and life processes.

NASA An acronym for National Aeronautics and Space Administration.

Nasal Turbinate Spongy, spiral-shaped bones in the nose passages.

NCQA An acronym for the National Committee for Quality Assurance, a not-for-profit organization dedicated to improving healthcare quality by measuring the performance of providers and health plans. NCQA is the developer of the HEDIS and PCMH standards.

NCVHS An acronym for National Committee on Vital and Health Statistics, an advisory panel within the U.S. Department of Health and Human Services, which selects national standards for HIPAA and recommends standards for the federal government initiatives on Electronic Health Records.

NDC An acronym for National Drug Code. The NDC is the standard identifier for human drugs. It is assigned and used by the pharmaceutical industry.

NDF-RT A nonproprietary terminology being developed by the Veterans Administration that classifies drugs by mechanism of action and physiologic effect.

NEC An acronym for Not Elsewhere Classified (diagnosis codes).

Negs (button) Auto Negative; a button that will automatically set all the findings (that are not already set) to "normal." The Negs button is operative only on Symptom or Physical Exam findings.

Neurological Disorders Disorders of the nervous system.

Nevi Moles on the skin; plural of nevus.

NHII An acronym for National Health Information Infrastructure, a plan to make EHR records available wherever the client is treated.

NHS An acronym for National Health Service, the national medical system in the United Kingdom.

NIC An acronym for Nursing Interventions Classification, which is a code set designed for codifying nursing interventions in any clinical setting.

NLM An acronym for the United States National Library of Medicine; a unit of the National Institute of Health, it is the world's largest medical library.

NMDS An acronym for Nursing Minimum Data Set, which defines the minimum set of basic data elements for nursing in a computerized client record.

NOC An acronym for Nursing Outcomes Classification, which is a code set used in conjunction with NIC for codifying the outcome of nursing interventions.

Nomenclature A system of names created by a recognized group or authority and used in a field of science. An EHR nomenclature is an organized list of medical phrases and codes that helps to standardize the way clinicians record information. These are also referred to as clinical vocabularies or clinical terminologies.

NOS An acronym for Not Otherwise Specified (diagnosis codes).

Note Textbox (entry detail) The Note textbox (in entry details) is used to enter or view a free-text note attached to the currently selected finding. Free text also may be added through a Note window, allowing easier entry of a longer note. The note dialog window can be invoked by clicking the Note button located beneath the right pane in the Student Edition software. (*See also* Free Text.)

Nursing Care Plan A plan of care based on one or more nursing diagnoses describing the planed interventions, nursing actions, and intended outcomes. This text describes three types of nursing care plans: standardized care plan is a formal care plan that specifies the nursing care for groups of clients with common needs. Also referred to as a Care Pathway or Critical Care pathway. An individualized care plan is tailored to meet the unique needs of a specific client—needs that are not addressed by the standardized plan. An interactive care plan is an individualized care plan that changes as the expected outcomes are met and the client's care needs change with improvement or deterioration of the client's condition.

OASIS An acronym for Outcome and Assessment Information Set, an assessment instrument required by CMS for home health agencies to assess clients' needs and plan for their home care.

OB Obstetrics is the field of specialty concerned with pregnancy, childbirth, and the period following.

Objective (chart) The clinician's observations and findings from the physical exam.

OCR (computer) An acronym for Optical Character Recognition, which is software that can analyze scanned document images, identify typed characters, and convert them into computer text.

Omaha System (codes) The Omaha System is the oldest standardized terminology for nursing documentation.

ONC An acronym for the Office of National Coordinator for Health Information Technology, an agency of the U.S. Department of Health and Human Services responsible for creating a national health information network and encouraging the use of EHR systems.

ONC-ATCB An acronym for organizations designated by the Office of the National Coordinator as Authorized Testing and Certification Body for purposes of certifying EHR systems.

Onset (entry detail) The Onset field (in entry details) is used to enter a number and a unit of time related to the onset of the currently selected finding. The time unit can be "second," "minute," "hour," "day" "week," "month," "year," or their plurals. A window with keypad for entering onset can be invoked by double-clicking the mouse in the onset field. Alternatively, a calendar in the window can be used to record a specific date of onset.

Order (button) Prefaces the highlighted finding with the prefix "Ordered" and records the finding in the Plan section. The button is enabled only when a finding is "orderable" but not a medication.

Otitis Media Inflammation of the middle ear, often accompanied by pain, fever, dizziness, or hearing abnormalities.

Otolaryngeal Ears, Nose, and Throat.

Outpatient A client who is examined or treated at a healthcare facility but is not hospitalized overnight. In this textbook, outpatient applies to all medical offices and clinics without overnight accommodation.

PAC(s) An acronym for Picture Archive and Communication System, a computer system that stores diagnostic images such as x-rays and CAT scans.

Pane (software) Two smaller windows within the Student Edition software, each capable of displaying and updating information. The left pane generally displays the nomenclature, or patient management tabs. The right pane generally displays the encounter note, outline view, or drawing tools; however, when using forms or flow sheets, the nomenclature tree may temporarily appear on the right to avoid covering a portion of the form or flow sheet.

Patient-Centered Medical Home An approach to providing comprehensive primary care in a healthcare setting that facilitates partnerships between individual clients, their personal physicians, and when appropriate, the client's family.

PC An acronym for Personal Computer, any computer capable of running applications without requiring connection to a server.

PCDS An acronym for Patient Care Data Set, which is a comprehensive set of nursing codes gathered from use in nine hospitals.

PDA An acronym for Personal Digital Assistant, a small handheld computer of a size that will fit in the palm of your hand.

PDF An acronym for Portable Document Format, a file format that retains the layout and fonts of the original document.

PE An abbreviation for Physical Exam. (*See also* Px.)

PEA A medical abbreviation for Pulseless Electrical Activity.

Pending Order A lab test or diagnostic procedure that has been ordered but for which no results have been received.

Peripheral Pulse The pulse in the periphery of the body (i.e., hand, foot, or neck).

Pertussis Whooping cough (vaccine).

PET Positron Emission Tomography combines CT (Computer Tomography) and nuclear scanning using a radioactive substance called a tracer, which is injected into a vein. A computer records the tracer as it collects in certain organs, then converts the data into a three-dimensional image of the organ, which can be used to detect or evaluate cancer.

PFSH An acronym for Past History, Family History, and Social History, obtained from client or other family member.

Pharynx The muscular and membranous cavity leading from the mouth and nasal passages to the larynx and esophagus.

PHI (HIPAA) An acronym for Protected Health Information; a client's personally identifiable health information (in any form) is protected by the HIPAA Privacy Rule.

Phlebotomist A medical technician who draws blood specimens.

PHR An acronym for Personal Health Record, an electronic health record owned and maintained by the client.

PIN An acronym for Personal Identification Number, a secret number used like a password.

Pitting Edema Edema in which pressing on the skin produces an indentation that remains for several seconds.

PKI An acronym for Public Key Infrastructure, which is used to secure messages or electronically sign documents.

Plan of Treatment Prescribed therapy, medication, orders, and instructions for treatment or management of the diagnosed condition.

PMS A medical abbreviation for Pre-menstrual Syndrome.

PNDS An acronym for Perioperative Nursing Data Set nursing codes.

POA Acronym for "present on admission," which is an indicator that a condition was present at the time of the order for inpatient admission. The POA indicator is required for each primary and secondary diagnosis on an inpatient.

Polydipsia Excessive, abnormal thirst.

Prefix (entry detail) The Prefix field (in entry details) is used to qualify a selected finding. The prefix will sometimes change the section of the note to which the finding is assigned. For example, penicillin normally appears under Medications. When the prefix "Ordered" is used, it will appear under Plan. If the prefix "Allergy to" is used, it will appear under Allergies.

Privacy Rule (HIPAA) Federal privacy protections for individually identifiable health information.

PRN A medical abbreviation for "as needed."

Problem List Acute conditions for which the client was recently seen as well as chronic conditions such as high blood pressure, diabetes, and so on, which are monitored at nearly every visit, and can affect decisions about medications and treatments for even unrelated illness.

Problem-Oriented Chart A method of documenting or viewing a client's chart by listing each problem or condition with the correlating symptoms, observations, and treatments related to that assessment.

Proctosigmoidoscopy *See* Sigmoidoscopy.

Prompt (button) Prompt stands for "prompt with current finding." Prompt is a software feature that generates a list of findings that are clinically related to the finding currently highlighted when the prompt button is clicked.

Protocol Standard plans of therapy used to treat a disease or condition.

PSA An acronym for Prostate-Specific Antigen, a test used to detect possible cancer of the prostate gland in men.

Psittacosis An infection acquired from raising birds.

Pulmonary Embolism Obstruction of the pulmonary artery or one of its branches by an abnormal particle such as a blood clot.

Purulent Discharge Pus or puslike discharge.

PVC An acronym for Pneumococcal Conjugate (vaccine).

Px An acronym for Physical Exam (same as PE). Also the Physical Exam tab in the software.

Radial Pulse The pulse in the radial artery measured at the wrist.

Radiologists Specialists who interpret x-rays, CAT scans, and other diagnostic tests.

RAI *See* Resident Assessment Instrument.

RAM An acronym for Random Access Memory, a measure of the quantity of computer memory.

Read Codes A nomenclature developed by Dr. James Read, later renamed Clinical Terms and merged into SNOMED-CT.

RELMA A free software program provided by Regenstrief Institute to assist with LOINC coding. *See also* LOINC.

Remote Access The ability to access the EHR from outside the medical facility network by using a direct-dial connection or a secure connection through the Internet.

Resectable Surgically removable.

Resident Assessment Instrument A form required by CMS for gathering information about nursing home residents to assess their needs and plan for their care. The RAI consists of three basic components: The Minimum Data Set (MDS) Version 3.0, the Care Area Assessment (CAA) process, and the RAI utilization guidelines.

Result (entry detail) The Result field (in entry details) is used to enter a result qualifier associated with the current finding. Examples include normal, abnormal, high, or low.

Review of Systems An inventory of body systems starting from the head down, often referred to as ROS. The body systems in a standard ROS are Constitutional symptoms, HEENT (Head, Eyes, Ears, Nose, Mouth, Throat), Cardiovascular, Respiratory, Gastrointestinal, Genitourinary, Musculoskeletal, Integumentary (skin and/or breast), Neurological, Psychiatric, Endocrine, Hematologic/Lymphatic, and Allergic/Immunologic.

Rhinitis Inflammation of the mucus membrane of the nose.

RHIO An acronym for Regional Health Information Organizations, entities formed to facilitate data exchange of client medical information in a region or state.

Rhonchi Rattling or snoring sounds heard in the chest when there is a partial bronchial obstruction.

RIS An acronym for Radiology Information System.

Risk Analysis (HIPAA) Identify potential security risks, and determine the probability of occurrence and magnitude of risks.

RNDx A Medcin prefix for a nursing diagnosis.

RNRx A Medcin prefix for a nursing intervention.

RNOx A Medcin prefix for a nursing order or nursing action.

ROS An acronym for Review of Systems. *See* Review of Systems.

ROS (button) A button that toggles On and Off with each click of the mouse. When On, the button changes color and symptom findings are recorded in the Review of Systems section; when Off, symptom findings are recorded in the History of Present Illness section.

RT An acronym for Respiratory Therapist.

Rx An abbreviation for Therapy (including prescriptions). Also the therapy tab in the software.

Rx (button) Invokes the prescription writer. The button is enabled only if the highlighted finding is a medication.

Rx Norm A nonproprietary vocabulary being developed by the NLM to codify drugs at the level of granularity needed in clinical practice.

Scanned Data (chart) Exam notes, letters, reports, and other documents that have been converted to an image by use of a scanner, then stored in the EHR. The data is accessible by a person viewing the chart, but the image contents cannot be used as data by the system for trend analysis, health maintenance, or similar purposes.

Scroll Bar (software) A scroll bar is a feature of most Windows software that automatically appears on the right of a list or text that is too long to fit in the window. The scroll bar has a button that can be moved by pressing the mouse button when dragging the mouse. The information in the window (or window pane) scrolls respective to the movement of the mouse.

Search (button) A word search used to quickly locate all findings in the nomenclature containing either matching words or synonyms of the search word.

Secure Messaging A recommended alternative to sending PHI in e-mail messages; secure messaging uses a secure Web page to read and write messages. The only message sent as e-mail is an alert to the receiving party that the actual message is waiting on the secure site. The contents of secure messages are stored in a secure server not in an e-mail system.

Security Rule (HIPAA) HIPAA security standards requiring implementation of appropriate security safeguards to protect health information stored in electronic form.

Sig Instructions for labeling a prescription (from Latin *signa*). Also timing interval in a care plan.

Sigmoidoscopy Examination of the rectum, colon, and sigmoid flexure using an illuminated, tubular instrument.

Sinusitis Inflammation of the sinus of the skull.

SNOMED An acronym for Systemized Nomenclature of Medicine had its origins in 1965 as Systemized Nomenclature of Pathology.

SNOMED-CT A medical nomenclature developed by the College of American Pathologists and United Kingdom's National Health Service. It is a merger of two previous coding systems, SNOMED and the Read codes, and has been recommended to become the core terminology for codified EHR in the United States.

SOAP A defined structure for documenting a client encounter by organizing the information into four sections. The acronym SOAP represents the first letter of each of the section titles: subjective, objective, assessment, and plan.

Social History (tab) A feature on the Patient Management tab that provides a list of the client's social and behavioral history items recorded in the EHR during all previous encounters.

Speech Recognition software Software that recognizes the patterns in human speech as words and turns them into computer text.

Spirometer An instrument that measures how much and how quickly air can enter and leave the lungs. Measurements may include VC (Vital Capacity), FVC (Forced Vital Capacity), PEFR (Peak Expiratory Flow Rate), MVV (Maximal Voluntary Ventilation), and FEV (Forced Expired Volume).

Spirometry An objective measurement useful in the diagnosis and management of asthma and other lung conditions. (*See* Spirometer.)

SSL An acronym for Secure Socket Layer that transparently encrypts and decrypts Web pages over the Internet.

Status (entry detail) The Status field (in entry details) is used to add the status of the currently selected finding.

Examples include worsening, improving, resolved, and similar designations.

Stress Test An electrocardiogram performed before, during, and after strenuous exercise, to measure heart function.

Subjective (chart) The client describes in his or her own words what the problem is, what the symptoms are, and what he or she is experiencing.

Sx An abbreviation for Symptoms—subjective evidence of disease or physical disturbance. Also the Symptom tab in the software.

Tablet PC A self-contained battery-operated computer similar to a laptop computer but using a special stylus and screen to replace the mouse, thus allowing the computer to be used as though the user was writing on a tablet.

Td An abbreviation for Tetanus and Diphtheria toxoids vaccine.

Telemonitors Biomedical devices worn by the client to capture vital signs or other data during the course of normal activity. The data is then downloaded or transmitted to the EHR.

Telemedicine Uses communication technology to deliver medical care to a client in another location, or through online consultation with that person's physician.

Teleradiology Uses communication technology to enable a radiologist in another location to interpret diagnostic images remotely.

Text Data (chart) Information stored in the EHR as word processing, blocks of text, or text reports. The data is searchable but neither codified nor standardized and is generally not indexed.

TIA A medical abbreviation for Transient Ischemic Attack, a brief incident of stroke-like symptoms caused by a temporary reduction or blockage of blood flow in the brain.

Toolbar A "toolbar" is row of icon buttons, the purpose of which is to allow quick access to commonly used functions. The Student Edition software has dynamic toolbars that change the selection of icons depending on the tab the user has selected, as well as special toolbars for functions such as annotated drawings and printing graphs.

Total Cholesterol A blood test that measures the total of all cholesterol in the blood, including both HDL (high density lipoprotein) and LDL (low density lipoprotein).

Transactions and Code Sets (HIPAA) HIPAA regulations requiring all covered entities to use standard EDI transaction formats and standard codes within those transactions for claims, remittance advice and payments, claim status, eligibility, referrals, enrollment, premium pay-

ments, claim attachments, report of injury, and retail drug claims.

Tree (software) A standard Windows software method of displaying hierarchical lists using small plus and minus symbols to indicate where additional hierarchical levels are hidden from view. The tree structure is used in the Student Edition Nomenclature pane. Clicking the mouse on the plus sign next to a finding will "expand the tree" to display additional related findings in an indented list. Clicking on the minus sign next to a finding will "collapse the tree," hiding all findings in the indented list below the selected finding. The purpose of the tree structure is to allow the user to quickly navigate extremely long lists by viewing only the level of hierarchy necessary.

Trend Analysis Comparing data from different dates, tests, or events to correlate the changes in the results with changes in the client's health.

Triage The screening of clients for allocation of treatment based on the urgency of their need for care. ER triage is often a simplified, organ-specific review of systems conducted by the triage nurse, based on the presenting complaint.

Tx An abbreviation for Tests (performed). Also a tab in the software.

URL an acronym for Universal Resource Locator, the address of a web site—for example: www.pearsonhighered.com.

U.S. Preventive Services Task Force An independent panel of experts in primary care and prevention sponsored by AHRQ that systematically reviews the evidence of effectiveness and develops recommendations for clinical preventive services based on the client's age, sex, and risk factors for disease. These recommendations are published by the AHRQ and are incorporated in EHR systems from several vendors.

UMDNS An acronym for Universal Medical Device Nomenclature System, which is used to identify the medical devices for ordering, inventory, or regulatory purposes, but does not provide for the codification of data from the devices.

UMLS An acronym for Unified Medical Language System from the National Library of Medicine. UMLS is not itself a medical terminology but, rather, a resource of software tools and data created from many medical nomenclatures to facilitate the development of EHR.

Uniform Identifiers (HIPAA) HIPAA regulations require all covered entities to adopt and use standard identification numbers for plans, providers, and employers in all HIPAA EDI transactions.

Unit (entry detail) The Unit field (in entry details) shows the currently selected unit for the currently selected finding, provided a standard unit exists. If more than one unit is available for selection, the selection will be shown in blue; otherwise, the selection will be shown in black.

URI An acronym for Upper Respiratory Infection. An infection affecting the nose, nasal passages, or upper part of the pharynx.

UTI A medical abbreviation for Urinary Tract Infection.

VA A common abbreviation for U.S. Department of Veteran Affairs.

Vaccine (tab) A feature on the Patient Management tab that provides a list of the client's immunizations that have been administered at the clinic.

Value (entry detail) The Value field (in entry details) is used to enter a numerical value for those findings that have a numeric value. (For example: blood pressure, weight, test results, and similar designations.) A window with keypad for entering numeric values can be invoked by double-clicking the mouse in the Value field.

Varicella Chickenpox (vaccine).

Vasoconstrictor An agent or drug that initiates or induces narrowing of the lumen (cavity) of blood vessels.

Venogram An imaging study where an x-ray is taken of the vein(s) after an opaque substance has been injected into it.

Vital Signs Functional measurements recorded at nearly every visit: temperature, respiration rate, pulse rate, and blood pressure. Most clinics measure height and weight as well.

Vital Statistics Statistics of birth, death, disease, and health of a population.

VPN An acronym for Virtual Private Network. Data sent over a public network is encrypted and decrypted without user intervention to attain a level of security similar to a private network.

Wellness Conditions Findings that are not disease related but, rather, used in health maintenance and preventative screening programs to keep healthy clients healthy. Wellness conditions are based on the age, sex, and history of the client. Examples of preventative recommendations based on wellness conditions include a mammogram for a healthy woman over 35; immunization vaccines at certain ages in children; and a colonoscopy for a healthy person with a family history of colorectal cancer.

WEP An acronym for Wired Equivalent Privacy, a protocol for securing the content of signals sent over a wireless network.

WHO An acronym for World Health Organization.

Wi-Fi An abbreviation for Wireless Fidelity, a type of fast wireless computer networking. *See also* Wireless Network.

Wireless Network A local area computer network using radio signals in place of wired network cables.

WNL (chart) An acronym for Within Normal Limits in medical charts.

Workstation A personal computer, usually connected to a main computer (server) via a network.

XML an acronym for eXtensible Mark-up Language, a file format similar to the hypertext mark-up language files, which contain fielded data with "tags" or names for the fields.

XPS an acronym for XML Paper Specification, a file format that retains the layout and fonts of the original document yet is viewable with a web browser.

X-Ray Traditionally an image made by the passage of short wave radiation through the body onto photographic film. Digital receptors are now able to replace film, allowing the image to be captured and stored in a computer without photo processing.

Index

Access
  client, to electronic health records, 490–491
  remote, 434–435
Advance Beneficiary Notice (ABN), 64, 65, 252
Agency for Healthcare Research and Quality (AHRQ),
      6, 490
Alerts, 61–65
American Academy of Family Physicians, 483
American Academy of Pediatrics, 483
American Health Information Management Association
      (AHIMA), 11, 422
American Nurses Association, 39, 40
  Clinical Care Classification system, 190–192
American Recovery and Reinvestment Act (ARRA), 6
Anatomical drawings, using, 367–383
Assessment instruments
  Outcome and Assessment Information Set (OASIS),
      389, 411–418
  Residential Assessment Instrument (RAI), 389, 390–408
  types of, 388–389
Association of Perioperative Registered Nurses, 40
Auto Negative (Negs) 151–154, 186

Bachman, John, 22–23
Bachman's Law and Bachman's Rule, 23
Billing. See Coding systems/nomenclatures
Biomedical devices, 56–57
Body mass index (BMI), 479–481
Brailer, David J., 6
Bush, George W., 6
Buttons
  basic, 73, 74, 75, 76, 78, 82, 83, 93
  Cite, 222–223, 238, 309, 343–344, 346
  Color, 372
  Delete, 373
  Details, 305
  Ellipsis, 344
  Exit, 373
  Font, 372
  FS Flow, 341, 346
  List size, 186, 260–261
  Lock, 371
  Medcin, 219, 238
  Mouse, 168
  Order, 298
  Outcome, 225, 238
  Print, 372
  Rx, 276, 298
  Save, 372
  Style, 371–372
  styles, 102–103
  Undelete, 373
  User images, 372

Care Area Assessment (CAA) process, 391
Care pathway, 196–200
Cataloging images, 42, 47–53
Catalog Pane, 45–46
CDISC (Clinical Data Interchange Standards
      Consortium), 56
Centers for Disease Control and Prevention, 476, 479, 480
  immunization schedules, 482–483
Certification Commission for Healthcare Information
      Technology (CCHIT), history of, 11–12
Certified EHR, 11–12
Charts
  See also Paper charts
  creating upon admission, 122–134
  inpatient versus outpatient, 19–22
Chief complaint, 100
Cite button, 222–223, 238, 309, 343–344
Client access to electronic health records, 490–491
Client-entered data, 58
  graphs, 487–488
  Internet workflow, using client-entered data, 439–448
Clinical Care Classification system (CCC), 38–39
  description of, 190–192
  model and flow, 216
  prefixes in Medcin, 191
Clinical quality measures (CQM), 12
Clinical notes, documentation of, 14
Clinton, Bill, 6
Closed Loop Safe Medication Administration, 271–272
CMS (Centers for Medicare & Medicaid Services), 9, 11,
      12, 65, 411, 412, 413, 418, 490
Coded data, 32, 33
Codified observations. See Findings
Coding systems/nomenclatures
  benefits of, 34, 58–67
  ICD-9-CM (International Classification of Diseases),
      285–286
  ICD-10, 285, 286
  LOINC®, 33, 38
  MEDCIN®, 33, 35–38
  nursing code sets, 38–41
  SNOMED-CT®, 33, 34–36
  standard, 33–41
  UMLS, 38

Acronyms Used in This Book

ABG	Arterial Blood Gas	DME	Durable Medical Equipment
ABN	Advance Beneficiary Notice	DOD	Department of Defense
ABN	Abnormal	DTaP	Diphtheria, Tetanus, Pertussis (vaccine)
ADL	Activities of Daily Living	DUR	Drug Utilization Review
ADT	Admission, Discharge and Transfer	DTV	Deep Vein Thrombosis
AHIMA	American Health Information Management Association	Dx	Diagnosis
AHRQ	Agency for Healthcare Research and Quality	ECG or EKG	Electrocardiogram
ALOS	Average Length of Stay	EDI	Electronic Data Interchange
AMA	Against Medical Advice	EHR	Electronic Health Record
AMI	Acute Myocardial Infraction	EMS	Emergency Medical Services
ANA	American Nurses Association	ENT	Ears, Nose, Throat
ANSI	American National Standards Institute	EPHI	Protected Health Information in Electronic form
ARRA	American Recovery and Reinvestment Act	EPs	Eligible Professionals
ADHD	Attention Deficit Hyperactivity Disorder	ER	Emergency Department or Emergency Room
BID	Twice Daily	FDA	Food and Drug Administration
BIPAP	Bilevel Positive Airway Pressure	FS Form	Flow Sheet (based on a) Form
BMI	Body Mass Index	FS Hx	Family and Social History
BMP	Basic Metabolic Panel	GI	Gastrointestinal
BP	Blood Pressure	GNA	Geriatric Nursing Assistants
CAA	Care Area Assessment	H&P	History and Physical
CAT	Computerized Axial Tomography	HAC	Hospital Acquired Condition
CBC	Complete Blood Count	HCAHPS	Hospital Consumer Assessment Healthcare Providers and Systems
CC	Chief Complaint	HDL-C	High-Density Lipoprotein (cholesterol test)
CCC	Clinical Care Classification system	HF	Hearth Failure
CCHIT	Certification Commission for Healthcare Information Technology	HEENT	Head, Eyes, Ears, Nose, (Mouth), and Throat
CCU	Critical Care Unit	HepB	Hepatitis B (vaccine)
CDC	Centers for Disease Control and Prevention	HHA	Home Health Agency
CDISC	Clinical Data Interchange Standards Consortium	HHS	U.S. Department of Health and Human Services
CDR	Clinical Data Repository	Hib	Haemophilus influenzae type B (vaccine)
CHF	Congestive Heart Failure	HIE	Health Information Exchange
CIS	Clinical Information Services	HIM	Health Information Management
CMS	Centers for Medicare and Medicaid Services	HIMSS	Health Information Management Systems Society
CNA	Certified Nursing Assistant	HIPAA	Health Insurance Portability and Accountability Act
CPOE	Computerized Provider Order Entry	HITECH	Health Information Technology for Economic and Clinical Health
CPR	Cardio-Pulmonary Resuscitation		
CPRI	Computer Based Patient Record Institute	HL7	Health Level 7
CPRS	Computerized Patient Record System	HPI	History of Present Illness
CQM	Clinical Quality Measures	Hx	History
CRNA	Certified Registered Nurse Anesthesiologist	ICD-9-CM	International Classification of Diseases, ninth revision, with clinical modifications
CT	Computed Tomography	ICD-10	International Classification of Diseases, tenth revision
CVA	Cerebrovascular Accident		
CVP	Cerebral Vascular Pressure	ICNP	International Classification for Nursing Practice
DAW	Dispense As Written	IMH	Instant Medical History
DICOM	Digital Imaging and Communications in Medicine	INR	International Normalized Ratio